Human Genomics

Human Genomics

Editor: Bryan Evans

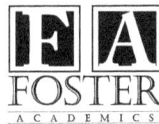

FOSTER
ACADEMICS

www.fosteracademics.com

www.fosteracademics.com

FA **FOSTER**
ACADEMICS

Cataloging-in-Publication Data

Human genomics / edited by Bryan Evans.
    p. cm.
Includes bibliographical references and index.
ISBN 978-1-63242-842-4
1. Human genome. 2. Genomics. 3. Human genetics. I. Evans, Bryan.
QH431 .H86 2019
611.018 166--dc23

Foster Academics,
118-35 Queens Blvd., Suite 400,
Forest Hills, NY 11375, USA

ISBN 978-1-63242-842-4 (Hardback)

Contents

Preface

This book was inspired by the evolution of our times; to answer the curiosity of inquisitive minds. Many developments have occurred across the globe in the recent past which has transformed the progress in the field.

The branch of science concerned with the evolution, structure, mapping, function and editing of genomes is known as genomics. The complete set of DNA of an organism, including all its genes is called a genome. Human genome refers to the set of nucleic acid sequences for humans, encoded as DNA, in a small DNA molecule found within individual mitochondria and 23 chromosome pairs in the cell nuclei. The human genome may be separated into the mitochondrial genome and the nuclear genome. Human genome includes both noncoding DNA and protein-coding DNA genes. The topics included in this book on human genomics are of utmost significance and bound to provide incredible insights to readers. It provides significant information of this discipline to help develop a good understanding of human genomics and related fields. Scientists, researchers and students actively engaged in this field will find this book full of crucial and unexplored concepts.

This book was developed from a mere concept to drafts to chapters and finally compiled together as a complete text to benefit the readers across all nations. To ensure the quality of the content we instilled two significant steps in our procedure. The first was to appoint an editorial team that would verify the data and statistics provided in the book and also select the most appropriate and valuable contributions from the plentiful contributions we received from authors worldwide. The next step was to appoint an expert of the topic as the Editor-in-Chief, who would head the project and finally make the necessary amendments and modifications to make the text reader-friendly. I was then commissioned to examine all the material to present the topics in the most comprehensible and productive format.

I would like to take this opportunity to thank all the contributing authors who were supportive enough to contribute their time and knowledge to this project. I also wish to convey my regards to my family who have been extremely supportive during the entire project.

Editor

Targeted next generation sequencing identifies novel NOTCH3 gene mutations in CADASIL diagnostics patients

Neven Maksemous, Robert A. Smith, Larisa M. Haupt and Lyn R. Griffiths[*]

Abstract

Background: Cerebral autosomal dominant arteriopathy with subcortical infarcts and leukoencephalopathy (CADASIL) is a monogenic, hereditary, small vessel disease of the brain causing stroke and vascular dementia in adults. CADASIL has previously been shown to be caused by varying mutations in the *NOTCH3* gene. The disorder is often misdiagnosed due to its significant clinical heterogeneic manifestation with familial hemiplegic migraine and several ataxia disorders as well as the location of the currently identified causative mutations. The aim of this study was to develop a new, comprehensive and efficient single assay strategy for complete molecular diagnosis of *NOTCH3* mutations through the use of a custom next-generation sequencing (NGS) panel for improved routine clinical molecular diagnostic testing.

Results: Our custom NGS panel identified nine genetic variants in *NOTCH3* (p.D139V, p.C183R, p.R332C, p.Y465C, p. C597W, p.R607H, p.E813E, p.C977G and p.Y1106C). Six mutations were stereotypical CADASIL mutations leading to an odd number of cysteine residues in one of the 34 *NOTCH3* gene epidermal growth factor (EGF)-like repeats, including three new typical cysteine mutations identified in exon 11 (p.C597W; c.1791C>G); exon 18 (p.C977G; c. 2929T>G) and exon 20 (p.Y1106C; c.3317A>G). Interestingly, a novel missense mutation in the *CACNA1A* gene was also identified in one CADASIL patient. All variants identified (novel and known) were further investigated using in silico bioinformatic analyses and confirmed through Sanger sequencing.

Conclusions: NGS provides an improved and effective methodology for the diagnosis of CADASIL. The NGS approach reduced time and cost for comprehensive genetic diagnosis, placing genetic diagnostic testing within reach of more patients.

Keywords: AmpliSeq Custom Panel, CADASIL, Next-generation sequencing, *NOTCH3*

Background

The stroke syndrome CADASIL [MIM 125310] (cerebral autosomal dominant arteriopathy with subcortical infarcts and leukoencephalopathy) disorder results in neuronal white matter abnormalities and is characterised by a variety of symptoms including, vascular degeneration, recurrent subcortical ischaemic strokes, progressive cognitive decline, dementia, migraine with aura (22 % of patients) and premature death [1]. The unique deposition of granular osmiophilic material (GOM) in systemic and brain vasculature

* Correspondence: lyn.griffiths@qut.edu.au
Genomics Research Centre, Institute of Health and Biomedical Innovation (IHBI), School of Biomedical Sciences, Queensland University of Technology (QUT), Q Block, 60 Musk Ave, Kelvin Grove Campus, Brisbane 4059, Queensland, Australia

differentiates CADASIL patients from those suffering similar hereditary vascular disorders [2]. CADASIL is often misdiagnosed due to its significant clinically heterogeneic manifestation with familial hemiplegic migraine and several ataxia disorders, as these disorders have an autosomal dominant mode of inheritance and share clinical characteristics such as hemiplegic migraine, migraine with typical aura and progressive ataxia [3–6]. Mutations implicated in CADASIL have been identified on chromosome 19, specifically within *NOTCH3* (MIM 600276), which encodes a transmembrane receptor primarily expressed in vascular smooth muscle cells. *NOTCH3* located at 19p13 is 33 exons long and spans approximately 7 kb [4]. Currently, at least 200 mutations resulting in an odd number of cysteine residues are known to be associated with CADASIL. These mutations all occur in exons 2–24 of *NOTCH3* that encode 34 epidermal growth factor (EGF)-like repeats in the extracellular domain of the NOTCH3 protein. The large number of exons combined with their high GC content makes comprehensive sequencing of this gene with traditional Sanger sequencing (SS) expensive and time consuming. With the advent of next-generation sequencing (NGS), the sequencing of target genes, regions, exomes or whole genomes, provides cost-effective, high-throughput screening suitable for molecular diagnostics enabling detection of a wide array of mutations with sensitivity and specificity. Here, we have performed targeted gene sequencing using a custom five-gene NGS panel [7], encompassing the coding sequences, 20–100 bp exon/intron boundaries and the 5′ and 3′UTR regions of *NOTCH3* in 44 patients.

Results

NGS-panel sequencing output

The sequencing output data from the Ion Torrent PGM was analysed using the Ion Torrent platform-specific software Torrent Suite V3.6 (Thermo Fisher Scientific, Scoresby, Victoria, Australia). The 44 samples were sequenced using seven different Ion 316 chips, to generate an average sequencing of 3,303,300 total reads, 477.4 Mb total bases sequenced, and 472.2 Mb with 99 % of bases aligned to the human complete genome (hg19) per Ion 316 chip. For all samples sequenced, the average read depth across the target region was 560.65×, while the average percentage of target bases covered at 20× or greater was 96 % and the average uniformity of coverage was 90.64 %.

Sequencing data analysis

Comprehensive screening for *NOTCH3* using the Ampli-Seq Custom NGS panel [7] (Thermo Fisher Scientific, Scoresby, Victoria, Australia) for targeted gene sequencing was conducted on 44 patients, previously screened for standard sequencing exons (3 and 4) and/or (2,11, 18 and 19) by SS and classified as being negative for known mutations.

Initial analysis using the IonReporter software (Thermo Fisher Scientific, Scoresby, Victoria, Australia) identified 42 variants scattered over *NOTCH3* among the 44 patients. An overview of all variants detected in our study is shown in Additional file 1: Table S1 online. Of these, nine particularly notable genetic variants were identified in 10 patients (22.7 %) out of the 44 subjects: five novel potential mutations (NOTCH3:NM_000435:exon4:c.416A>T:p.D139V, exon1 1:c.1791C>G:p.C597W and c.1820G>A: p.R607H, exon18: c.2929T>G,: p.C977G; and exon20: c.3317A>G: p.Y1106C); three previously reported disease-causing missense mutations (NOTCH3:NM_000435:exon4:c.547T>Cp.C183R [8], exon 6:c.994C>T, p.R332C [9, 10]; and exon9: c.1394A>G: p.Y465R [11]) and one novel synonymous genetic variant

in NOTCH3:NM_000435:exon16:c.2439G>A: p.E813E [Tables 1 and 2]. Clinical information for all samples was not available [see Additional file 2: Table S2]; however, the following clinical parameters were attributed to the relevant samples in our cohort: (i) white matter abnormalities were seen in patients with E813E, C183R and R332C mutations; (ii) positive skin biopsy signs were reported in patients with C977G, Y1106C, Y465C and C183R and (iii) a family history of dementia and/or stroke was reported in patients with E813E, C977G, Y1106C, C183R, R332C and R465C mutations.

Molecular genetic testing using the custom NGS panel encompassing five genes (*NOTCH3*, *CACNA1A*, *ATP1A2*, *SCN1A* and *TRESK* genes) identified two remarkable variants in case C-36 (CACNA1A:NM_023035:c.832G>T:-p.A278S and SCN1A:NM_006920:c.3924A>T: p.E1308D [Table 1]). These mutations correspond to highly conserved amino acid residues according to four in silico prediction tools (PhyloP of score of >2.0, PolyPhen2 HVar of score >0.7, and MutationTaster with a damaging effect and GERP++ score above 5).

In addition to these variants, nine rare single nucleotide polymorphisms (SNPs) in the *NOTCH3* gene with minor allele frequency (MAF) ≤0.1 % were observed in nine patients with no other causative mutation found in *NOTCH3* [Additional file 1: Table S1 online and Table 3]. One patient (case C-3) was shown to carry two rare amino acid changing variants p.S497L and p.A1020P in exons 9 and 19 of *NOTCH3*, respectively. All nine SNPs were further assessed by seven in silico prediction programmes with three of these variants (p.S497L, p.P496L and p.Y220Y) shown to have a damaging effect by MutationTaster.

All variants detected by NGS and reported in this study were visually confirmed using Integrative Genomics Viewer (IGV v2.3) software [12] and compared with NCBI reference sequences [13]. In order to verify the accuracy of potential novel mutations identified by NGS, SS was performed for all samples with the five non-synonymous variants along with the synonymous new variant showing complete consistency (100 %) between the two methods [Fig. 1].

Analyses of the potential functional significance of the six novel *NOTCH3* genetic variants identified the C597W, C977G and Y1106C missense mutations to be pathogenic by six of the seven genetic prediction software programmes (PhyloP, SIFT, PolyPhen2, MutationTaster, AGVGD and PhD-SNP) [Table 1].

Finally, we compared the potential functional significance of the three known pathogenic missense mutations (C183R, R332C and Y465C) with the six novel genomic variants identified using the same seven in silico software programmes. The C183R and R332C mutations showed a high potential damaging effect when analysed by all seven programmes used; in contrast, the

Table 1 Variants of unknown significance of *NOTCH3*, *CACNA1A* and *SCN1A* genes identified in eight suspicious CADASIL patients. RefSeq NM_000435, NM_001127221 and NM_001165963

Sample ID	Gene	Gender	Age	Exon	EGF-repeat	Codon change (FWD)	Protein change	PhyloP	SIFT	PolyPhen2 HVar	MutationTaster	GERP++	AGVGD	PhD-SNP
C-11	NOTCH3	F	42	4	3	c.416A>T	p.Asp139Val	C (1.89)	T (0.06)	P (0.499)	D	5.02	C65	Non-neutral
C-4	NOTCH3	M	67	11	15	c.1791C>G	p.Cys59Trp	N (0.434)	D (0)	D (1.0)	D	2.25	C65	Non-neutral
C-15	NOTCH3	F	52	11	15	c.1820G>A	p.Arg607His	C (2.21)	T (0.54)	B (0.0.026)	D	3.22	C25	Neutral
C-24	NOTCH3	M	54	16	21	c.2439G>A	p.Glu813Glu	–	–	–	D (splice site changes)	–	–	–
C-10 and C-44	NOTCH3	F	74, 52	18	25	c.2929T>G	p.Cys977Gly	C (2.04)	D (0)	D (1.0)	D	5.36	C65	Non-neutral
C-6	NOTCH3	F	51	20	28	c.3317A>G	p.Tyr1106Cys	C (1.92)	D (0)	D (0.998)	D	5.08	C65	Non-neutral
C-36	CACNA1A	M	60	6	–	c.832G>T	p.Ala278Ser	C (2.46)	T (0.13)	D (0.963)	D	5.27	NA	Neutral
C-36	SCN1A	M	60	20	–	c.3924A>T	p.Glu1308Asp	C (2.08)	T (0.37)	P (0.727)	D	5.46	NA	Neutral

PhyloP, SIFT, Polyphen-2, MutationTaster, GERP++, AGVGD and PhD-SNP are functional prediction scores in which increasing values indicate a more damaging effect except SIFT score <0.05 has damaging effect

Abbreviations: C conserved, *N* not-conserved or neutral, *D* damaging or deleterious, *P* possible damaging, *T* tolerated, *B* benign, *NA* not applicable

Table 2 Variants of known *NOTCH3* mutations identified in three patients by NGS. RefSeq NM_000435.2

Sample ID	Gender	Age	Exon	EGF-repeat	Codon change	Protein change	PhyloP	SIFT	PolyPhen2 HVar	MutationTaster	GERP++	AGVGD	PhD-SNP	Snp138
C-20	F	54	4	4	c.547T>C	p.Cys183Arg	C (1.82)	D (0)	D (1)	D	4.32	C65	Non-neutral	
C-42	F	47	6	8	c.994C>T	p.Arg332Cys	C (2.46)	D (0.03)	D (1)	D	4.6	C65	Non-neutral	rs137852641
C-14	M	33	9	11	c.1394A>G	p.Tyr465Cys	N (−0.833)	T (0.08)	P (0.886)	D	−4.41	C65	Non-neutral	

PhyloP, SIFT, Polyphen-2, MutationTaster, GERP++, AGVGD and PhD-SNP are functional prediction scores in which increasing values indicate a more damaging effect except SIFT score <0.05 has damaging effect
Abbreviations: C conserved, *N* not-conserved or neutral, *D* damaging or deleterious, *P* possible damaging, *T* tolerated

Table 3 Rare variants identified by NGS in the *NOTCH3* gene. RefSeq NM_000435.2

Patient ID	Locus.	Ref	Location	Codon change	Protein change	PhyloP	SIFT	PolyPhen	LRT	MutationTaster	GERP++	AGVGD	PhD-SNP	dbSNP	MAF
C31	chr19:15281342	T	Ex27	c.4914A>G	WT (p.Glu1638Glu)	0.25				Poly				rs149222385	0.001
C13, C28, C33	chr19:15290236	G	Ex21	c.3399C>A	p.His1133Gln	-2.55	D	P (0.68)	NA	Poly	-8.6	C15	Neutral	rs112192217	0.005
C3, C12	chr19:15291576	C	Ex19	c.3058G>C	p.Ala1020Pro	0.57	T (0.19)	B (0.054)	N (0.006)	Poly	1.44	C25	Neutral	rs35769976	0.083
C3	chr19:15296513	C	In12			0.5				Poly				rs147014533	0.006
C3	chr19:15299048	G	Ex9	c.1490C>T	p.Ser49Leu	2.35	T (0.33)	B (0.036)	N (0.018)	D	5.04	C65	Neutral	rs114207045	0.006
C34	chr19:15299051	G	Ex9	c.1487C>T	p.Pro496Leu	2.35	T (0.1)	p (0.883)	N (0.007)	D	5.04	C65	Disease	rs11670799	0.005
C9	chr19:15302790	G	Ex4	c.660C>T	WT (p.Tyr220Tyr)	-1.85				D				rs114457076	0.001
C3	chr19:15308287	G	In2			-0.16				Poly				rs188132716	0.006
C16	chr19:15308288	G	In2			-0.98				Poly				rs202151374	0.003

PhyloP, SIFT, Polyphen-2, Mutation Taster, GERP++, AGVGD, and PhD-SNP are functional prediction scores in which increasing values indicate a more damaging effect except SIFT score <0.05 has damaging effect

Abbreviations: B benign, *C* conserved, *D* damaging or deleterious, *Ex* exon, *In* intron, *NA* not applicable, *N* not-conserved or neutral, *P* possible damaging, *Poly* polymorphic, *T* tolerated, *WT* wild type

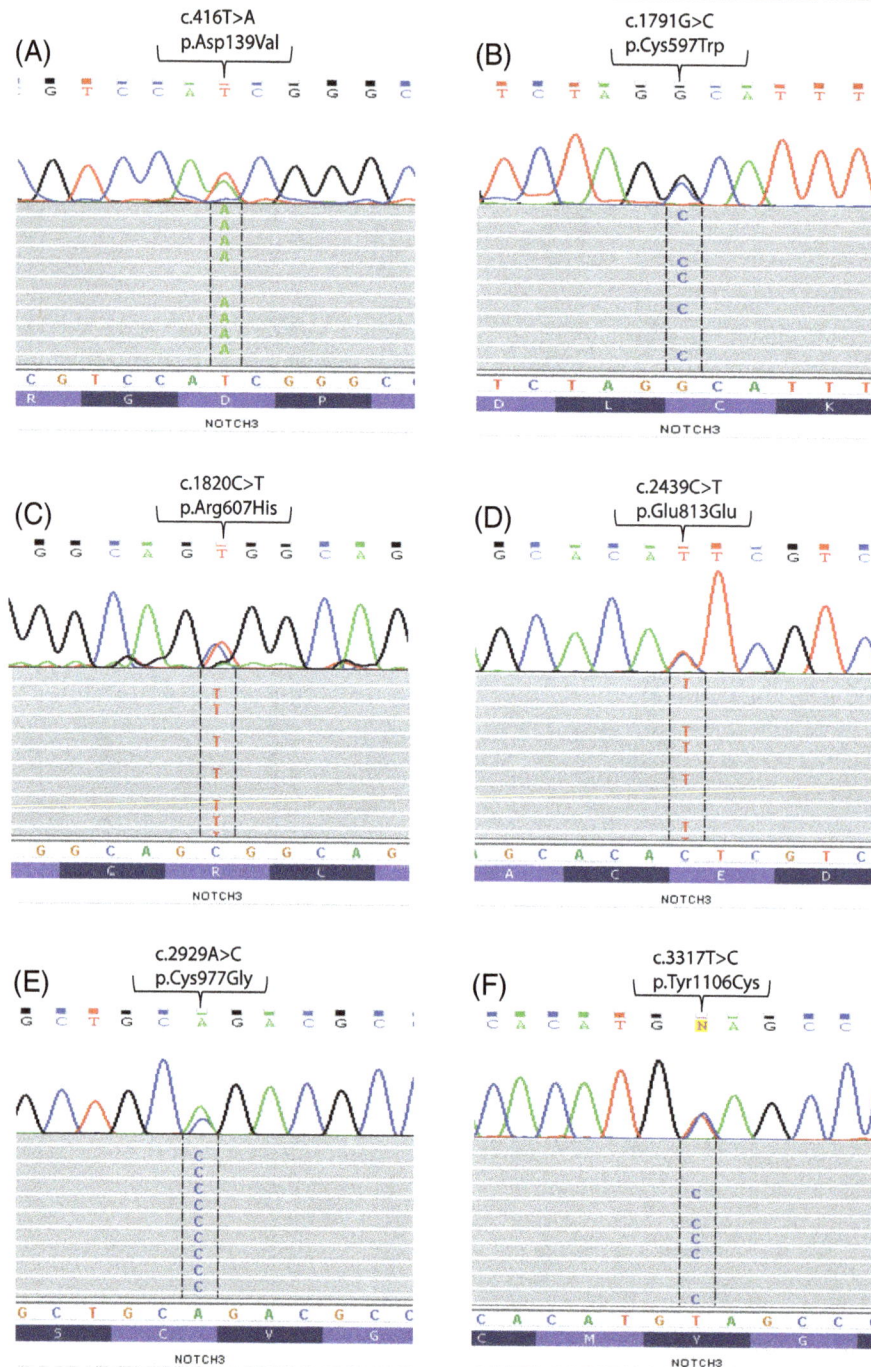

Fig. 1 Sequences (reverse complement) of the six novel genetic variants in *NOTCH3* identified by NGS. The figure shows the six heterozygous exonic point variants: **a** p.D139V in exon 4, **b** p.C597W in exon 11, **c** p.R607H in exon 11, **d** synonymous variant p.E813E in exon 16, **e** p.C977G in exon 18 and **f** p.Y1106C in exon 20 identified in this study. Only bases non-concordant with consensus sequence are displayed in the target reads with the integrative genomics viewer IGV [12]. The normal nucleotide and protein sequences are depicted at the *bottom* and *top* of the figure

Y465C mutation showed a tolerated or benign effect in four of the seven in silico programmes [Table 2].

Discussion

Molecular genetic testing is an essential tool for accurate CADASIL diagnosis. Several diagnostic approaches have been used for CADASIL, in particular the use of skin biopsy to detect unusual NOTCH3 expression. However, despite the widespread use of biopsy testing, the low sensitivity of this method in CADASIL diagnosis has been reported [14]. In addition, previous work by Markus et al. tested the sensitivity of single strand conformation polymorphism (SSCP) analysis for detecting NOTCH3 mutations, with an effective success rate of 80 to 85 % [14]. More recently, He et al. reported that varying and population-dependant results in the effectiveness of using the pre-genetic "CADASIL scale" screening tool which evaluates clinical presentations and neuroimaging data in an effort to minimise NOTCH3 gene testing [15, 16]. As such, current diagnosis relies on the screening of all exons by sequencing to identify mutations in NOTCH3.

We have previously demonstrated the efficiency of our NGS panel for detecting known and novel mutations in a cohort of episodic ataxia patients and increasing the rate of mutation detection by 48 % [7]. We have now utilised this custom targeted massively parallel NGS panel to examine the coding sequences, intron/exon boundaries including 20–100 bases of flanking intronic nucleotides and the 5′ and 3′ UTR regions of NOTCH3 in a cohort of 44 patients with clinically suspicious CADASIL.

Targeted gene sequencing analysis efficiently identified nine novel genetic variants in NOTCH3, of which five non-synonymous mutations (p.D139V, p.C597W, p.R607H, p.C977G and p.Y1106C) and one synonymous variant (p.E813E) have not been previously described. In addition, three missense mutations previously reported as pathogenic (C183R [8], R332C [9, 10] and Y465C [11]) but not previously identified in our diagnostics cohort were also detected [17]. In total, six typical CADASIL mutations involving cysteine alterations were identified in seven patients (15.9 %) out of 44 subjects, a detection rate higher than previously reported by Fernandez et al. and Bianchi et al. [18, 19].

Interestingly, previous studies have revealed differences in the spectrum of NOTCH3 mutations between Asian and Italian populations and populations of Caucasian ethnicity [18, 20, 21]. Our results also showed no evidence of strong clustering of NOTCH3 mutations in specific exons. The variants identified in this study occur in seven different exons (4, 6, 9, 11, 16, 18 and 20) within the EGF-like repeat regions of the gene. The patient cohort encompasses different ethnic backgrounds, reflecting the diversity of the Australian population. This highlights the potential confounding factor in nations of multiple ethnic backgrounds, where mutations may occur at multiple sites making molecular diagnosis difficult and time consuming if using traditional SS methodologies. While exonic clustering in ethnic groups is likely due to founder effects, de novo mutations resulting in mutations in ethnically homogenous populations are possible. In this instance, the use of SS may still miss mutations in a proportion of patients suggesting that screening of all coding regions in NOTCH3 is of benefit for the comprehensive molecular diagnosis of CADASIL.

Six of the missense mutations identified were stereotypical CADASIL mutations, resulting in a loss or gain of one of the six cysteine residues (4, 8, 11, 15, 25 and 28) of the EGF-like repeats located in the extracellular domain of NOTCH3 [4]. Any mutation within the cysteine residues (a gain or loss) leads to an odd number of cysteine residues and result in impaired dimerisation of NOTCH3 or formation of inappropriate disulphide bonds causing aberrant NOTCH3 signaling [22, 23]. As such, these three mutations (p.C597W, p.C977G and p.Y1106C) were considered to be disease-causing and associated with the pure and typical pathogenetic mechanisms of CADASIL [4, 24]. The substitution of the p.C597S has been previously identified in an Arabic family [25], while the substitution of p.C977S has been reported in a Chinese patient [26] with both mutations found to be associated with CADASIL pathogenesis.

We also observed two novel amino acid substitutions (p.D139V and p.R607H) not directly involving cysteine residues, predicted to be possibly damaging and benign, respectively. As discussed by Roy et al. [17], there is some controversy over the classification non-cysteine residue altering variants and their significance to CADASIL. Several NOTCH3 alterations that do not affect cysteine residues have been reported in families with CADASIL, which may involve other disruptions to protein function, though these may result in changes that effectively change cysteine residue availability [27–32]. It is worth noting that the predicted score for p.D139V by the SIFT programme (0.06) was more deleterious than the known pathogenic mutation p.Y465C, with a score of 0.08, technically considered to be benign. A SIFT score from 0 to 0.05 indicates that the amino acid change has a damaging effect. Further investigation of this mutation is warranted to determine the effect of these non-cysteine affecting changes on NOTCH3 function as well as on mediating signal transduction for vascular development and inducing the pathology of CADASIL. This provides new insights into the diagnosis of and pathomechanisms causing CADASIL.

The last novel synonymous variant we identified (p.E813E) was predicted by the MutationTaster programme to cause the gain of an RNA splicing donor site. This gain may result in altered protein function and therefore, despite being silent, this variant could be a real mutation causing CADASIL. Direct functional evaluation of NOTCH3 in this patient is needed to confirm this hypothesis, but such studies were not able to be performed at this time.

The in silico analysis tools to analyse the detected variants also revealed some interesting potential ramifications of the previously identified p.Y465C mutation. In 2003, Razvi et al. described this amino acid substitution as a mutation causing CADASIL [11]. In contrast, during our analysis, the computational tools predicted this amino acid change as tolerated or benign. The PhyloP score of 0.0272 and SIFT score of 0.08 (damaging score <0.05) suggest this amino acid is not conserved. The mutation is a classical CADASIL mutation; however, as stated by Joutel et al. "mutations can be unambiguously classified as pathogenic when they lead to an uneven number of cysteine residues in one of the 34 EGFR domains constituting the extracellular domain of the receptor" [24]. This discrepancy between evolutionary conservation and functional correlation models suggests caution when using functional prediction software in assigning a role to missense mutations involving cysteine residues in NOTCH3. The in vivo effect of amino acid substitutions should be the final arbiter for precisely describing their role in causing CADASIL, but as such tests are laborious to undertake, they are rarely performed for diagnoses. Careful consideration of the symptomatic profile may be useful in such cases and in the future when sufficient mutation data has accumulated offering clinicians more precision in ascribing the functional role of mutations in CADASIL.

Interestingly, in this study, patient C-36 demonstrated compound heterozygosity for two missense mutations in the CACNA1A and SCN1A genes (not normal target genes for CADASIL screening) [Table 1]. Mutations within these two ion channel genes are associated with various autosomal dominant disorders: hemiplegic migraine, episodic ataxia type 2, spinocerebellar ataxia type 6 and epilepsy with previously reported overlapping symptoms among these disorders [33–35]. It is worth noting that the p.E1297D mutation in SCN1A gene was previously reported in an Italian family with idiopathic childhood epilepsy [36]. The linkage between CACNA1A and SCN1A gene mutations and CADASIL has not previously been reported; therefore, an ongoing study in our lab will investigate the effect of these two variants/genes on CADASIL disease pathophysiology.

In terms of the clinical classification of the detected genetic variants, the full available evidence needs to be considered. Typical CADASIL mutations involve the addition or elimination of a cysteine residue in one of the 34 NOTCH3 gene epidermal growth factor (EGF)-like repeats, resulting in mismatched disulphide bridging and altered protein function, a hypothesis which has been borne out by observational and functional studies [37, 38]. Under the current American College of Medical Genetics and Genomics (ACMG) guidelines for variant classification, functional studies supporting a damaging effect for a variant on gene function constitute strong evidence for pathogenicity. Each of the cysteine altering variants also has multiple moderate and supporting lines of evidence. These include presence in a disease-associated functional domain; presence at a loci where

another pathogenic mutation is known (as determined by searching HGMD, LOVD and VEP databases); absence from controls in population databases (1000 Genomes, dbSNP, ExAC); being the kind of variant (missense SNV) associated with the disease; presence in an individual with a clear phenotype; cosegregation with disease in family members (only for patients C-10 and C-44) and multiple in silico analyses predicting pathogenicity. This combination of evidence is sufficient to characterise them as pathogenic or disease-causing mutations according to the ACMG guidelines [39].

For the non-cysteine altering NOTCH3 variants, there is less information available. Family segregation analysis and clinical information were not available for patients C-11 (p.D39V) or C-15 (p. R607H). Despite being novel amino acid changing variants in loci where disease-causing mutations are known to exist and/or functional domains, there is insufficient strength of evidence to classify either variant as pathogenic or likely pathogenic. Additionally, both these patients had complex phenotypes that do not precisely map to CADASIL, and share features of episodic ataxia or familial hemiplegic migraine, indicating a potential overlapping pathophysiology or comorbidities with these disorders. Thus, these variants should be classified as variants of uncertain significance (VOUS) according to the ACMG guidelines. Patient C-24 with the synonymous variant (p.E318E) had family history indicative of CADASIL, but no other supporting evidence, though neither does the variant have any criteria for being classified as benign. This variant has also been classified as a VOUS.

Patient C-36, who bears variants in both CACNA1A and SCN1A also, had no family members available for further investigation. Neither variant has sufficient evidence to indicate direct pathogenicity, despite being in regions of these genes known to harbour disease-causing mutations. Additionally, their presence in a gene which causes symptoms overlapping with CADASIL indicates a possible complex pathophysiology that requires more research. Hence, these variants have been classified as VOUS [39].

Finally, nine rare variants were identified in nine patients with no other causative mutation in NOTCH3 [Table 3]. Of these, three amino acid changing variants (p.S497L, p.A1020P and p.H1133Q) were recently reported by Abramycheva et al. [15] as normal polymorphisms in Russian CADASIL patients. However, in this study, patient C-3 was found to carry non-cysteine NOTCH3 gene variants (p.S496L and p.A1020P). As yet, a comparison of the effect of these two non-cysteine variants on the pathogenic mechanisms of CADASIL or CADASIL-like phenotype [16] to a single non-cysteine variant on disease pathogenesis has not been functionally tested.

We have identified classical CADASIL-causing mutations as well as a number of amino acid changing variants that have uncertain causative effects on this disease. The study of a larger population cohort of cases including symptomatic detail will likely provide more clinical and molecular information about their impact as well as the potential effect of any rare SNPs. Most interestingly, our results indicate that there may be other CADASIL gene/genes yet to be identified for inclusion in future diagnostic arrays.

Conclusions

NGS technologies provide an effective method for CADASIL and related disease diagnosis. Sequencing large but targeted regions of interest of pooled DNA from multiple samples is a promising tool for the discovery of both known and novel variants associated with disease. Compared with traditional SS, the NGS platform provides increased accuracy along with reduced time and assay costs necessary to perform routine genetic diagnosis of CADASIL in ethnically heterogeneous populations, putting such testing within reach of more patients.

Materials and methods
Patients

Forty-four patients with a suspected clinical diagnosis of CADASIL were re-screened using the NGS approach. Patients referred to the Genomics Research Centre (GRC) diagnostic laboratory for CADASIL molecular testing through neurologists from Australia and New Zealand and showed no mutations when using SS in our standard exon sequencing (3 and 4) at the first stage and (2, 11, 18 and 19) second stage [17]. Re-sequencing of the 44 patients was based on the clinical information had provided (i.e. positive skin biopsy results for CADA-SIL or white matter changes in their MRI) indicating that CADASIL-causing mutations may be present.

Molecular analysis
Ion AmpliSeq custom panel design

The AmpliSeq design target used in this report comprised the coding exons, exon/intron junctions and UTR regions of the *NOTCH3* gene. The Ampliseq automated primer design tool (http://www.ampliseq.com) was used to design primers covering 92.79 % of the desired target area (8071 bp) aligned to the reference human genome (hg 19). The missing regions include a 175 bp region in exon 1 (position 15311617-15311792 on chromosome 19) and a 407 bp region in exon 24 (position 15288427-15288834 on chromosome 19). The remainder of the 33 exons in the *NOTCH3* gene were included at 100 % coverage.

Library preparation

Genomic DNA was previously purified from peripheral blood samples using standard extraction conditions using Qiagen QIAamp DNA Blood Midi Kits as recommended by the manufacturer. The Qubit dsDNA High Sensitivity (HS) Assay Kit (Thermo Fisher Scientific, Scoresby, Victoria, Australia) was used to ensure accuracy of DNA concentration input (10 ng/μL) to NGS library construction.

Library preparation was performed using the Ion Ampli-Seq library kit 2.0 (Thermo Fisher Scientific, Scoresby, Victoria, Australia) according to the standard protocol (Cat. no. 4480441, Rev. 4.0). Briefly, for the multiplex PCR amplification, 10 ng of each genomic DNA sample was amplified using the optimised modification method generated in our laboratory allowing each primer pool to be amplified as a 5-μL reaction, rather than a 20-μL reaction (protocol is available upon request). This was performed using 1 μL of 5× Ion AmpliSeq HiFi Master Mix, 2.5 μL of 2× AmpliSeq Custom primer pool, 0.5 μL nuclease-free water and 1 μL (10 ng/μL) of DNA. The reaction mix was heated for 2 min at 99 °C for enzyme activation, followed by 18 two-step cycles of 99 °C for 15 s and 60 °C for 4 min, ending with a holding period at 10 °C.

After cycling, the two 5 μL/reaction pools for each sample were combined into a single well with a total volume 10 μL. The pooled amplified samples were partially digested using 1 μL FuPa enzyme per sample at 50 °C for 10 min and 55 °C for 10 min followed by enzyme inactivation at 60 °C for 20 min. To enable multiple sample libraries to be loaded per chip, 2 μL of a unique diluted Barcode Adapter mix including Ion Xpress Barcode (numbered 1-16) and Ion P1 Adaptor at standard volumes was ligated to the end of the digested amplicons using 1 μL DNA ligase for 30 min at 22 °C followed by ligase inactivation for 10 min at 72 °C. The resulting unamplified adaptor-ligated libraries were purified using the 22.5 μL Agencourt AMPure XP system (Beckman Coulter, Brea, CA, USA) followed by addition of 75 μL freshly prepared 70 % ethanol to each library.

After purification, the amplicon libraries were further amplified to enrich material for accurate quantification using 25 μL Platinum PCR SuperMix High Fidelity and 1 μL of library Amplification Primer Mix (Ion AmpliSeq library kit 2.0, Thermo Fisher Scientific, Scoresby, Victoria, Australia), at 98 °C for 2 min followed by five two-step cycles of 98 °C for 15 s and 60 °C for 1 min. The amplified amplicon libraries were then purified using 12.5 μL Agencourt AMPure XP Reagent followed by a second purification step with 30 μL AMPure XP and 75 μL of freshly prepared 70 % ethanol added to each library. The concentration and size of amplicons was then determined using an Agilent BioAnalyzer DNA High-Sensitivity chip (Agilent Technologies, Santa Clara,

CA, USA), according to manufacturers' instructions. After quantification, each library was diluted to a concentration of ~10 pM prior to template preparation. Subsequently, libraries ($n = 16$) were pooled in equimolar amounts prior to further processing.

Template preparation (emulsion PCR) and sequencing

Emulsion PCR, emulsion breaking and enrichment (template preparation) were performed using the Ion PGM OT2 200 Template Kit (Thermo Fisher Scientific, Scoresby, Victoria, Australia), according to the manufacturers' instructions (part no. 4480974 Rev. 4.0).

After preparation of the ISPs, sequencing was performed with an Ion Torrent Personal Genome Machine (PGM) system using Ion Sequencing 200 Kit V2 and an Ion 316 Chip (Thermo Fisher Scientific, Scoresby, Victoria, Australia) according to the manufacturers' procedures (Cat. no.4482006 Rev.1.0).

Bioinformatic analyses

The Ion Torrent PGM sequence data was mapped to the complete human genome (hg19) by the Ion Torrent Suite software and Torrent Server along with Torrent Mapping Alignment Program optimised to Ion Torrent data. The bam format file generated by Torrent Suite was uploaded and visualised for human examination using Integrative Genomics Viewer (IGV) 2.3 software [12]. The Ion Reporter software 4.0 (Thermo Fisher Scientific, Scoresby, Victoria, Australia) was used to analyse data from Torrent PGM. The software identifies variants and performs automated annotation on Ion PGM data. Variants were classified into simple categories, summarised into a report which included links to appropriate databases for known variants.

DNA and protein sequences from NGS and SS were compared with the NCBI reference sequences [13] and the UCSC genome browser [40]. All rs ID numbers, locations, allele frequencies and genotypes for all variants were determined based on SNPs reported in the dbSNP database [41] and further analysed in the 1000 Genomes data set. To predict the effect of non-synonymous single nucleotide substitutions on protein structure, function or phenotype, we used the wANNOVAR programme [42, 43] which included the use of five functional prediction software programmes for non-synonymous variants (PhyloP [44], SIFT [45], PolyPhen2 [46], MutationTaster [47] and GERP++ [48]). In silico prediction programmes including AGVGD [49] and PhD-SNP [50] were also used to predict causative variants. For synonymous variants and variants in non-coding regions, the MutationTaster [47] software alone was used. All variants detected were examined for associated information in the public databases (at a minimum, dbSNP, OMIM, LOVD, 1000 Genomes and HGMD) and in the published literature.

Sanger sequencing (SS)

All detected novel mutations by NGS were further investigated by SS. Molecular analysis of the *NOTCH3* gene was performed according to a previously described protocol [17]. Briefly, genomic DNA was extracted using Qiagen QIAamp DNA Blood Midi kits. DNA was amplified by PCR to screen the exons containing novel mutations and was performed with the primers shown in Additional file 3: Table S3 online. PCR amplification for all exons were conducted as previously described [17], and cycling protocols is available for all exons upon request. PCR products were purified using Affymetrix ExoSap-IT reagent (ExoSap-IT, USB Corporation, Staufen, Germany) and directly sequenced for both sense and antisense strands using Big Dye Terminator V3.1 (Applied Biosystems, Foster City, CA, USA) on an ABI 3500 Genetic Analyser (Applied Biosystems) according to established procedures. Sequences were analysed with Chromas 2.33 software (Technelysium, Brisbane, Queensland, Australia).

Abbreviations

CADASIL: Cerebral autosomal dominant arteriopathy with subcortical infarcts and leukoencephalopathy; DNA: Deoxyribonucleic acid; EGF: Epidermal growth factor; GERP: Genomic evolutionary rate profiling; GOM: Granular osmiophilic material; GRC: The Genomics Research Centre; IGV: Integrative Genomics Viewer; NATA: National Association of Testing Authorities, Australia; NCBI: National Centre for Biotechnology Information; NGS: Next-generation sequencing; *NOTCH3*: Notch, Drosophila, Homolog of, 3; PCR: Polymerase chain reaction; PGM: Personal Genome Machine; SNPs: Single nucleotide polymorphisms; UTR: Untranslated region

Acknowledgements

The authors express their gratitude to all neurologists for referring patients and supplying clinical data to our NATA accredited diagnostic lab at the Genomics Research Centre, IHBI, QUT. We thank A/Prof Rod Lea and Dr Miles Benton for help with bioinformatic analysis, interpretation and advice.

Funding

Neven Maksemous was supported by a QUT Postgraduate Scholarship. This work was supported by an Australian International Science Linkages grant and by infrastructure purchased with Australian Government EIF Super Science Funds as part of the Therapeutic Innovation Australia - Queensland Node project and by the Migraine Research Foundation, NY, USA.

Authors' contributions

NM performed the experimental, sequence analysis research, data analysis and drafted the manuscript with input from all authors. LMH contributed to the interpretation of the data, read, edited and approved the manuscript. LRG and RAS conceived the project, supervised research and analysis, read, edited and approved the manuscript.

Competing interests

The authors declare that they have no competing interests.

References

1. Chabriat H, et al. Clinical spectrum of CADASIL: a study of 7 families. Cerebral autosomal dominant arteriopathy with subcortical infarcts and leukoencephalopathy. Lancet. 1995;346(8980):934–9.
2. Ruchoux MM, et al. Presence of ultrastructural arterial lesions in muscle and skin vessels of patients with CADASIL. Stroke. 1994;25(11):2291–2.
3. Chabriat H, et al. Autosomal dominant migraine with MRI white-matter abnormalities mapping to the CADASIL locus. Neurology. 1995;45(6):1086–91.
4. Joutel A, et al. Notch3 mutations in CADASIL, a hereditary adult-onset condition causing stroke and dementia. Nature. 1996;383(6602):707–10.
5. Thomsen LL, Olesen J, Russell MB. Increased risk of migraine with typical aura in probands with familial hemiplegic migraine and their relatives. Eur J Neurol. 2003;10(4):421–7.
6. Vedeler C, Bindoff L. A family with atypical CADASIL. J Neurol. 2011;258(10):1888–9.
7. Maksemous N, et al. Next-generation sequencing identifies novel CACNA1A gene mutations in episodic ataxia type 2. Mol Genet Genomic Med. 2016;4(2):211–22.
8. Dichgans M, et al. Small in-frame deletions and missense mutations in CADASIL: 3D models predict misfolding of Notch3 EGF-like repeat domains. Eur J Hum Genet. 2000;8(4):280–5.
9. Oliveri RL, et al. A novel mutation in the Notch3 gene in an Italian family with cerebral autosomal dominant arteriopathy with subcortical infarcts and leukoencephalopathy: genetic and magnetic resonance spectroscopic findings. Arch Neurol. 2001;58(9):1418–22.
10. Tang SC, et al. Arg332Cys mutation of NOTCH3 gene in the first known Taiwanese family with cerebral autosomal dominant arteriopathy with subcortical infarcts and leukoencephalopathy. J Neurol Sci. 2005;228(2):125–8.
11. Razvi SS, et al. Diagnostic strategies in CADASIL. Neurology. 2003;60(12):2019–20. author reply 2020.
12. Thorvaldsdottir H, Robinson JT, Mesirov JP. Integrative Genomics Viewer (IGV): high-performance genomics data visualization and exploration. Brief Bioinform. 2013;14(2):178–92.
13. Pruitt KD, et al. NCBI Reference Sequences (RefSeq): current status, new features and genome annotation policy. Nucleic Acids Res. 2012;40(Database issue):D130–5.
14. Markus HS, et al. Diagnostic strategies in CADASIL. Neurology. 2002;59(8):1134–8.
15. Abramycheva N, et al. New mutations in the Notch3 gene in patients with cerebral autosomal dominant arteriopathy with subcortical infarcts and leucoencephalopathy (CADASIL). J Neurol Sci. 2015;349(1-2):196–201.
16. He D, et al. The comparisons of phenotype and genotype between CADASIL and CADASIL-like patients and population-specific evaluation of CADASIL scale in China. J Headache Pain. 2016;17:55.
17. Roy B, et al. Two novel mutations and a previously unreported intronic polymorphism in the NOTCH3 gene. Mutat Res. 2012;732(1-2):3–8.
18. Bianchi S, et al. CADASIL in central Italy: a retrospective clinical and genetic study in 229 patients. J Neurol. 2015;262(1):134–41.
19. Fernandez A, et al. A next-generation sequencing of the NOTCH3 and HTRA1 Genes in CADASIL Patients. J Mol Neurosci. 2015;56(3):613–6.
20. Adib-Samii P, et al. Clinical spectrum of CADASIL and the effect of cardiovascular risk factors on phenotype: study in 200 consecutively recruited individuals. Stroke. 2010;41(4):630–4.
21. Kim YE, et al. Spectrum of NOTCH3 mutations in Korean patients with clinically suspicious cerebral autosomal dominant arteriopathy with subcortical infarcts and leukoencephalopathy. Neurobiol Aging. 2014;35(3):726 e1–6.
22. Joutel A, et al. Pathogenic mutations associated with cerebral autosomal dominant arteriopathy with subcortical infarcts and leukoencephalopathy differently affect Jagged1 binding and Notch3 activity via the RBP/JK signaling Pathway. Am J Hum Genet. 2004;74(2):338–47.
23. Wang W, et al. Notch3 signaling in vascular smooth muscle cells induces c-FLIP expression via ERK/MAPK activation. Resistance to Fas ligand-induced apoptosis. J Biol Chem. 2002;277(24):21723–9.
24. Joutel A. Loss-of-function mutation in the NOTCH3 gene: simply a polymorphism? Hum Mutat. 2013;34(11):v.
25. Bohlega S. Novel mutation of the notch3 gene in arabic family with CADASIL. Neurol Int. 2011;3(2):e6.
26. Lee YC, et al. Cerebral autosomal dominant arteriopathy with subcortical infarcts and leukoencephalopathy: two novel mutations in the NOTCH3 gene in Chinese. J Neurol Sci. 2006;246(1-2):111–5.
27. Brass SD, et al. Case records of the Massachusetts General Hospital. Case 12-2009. A 46-year-old man with migraine, aphasia, and hemiparesis and similarly affected family members. N Engl J Med. 2009;360(16):1656–65.
28. Kim Y, et al. Characteristics of CADASIL in Korea: a novel cysteine-sparing Notch3 mutation. Neurology. 2006;66(10):1511–6.
29. Mazzei R, et al. A novel Notch3 gene mutation not involving a cysteine residue in an Italian family with CADASIL. Neurology. 2004;63(3):561–4.
30. Santa Y, et al. Genetic, clinical and pathological studies of CADASIL in Japan: a partial contribution of Notch3 mutations and implications of smooth muscle cell degeneration for the pathogenesis. J Neurol Sci. 2003;212(1-2):79–84.
31. Scheid R, et al. Cysteine-sparing notch3 mutations: cadasil or cadasil variants? Neurology. 2008;71(10):774–6.
32. Uchino M, et al. Cerebral autosomal dominant arteriopathy with subcortical infarcts and leukoencephalopathy (CADASIL) and CADASIL-like disorders in Japan. Ann N Y Acad Sci. 2002;977:273–8.
33. Herman-Bert A, et al. Mapping of spinocerebellar ataxia 13 to chromosome 19q13.3-q13.4 in a family with autosomal dominant cerebellar ataxia and mental retardation. Am J Hum Genet. 2000;67(1):229–35.
34. Ophoff RA, et al. Familial hemiplegic migraine and episodic ataxia type-2 are caused by mutations in the Ca2+ channel gene CACNL1A4. Cell. 1996;87(3):543–52.
35. Wallace RH, et al. Neuronal sodium-channel alpha1-subunit mutations in generalized epilepsy with febrile seizures plus. Am J Hum Genet. 2001;68(4):859–65.
36. Orrico A, et al. Mutational analysis of the SCN1A, SCN1B and GABRG2 genes in 150 Italian patients with idiopathic childhood epilepsies. Clin Genet. 2009;75(6):579–81.
37. Arboleda-Velasquez JF, et al. CADASIL mutations impair Notch3 glycosylation by Fringe. Hum Mol Genet. 2005;14(12):1631–9.
38. Opherk C, et al. CADASIL mutations enhance spontaneous multimerization of NOTCH3. Hum Mol Genet. 2009;18(15):2761–7.
39. Richards S, et al. Standards and guidelines for the interpretation of sequence variants: a joint consensus recommendation of the American College of Medical Genetics and Genomics and the Association for Molecular Pathology. Genet Med. 2015;17(5):405–24.
40. Dreszer TR, et al. The UCSC Genome Browser database: extensions and updates 2011. Nucleic Acids Res. 2012;40(Database issue):D918–23.
41. Sherry ST, et al. dbSNP: the NCBI database of genetic variation. Nucleic Acids Res. 2001;29(1):308–11.
42. Chang X, Wang K. wANNOVAR: annotating genetic variants for personal genomes via the web. J Med Genet. 2012;49(7):433–6.
43. Wang K, Li M, Hakonarson H. ANNOVAR: functional annotation of genetic variants from high-throughput sequencing data. Nucleic Acids Res. 2010;38(16):e164.
44. Pollard KS, et al. Detection of nonneutral substitution rates on mammalian phylogenies. Genome Res. 2010;20(1):110–21.
45. Ng PC, Henikoff S. Predicting deleterious amino acid substitutions. Genome Res. 2001;11(5):863–74.
46. Adzhubei IA, et al. A method and server for predicting damaging missense mutations. Nat Methods. 2010;7(4):248–9.
47. Schwarz JM, et al. MutationTaster evaluates disease-causing potential of sequence alterations. Nat Methods. 2010;7(8):575–6.
48. Davydov EV, et al. Identifying a high fraction of the human genome to be under selective constraint using GERP++. PLoS Comput Biol. 2010;6(12):e1001025.
49. Tavtigian SV, et al. Comprehensive statistical study of 452 BRCA1 missense substitutions with classification of eight recurrent substitutions as neutral. J Med Genet. 2006;43(4):295–305.
50. Capriotti E, Calabrese R, Casadio R. Predicting the insurgence of human genetic diseases associated to single point protein mutations with support vector machines and evolutionary information. Bioinformatics. 2006;22(22):2729–34.

2

The peptidylglycine-α-amidating monooxygenase (*PAM*) gene rs13175330 A>G polymorphism is associated with hypertension in a Korean population

Hye Jin Yoo[1,2†], Minjoo Kim[3†], Minkyung Kim[3], Jey Sook Chae[3], Sang-Hyun Lee[4] and Jong Ho Lee[1,2,3*]

Abstract

Background: Peptidylglycine-α-amidating monooxygenase (PAM) may play a role in the secretion of atrial natriuretic peptide (ANP), which is a hormone involved in the maintenance of blood pressure (BP). The objective of the present study was to determine whether *PAM* is a novel candidate gene for hypertension (HTN).

Results: A total of 2153 Korean participants with normotension and HTN were included. Genotype data were obtained using the Korean Chip. The rs13175330 polymorphism of the *PAM* gene was selected from the ten single nucleotide polymorphisms (SNPs) most strongly associated with BP. The presence of the G allele of the *PAM* rs13175330 A>G SNP was associated with a higher risk of HTN after adjustments for age, sex, BMI, smoking, and drinking [OR 1.607 (95% CI 1.220–2.116), $p = 0.001$]. The rs13175330 G allele carriers in the HTN group treated without antihypertensive therapy (HTN w/o therapy) had significantly higher systolic and diastolic BP than the AA carriers, whereas the G allele carriers in the HTN group treated with antihypertensive therapy (HTN w/ therapy) showed significantly higher diastolic BP. Furthermore, rs13175330 G allele carriers in the HTN w/o therapy group had significantly increased levels of insulin, insulin resistance, and oxidized low-density lipoprotein (LDL) and significantly decreased LDL-cholesterol levels and LDL particle sizes compared to the AA carriers.

Conclusion: These results suggest that the *PAM* rs13175330 A>G SNP is a novel candidate gene for HTN in the Korean population. Additionally, the *PAM* rs13175330 G allele might be associated with insulin resistance and LDL atherogenicity in patients with HTN.

Keywords: Hypertension, Genetic polymorphisms, Genetic association, Peptidylglycine-α-amidating monooxygenase, Atrial natriuretic peptide, LDL atherogenicity

Background

Hypertension (HTN) is a significant contributor to the global burden of heart disease, stroke, kidney failure, and premature mortality and disability [1, 2]. HTN is a complex trait that is caused by both genetic and environmental factors [3]. Evidence from family studies indicates that more than 30% of blood pressure (BP) variation can be attributed to genetics [4, 5]. Recently, genome-wide association studies (GWASs) have identified more than 50 single nucleotide polymorphisms (SNPs) associated with an increased risk of HTN [6–8].

The neuroendocrine processing enzyme peptidylglycine-α-amidating monooxygenase (PAM) is highly concentrated in the atrium and may play a role in the secretion of atrial natriuretic peptide (ANP), which is a hormone involved in BP maintenance and fluid homeostasis [9–11]. Indeed, PAM and pro-ANP (the bioactive form of ANP) are the predominant membrane-associated proteins in atrial secretory granules [12]. Because close relationships exist

* Correspondence: jhleeb@yonsei.ac.kr

†Equal contributors

[1]National Leading Research Laboratory of Clinical Nutrigenetics/Nutrigenomics, Department of Food and Nutrition, College of Human Ecology, Yonsei University, 50 Yonsei-ro, Seodaemun-gu, Seoul 03722, South Korea

[2]Department of Food and Nutrition, Brain Korea 21 PLUS Project, College of Human Ecology, Yonsei University, Seoul 03722, South Korea

Full list of author information is available at the end of the article

between ANP and BP and between ANP and PAM [9–11], specific *PAM* SNP genotypes in humans may be associated with BP alterations.

Since 2014, the Korean Chip (K-CHIP), which includes 833,535 SNPs and uses an oligomer as a probe, has been developed by the Korea Biobank Array project as a low-cost customized chip that is optimized for genetic studies of diseases and complex traits in Koreans (Additional file 1: Table S1). Since whole-genome sequencing requires very high calculation capacity and cost and commercial chips are designed for Western populations, whose genomic variants differ from Asian populations, the K-CHIP is more suitable for the discovery and identification of Korean population-specific SNPs related to disease occurrence [13, 14]. Although the K-CHIP has only been released recently, several published studies have used the K-CHIP [15, 16]. These studies have gained international recognition; thus, the K-CHIP has been shown to be an appropriate tool for analyzing SNPs associated with diseases in a Korean population.

To the best of our knowledge, this study was the first to investigate HTN-related SNPs using the K-CHIP in a Korean population. Therefore, the objective of the present study was to explore HTN-related SNPs using the K-CHIP, to identify the SNP most strongly associated with BP, and to determine whether *PAM* is a novel candidate gene for HTN among the Korean population.

Methods

Study population

A total of 2153 Korean male and female adult participants (male, $n = 866$; female, $n = 1287$; aged 20–86 years; median = 50 years) with nondiabetic normotension (systolic BP < 140 mmHg and diastolic BP < 90 mmHg) and HTN (systolic BP ≥ 140 mmHg or diastolic BP ≥ 90 mmHg) were recruited for this study from the Health Service Center (HSC) during routine checkups at the National Health Insurance Corporation Ilsan Hospital in Goyang, Korea (January 2010–March 2015). Based on the data screened from the HSC, potential subjects with HTN were referred to the Department of Family Medicine or Internal Medicine, where their health and BP were rechecked. Finally, subjects who did not meet the exclusion criteria were all included as study participants. The exclusion criteria were a current diagnosis and/or a history of diabetes, cardiovascular disease, liver disease, renal disease, pancreatitis, cancer, or any life- and health-threatening diseases; pregnancy or lactation; and regular use of any medication except HTN therapy. The aim of the study was carefully explained to all participants, whom provided written informed consent. The Institutional Review Board of Yonsei University and the National Health Insurance Corporation Ilsan Hospital approved the study protocol, which complied with the Declaration of Helsinki.

Anthropometric measurements

Body weight (UM0703581; Tanita, Tokyo, Japan) and height (GL-150; G-Tech International, Uijeongbu, Korea) were measured in lightly clothed subjects without shoes, and body mass index (BMI) values were calculated (kg/m^2). Waist circumference was measured directly on the skin at the umbilical level after normal expiration with the subject in an upright standing position. Hip circumference was measured at the protruding part of the hip in standing subjects using a plastic measuring tape with measurements to the nearest 0.1 cm. Waist to hip ratio values were obtained by dividing the waist circumference by the hip circumference. Systolic and diastolic BP were measured using a random-zero sphygmomanometer (HM-1101, Hico Medical Co., Ltd., Chiba, Japan) with appropriately sized cuffs after a rest period of at least 20 min in a seated position. BP was measured three times in both arms. The differences among the three systolic BP measurements were always less than 2 mmHg. Participants were instructed not to smoke or drink alcohol for at least 30 min before each BP measurement.

Sample collection

Fasting venous blood specimens were collected following an overnight fast of at least 12 h. The samples were collected in EDTA-treated tubes and serum tubes (BD Vacutainer; Becton, Dickinson and Company, Franklin Lakes, NJ, USA). The samples were placed in an ice box that was protected from light within approximately 30 min and then centrifuged (1200 rpm for 20 min at 4 °C) within 3 h to obtain plasma and serum. The plasma and serum aliquots were stored at – 80 °C prior to analysis.

Serum fasting lipid profiles

The serum fasting triglyceride (TG) and total-cholesterol (TC) levels were measured using enzymatic assays with the TG and CHOL Kits (Roche, Mannheim, Germany), respectively. Serum fasting high-density lipoprotein (HDL)-cholesterol was measured using a selective inhibition method with the HDL-C Plus Kit (Roche, Mannheim, Germany). The resulting color reactions of the assays were monitored using a Hitachi 7600 autoanalyzer (Hitachi, Tokyo, Japan). The Friedewald formula was used to indirectly calculate low-density lipoprotein (LDL)-cholesterol levels as follows: LDL-cholesterol = TC – [HDL-cholesterol + (TG/5)].

Serum fasting glucose, insulin, and insulin resistance (IR)

The serum fasting glucose level was measured using the hexokinase method with the GLU Kit (Roche, Mannheim, Germany), and the resulting color reaction was monitored with the Hitachi 7600 autoanalyzer (Hitachi, Tokyo, Japan). Serum fasting insulin was measured with an immunoradiometric assay using the Insulin IRMA

Kit (DIAsource, Louvain, Belgium), and the resulting color reaction was monitored with an SR-300 system (Stratec, Birkenfeld, Germany). The homeostatic model assessment (HOMA) equation was used to calculate the IR as follows: HOMA-IR = [fasting insulin (μIU/mL) $\times$ fasting glucose (mg/dL)]/405.

Plasma LDL particle size and oxidized (ox)-LDL level

Plasma LDL particles were isolated by sequential flotation ultracentrifugation, and the particle size distribution (1.019–1.063 g/mL) was assessed using a pore-gradient lipoprotein system (CBS Scientific Company, San Diego, CA, USA) on commercially available non-denaturing gels containing a linear 2–16% acrylamide gradient (CBS Scientific Company, San Diego, CA, USA). Latex bead (30 nm)-conjugated thyroglobulin (17 nm), ferritin (12.2 nm), and catalase (10.4 nm) standards were used to measure the relative band migration rates. The gels were scanned using a GS-800 Calibrated Imaging Densitometer (Bio-Rad Laboratories, Hercules, CA, USA). Plasma ox-LDL was estimated using an enzyme immunoassay (Mercodia AB, Uppsala, Sweden), and the resulting color reaction was determined at 450 nm on a Wallac Victor2 multilabel counter (Perkin-Elmer Life Sciences, Boston, MA, USA).

Affymetrix axiom™ KORV1.0–96 array hybridization and SNP selection

A total of 2167 samples were genotyped according to the manufacturer's protocol included in the Axiom® 2.0 Reagent Kit (Affymetrix Axiom® 2.0 Assay User Guide; Affymetrix, Santa Clara, CA, USA). Approximately 200 ng of genomic DNA (gDNA) was amplified and randomly fragmented into 25- to 125-base pair (bp) fragments. The initial gDNA amplification was performed in a 40-μL reaction volume containing 20 μL of genomic DNA at a 10 ng/μL concentration and 20 μL of the denaturation master mix. The initial amplification reaction included a 10-min incubation at room temperature; then, the incubated products were amplified with 130 μL of Axiom 2.0 Neutral Soln, 225 μL of Axiom 2.0 Amp Soln, and 5 μL of Axiom 2.0 Amp Enzyme. The amplification reactions were performed for 23 $\pm$ 1 h at 37 °C. The amplification products were analyzed in an optimized reaction to amplify fragments between 200 and 1100 bp in length. A fragmentation step reduced the amplified products to segments of approximately 25–50 bp in length, which were end-labeled using biotinylated nucleotides. Following hybridization, the bound target was washed under stringent conditions to remove non-specific background and to minimize the background noise caused by random ligation events. Each polymorphic nucleotide was investigated via a multicolor ligation event conducted on the array surface. After ligation, the arrays were stained and imaged using the GeneTitan MC Instrument (Affymetrix, Santa Clara, CA, USA). The images were analyzed using the Genotyping Console™ Software (Affymetrix, Santa Clara, CA, USA). Genotype data were produced using the K-CHIP, which is available through the K-CHIP consortium. The K-CHIP was designed by the Center for Genome Science at the Korea National Institute of Health (4845–301, 3000–3031).

Samples with the following thresholds were excluded: sex inconsistency, markers with a high missing rate (> 5%), individuals with a high missing rate (> 10%), a minor allele frequency < 0.01, and a significant deviation from the Hardy-Weinberg equilibrium (HWE) ($p <$ 0.001). Additionally, SNPs that were in linkage disequilibrium (LD, $r^2 \geq 0.5$) were excluded. The remaining 394,222 SNPs and 2159 samples were included in the subsequent association analysis.

Statistical analysis

HWE and the associations between SNPs and BP were analyzed with PLINK version 1.07 (http://zzz.bwh.harvard.edu/plink/); the associations were assessed using the linear regression analysis method. Descriptive statistical analyses were conducted using SPSS version 23.0 (IBM, Chicago, IL, USA). For the *PAM* rs13175330 polymorphism, because of the small number of rare allele homozygotes (GG), we pooled heterozygotes (AG) and rare allele homozygotes to increase the statistical power. Logarithmic transformation was used for skewed variables, and data are expressed as the mean $\pm$ standard error (SE). A two-tailed p value < 0.05 was considered statistically significant. An independent t test was performed on continuous variables to compare values between the normotensive group and each hypertensive subgroup and to compare the values between the genotypes within the normotensive group and each hypertensive subgroup. Frequencies were tested with a chi-square test. The association of HTN with a *PAM* rs13175330 genotype was calculated using the odds ratio (OR) [95% confidence intervals (CIs)] of a logistic regression model with adjustments for confounding factors.

Results

As mentioned above, 394,222 SNPs and 2159 samples were included in the analysis. The ten SNPs that were most strongly associated with BP were selected from the linear regression analysis to assess the association between SNPs and BP. Among them, we identified rs13175330 in the *PAM* gene. The first systolic and diastolic BP-related SNP did not have a reference SNP ID in the SNP database; therefore, we conducted an association analysis using rs13175330, which was the second diastolic BP-related SNP and the seventh systolic BP-related SNP (Additional file 1: Table S2). Among the 2159 genotyped subjects, 6 subjects did not possess a *PAM* variant; thus, only 2153 subjects were included in the final sample.

This was a large study with many samples, and the samples were run on multiple assay plates; thus, we checked inter-and intra-assay coefficient of variability (CV) to reduce multiple assay error although the experiments were not repeated. The mean inter- and intra-assay CV (%) of each variable was as follows (inter-assay CV; intra-assay CV): triglyceride (2.18; 0.95), total-cholesterol (1.19; 1.29), HDL-cholesterol (1.13; 1.16), LDL-cholesterol (0.98; 0.65), glucose (1.01; 0.71), insulin (4.25; 3.55), LDL particle size (2.29; 3.88), and ox-LDL (0.96; 6.78).

Clinical and biochemical characteristics according to the presence of hypertension

A total of 2153 subjects were divided into a normotensive control group (*n* = 1610) and an HTN group (*n* = 543). The HTN group was stratified according to their antihypertensive therapy [patients with HTN without antihypertensive therapy (HTN w/o therapy), *n* = 377; and patients with HTN with antihypertensive therapy (HTN w/ therapy), *n* = 166]. The clinical and biochemical characteristics of each group are shown in Table 1. Patients in the HTN group and all of the HTN subgroups were significantly older and heavier and had significantly higher systolic and diastolic BP, TG, glucose,

insulin, and HOMA-IR indices than the normotensive controls (Table 1). Conversely, the HTN group and all of the HTN subgroups had significantly decreased HDL-cholesterol levels compared with the normotensive controls (Table 1). Ox-LDL was significantly increased in the HTN and HTN w/o therapy groups but not in the HTN w/ therapy group compared to the normotensive controls (Table 1).

Distribution of the *PAM* rs13175330 A>G polymorphism

The genotype distributions of the *PAM* rs13175330 A>G polymorphism were in HWE in the entire population. Among the 1610 normotensive controls, 1377 subjects (85.5%) had the AA genotype, 228 subjects (14.2%) had the AG genotype, and 5 subjects (0.3%) had the GG genotype. The allele frequency of the G allele was 0.074 in the normotensive controls. Conversely, among the 543 patients with HTN, 434 subjects (79.9%) had the AA genotype, 102 (18.8%) subjects had the AG genotype, and 7 (1.29%) subjects had the GG genotype. The allele frequency of the G allele was 0.107 in the HTN group. The distribution of the *PAM* rs13175330 A>G genotype ($p = 0.001$) and the allele frequencies ($p = 0.001$) in the HTN group differed significantly from the values obtained in the normotensive controls (Additional file 1: Table S3).

Table 1 Clinical and biochemical characteristics in the normotensive controls and HTN patient subgroups according to the antihypertensive therapy

	Normotensive controls (*n* = 1610)		HTN group (*n* = 543)					
			Total (*n* = 543)		HTN w/o therapy (*n* = 377)		HTN w/ therapy (*n* = 166)	
Age (years)	48.0	± 0.27	54.4	± 0.50[***]	53.0	± 0.61[***]	57.7	± 0.83[***]
Weight (kg)	63.0	± 0.25	68.1	± 0.51[***]	68.9	± 0.64[***]	66.3	± 0.81[***]
BMI (kg/m²)	23.7	± 0.07	25.4	± 0.14[***]	25.4	± 0.17[***]	25.2	± 0.22[***]
Waist (cm)	83.5	± 0.19	87.9	± 0.37[***]	87.9	± 0.46[***]	88.0	± 0.63[***]
Waist hip ratio	0.88	± 0.00	0.90	± 0.00[***]	0.90	± 0.00[***]	0.91	± 0.00[***]
Systolic BP (mmHg)	116.4	± 0.29	138.5	±0.66[***]	145.2	± 0.62[***]	123.2	± 0.79[***]
Diastolic BP (mmHg)	72.7	± 0.22	87.4	± 0.46[***]	91.8	± 0.42[***]	77.4	± 0.66[***]
Triglyceride (mg/dL)[a]	119.6	± 1.84	148.6	± 3.76[***]	151.2	± 4.79[***]	142.8	± 5.72[***]
Total-cholesterol (mg/dL)[a]	198.1	± 0.90	198.3	± 1.54	200.2	± 1.87	193.9	± 2.68
HDL-cholesterol (mg/dL)[a]	53.9	± 0.34	50.4	± 0.55[***]	50.3	± 0.65[***]	50.5	± 1.03[**]
LDL-cholesterol (mg/dL)[a]	121.1	± 0.82	119.1	± 1.42	120.7	± 1.77	115.4	± 2.31
Glucose (mg/dL)[a]	95.6	± 0.51	103.9	± 1.11[***]	103.9	± 1.40[***]	103.9	± 1.73[***]
Insulin (μIU/dL)[a]	9.09	± 0.12	9.84	± 0.25[*]	10.1	± 0.33[*]	9.73	± 0.35[*]
HOMA-IR[a]	2.15	± 0.03	2.55	± 0.09[***]	2.65	± 0.12[***]	2.44	± 0.09[***]
LDL particle size (nm)[a]	23.9	± 0.03	24.0	± 0.05	23.9	± 0.06	24.0	± 0.08
Oxidized LDL (U/L)[a]	46.1	± 0.53	48.3	± 0.97[*]	50.8	± 1.15[***]	43.7	± 1.75

Mean ± SE

HTN hypertension, *HTN w/o therapy* HTN group treated without antihypertensive therapy, *HTN w/ therapy* HTN group treated with antihypertensive therapy, *BMI* body mass index, *BP* blood pressure, *HDL* high-density lipoprotein, *LDL* low-density lipoprotein, *HOMA-IR* homeostatic model assessment of insulin resistance

[*]$p < 0.05$, [**]$p < 0.01$, and [***]$p < 0.001$ derived from an independent *t* test between the normotensive controls and each HTN subgroup

[a]Tested following logarithmic transformation

Increased HTN risk associated with the *PAM* rs13175330 A>G polymorphism

Table 2 shows the unadjusted and adjusted odds ratios (OR) for all patients with HTN according to their *PAM* rs13175330 genotype. The presence of the GG genotype of the *PAM* rs13175330 A>G SNP was associated with a higher risk of HTN [OR 4.192 (95% CI 1.325–13.263), $p = 0.015$] (Table 2). The significance of the association remained after adjustments for confounding factors, including age, sex, BMI, smoking, and drinking [OR 7.826 (95% CI 2.228–27.484), $p = 0.001$]. Moreover, the rs13175330 G allele was associated with a higher risk of HTN before [OR 1.484 (95% CI 1.154–1.909), $p = 0.002$] and after adjustments for the confounding factors [OR 1.607 (95% CI 1.220–2.116), $p = 0.001$] (Table 2).

Association between BP and the *PAM* rs13175330 A>G genotype

No significant genotype-related differences were observed among the normotensive controls or HTN subjects treated with/without antihypertensive therapy according to the *PAM* rs13175330 A>G genotype with respect to age, sex, BMI, smoking, and drinking (data not shown). In the normotensive controls, rs13175330 G allele carriers tended to have higher systolic BP than the AA carriers ($p = 0.056$) (Table 3). In the HTN w/o therapy group, rs13175330 G allele carriers had significantly higher systolic BP ($p = 0.036$) and diastolic BP ($p = 0.048$) than the AA carriers. Additionally, the rs13175330 G allele carriers in the HTN w/ therapy group had significantly higher diastolic BP ($p < 0.001$); however, no significant difference in systolic BP between rs13175330 G allele and AA carriers was observed in the HTN w/ therapy group (Table 3).

Table 2 Unadjusted and adjusted OR for all patients with HTN according to the *PAM* rs13175330 genotypes

PAM rs13175330	HTN group ($n = 543$) OR (95% CI)	p values
Model 1		
A[‖] compared with G	1.498 (1.186, 1.892)	0.001
AA + AG[‖] compared with GG	4.192 (1.325, 13.263)	0.015
AA[‖] compared with AG + GG	1.484 (1.154, 1.909)	0.002
Model 2		
A[‖] compared with G	1.642 (1.272, 2.121)	< 0.001
AA + AG[‖] compared with GG	7.826 (2.228, 27.484)	0.001
AA[‖] compared with AG + GG	1.607 (1.220, 2.116)	0.001

[‖]Reference
CI confidence interval, *Model 1* unadjusted, *Model 2* adjusted for age, sex, BMI, smoking, and drinking, *OR* odds ratio, *HTN* hypertension, *PAM* peptidylglycine-α-amidating monooxygenase

Lipid profiles, insulin levels, LDL particle sizes, and ox-LDL levels according to the *PAM* rs13175330 A>G genotype

In the HTN w/o therapy group, rs13175330 G allele carriers had significantly higher insulin levels ($p = 0.001$), HOMA-IR indices ($p = 0.002$), and ox-LDL levels ($p = 0.046$) than the AA carriers (Table 3) but significantly lower LDL-cholesterol levels ($p = 0.039$) and smaller LDL particle sizes ($p = 0.003$) than the AA carriers. These genotype effects on the lipid profile, insulin level, LDL particle size, and ox-LDL level were not observed in the normotensive controls or the HTN w/ therapy group (Table 3).

Discussion

To conduct statistical analysis, we pooled heterozygotes (AG) and rare allele homozygotes (GG) because the number of rare allele homozygotes was too small. Even though there are statistical procedures that can handle unbalanced sample size across compared groups, immoderate unbalanced samples can cause problems [17]. In many cases, a sample size of groups stratified by a genotype is unbalanced due to rare allele frequency. To solve the problem, researchers (1) should anticipate the number of study participants via estimation of genotype frequency according to allele frequency or (2) should balance the number of study participants across groups through a prescreening of genotypes [17]. However, in both cases, if rare allele frequency of a SNP in which researchers are interested is too low, the number of study participants increases too much and the loss of time and cost associated with genotype prescreening will be huge [17]. Therefore, as the other strategy for balancing sample size across the groups, we combined AG and GG genotypes; it is more balanced for statistical purposes [17] rather than analyzing the subjects according to the rs13175330 genotypes (AA vs. AG vs. GG).

The major finding of this study was that the minor G allele frequency of *PAM* rs13175330 A>G was significantly higher in the patients with HTN than in the normotensive controls, suggesting an association between *PAM* rs13175330 A>G and HTN. There are no previous publications regarding a relationship between polymorphisms of *PAM* and HTN development and the effects of PAM dysfunction caused by *PAM* polymorphisms on the risk of HTN; thus, this is the first study to suggest that the *PAM* rs13175330 G allele is related to an increase risk of HTN.

PAM rs13175330 A>G is an intronic SNP. Introns have several functions including regulation of alternative splicing and gene expression [18]; via regulating a rate of transcriptional elongation, RNA processing, or RNA turnover, intronic regions can influence RNA levels [19]. Studies support that intronic SNPs do affect RNA splicing [20] and mRNA expression [19, 21]. Finally, Zhou et al. [22] reported that an intronic SNP in *CD44* intron 1 is associated with breast cancer development. Many evidences prove that an intronic SNP can be a novel

Table 3 Clinical and biochemical characteristics in the normotensive controls and HTN patient subgroups according to the PAM rs13175330 genotype

PAM rs13175330	Normotensive controls (n = 1610)				HTN group (n = 543)							
					HTN w/o therapy (n = 377)				HTN w/ therapy (n = 166)			
	AA (n = 1377)		G allele (n = 233)		AA (n = 305)		G allele (n = 72)		AA (n = 129)		G allele (n = 37)	
Systolic BP (mmHg)	116.2	± 0.31	117.7	± 0.74[†]	144.6	± 0.68	147.9	± 1.46[*]	123.2	± 0.90	123.4	± 1.70
Diastolic BP (mmHg)	72.6	± 0.23	73.3	± 0.58	91.4	± 0.45	93.8	± 1.11[*]	75.7	± 0.63	83.3	± 1.67[***]
Triglyceride (mg/dL)[a]	119.4	± 2.02	121.1	± 4.29	148.2	± 5.10	163.9	± 12.7	141.3	± 6.79	148.4	± 9.93
Total-cholesterol (mg/dL)[a]	198.0	± 0.96	198.6	± 2.53	201.7	± 2.06	194.1	± 4.43	193.8	± 3.01	194.5	± 5.97
HDL-cholesterol (mg/dL)[a]	54.0	± 0.37	53.5	± 0.84	50.3	± 0.73	50.4	± 1.45	50.7	± 1.20	49.7	± 1.98
LDL-cholesterol (mg/dL)[a]	121.1	± 0.88	121.1	± 2.20	122.7	± 1.99	112.0	± 3.71[*]	115.5	± 2.66	115.1	± 4.63
Glucose (mg/dL)[a]	95.5	± 0.55	96.5	± 1.47	103.7	± 1.49	104.8	± 3.76	105.7	± 2.08	97.5	± 2.56[*]
Insulin (μIU/dL)[a]	9.07	± 0.13	9.26	± 0.28	9.60	± 0.33	12.1	± 0.99[**]	9.56	± 0.38	10.4	± 0.79
HOMA-IR[a]	2.14	± 0.04	2.21	± 0.08	2.50	± 0.11	3.29	± 0.41[**]	2.45	± 0.11	2.40	± 0.17
LDL particle size (nm)[a]	23.9	± 0.04	24.0	± 0.06	24.0	± 0.07	23.5	± 0.12[**]	24.0	± 0.09	23.9	± 0.17
Oxidized LDL (U/L)[a]	45.9	± 0.56	47.4	± 1.53	49.8	± 1.27	55.0	± 2.70[*]	43.7	± 2.09	43.7	± 2.85

Mean ± SE

HTN hypertension, HTN w/o therapy HTN group treated without antihypertensive therapy, HTN w/ therapy HTN group treated with antihypertensive therapy, BP blood pressure, HDL high-density lipoprotein, LDL low-density lipoprotein, HOMA-IR homeostatic model assessment of insulin resistance, PAM peptidylglycine-α-amidating monooxygenase

[†]$p < 0.1$, [*]$p < 0.05$, [**]$p < 0.01$, and [***]$p < 0.001$ derived from an independent t test within the normotensive controls and each HTN subgroup
[a]Tested following logarithmic transformation

candidate gene for a certain disease (in case of the present study, HTN) through various mechanisms. Likewise, our data in Tables 2 and 3 support that the PAM rs13175330 G allele is associated with a higher risk of HTN development compared with the AA genotype although it is an intronic SNP.

The primary function of the neuroendocrine processing enzyme PAM in the atrium may be to package ANP, a hormone involved in the control of BP and the regulation of sodium and water excretion [10, 11], into atrial secretory granules for storage. Additionally, PAM possibly functions in the presence of activated ANP, which results from the proteolytic processing of pro-ANP [9]. The exact mechanism underlying the association between PAM rs13175330 A>G and HTN is unknown; thus, it is difficult to ascertain which function of PAM listed in Additional file 1: Table S4 (NCBI gene database; http://www.ncbi.nlm.nih.gov/gene/) is related to BP alteration and HTN development. However, since PAM and pro-ANP are the predominant membrane-associated proteins in atrial secretory granules [12] and PAM plays a role in ANP secretion [9], the PAM rs13175330 polymorphism may be involved in the dysregulation of ANP secretion and thus cause HTN. Indeed, the significance of the present observations is underscored by the identification of a human polymorphism in the PAM locus that is associated with altered systolic and diastolic BP. The present study showed that normotensive control PAM rs13175330 G allele carriers showed a trend toward increased systolic BP, whereas PAM rs13175330 G allele carriers in the HTN w/o therapy group had significantly higher

systolic and diastolic BP than the AA carriers. Moreover, in the HTN w/ therapy group, rs13175330 G allele carriers also showed significantly increased diastolic BP even though antihypertensive medication significantly lowered systolic and diastolic BP in both AA and G allele carriers compared to those in the HTN w/o therapy group (p values of systolic and diastolic BP between AA carriers in the HTN w/o therapy and HTN w/ therapy groups: both $p < 0.001$; p values of systolic and diastolic BP between G allele carriers in the HTN w/o therapy and HTN w/ therapy groups: both $p < 0.001$). As shown in Table 2, G allele carriers had a significantly high risk of HTN development; therefore, alteration of BP can be partially explained by PAM dysfunction due to the PAM rs13175330 polymorphism.

PAM gene polymorphisms affect not only BP but also other HTN-related risk factors. Recently, two missense variants in PAM (p.Asp563Gly and p.Ser539Trp) were reported to be associated with a high risk of type 2 diabetes [23]. Additionally, Czyzk et al. [12] showed that 10-month-old PAM-heterozygous mice had mild but significant glucose intolerance compared to wild-type mice. Although the PAM rs13175330 A>G SNP found in this study was different from those SNPs, rs13175330 G allele carriers showed significantly higher insulin and HOMA-IR indices than the AA carriers in the HTN w/o therapy group. Moreover, PAM rs13175330 G allele carriers showed significantly smaller LDL particle sizes and higher ox-LDL levels than the AA carriers in the HTN w/o therapy group even though the G allele carriers had significantly lower

LDL-cholesterol levels. Thus, the rs13175330 G allele may be associated with worse atherogenicity of LDL-cholesterol. To verify associations between *PAM* genotypes and each variable involved in HTN development (HOMA-IR, LDL particle size, and ox-LDL), we performed a logistic regression analysis (data not shown). The G allele carriers in the HTN group were significantly associated with high HOMA-IR before adjustment for confounding factors including age, sex, BMI, smoking, and drinking [OR 1.110 (95% CI 1.007–1.224), $p = 0.036$]; after adjustment for confounding factors, only tendency was remained [OR 1.094 (95% CI 0.993–1.205), $p = 0.069$]. LDL particle size was significantly small in the G allele carriers before [OR 0.579 (95% CI 0.390–0.861), $p = 0.007$] and after [OR 0.529 (95% CI 0.349–0.800), $p = 0.003$] adjustment. Ox-LDL did not show any association with *PAM* rs13175330 genotypes. In summary, HOMA-IR and LDL particle size are associated with HTN development along with the *PAM* rs13175330 polymorphism. Thus, the increased risk of HTN in the *PAM* rs13175330 G allele carriers can be partially explained by the association between the *PAM* rs13175330 mutation and alteration of glucose tolerance and atherogenicity of LDL-cholesterol.

Taken together, our results indicated a genotype effect from the *PAM* rs13175330 A>G SNP on systolic and diastolic BP, insulin level, the HOMA-IR index, LDL particle size, and ox-LDL level in the HTN w/o therapy group. Since type 2 diabetes [24], decreased LDL particle size [25], and increased ox-LDL level [26] are well-known atherogenic traits related to HTN, these results suggest that the *PAM* gene polymorphism may be involved in HTN development via complex mechanisms, including PAM dysfunction, alterations of glucose tolerance, and atherogenicity of LDL-cholesterol.

Our results share the limitations of cross-sectional observational studies, because we evaluated only associations rather than prospective predictions. Since we verified only the relationship between the *PAM* rs13175330 polymorphism and the risk of HTN, exact mechanisms regarding HTN development by the rs1317530 SNP cannot be fully explained; thus, further studies are needed to demonstrate an association between PAM dysfunction due to the *PAM* rs13175330 polymorphism and HTN. Additionally, we specifically focused on a representative group of Korean subjects in the present study. Therefore, our results cannot be generalized to other ethnic, age, or geographic groups. Moreover, the IR in the HTN group could exaggerate other cardiometabolic syndrome phenotypes and should be considered when interpreting the present findings. Despite these limitations, our results show an interesting association between the *PAM* rs13175330 G allele and an increased risk of HTN.

Conclusions
Although *PAM* has diverse functions (Additional file 1: Table S4), there are a lack of studies on the association between PAM dysfunction due to *PAM* polymorphisms and diseases. Therefore, the findings in the present study are valuable, as this study reported associations between *PAM* polymorphisms and HTN for the first time. Our study suggests that the *PAM* rs13175330 A>G SNP is a novel candidate gene for HTN among the Korean population. Additionally, the *PAM* rs13175330 G allele may be associated with IR and LDL atherogenicity in patients with HTN. To verify the exact *PAM* rs131753301 polymorphism-related mechanisms underlying HTN development, further studies are required.

Abbreviations
ANP: Atrial natriuretic peptide; BMI: Body mass index; bp: Base pair; BP: Blood pressure; CV: Coefficient of variability; gDNA: Genomic DNA; GWAS: Genome-wide association study; HDL: High-density lipoprotein; HOMA: Homeostatic model assessment; HTN: Hypertension; HWE: Hardy-Weinberg equilibrium; IR: Insulin resistance; K-CHIP: Korean Chip; LDL: Low-density lipoprotein; OR: Odds ratio; Ox-: Oxidized; PAM: Peptidylglycine-α-amidating monooxygenase; SNP: Single nucleotide polymorphism; TC: Total cholesterol; TG: Triglyceride

Acknowledgements
The genotype data were generated using the Korean Chip (K-CHIP), which is available through the K-CHIP consortium. The K-CHIP was designed by the Center for Genome Science at the Korea National Institute of Health, Korea (4845-301, 3000-3031).

Funding
This study was funded by the Bio-Synergy Research Project (NRF-2012M3A9C4048762) and the Mid-Career Researcher Program (NRF-2016R1A2B4011662) of the Ministry of Science, ICT and Future Planning through the National Research Foundation of Korea in the Republic of Korea.

Authors' contributions
All authors contributed to the conception and design of the study. HJY, MJK, and JHL contributed to the acquisition, analysis, and interpretation of the data and preparation of the manuscript. MKK, JSC, and S-HL contributed to the acquisition and analysis of the data. All authors contributed to the critical revisions of the paper and have approved the manuscript for publication.

Competing interests
The authors declare that they have no competing interests.

Author details
[1]National Leading Research Laboratory of Clinical Nutrigenetics/Nutrigenomics, Department of Food and Nutrition, College of Human Ecology, Yonsei University, 50 Yonsei-ro, Seodaemun-gu, Seoul 03722, South Korea. [2]Department of Food and Nutrition, Brain Korea 21 PLUS Project, College of Human Ecology, Yonsei University, Seoul 03722, South Korea. [3]Research Center for Silver Science, Institute of Symbiotic Life-TECH, Yonsei University, Seoul 03722, South Korea. [4]Department of Family Practice, National Health Insurance Corporation, Ilsan Hospital, Goyang 10444, South Korea.

References
1. World Health Organization. A global brief on hypertension. Geneva: WHO Press; 2013.
2. Lim SS, Vos T, Flaxman AD, Danaei G, Shibuya K, Adair-Rohani H, et al. A comparative risk assessment of burden of disease and injury attributable to 67 risk factors and risk factor clusters in 21 regions, 1990-2010: a systematic analysis for the global burden of disease study 2010. Lancet. 2012;380:2224–60.

3. Xi B, Cheng H, Shen Y, Zhao X, Hou D, Wang X, et al. Physical activity modifies the associations between genetic variants and hypertension in the Chinese children. Atherosclerosis. 2012;225:376–80.

4. El Shamieh S, Visvikis-Siest S. Genetic biomarkers of hypertension and future challenges integrating epigenomics. Clin Chim Acta. 2012;414:259–65.

5. Van Rijn MJ, Schut AF, Aulchenko YS, Deinum J, Sayed-Tabatabaei FA, Yazdanpanah M, et al. Heritability of blood pressure traits and the genetic contribution to blood pressure variance explained by four blood-pressure-related genes. J Hypertens. 2007;25:565–70.

6. Levy D, Ehret GB, Rice K, Verwoert GC, Launer LJ, Dehghan A, et al. Genome-wide association study of blood pressure and hypertension. Nat Genet. 2009;41:677–87.

7. Padmanabhan S, Melander O, Johnson T, Di Blasio AM, Lee WK, Gentilini D, et al. Genome-wide association study of blood pressure extremes identifies variant near UMOD associated with hypertension. PLoS Genet. 2010;6:e1001177.

8. International consortium for blood pressure genome-wide association studies. Genetic variants in novel pathways influence blood pressure and cardiovascular disease risk. Nature. 2011;478:103–9.

9. O'Donnell PJ, Driscoll WJ, Bäck N, Muth E, Mueller GP. Peptidylglycine-alpha-amidating monooxygenase and pro-atrial natriuretic peptide constitute the major membrane-associated proteins of rat atrial secretory granules. J Mol Cell Cardiol. 2003;35:915–22.

10. Thibault G, Amiri F, Garcia R. Regulation of natriuretic peptide secretion by the heart. Annu Rev Physiol. 1999;61:193–217.

11. Sagnella GA. Atrial natriuretic peptide mimetics and vasopeptidase inhibitors. Cardiovasc Res. 2001;51:416–28.

12. Czyzyk TA, Ning Y, Hsu MS, Peng B, Mains RE, Eipper BA, et al. Deletion of peptide amidation enzymatic activity leads to edema and embryonic lethality in the mouse. Dev Biol. 2005;287:301–13.

13. Department of Infectious Disease Control, Korea Centers for Disease Control & Prevention (KCDC). Public health weekly report, PHWR 2015: Vol. 8 No. 29. In: The Korea Biobank Array Project. Korea Centers for Disease Control & Prevention. 2015. http://www.cdc.go.kr/CDC/info/CdcKrInfo0301.jsp?menuIds=HOME001-MNU1154-MNU0005-MNU0037&q_type=&year=2015&cid=64288&pageNum=. Accessed 6 Nov 2017.

14. Korea Centers for Disease Control & Prevention (KCDC). Korean Chip project. 2017. http://cdc.go.kr/CDC/eng/contents/CdcEngContentView.jsp?cid=74266&menuIds=HOME002-MNU0576-MNU0586. Accessed 6 Nov 2017.

15. Kim M, Kim M, Yoo HJ, Yun R, Lee SH, Lee JH. Estrogen-related receptor γ gene (ESRRG) rs1890552 A>G polymorphism in a Korean population: association with urinary prostaglandin $F_{2\alpha}$ concentration and impaired fasting glucose or newly diagnosed type 2 diabetes. Diabetes Metab. 2017;43:385–8.

16. Kim M, Yoo HJ, Kim M, Seo H, Chae JS, Lee SH, et al. Influence of estrogen-related receptor γ (ESRRG) rs1890552 A > G polymorphism on changes in fasting glucose and arterial stiffness. Sci Rep. 2017;7:9787.

17. Roth SM. Genetics primer for exercise science and health. In: Roth SM, editor. Issues in study design and analysis. Champaign: Human Kinetics Publishers; 2007. p. 89–90.

18. Jo BS, Choi SS. Introns: the functional benefits of introns in genomes. Genomics Inform. 2015;13:112–8.

19. Wang D, Guo Y, Wrighton SA, Cooke GE, Sadee W. Intronic polymorphism in CYP3A4 affects hepatic expression and response to statin drugs. Pharmacogenomics J. 2011;11:274–86.

20. Wang D, Sadee W. CYP3A4 intronic SNP rs35599367 (CYP3A4*22) alters RNA splicing. Pharmacogenet Genomics. 2016;26:40–3.

21. Xia Z, Yang T, Wang Z, Dong J, Liang C. GRK5 intronic (CA)n polymorphisms associated with type 2 diabetes in Chinese Hainan Island. PLoS One. 2014;9:e90597.

22. Zhou J, Nagarkatti PS, Zhong Y, Creek K, Zhang J, Nagarkatti M. Unique SNP in CD44 intron 1 and its role in breast cancer development. Anticancer Res. 2010;30:1263–72.

23. Steinthorsdottir V, Thorleifsson G, Sulem P, Helgason H, Grarup N, Sigurdsson A, et al. Identification of low-frequency and rare sequence variants associated with elevated or reduced risk of type 2 diabetes. Nat Genet. 2014;46:294–8.

24. Mehta JL, Rasouli N, Sinha AK, Molavi B. Oxidative stress in diabetes: a mechanistic overview of its effects on atherogenesis and myocardial dysfunction. Int J Biochem Cell Biol. 2006;38:794–803.

25. Maruyama T, Imamura K, Teramoto T. Assessment of LDL particle size by triglyceride/HDL-cholesterol ratio in non-diabetic, healthy subjects without prominent hyperlipidemia. J Atheroscler Thromb. 2003;10:186–91.

26. Witztum JL, Steinberg D. Role of oxidized low density lipoprotein in atherogenesis. J Clin Invest. 1991;88:1785–92.

3

Navigating the dynamic landscape of long noncoding RNA and protein-coding gene annotations in GENCODE

Saakshi Jalali[1,2], Shrey Gandhi[1] and Vinod Scaria[1,2]*

Abstract

Background: Our understanding of the transcriptional potential of the genome and its functional consequences has undergone a significant change in the last decade. This has been largely contributed by the improvements in technology which could annotate and in many cases functionally characterize a number of novel gene loci in the human genome. Keeping pace with advancements in this dynamic environment and being able to systematically annotate a compendium of genes and transcripts is indeed a formidable task. Of the many databases which attempted to systematically annotate the genome, GENCODE has emerged as one of the largest and popular compendium for human genome annotations.

Results: The analysis of various versions of GENCODE revealed that there was a constant upgradation of transcripts for both protein-coding and long noncoding RNA (lncRNAs) leading to conflicting annotations. The GENCODE version 24 accounts for 4.18 % of the human genome to be transcribed which is an increase of 1.58 % from its first version. Out of 2,51,614 transcripts annotated across GENCODE versions, only 21.7 % had consistency. We also examined GENCODE consortia categorized transcripts into 70 biotypes out of which only 17 remained stable throughout.

Conclusions: In this report, we try to review the impact on the dynamicity with respect to gene annotations, specifically (lncRNA) annotations in GENCODE over the years. Our analysis suggests a significant dynamism in gene annotations, reflective of the evolution and consensus in nomenclature of genes. While a progressive change in annotations and timely release of the updates make the resource reliable in the community, the dynamicity with each release poses unique challenges to its users. Taking cues from other experiments with bio-curation, we propose potential avenues and methods to mend the gap.

Keywords: GENCODE, Long noncoding RNAs, Transcripts, Annotations

Introduction

The last decade has seen a tremendous improvement in our ability to understand the human genome and its transcriptional output at a much higher resolution than previously possible. This has largely been possible due to the availability of technologies which have enabled the annotation of transcripts at much higher depths and resolution. A number of systematic efforts to annotate the transcriptome in the human are also worth mentioning. The earliest and most comprehensive approaches have been the H-invitational database consortium which aimed at assembling complementary DNA (cDNA) sequence information on the human genome through a global collaborative effort. This was followed by approaches including tiling arrays to characterize the transcriptional potential of the genome. Further, recent developments in deep sequencing approaches have greatly increased the resolution and facilitated the understanding of the transcriptome. Consequently, there has been the discovery of a significantly large number of novel gene loci in the genome. A large number of databases, including the ENCODE consortium, has made available gene annotations for the human genome by integrating data from the systematic explorations [1].

* Correspondence: vinods@igib.res.in
[1]GN Ramachandran Knowledge Center for Genome Informatics, CSIR Institute of Genomics and Integrative Biology (CSIR-IGIB), Mathura Road, Delhi 110 025, India
[2]Academy of Scientific and Innovative Research (AcSIR), CSIR-IGIB South Campus, Mathura Road, Delhi 110025, India

The efforts of the GENCODE consortium has been one of the most comprehensive and standardized approach for gene annotation and widely used by the community [1]. The initial efforts of GENCODE in the year 2008 (version 1) annotated 36,247 genes and 83,725 transcripts [2, 3] and subsequent versions of data show the annotations improve over time. The annotations were based on computational analysis, manual annotation, and experimental validation of genes and transcripts. The current release GENCODE Version 24 (V24) released in 2015 for humans has in total 60,554 genes annotated as protein-coding genes (19,815), long noncoding RNA genes (15,941), and small noncoding RNA genes (9882). It is also one of the most comprehensive annotations for long noncoding RNA genes.

Widely used by the community and constantly updated, with an average of three updates every year, we were motivated in understanding how the database evolved in the annotations, as this would provide a snapshot of the dynamic evolution of human gene annotations and specifically the long noncoding RNA annotations. We were interested in exploring both the different classes of annotations and the relative number of genes/transcripts in each annotation version towards understanding how the different gene classes and annotations evolved over time in the last decade.

We systematically analyzed the different annotations of genes/transcripts over different versions of GENCODE, starting with the first release till the latest release (V24) for the Human genome. While GENCODE serves as a major source of long noncoding RNA (lncRNA) annotations and has over time significantly and systematically catalogued the growth of lncRNA annotations, our analysis suggests a significant dynamism in gene annotations, reflective of the evolution and consensus in nomenclature of genes. We also find a number of cases where such dynamism in annotation has contributed to misannotation and in some cases results

which might be highly inconsistent. An overview of the dynamism in annotation and the different facets thereof are presented.

Results

Data compendium of transcripts in the human genome

Through data integration of transcript information from a total of 24 versions of GENCODE from years 2008 to 2015, we assembled a large compendium of a total of 2,51,614 transcripts. The growth of GENCODE has been consistent over the different versions. The initial version started with an annotation of 87,852 transcript annotations of which 43,415 were protein-coding, while 44,437 belonged to other biotypes. The most recent version of GENCODE (V24) annotates 1,99,005 transcripts, out of which 79,865 are protein-coding while 1,19,140 belong to other RNA biotypes. The most recent annotation as per GENCODE V24 estimates approximately 4.18 % of the human genome to be transcribed, significantly up from the estimate of 2.6 % in the first version. The summary of the gene and transcript numbers, the percentage of genome transcribed as annotated in each of the versions, and their growth over the different versions is summarized in Fig. 1.

The compendium of protein-coding and long noncoding RNA annotations

Of the entire compendium of 2,51,614 transcripts, a total of 1,14,114 transcripts were annotated as protein-coding, while a total of 1,20,864 transcripts were annotated as lncRNA biotype, in at least one of the 28 versions of GENCODE. The overlaps between these annotations revealed, a total of 11,069 transcripts had potential moonlighting identities, as shown by clashing annotations in one or the other release of the data resource. The transcripts and their overlapping annotations are summarized in Additional file 1: Figure S1.

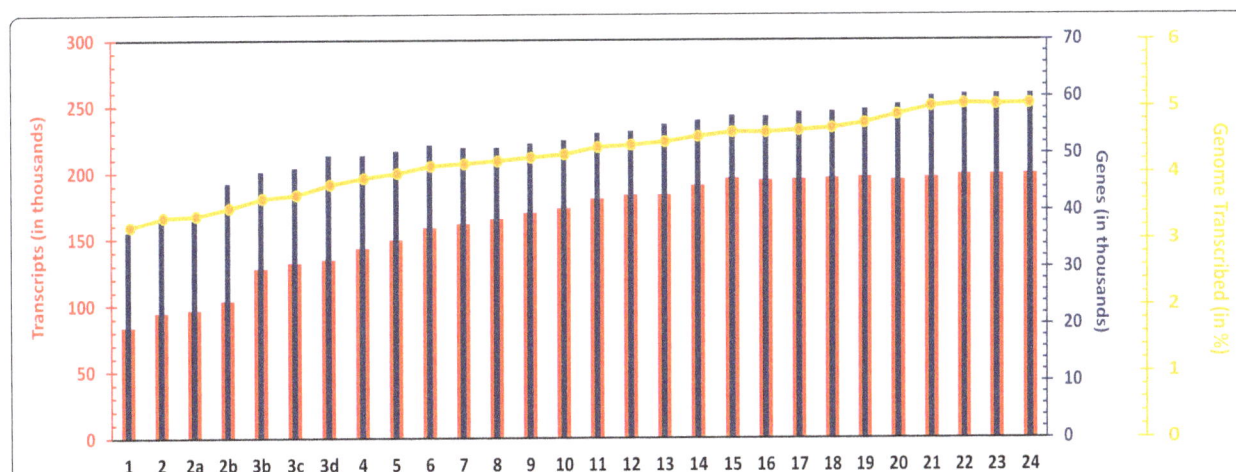

Fig. 1 The data compendium of genes and transcripts in Human genome. The X-axis represents GENCODE versions 1-24. The Primary Y-axis (red) represents the number of transcripts (in thousand); the Secondary Y-axis (blue) represents the number of genes (in thousand) and the tertiary Y-axis (yellow) shows percentage of the genome transcribed across GENCODE versions

Growth of the compendium over time

Over years and versions, the compendium has seen significant addition of transcript annotations, with an average of 6277 additions in every new version. The largest addition to the catalog was with the V3b version in the year 2009, which saw an addition of a whopping 26,715 transcripts to the compendium. This accounted for a significant 20.91 % addition of transcript annotations to the compendium. Of these, a total of 20,499 were protein-coding transcripts, while 3096 were lncRNAs. The update also saw a deletion of 7087 transcript annotations.

While the most significant addition to the protein-coding transcript annotations occurred in V3b, the most significant addition to the lncRNA annotations happened in V4, which saw an addition of 8897 new lncRNA transcript annotations.

The consistent updates to the GENCODE compendium also saw deletion of entries in every update. On an average, 2160 transcript annotations were deleted from the database with every version. The largest deletion of transcript annotations occurred with the V20 update of the compendium in the year 2014. This update accounted for the deletion of 11,410 transcript annotations from the compendium, of which 6727 were protein-coding and 3623 were lncRNAs.

The most significant deletion of protein-coding transcript annotations occurred with V20 which saw the deletion of 6727 transcript annotations, while the most significant deletion of lncRNA annotations occurred in the V4 update which saw the deletion of 4149 transcripts. V20 was close behind with a deletion of 3623 lncRNA transcript annotations. The detail for each version is specified in Table 1.

Consistency in annotations for protein-coding and long noncoding RNAs

Of the total number of transcripts, a total of 54,840 consistently maintained their annotations across all the GENCODE versions. Of these, 32,458 were protein-coding transcripts, while 22,382 belonged to other RNA biotypes. Out of the consistent transcript annotations throughout the versions, 19,520 belonged to lncRNAs. The dynamicity of the GENCODE compendium is summarized in Fig. 2.

Dynamicity of the lncRNA compendium and transformation of annotations

Out of this compendium, a total of 1,37,909 were annotated as noncoding RNA in one of the versions of GENCODE, of which a significant number amounting to 29,512 transcripts were systematically and consistently annotated as lncRNAs in all of the 24 versions. This accounted for 24.41 % of the total lncRNA annotations.

Of the total of 10,718 transcripts which had fleeting identities, a significant number of annotations were from a protein-coding biotype to lncRNA, which accounted to 6560 transcripts, while the reverse accounted for 5463 transcripts in total. A total of 650 lncRNA transcript annotations reversed back after moonlighting as a protein-coding transcript, while 688 protein-coding transcripts reverted back after moonlighting as an lncRNA.

This dynamic nature of transcript biotypes was consistently observed across all the updates to the GENCODE compendium. The most significant change in the protein-coding transcript annotations happened in V3b leading to 20,499 transformations. In V4, had the most significant change in the lncRNA annotations wherein 10,044 transcripts changed their annotations to lncRNA while simultaneously 4498 lncRNA transcripts mutated their annotations to other biotypes. The largest change from the protein-coding transcripts to other biotypes occurred with V20 update of the compendium in 2014 which accounted for 7212 transcripts. The detail for each version is specified in Table 2.

Differences in the biotypes and annotations between versions of GENCODE

We evaluated the dynamicity in the biotypes under which the transcripts were annotated in different versions of GENCODE. Our analysis revealed a total of 70 biotypes were considered in total for annotation of transcripts. Only a small proportion (17) of their entire compendium of biotypes was systematically used in all the versions of GENCODE. A subset of 9 (Ambiguous ORF, scRNA pseudogene, Mt tRNA pseudogene, snRNA pseudogene, snoRNA pseudogene, rRNA pseudogene, miRNA pseudogene, misc RNA pseudogene) biotypes were dropped after v12, while 12 (ncRNA host, Disrupted domain, TR pseudogene, Artifact, scRNA, TR gene, IG gene, V segment, transcribed pseudogene, J segment, C segment) biotypes were used only in the earlier versions of GENCODE. The presence and absence of all biotypes across various versions of GENCODE are summarized in Fig. 3.

Impact of dynamicity of the lncRNA compendium

We also evaluated the impact of the dynamicity of annotations. Our analysis revealed a total of 1,96,988 transcripts had a dynamic annotation in at least one of the versions of GENCODE. This accounted for a total of 78.29 % of all the transcript annotations in GENCODE.

We closely examined a few candidates which had a significant dynamicity in its annotation (as shown in Additional file 2: Figure S2). We selected candidates which over versions of GENCODE have been dynamically annotated as a protein-coding or long noncoding RNA. One such candidate is C3orf10 (ENST00000256463). C3orf10 gene encodes for a 9-kD protein which plays a role in regulation of actin and microtubule organization. This gene encodes for ENST00000256463 which was annotated as

Table 1 Census of transcripts and their biotypes across all GENCODE versions

S.No	GENCODE versions	Freeze year	No. of Havana transcripts	No. of Ensembl transcripts	Total transcripts	No. of Havana converted to Ensembl ID	Total number of unique transcript IDs which were considered	No. of biotypes	No. of lncRNA biotypes
1	1	2008	67,432	16,293	83,725	66,579	87,852	37	14
2	2	2009	79,899	14,505	94,404	76,890	98,855	36	14
3	2a	2009	83,049	13,352	96,401	81,833	1,01,088	35	14
4	2b	2009	83,049	20,570	10,3619	81,833	1,08,145	39	14
5	v3b	2009	7896	1,19,809	1,27,705	7669	1,27,773	38	14
6	v3c	2009	0	13,2067	1,32,067	0	1,31,891	37	14
7	v3d	2009	0	1,34,266	1,34,266	0	1,34,267	38	15
8	4	2010	0	1,42,637	1,42,637	0	1,42,467	41	15
9	5	2010	0	1,48,880	1,48,880	0	1,48,710	43	15
10	6	2010	0	1,58,489	1,58,489	0	1,58,321	44	16
11	7	2010	0	1,61,375	1,61,375	0	1,61,214	44	16
12	8	2011	0	1,65,067	1,65,067	0	1,64,906	46	18
13	9	2011	0	1,69,419	1,69,419	0	1,69,257	50	20
14	10	2011	0	1,72,975	1,72,975	0	1,72,810	51	20
15	11	2011	0	1,80,272	1,80,272	0	1,80,107	51	19
16	12	2011	0	1,83,086	1,83,086	0	1,82,921	50	19
17	13	2012	0	1,82,967	1,82,967	0	1,82,798	41	18
18	14	2012	0	1,90,051	1,90,051	0	1,89,882	41	18
19	15	2012	0	1,95,433	1,95,433	0	1,95,264	40	17
20	16	2012	0	1,94,034	1,94,034	0	1,93,865	40	17
21	17	2013	0	1,94,871	1,94,871	0	1,94,702	38	15
22	18	2013	0	1,95,584	1,95,584	0	1,95,418	38	14
23	19	2013	0	1,96,520	1,96,520	0	1,96,354	38	14
24	20	2014	0	1,94,334	1,94,334	0	1,94,173	38	14
25	21	2014	0	1,96,327	1,96,327	0	1,96,165	43	17
26	22	2014	0	1,98,442	1,98,442	0	1,98,278	47	17
27	23	2015	0	1,98,619	1,98,619	0	1,98,455	45	16
28	24	2015	0	1,99,169	1,99,169	0	1,99,005	47	18

protein coding in V1 then as an lncRNA in V2-V2a and V3c-V6 and later again annotated as protein coding and further dropped from the database since version 20. In addition to inconsistency to the annotation type, it also had different gene names across versions the name of this transcript also changed: C3orf10 (V1-V8) -> AC034193.5 (V2-V3b) -> BRK1 (V9-V19). There were also few transcripts which had consistently same name such as ENST00 000436930: FER1L5 (V1-V24), ENST00000366438: ATAD 2B (V1-V24) across the entire version with varying annotations. While few transcripts such as ENST00000334998: RP1-163 M9.4 (V1-V2b) -> MST1P9 (V3b-V14) -> MST1L (V15) -> current status does not exist, ENST000 00339140: RP11-167P23.5 (V1-2b) -> FOXR2 (2b-V24), ENST00000408914: RIMKLP (V1-V3d) -> RIMKLB2 (V4-

V5) -> RIMKLBP1 (V6-V24) and had both inconsistent name as well as biotype.

Another example from our analysis is AC074389.6 gene which encodes for a single transcript (ENST00000382528) according to GENCODE annotations. It was annotated as protein coding in V1- 20 and this transcript is annotated as lincRNA from V21. This gene was identified as a novel bioactive peptide in year 2006 derived from precursor proteins which can be used as targets for drug interventions. To identify this new gene, the human genome National Center for Biotechnology Information (NCBI) 33 assembly, July 1, 2003, was used as reference and novelty of peptide sequence was confirmed using Universal Protein Resource (UNIPROT) [4]. Expression profile studies were also conducted to show their presence in various tissues [5].

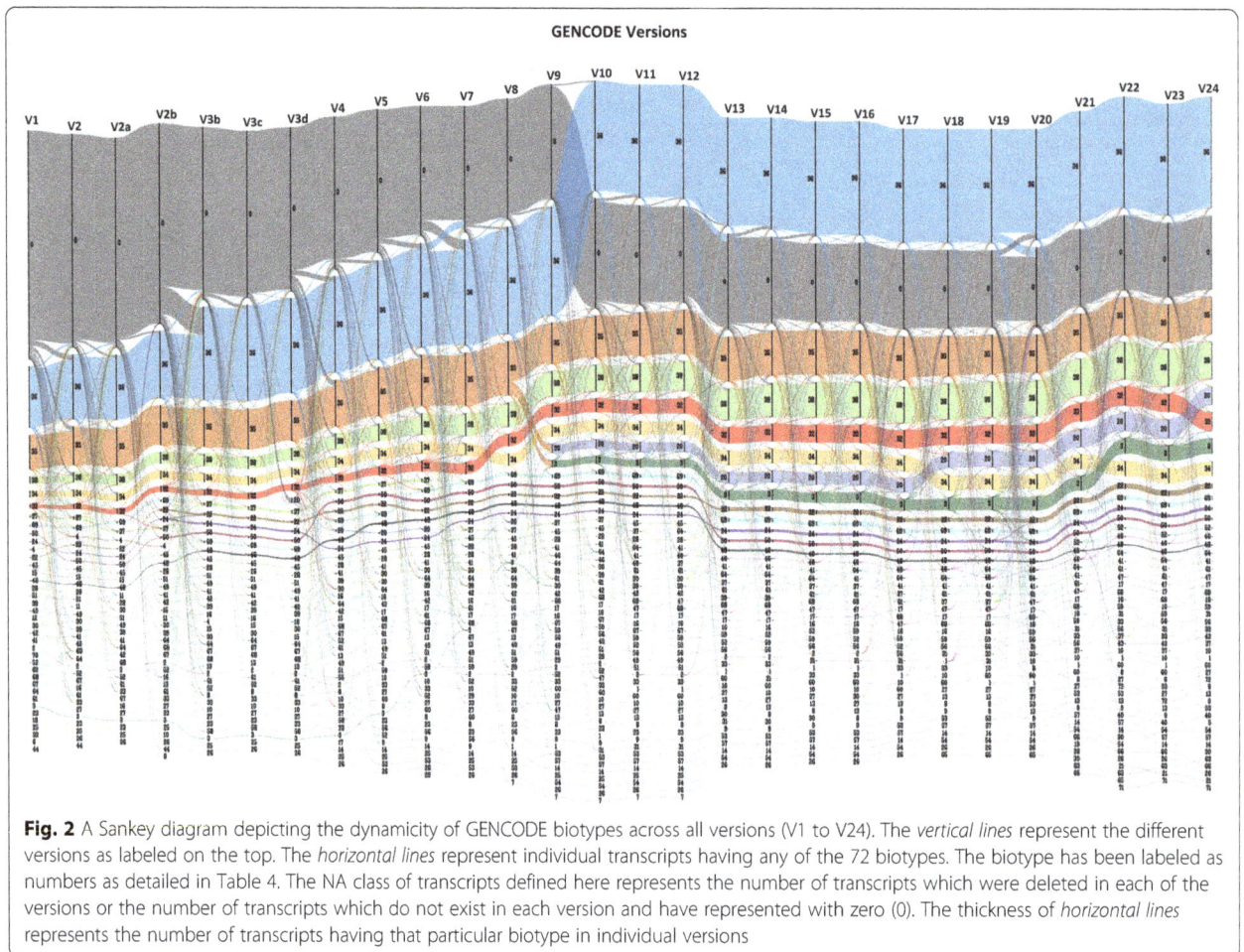

Fig. 2 A Sankey diagram depicting the dynamicity of GENCODE biotypes across all versions (V1 to V24). The *vertical lines* represent the different versions as labeled on the top. The *horizontal lines* represent individual transcripts having any of the 72 biotypes. The biotype has been labeled as numbers as detailed in Table 4. The NA class of transcripts defined here represents the number of transcripts which were deleted in each of the versions or the number of transcripts which do not exist in each version and have represented with zero (0). The thickness of *horizontal lines* represents the number of transcripts having that particular biotype in individual versions

Recently, Wang et al. reported this transcript to be expressed as an Lnc-RI lncRNA, and the same was shown through experimental validation to be ubiquitously expressed [6]. These contrasting reports highlight the genuine concern which arises due to frequent and ever changing landscape of GENCODE annotations.

The transcript ENST00000413529, encoded by the gene SDHAP3, was the most inconsistent transcript across the entire GENCODE compendium, which witnessed a total of nine transitions and was assigned six different biotypes during its short lived journey (V3b-19) Additional file 3: Figure S3.

Using HGNC (The HUGO Gene Nomenclature Committee) [7], one of the largest consortium of the human genes, we wanted to check the existence of the deleted genes in the present GENCODE(V24). The total human gene list extracted from HGNC consisted of 39,777 loci, and there were total of 56,095 GENCODE genes which were present in the earlier GENCODE versions but got eliminated in the current version (V24). When we overlapped the current HGNC genes with the genes deleted in V24, we found 285 genes to be common, out of

which, 35 were lncRNAs. The same is depicted in Additional file 4: Figure S4.

Discussion

The GENCODE compendium of transcript annotations has undoubtedly significantly enhanced the accessibility to a standardized set of genome annotations and accelerated the experimental annotation and understanding of gene functions, especially long noncoding RNA functions. Though there have been a number of databases [8] systematically annotating various aspects of lncRNAs including their functions, interactions etc., all the databases have been lacking continuous updates. GENCODE fills in this gap by covering and integrating the latest in terms of gene and transcript annotation, methodologies, and standards. Notwithstanding the limitations of the resource, which primarily arise from the changing landscape of technologies, definitions and methods for transcriptome analysis, GENCODE still provides one of the most comprehensive and well-accepted compendium of transcript annotations widely used and followed in literature.

Table 2 Details of all the biotypes used in GENCODE and their respective codes as used in our study

Biotype name	Code given
3 prime overlapping ncrna	1
Ambiguous orf	2
Antisense	3
Artifact	4
Bidirectional promoter lncrna	5
C segment	6
Disrupted domain	7
IG C gene	8
IG C pseudogene	9
IG D gene	10
ig gene	11
IG gene	12
IG J gene	13
IG J pseudogene	14
IG pseudogene|ig pseudogene	15
IG V gene	16
IG V pseudogene	17
J segment	18
Known ncrna	19
lincRNA	20
macro lncRNA	21
miRNA	22
miRNA pseudogene	23
misc RNA	24
misc RNA pseudogene	25
Mt rRNA	26
Mt tRNA	27
Mt tRNA pseudogene	28
ncrna host	29
Non-coding	30
Non-stop decay	31
Nonsense-mediated decay	32
Polymorphic pseudogene	33
Processed pseudogene	34
Processed transcript	35
Protein coding	36
Pseudogene	37
Retained intron	38
Retrotransposed	39
Ribozyme	40
rRNA	41
rRNA pseudogene	42
scaRNA	43

Table 2 Details of all the biotypes used in GENCODE and their respective codes as used in our study *(Continued)*

scRNA	44
scRNA pseudogene	45
Sense intronic	46
Sense overlapping	47
snoRNA	48
snoRNA pseudogene	49
snRNA	50
snRNA pseudogene	51
TEC|tec	52
TR C gene	53
TR D gene	54
TR gene	55
TR J gene	56
TR J pseudogene	57
TR pseudogene	58
TR V gene	59
TR V pseudogene	60
Transcribed processed pseudogene	61
Transcribed pseudogene	62
Transcribed unitary pseudogene	63
Transcribed unprocessed pseudogene	64
Translated processed pseudogene	65
Translated unprocessed pseudogene	66
tRNA pseudogene	67
Unitary pseudogene	68
Unprocessed pseudogene	69
V segment	70
Vaultrna	71
sRNA	72

A major limitation of the field has been the inconsistency in the nomenclature of transcript/gene biotypes which significantly adds confusion in the classification and long-term annotation of transcripts, especially lncRNAs. Our analysis of GENCODE suggests that a significant number of 52 biotype annotations were dropped at one point or the other between different versions of GENCODE, which affects a total of 1,96,799 transcript annotations while 17 biotypes remained constant across all GENCODE version for 54,815 transcripts.

In a very dynamic technological and knowledge landscape, it would be imperative for resources to closely integrate the long tail of annotations. It is humanly impossible for organizations to systematically track the growing corpus of literature in the field (Additional file 5: Figure S5), which presently adds over 1000 new publications per year. Therefore, it is imperative to dynamically interlink publications

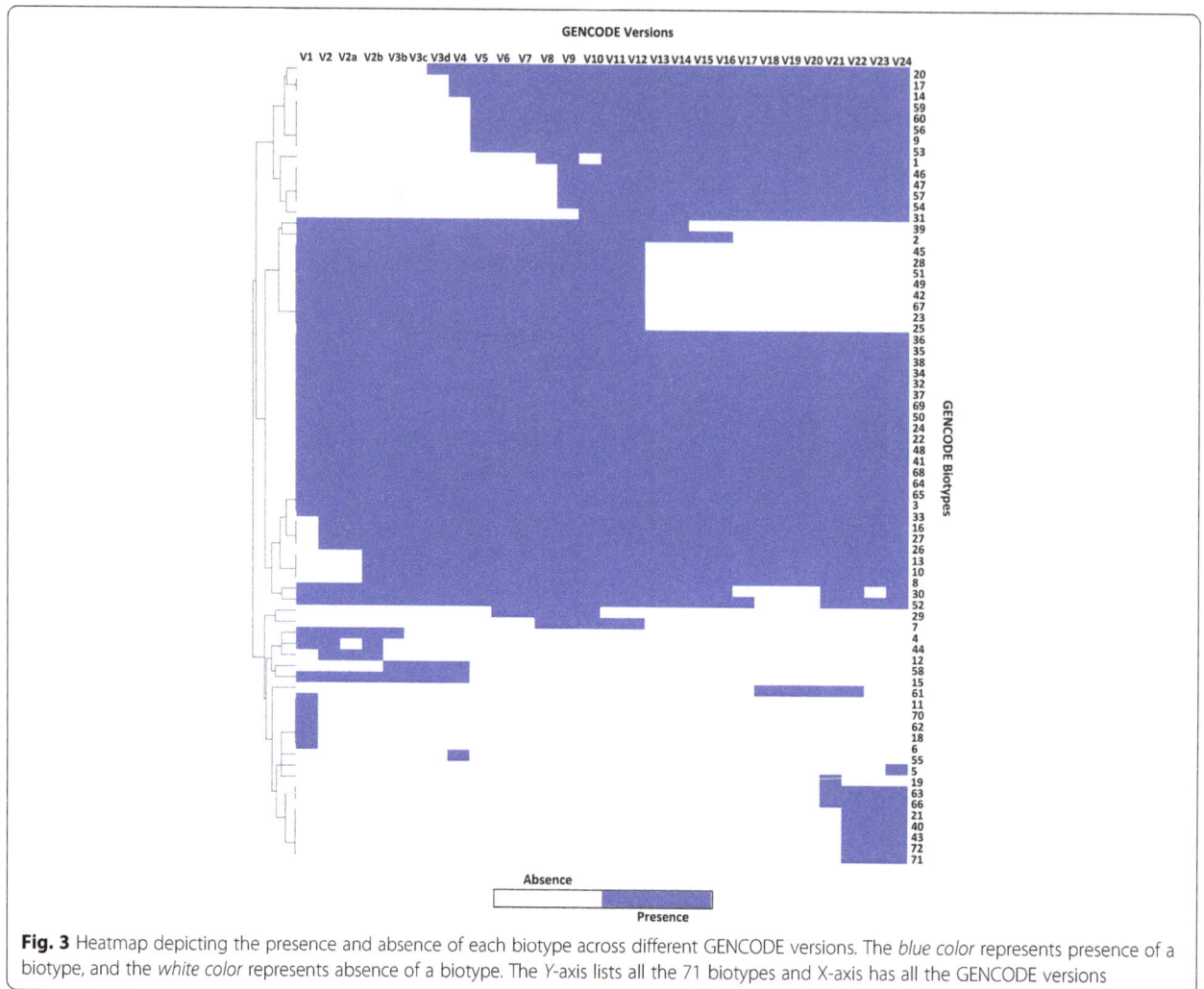

Fig. 3 Heatmap depicting the presence and absence of each biotype across different GENCODE versions. The *blue color* represents presence of a biotype, and the *white color* represents absence of a biotype. The *Y*-axis lists all the 71 biotypes and *X*-axis has all the GENCODE versions

and resources related to the field as has been extensively built for protein-coding genes [7].

Another major gap in the field has been the lack of interoperable databases annotating different biological aspects of lncRNAs. Apart from the standard Ensembl IDs followed by GENCODE and used by many other databases, only a small proportion of the lncRNAs 1.46 % of the entire compendium of lncRNAs have also been annotated and provided an HGNC gene symbol. Apart from the standard HGNC gene nomenclature, many publications and resources cite a variety of other nomenclatures, which adds to the confusion and inability to cross-link resources, publications, and analysis results. This major limitation stems from that fact that there has been a lack of standard and consensus standards for nomenclature of lncRNAs. Such standards for nomenclature and annotation of many other noncoding classes including miRNAs have ensured accordance in nomenclature which in turn maintains the compatibility between resources, databases, and citations in publications [7, 9, 10].

A number of resources and databases on lncRNAs have emerged in the recent years and has been comprehensively reviewed by Jalali and co-workers [11]. The resources encompass a variety of biological relationships, interactions, and functionalities. Nevertheless, the integration of the resources into a common platform has been a tedious task due to the variability in annotation standards, version of the annotations used, and lack of interoperability between the resources. The immediate goal would be to enable these complementary resources to be interoperable. The availability of common standards for nomenclature and annotation would enable the resources to be systematically integrated which would in turn enable timely updates. This would facilitate experimental as well as computational biologists wade through the unchartered waters quickly, and effectively.

The update in this ever-growing field has been fast outpacing the efforts by individual groups or laboratories to be able to systematically curate the information in a comprehensive way. Different attempts to fill in the gap of the long tail of bio-curation has emerged in the recent years, including Wiki-based systems for systematic and real-time annotation and curation of biological information. Such resources have been extensively developed not just for model systems but also for noncoding RNA databases. This could be complemented by efforts to automatically tag and annotate data from publications and resources using machine learning approaches developed recently [12].

Conclusion

In summary, our analysis of one of the most comprehensive resource of lncRNAs suggest the dynamic progression of the field in terms of both the number of annotations as well as the changing view of the classification of lncRNAs. While a dynamic change in annotations and a timely release of the updates make the resource unique, popular, and therefore widely used by the community, the dynamicity poses unique challenges to the community. Taking cues from other domains of bio-curation, we propose modalities to mend the gap.

Methods
GENCODE annotation

We downloaded the annotation data in form of Gene Transfer File (GTF) files from the GENCODE database and extracted all the transcript IDs along with their corresponding biotypes across all the versions from V1 to V24. GENCODE consortium has not made available Version 3a publically, hence not included in our study. The census for transcripts and biotypes across versions is detailed in Table 1. There are 28 GENCODE releases in our analyses consisting of genomic elements such as genes, transcripts, Coding sequence (CDS), untranslated regions (UTRS), and Exons annotated by Ensembl and Havana (Human and Vertebrate Analysis and Annotation). These were classified into 71 different biotypes as listed in Table 2 across all versions.

Analysis of consistency of transcripts across GENCODE versions

We extracted all the transcript identifiers comprising of both ENST (Ensembl) and\or OTTHUMT(Havana) IDs along with their transcript type. V1 consisted of only annotations for exons with no separate records for the other genomic elements such as genes, transcripts, or CDS. Hence, we directly used the transcript IDs as assigned to these exons for further analysis.

GENCODE assigned ENSTR/ENSTRR identifiers for pseudo autosomal regions of Y chromosome which are same for the X and Y chromosomes. For our analysis, we replaced all such transcripts with their respective ENST0 IDs in order avoid duplicate entries. We replaced 218 ENST0 IDs with their respective ENSTR /ENSTRR IDs if they had the same ENST identifier and biotype in a particular version.

Moreover, the earlier versions (V1 to 2c) of GENCODE consisted of either OTTHUMT or ENST identifiers for all transcripts. From V3b, GENCODE started to assign both the identifiers to most of the transcripts with an exception of a few which were assigned only IDs prefixed with OTTHUMT. After V3c the OTTHUMT prefixed IDs were systematically phased out as the main identifier, with each transcript having an ENST prefixed ID along with its corresponding OTTHUMT prefixed identifier. 77,193 OTTHUMT prefixed IDs had single ENST prefixed ID throughout their lifetime and hence were replaced with their respective ENST prefixed IDs. While 1982 OTTHUMT prefixed IDs had more than one ENST IDs in the same version therefore such OTTHUMT prefixed IDs were duplicated by assigning them both the Ensembl prefixed IDs while keeping their biotypes intact.

Another set of 3188 OTTHUMT prefixed IDs having more than one ENST prefixed IDs assigned to them across versions were replaced with respective IDs in that version by keeping the biotype of OTTHUMT prefixed ID intact. In addition, for 3272 OTTHUMT prefixed IDs there existed no ENST prefixed ID hence we kept them as it is.

All these transcripts IDs along with their assigned biotypes were organized into compiled record of total annotations. Those transcripts which did not have any biotype assigned to them in GENCODE versions were given a hypothetical code NA (not assigned). All the computation was performed by using custom shell and Perl scripts.

Analysis of consistency of lncRNA transcripts across GENCODE versions

To analyze the distribution and dynamism of lncRNA annotations across the GENCODE versions, we compared the lncRNA biotypes assigned by GENCODE. We made a comprehensive list of all the lncRNA biotypes or transcript biotypes used and dropped across the different versions (as listed in Table 3). While considering lncRNA as a class, we clubbed 23 sub-biotypes, namely 3 prime overlapping ncrna, TEC, Ambiguous orf, Antisense, Bidirectional promoter lncrna, Disrupted domain, Known ncrna, lincRNA, macro lncRNA, misc RNA, ncrna host, Non coding, Processed pseudogene, Processed transcript, Pseudogene, Retained intron, Retrotransposed, Sense intronic, Sense overlapping, Transcribed processed pseudogene, Transcribed unprocessed pseudogene, Unitary pseudogene, and Unprocessed pseudogene. From the compiled record of complete annotations, we extracted the transcripts belonging to these lncRNA subclasses and named it as lncRNA annotations.

Table 3 Number of transcripts added or deleted in each version of GENCODE

GENCODE version	Transcripts added	lncRNAs added	PC transcripts added	Transcripts deleted	lncRNAs deleted	PC transcripts deleted
1	–	–	–	–	–	–
2	13,568	7455	4156	2565	357	1690
2a	5580	3195	1769	3347	1756	1326
2b	7069	1243	1606	12	7	0
v3b	26,715	2924	19,998	7087	1666	1674
v3c	4978	1606	2643	860	169	143
v3d	3581	3481	96	1206	192	967
4	15,138	8897	3786	6937	4149	1481
5	7065	3820	2443	822	323	221
6	10,409	5527	3838	798	156	616
7	11,285	3234	7524	8392	2519	5834
8	5036	2750	1784	1344	61	1268
9	4568	2551	1582	217	67	146
10	3684	2171	1169	131	28	102
11	7817	4801	2290	520	463	56
12	3243	1808	1096	429	237	155
13	6734	3393	1391	6857	120	5272
14	7291	4013	2543	207	118	77
15	5749	3237	2079	367	214	107
16	628	451	132	2027	1052	812
17	1469	1194	206	632	340	185
18	1055	778	158	339	204	109
19	1378	1147	192	442	234	176
20	9229	3676	4238	11,410	3623	6727
21	2218	1709	432	226	119	97
22	2873	1630	751	760	268	320
23	350	212	104	173	117	52
24	758	473	206	208	71	105

Visualization

The distribution of all the transcripts in conjunction with their biotypes across the GENCODE versions from the compiled record for total annotations was visualized using an open web app, RAW [13]. A custom vector-based visualization based D3.js library through an interactable interface was used. The dynamicity of GENCODE annotations across all versions was depicted in form of a Sankey diagram (Fig. 2). In addition, we plotted a Sankey using lncRNA annotations file, as depicted in Fig. 4. Here, we considered four categories, namely lncRNA, protein coding, NA, and others (which included all other biotypes).

We also explored the disparity of biotypes across the GENCODE annotations. Hence, we considered the all the biotypes across different versions and plotted them in form of a heatmap. We observed many biotypes which were eliminated completely while few were retained throughout (Fig. 3).

Comparison across GENCODE versions

We calculated the number of transitions which each transcript went through during their lifetime which has been outlined in the Table 4. We also computed the various biotypes which each transcript was assigned and compiled this information in Table 5.

A compilation of the number of transcripts which were added and deleted in each version of GENCODE was derived from the compiled record of complete annotations. We also did this for both lncRNA and protein-coding transcripts which has been added/deleted, and the same has been outlined in the Table 1.

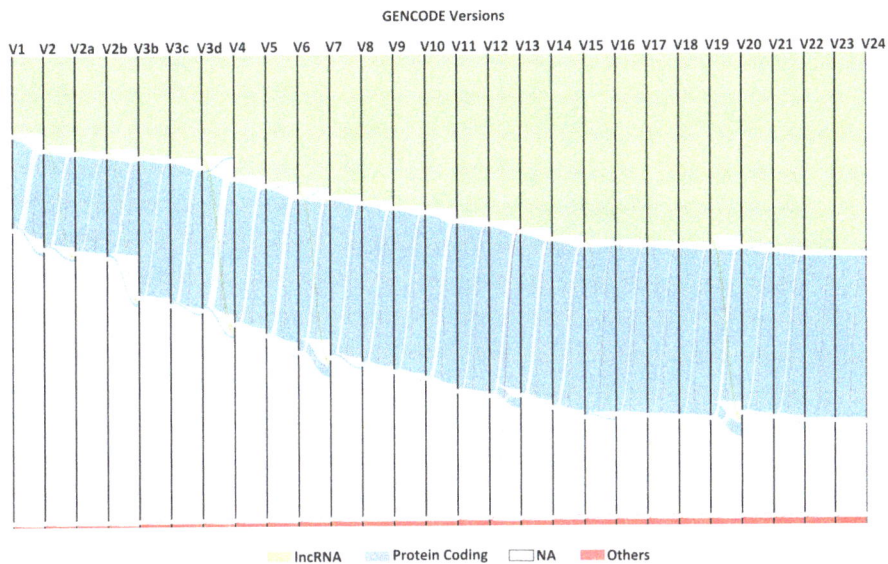

Fig. 4 A Sankey diagram depicting the dynamicity of GENCODE lncRNAs and protein-coding biotypes across all versions (V1 to V24). The lncRNA class considered here covers 23 sub-biotypes which includes 3 prime overlapping ncrna, TEC, Ambiguous orf, Antisense, Bidirectional promoter lncrna, Disrupted domain, Known ncrna, lincRNA, macro lncRNA, misc RNA, ncrna host, Non coding, Processed pseudogene, Processed transcript, Pseudogene, Retained intron, Retrotransposed, Sense intronic, Sense overlapping, Transcribed processed pseudogene, Transcribed unprocessed pseudogene, Unitary pseudogene, Unprocessed pseudogene. The protein-coding class represents the number of transcripts having protein-coding biotype. The NA class of transcripts defined here represents the number of transcripts which were deleted in each of the versions or the number of transcripts which do not exist in each version. While the others category comprises rest of biotypes

While the above table depicted the number of added/deleted transcripts, we also wanted to highlight the different transitions which these protein-coding and lncRNA transcripts went through across the GENCODE versions. Thus, on similar lines, we also produced a table outlining the switching of these transcripts which has been demonstrated in the Table 6.

We also analyzed the abundance of publications for long non coding RNAs over last decade, for which we derived the year wise publication list from Pubmed by searching keyword "lncRNA." The graph shown in Additional file 3: Figure S3 gives a brief layout of the number of publication per year.

Table 4 Summary of the number of biotypes assigned to each of the transcripts

No. of biotypes assigned to the transcript	No. of transcripts
1	54,840
2	1,74,779
3	20,528
4	1945
5	256
6	41
7	5

Comparison with HGNC

HGNC is the largest and one of the most reliable sources for which assigns unique and standardized nomenclature for human genes created as part of the Human Genome Organization (HUGO) [7]. We wanted to verify whether the genes which do not exist in the present GENCODE version are still present in HGNC. Thus, we extracted all the HGNC genes having approved HGNC IDs (up till last updated: 05/07/16 04:51:01) and checked their presence in last V24.

Table 5 Summary of the number of transitions each transcript went through

No. of transitions	No. of transcripts
0	54,840
1	1,33,630
2	55,951
3	6420
4	1125
5	283
6	95
7	35
8	12
9	3

Table 6 Switching of transcripts across versions

GENCODE version	Transcripts added	Transformed to lncRNAs	Transformed to PC transcripts	Transcripts deleted	Transformed from lncRNAs transcripts	Transformed from PC transcripts
1	–	–	–	–	–	–
2	13,568	7781	4336	2565	580	2000
2a	5580	3296	5354	3347	1834	96
2b	7069	1261	1687	12	7	0
v3b	26,715	3096	20,499	7087	2255	2049
v3c	4978	1611	2665	860	194	162
v3d	3581	3722	96	1206	189	1210
4	15,138	10,044	4073	6937	4498	2717
5	7065	4078	2662	822	593	521
6	10,409	6141	4261	798	714	1266
7	11,285	3874	8325	8392	3292	6519
8	5036	2933	1868	1344	155	1508
9	4568	2762	1677	217	178	282
10	3684	2284	1257	131	119	235
11	7817	5028	2530	520	855	322
12	3243	2069	1273	429	469	428
13	6734	4244	1679	6857	557	5660
14	7291	4314	2927	207	631	415
15	5749	3364	2201	367	384	278
16	628	649	311	2027	1271	1019
17	1469	1480	415	632	677	474
18	1055	940	385	339	481	275
19	1378	1289	474	442	582	334
20	9229	4125	4861	11,410	4324	7212
21	2218	2263	535	226	231	618
22	2873	1820	838	760	390	503
23	350	277	195	173	231	112
24	758	527	300	208	197	165

Data availability

The detailed methodology along with all the associated content used in our analysis is available as a GitHub repository (https://github.com/vinodscaria/Gencode-moonlighting/blob/master/README.md). All other relevant data are within the paper and its supporting information.

Additional files

Additional file 1: Figure S1. Venn diagram representing the moonlighting

Additional file 2: Figure S2. Heatmap depicting transitions of the six candidate transcripts from Protein-coding biotype to lncRNA biotype or

Additional file 3: Figure S3. The transition of ENST00000413529 (SDHAP3)

Additional file 4: Figure S4. Common and unique annotated genes of absent in GENCODE V24 and HGNC. Venn diagram shows intersection

Additional file 5: Figure S5. Growth of literature in the field of lncRNAs. The number of publications for each year was retrieved using keyword "lncRNA" from PubMed. The data for 2016 is incomplete at the time of writing

Acknowledgements

The authors also acknowledge constructive criticism and editorial help from Remya Koshy and Ambily Sivadas which significantly improved the readability and perspective of the article.

Funding

The authors acknowledge funding from CSIR India through Grant BSC0123 (GENCODE-C).

Authors' contributions

VS conceptualized the analysis. Data analysis was performed by SJ and SG. SJ and SG prepared the data summaries and visualization. SJ, SG, and VS wrote the manuscript. All authors reviewed the manuscript. All authors read and approved the final manuscript.

Competing interests

The authors declare that they have no competing interests.

References

1. ENCODE Project Consortium TEP. The ENCODE (ENCyclopedia Of DNA Elements) Project. Science. 2004;306:636–40.
2. Harrow J, Denoeud F, Frankish A, Reymond A, Chen C-K, Chrast J, et al. GENCODE: producing a reference annotation for ENCODE. Genome Biol. 2006;7:S4.
3. GENCODE Project. GENCODE Data. ftp://ftp.sanger.ac.uk/pub/gencode/ Gencode_human (2015). Accessed 19 Feb 2016.
4. UniProt Consortium TU. UniProt: a hub for protein information. Nucleic Acids Res. 2015;43:D204–12.
5. Jung E, Dittrich W, Scheidler S. Coding genes with a single exon for new bioactive peptides [Internet]. Google Patents; 2008. Available from: http:// www.google.com.gt/patents/WO2008074424A3?cl=en.
6. Wang Z-D, Shen L-P, Chang C, Zhang X-Q, Chen Z-M, Li L, et al. Long noncoding RNA lnc-RI is a new regulator of mitosis via targeting miRNA-210-3p to release PLK1 mRNA activity. Sci Rep. 2016;6:25385.
7. Gray KA, Yates B, Seal RL, Wright MW, Bruford EA. Genenames.org: the HGNC resources in 2015. Nucleic Acids Res. 2015;43:D1079–85.
8. Fritah S, Niclou SP, Azuaje F. Databases for lncRNAs: a comparative evaluation of emerging tools. RNA. 2014;20:1655–65.
9. Wright MW, Povey S, Lovering R, Bruford E, Wright M, Lush M, et al. A short guide to long non-coding RNA gene nomenclature. Hum Genomics BioMed Central. 2014;8:7.
10. Genome Information Integration Project And H-Invitational 2 GIIPAH-I, Yamasaki C, Murakami K, Fujii Y, Sato Y, Harada E, et al. The H-Invitational Database (H-InvDB), a comprehensive annotation resource for human genes and transcripts. Nucleic Acids Res. 2008;36:D793–9.
11. Jalali S, Kapoor S, Sivadas A, Bhartiya D, Scaria V. Computational approaches towards understanding human long non-coding RNA biology. Bioinformatics. 2015;31:2241–51.
12. Tarca AL, Carey VJ, Chen X, Romero R, Drăghici S. Machine learning and its applications to biology. PLoS Comput Biol. 2007;3:e116.
13. Caviglia G, Mauri M, Azzi M, Uboldi G: DensityDesign Research Lab, RAW App. http://raw.densitydesign.org/ (2014). Accessed 17 May 2016.

4

The *NF1* somatic mutational landscape in sporadic human cancers

Charlotte Philpott, Hannah Tovell, Ian M. Frayling, David N. Cooper and Meena Upadhyaya[*]

Abstract

Background: Neurofibromatosis type 1 (NF1: Online Mendelian Inheritance in Man (OMIM) #162200) is an autosomal dominantly inherited tumour predisposition syndrome. Heritable constitutional mutations in the *NF1* gene result in dysregulation of the RAS/MAPK pathway and are causative of NF1. The major known function of the *NF1* gene product neurofibromin is to downregulate RAS. NF1 exhibits variable clinical expression and is characterized by benign cutaneous lesions including neurofibromas and café-au-lait macules, as well as a predisposition to various types of malignancy, such as breast cancer and leukaemia. However, acquired somatic mutations in *NF1* are also found in a wide variety of malignant neoplasms that are not associated with NF1.

Main body: Capitalizing upon the availability of next-generation sequencing data from cancer genomes and exomes, we review current knowledge of somatic *NF1* mutations in a wide variety of tumours occurring at a number of different sites: breast, colorectum, urothelium, lung, ovary, skin, brain and neuroendocrine tissues, as well as leukaemias, in an attempt to understand their broader role and significance, and with a view ultimately to exploiting this in a diagnostic and therapeutic context.

Conclusion: As neurofibromin activity is a key to regulating the RAS/MAPK pathway, *NF1* mutations are important in the acquisition of drug resistance, to BRAF, EGFR inhibitors, tamoxifen and retinoic acid in melanoma, lung and breast cancers and neuroblastoma. Other curiosities are observed, such as a high rate of somatic *NF1* mutation in cutaneous melanoma, lung cancer, ovarian carcinoma and glioblastoma which are not usually associated with neurofibromatosis type 1. Somatic *NF1* mutations may be critical drivers in multiple cancers. The mutational landscape of somatic *NF1* mutations should provide novel insights into our understanding of the pathophysiology of cancer. The identification of high frequency of somatic *NF1* mutations in sporadic tumours indicates that neurofibromin is likely to play a critical role in development, far beyond that evident in the tumour predisposition syndrome NF1.

Keywords: NF1, Sporadic tumours, Somatic mutations, Cancer, Melanoma, Lung cancers, Glioblastoma, Leukaemia, Breast cancer, Phaeochromocytoma

Background

Neurofibromatosis type 1 (NF1: Online Mendelian Inheritance in Man (OMIM) #162200) is an autosomal dominantly inherited tumour predisposition syndrome. Affecting 1/3000–4000 individuals worldwide, it results from constitutional mutations of the *NF1* gene, lo\cated on the long arm of human chromosome 17 [1–4]. A variety of characteristic clinical features are associated with NF1, including hyperpigmentary abnormalities of the skin (café-au-lait macules (CALMs) and inguinal/axillary freckling, iris hamartomas (Lisch nodules) and the growth of benign peripheral nerve sheath tumours (neurofibromas) in the skin. Neurofibromas can be divided into several different subtypes and are associated with a variety of clinical complications. Cutaneous neurofibromas are small, discrete dermal tumours observed in most, but not all, adult NF1 patients [5]. The generally much larger plexiform neurofibromas (PNFs), a more diffuse tumour type, are present in 30–50% of NF1 patients. Importantly, some 10–15% of these benign PNFs subsequently develop into aggressive malignant peripheral nerve sheath tumours (MPNSTs) which are the main cause of morbidity in NF1 [6–8]. A number of other tumours are also associated with NF1, including optic gliomas, juvenile myelomonocytic leukaemia (JMML), benign

* Correspondence: Upadhyaya@cardiff.ac.uk
Division of Cancer and Genetics, Institute of Medical Genetics, Cardiff University, Heath Park, Cardiff CF14 4XN, UK

or malignant phaeochromocytomas, gastrointestinal stromal tumours, glomus tumours, juvenile xanthogranulomas, rhabdomyosarcomas and lipomas.

NF1 is a tumour suppressor gene; in order for a particular cell to become cancerous, both alleles of a tumour suppressor gene must be mutated. This concept, known as the 'two-hit' hypothesis, was first proposed by Knudson, and the majority of NF1-associated tumours exhibit biallelic inactivation of *NF1* [9, 10].

The *NF1* gene is spread over a large locus (350 kbp) at 17q11.2. It contains 61 exons, including four alternatively spliced exons, and is transcribed into a 12 kbp messenger RNA (mRNA) containing an open reading frame of 8454 nucleotides [11]. Curiously, intron 27b, the largest intron of *NF1* at 61 kbp, contains three embedded genes, *OMGP*, *EVI2B* and *EVI2A*, that are all transcribed in the opposite orientation to *NF1* but whose protein products appear to have little or no interaction with neurofibromin [11].

Neurofibromin: the *NF1* gene product

Neurofibromin is a 2818 amino acid, multidomain protein. Although ubiquitously expressed, its highest levels are to be found in cells of the central nervous system (CNS), where it is often found in association with tubulin. Neurofibromin is a member of a large family of evolutionarily conserved proteins: the mammalian Ras-GTPase-activating protein (GAP)-related proteins, and its most highly conserved region is the centrally located GAP-related domain (GRD), which is encoded by exons 20–27a. The best understood function of neurofibromin is its role in tightly regulating cellular levels of activated RAS proteins. All RAS proteins exist in two cellular states, the majority being found in their inactive GDP-bound form, with only a very small fraction present in their metabolically active GTP-bound form. Only in their GTP-bound form are RAS proteins able to upregulate the many downstream effector proteins that form part of the RAS/RAF/MAPK signalling pathway [12–16]. The key role of neurofibromin is to downregulate the activated GTP-bound RAS by stimulating the low intrinsic GTPase activity of the RAS proteins themselves, thereby promoting the conversion of active RAS-GTP into its inactive RAS-GDP state. Hence, any loss of neurofibromin functionality, due to inactivating mutations in *NF1*, will result in sustained intracellular levels of active RAS-GTP, resulting in prolonged activation of the RAS/RAF/MAPK signalling pathway and ultimately a loss of growth control and increased cellular proliferation.

Increased active RAS-GTP levels also stimulate the PI3K/AKT/mTOR signalling pathway which protects cells from apoptosis. In the absence of functional neurofibromin, the pathway can become constitutively activated resulting in an increase in cell proliferation and

survival. The RAF/MAPK and PI3K/AKT pathways both activate mTOR signalling, a process found to be highly regulated in neurofibromas whereby mTOR pathway activation occurs in the absence of growth factors, in both NF1 tumours and neurofibromin-deficient cultured cells. Indeed, the mTOR pathway is constitutively activated in neurofibromin-deficient primary cells and tumours, and is regulated by phosphorylation and inactivation of the *TSC2*-encoded protein tuberin by AKT, ERK and RSK [13, 17]. It has also been suggested that increased RAS activity in brain cells may be associated with NF1-related learning deficiencies; it may result in long-term impairment as a result of increased GABA-mediated inhibition [18]. Neurofibromin levels and therefore Ras signalling can also be affected by mechanisms other than *NF1* mutation including ubiquitination [19].

Neurofibromin is known to associate with a large number of proteins, including tubulin, kinesin, protein kinases A and C, syndecan, caveolin, cytokeratin intermediate filaments and the amyloid precursor protein, although the biological significance of these protein-protein interactions is largely unknown. The diversity of protein associations does however emphasize the point that neurofibromin is likely to have many functions other than merely functioning as a GAP protein [14, 20]. Nonetheless, to date, only the function of the GAP-related domain of neurofibromin is fully understood, so it is to be hoped that new molecular studies will reveal additional functional properties of neurofibromin [21].

Mutation analysis of the *NF1* gene

The germline mutation rate of *NF1* is some 10-fold higher than that observed for most other inherited disease genes, with more than half of NF1 cases attributed to de novo mutations [7]. Currently, over 2600 different inherited mutations in *NF1* have been reported in the Human Gene Mutation Database (HGMD®) as a cause of NF1, varying in size from large genomic deletions spanning several megabases to single base-pair substitutions that alter an encoded amino acid or the function of a splice site [22–26]. There is, however, no evidence of any localized mutation clustering within *NF1*. Whilst the constitutional *NF1* mutational spectrum is well defined with missense/nonsense (27.7%), splicing (16.3%), microdeletions (26.9%), microinsertions (11.1%), indels (2.0%), gross deletions (>20 bp; 13.3%), gross insertions (>20 bp; 2.0%), complex rearrangements (0.6%) and a couple of putative regulatory mutations, there is no evidence of any localized mutation clustering within *NF1* [27, 28]. The majority (>80%) of constitutional *NF1* mutations are inactivating, predicted to result in almost complete absence of the transcript or protein [25]. Approximately 5–10% of all heritable *NF1* mutations involve gross DNA alterations, mainly genomic deletions spanning the whole gene and flanking region, as well as intragenic multi-exon rearrangements [29]. Constitutional mutations have not been identified in any of the four alternatively spliced exons in research studies, but this may be due to ascertainment bias, as the majority of clinical laboratories that analyse *NF1* do not screen these alternative exons for mutations.

A subset of the many *NF1* splicing mutations, i.e. deep intronic mutations, result in the creation of novel acceptor/donor splice sites. These may give rise to the inclusion of a novel cryptic exon into the transcribed mRNA, leading to the production of an aberrant neurofibromin protein. Such mutations account for ~2% of all reported constitutional *NF1* mutations [30].

To date, only three NF1 families with gonadal or germline mosaicism have been reported [31–33]. In such families, only a small proportion of the germ cells, whether sperm or ova, will carry the new *NF1* mutation, but this can nevertheless result in more than one affected child being produced by clinically normal parents [34].

A major challenge for clinicians and geneticists dealing with NF1 is the successful identification and characterization of causative *NF1* mutations in their patients. This problem relates to a number of features of the *NF1*, including its large genomic size (~350 kbp) and complexity (61 exons), the absence of any obvious mutational hotspots or recurrent mutations, and the wide spectrum of mutation types observed. Indeed, the lack of mutational clustering and the paucity of recurrent mutations necessitates analysis of the entire *NF1* gene in the search for potential pathogenic mutations. Furthermore, given the broad spectrum of known *NF1* mutations, no single mutation detection test can, as yet, successfully identify all such mutation types [35]. Furthermore, some 30% of all *NF1* mutations are predicted to cause aberrant splicing, and for this reason, the analysis of both RNA and DNA from patients in mutation screening protocols is clearly required [25]. Whilst the majority of *NF1* splicing mutations occur within consensus acceptor and donor splice site sequences, a number of missense, nonsense, and even 'silent' mutations may also result in aberrant splicing, which are often only identifiable by screening a patient's RNA [25]. As well as the challenges in collection and analysis of patient mRNA, a frequent issue is the difficulty in interpreting the clinical diagnostic significance of putative *NF1* missense mutations, as this may require a family segregation study and/or in vitro functional analysis to determine the pathogenicity (or otherwise) of the variant in question [25, 36].

Furthermore, many highly homologous *NF1* pseudogene sequences are scattered throughout the human genome and can often interfere with PCR-based diagnostic tests. This emphasizes the need for the careful selection of PCR primers to avoid non-specific amplification of these pseudogene sequences.

The spatial distribution of *NF1* microdeletions is strongly influenced by the presence of a number of low-copy repeats (LCRs) spanning the 17q11.2 region that encompasses the *NF1* gene. Indeed, studies into *NF1* microdeletions have provided a general model to understand the different mutational mechanisms underlying large genomic rearrangements associated with inherited diseases [37].

The *NF1* mutation detection rate in classical NF1 patients can be up to 95%. However, somatic mutation detection is more challenging, largely because of the cellular heterogeneity which is characteristic of tumour tissue [38]. Mutations in multiple genes encoding the components of the RAS/MAPK pathway predispose patients to develop clinical features that overlap with those of NF1, e.g. Legius syndrome, Noonan syndrome inter alia, and the majority of these conditions are associated with tumours [39].

Tumour biology

All cancers originate from a single cell that starts to behave abnormally due to acquired somatic mutations in its genome. These somatic mutations may be the consequence of impaired DNA replication machinery, exogenous or endogenous mutagen exposures, enzymatic modification of DNA or defective DNA repair.

A subset of these somatic changes, termed 'driver mutations', confer a selective growth advantage and are implicated in cancer development, whereas the remainder are considered to be 'passengers' [40]. The Cancer Genome Atlas (TCGA), International Cancer Genome Consortium (ICGC), Catalogue of Somatic Mutations in Cancer (COSMIC) and cBioPortal for Cancer Genomics collectively represent the results of large-scale sequencing of cancers, thereby capturing many of the genomic alterations driving malignancy [41–44]. The cBio Cancer Genomics Portal is an open-access resource for the interactive exploration of multidimensional cancer genomics data sets, currently providing access to data from more than 5000 tumour samples from 147 cancer studies [44–46]. It contains data on somatic *NF1* mutations in different types of tumour including melanoma (desmoplastic, skin cutaneous and uveal), breast carcinoma, neuroendocrine prostate cancer, glioblastoma, lung adenocarcinoma and squamous cell carcinoma, urothelial carcinoma, uterine carcinoma, adenoid and ovarian serous cystadenocarcinoma, paraganglioma, phaeochromocytoma, pancreatic cancer, adrenocortical carcinoma, stomach adenocarcinoma, sarcoma, oesophageal cancer, rhabdomyosarcoma and many more. In this review, we detail the frequency of somatic *NF1* mutations in many non-NF1-associated sporadic cancers including melanoma, glioblastoma, neuroblastoma, breast cancer, ovarian serous carcinoma, paraganglioma and phaeochromocytoma, lung adenocarcinoma, lung squamous cell carcinoma, bladder, colorectal and leukaemia. Further, it is anticipated that with the advent of powerful sequencing technologies, combined with precise microdissection of tissue, somatic *NF1* mutations will be identified in additional tumour types. Somatic *NF1* mutations are important not only because they may be drivers but also because they may contribute to resistance to therapy [47]. Elucidation of the mutational landscape of somatic *NF1* mutations in a large number of sporadic tumours, their role in the initiation and progression of tumours and how they can confer resistance or sensitivity to a therapeutic intervention may provide further insight into the mechanisms underlying tumour development and ultimately aid the development and targeting of therapies.

The frequency of somatic *NF1* mutations in different sporadic tumour types derived from the literature is given in Table 1. The cBioPortal for Cancer Genomics provides a web resource for exploring, visualizing and analysing multidimensional cancer genomics data and provides graphical summaries of gene-level data from multiple platforms, shown in Fig. 1 [45].

Main body

Melanoma

Melanoma is a skin cancer that arises from melanocytes. Although the precise causes of melanomas are still not fully understood, environmental exposure to ultraviolet (UV) radiation from sunlight or tanning lamps certainly increases

Table 1 Frequency of somatic *NF1* mutations in different human neoplasms

Neoplasm	Frequency of somatic NF1 mutations	References
Cutaneous melanoma	12–30%	[49–51, 58]
Desmoplastic melanoma	45–90%	[60, 61]
Lung adenocarcinoma	7–11.8%	[65–67, 166, 176, 177]
Lung squamous cell carcinoma	10.3–11%	[72, 177]
Acute myeloid leukaemia	3.5–23.6%	[82–85]
T cell acute lymphoblastic leukaemia	3%	[88]
Breast cancer	2.5–27.7%	[106, 177]
Ovarian carcinoma	12–34.4%	[113, 115, 170, 177–180]
Paraganglioma/ phaeochromocytoma	21–26%	[121, 124, 177]
Neuroblastoma	2.2–6%	[130]
Glioblastoma	14–23%	[132, 134, 177]
Colon adenocarcinoma	3.8–6.25%	[143, 177]
Bladder transitional cell carcinoma	6–14%	[149, 167, 177]

the risk of developing melanoma. Although NF1 is associated with pigmentary abnormalities such as CALMs, malignant melanoma is not a tumour type associated with NF1.

Somatic mutation analysis of melanoma by next-generation sequencing has been performed at multiple centres leading to the identification of several different pathways thought to be involved in the initiation and progression of melanoma.

The direct involvement of *NF1* in melanoma was first reported by Andersen and colleagues in 1993 who identified a homozygous *NF1* deletion in one of eight malignant melanoma cell lines which resulted in the loss of detectable *NF1* mRNA and neurofibromin protein [48]. Furthermore, the apparent absence of neurofibromin and *NF1* mRNA was recorded in a primary melanoma. This led to their proposal that *NF1* may function as a tumour suppressor gene in the development or progression of malignant melanoma. Many subsequent studies have identified additional somatic *NF1* mutations in melanoma in 12–30% of cases [45, 49–55].

RAS/MAPK pathway dysregulation has been identified as a key culprit in non-familial melanoma, leading to the discovery of *BRAF* and *NRAS* as the most commonly mutated genes [56]. Indeed, *BRAF* mutations occur in 50–70% of all cutaneous malignant melanomas, whilst *NRAS* alterations only occur in 19–28% of tumours. In both cases, these gene lesions result in constitutive activation of the MAPK pathway and are believed to be early somatic events associated with melanoma initiation [56, 57]. The high frequency of *BRAF* and *NRAS* mutations in melanomas has recently been confirmed by high-throughput next-generation sequencing (NGS) analysis which also identified additional driver mutations, including a recurrent *RAC* mutation, which is the third most frequent activating mutation in sun-exposed melanomas after *BRAF* and *NRAS* mutations [50, 51].

Inactivating *NF1* mutations have been detected in approximately 13% of melanomas, alongside mutations in other tumour suppressor genes, including *TP53*, *ARID2*, *PTEN*, *CDKN2A*, *MAP2K1* and *RB1* [51]. The impact on *NRAS* is however non-uniform, with some *NF1* mutant melanomas exhibiting full *NRAS* activation (i.e. the same activation level as oncogenic *NRAS* mutations), whereas others exhibit only partial activation [51]. In a mouse melanoma model, *NF1* mutations cooperate with *BRAF* mutations in the pathogenesis of melanoma by preventing oncogene-induced senescence, an indication that NF1 plays a key role in early melanoma development [58]. In both mouse tumour models and A375 human melanoma cell lines, Maertens and colleagues have shown that resistance to treatment was enhanced by further suppression of *NF1* by small hairpin RNA (shRNA). Furthermore, they observed that resistance to the BRAF inhibitor PLX4720 was attenuated by reconstitution of

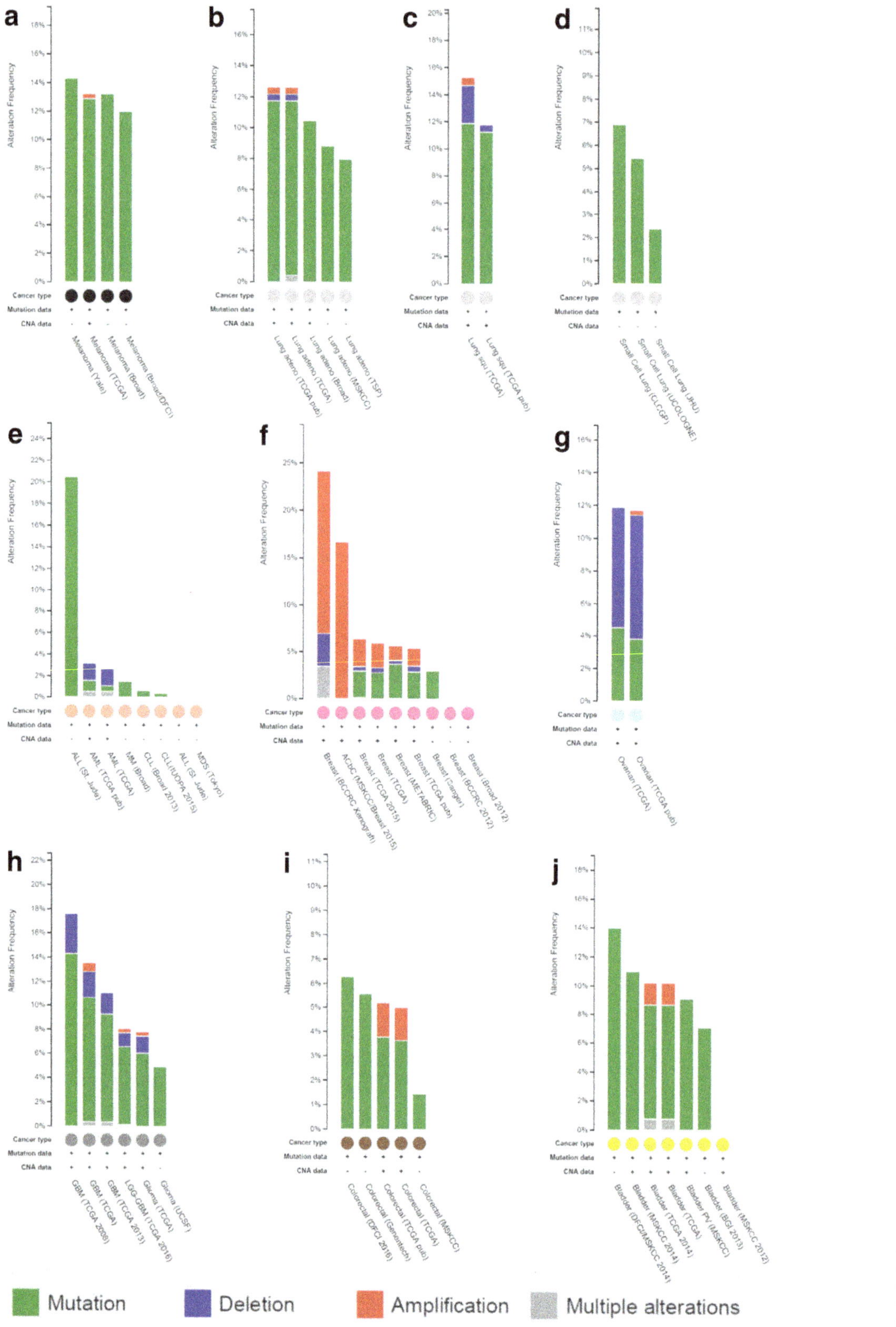

Fig. 1 (See legend on next page.)

NF1 in these cells [58]. Using RNA interference (RNAi) screening techniques, Whittaker and colleagues confirmed that *NF1* mutation is a key mechanism in BRAF inhibitor resistance. An RNAi screen, targeting more than 16,500 genes in a BRAF inhibitor-sensitive melanoma cell line, identified NF1 as the highest ranking protein affected by BRAF inhibition, and that, *NF1* knockdown abrogated the growth inhibitory effects of BRAF inhibition [53]. Indeed, it was found that *NF1* suppression led to a 31-fold increase in resistance to PLX4720, as well as a partial (7-fold) resistance to MEK inhibition, demonstrating that human melanoma samples with innate resistance to BRAF inhibition and sensitivity to a MEK inhibitor harboured *NF1* mutations [53].

Importantly, *NF1* mutations have been found in melanomas that lack both *BRAF* and *NRAS* mutations, with 25–30% of such melanomas found to harbour deleterious *NF1* mutations, thus implying that *NF1* inactivation has conferred aberrant MAPK pathway activation in these tumours [50, 51]. *BRAF/NRAS* wild-type and *NF1* mutant melanomas are strongly associated with UV damage, as evidenced clinically by the higher degree of solar elastosis and, at a molecular level, by a high proportion of C > T transitions at pyrimidine dimers and more frequent tandem CC>TT transitions [59].

A recent study based on 213 human melanoma samples identified three frequently mutated genes: *BRAF*, *NRAS* and *NF1*, with frequencies of 38.5, 28.6 and 12.2%, respectively [49]. Whilst known recurrent activating mutations were identified in *BRAF* and *NRAS*, a high number of inactivating mutations were identified in *NF1*. Notably, almost half (26/56) of *BRAF* and *NRAS* wild-type melanomas had an *NF1* mutation, most identified by loss of heterozygosity (LOH). Furthermore, *NF1* mutation-containing melanomas also harboured significantly more somatic mutations across all loci and occurred in significantly older patients, although they were associated with similar overall patient survival rates as compared to *BRAF* or *RAS* mutant or *BRAF-RAS-NF1* wild-type melanoma. In addition, all 26 *NF1* mutant *BRAF-RAS* wild-type melanomas carried mutations in other known RASopathy genes, including *RASA2*, *PTPN11*, *SOS1*, *RAF1* and *SPRED1* [49]. In contrast to Whittaker and colleagues, Krauthammer et al. also

found that 6/10 *NF1* mutant cell lines were highly sensitive to a MEK inhibitor, whereas the other four were highly resistant, clearly indicating that *NF1* suppression is not always associated with either sensitivity or resistance to MEK inhibitor [49, 53].

Desmoplastic melanoma

The highest frequency of somatic *NF1* mutations were found in desmoplastic melanomas (14/15) [60]. These melanomas are characterized by their higher propensity for local recurrence and less frequent metastatic spread to regional lymph nodes. The high frequency of *NF1* mutations in desmoplastic melanomas appears to indicate an important role for neurofibromin in the specific biology of this type of melanoma. Another recent study screened 20 desmoplastic melanomas by exome sequencing for alterations in the MAPK and PI3K signalling pathways, i.e. mutations in *CBL*, *ERBB2*, *MAP2K1*, *MAP3K1*, *BRAF*, *EGFR*, *PTPN11*, *MET*, *RAC1*, *SOS2*, *NRAS* and *PIK3C*, which were found in 15/20 (75%), with *NF1* mutations being found in 9/20 (45%) [61].

Uveal melanoma

Melanoma of the uveal tract (i.e. iris, ciliary body and choroid) is rarer than cutaneous melanoma but is nevertheless the most common primary intraocular malignancy in adults, with inactivating mutations found in approximately 60% (23/38) of uveal melanomas [62]. Intriguingly, whilst not malignant, the Lisch nodules characteristic of NF1 is hamartomatous uveal melanocytic proliferations of the iris.

Mucosal melanoma

Mucosal melanoma differs from cutaneous melanoma in terms of its molecular profile, with less frequent *BRAF* and more frequent *KIT* mutations but also has a poor prognosis. In a recent study [63] of a cohort of 75 tumours from patients with a mucosal melanoma, *NF1* and *RAS* mutations were identified in 18.3 and 16.9% samples, respectively, whereas 8.4 and 7% of tumour samples harboured *BRAF* and *KIT* mutations [63]. This study demonstrates that *NF1* is the most frequently occurring driver mutation in mucosal melanoma.

Lung cancer

Lung cancer is responsible for about 10% of all cancer cases worldwide; the vast majority of which has been attributed to tobacco smoking [64]. The two main types are non-small cell lung cancer (NSCLC) in 80–90% cases and small cell lung cancer (SCLC) found in 10–15% of patients. NSCLC has multiple subtypes, including adenocarcinoma (ADC), squamous cell carcinoma (SqCC) and undifferentiated (large cell) lung carcinoma.

Adenocarcinoma

Approximately 40% of NSCLC are ADC, and several studies have reported somatic NF1 mutations in some 7–11% of ADC [65–68]. The high mortality rate characteristic of this tumour type is due in part to the frequent presentation of such tumours at a locally advanced or metastatic stage and the lack of an effective advanced stage treatment [65, 69]. A number of potential novel therapeutic targets have been identified, including the activating mutations in KRAS, BRAF, ERBB2 and PIK3CA; the translocations in RET and ROS1; and the loss of function or deletions of TP53, NF1, CDKN2A and KEAP1 [65, 70]. Whilst NF1 mutations were only found in 7% (13/188) of sporadic lung ADC [65], further analysis found that biallelic inactivation at the NF1 locus may be present in as many as 23% (3/13), although it is not known whether these lesions occurred in cis or in trans [65]. Similarly, Imielinski et al. identified somatic NF1 mutations in 10.9% (20/183) of lung ADC, of which half were found to be truncating mutations, resulting in a complete loss of function [66].

In addition to NF1 being recurrently mutated in a subset of sporadic lung ADC patients, the MAPK pathway also appears to be an important regulatory pathway involved in tumorigenesis [65]. The TCGA research network examined the genomes, RNA and some protein from 230 previously untreated lung ADC and matched normal samples [41, 67]. In three quarters of the samples, the group identified mutations in NF1 and other genes that activate the RTK/RAS/RAF cell signalling pathway. This study not only identified loss-of-function NF1 defects but also demonstrated that NF1 mutations (as well as KEAP1 and TP53 mutations) are far more frequent in the BRAF-RAS oncogene-negative subset of lung ADC. Additionally, TCGA and other groups have identified genes such as TP53, KRAS, STK11 (LKB1), EGFR and NF1 to be significantly mutated in ADC [67].

Markedly reduced NF1 mRNA expression in ADC has been found to confer both an intrinsic and an acquired resistance to EGFR inhibitors [71]. By performing a genome-wide siRNA screen of both a human lung cancer cell line and a murine mutant EGFR-driven lung ADC, this revealed reduced NF1 mRNA expression in both, and furthermore, whilst the EGFR inhibitor erlotinib failed to

fully inhibit RAS-ERK signalling when neurofibromin levels were reduced, treatment of neurofibromin-deficient lung cancers with MEK inhibitor restored sensitivity to erlotinib [71].

In a recent study of 591 NSCLC, 60 had NF1 mutations (10%) whilst 141 (24%) harboured KRAS mutations [68]. Approximately 25% of the NF1 mutations co-occurred with mutations in known oncogenes: BRAF, ERBB2, KRAS, HRAS and NRAS. Therapeutic strategies targeting KRAS activation, including the use of inhibitors of MAP kinase signalling, may warrant investigation in NF1 mutant tumours. Additional tumour suppressor inactivation pattern studies may help to inform novel treatment strategies.

Squamous cell carcinoma

According to the TCGA, somatic NF1 changes are present in approximately 12% of squamous cell lung cancers (SqCC), of which four distinct subtypes have been identified: classical, primitive, basal and secretory expression [72]. The basal expression subtype was found to harbour NF1 alterations, suggesting a potential direction for the treatment of such tumours. The information from the TCGA studies has highlighted the involvement of NF1 in both lung ADC and SqCC and served to improve our understanding of the genetic pathways that lead to lung cancer [72].

Transcriptome analysis of 153 tumour samples, including ADC, SqCC, large cell lung cancer, adenoid cystic carcinomas and derived cell lines, has been integrated with the data from The Cancer Genome Atlas and other published sources [73]. This confirms the previously reported CD74-NRG1 fusion and also suggests that the NRG1, NF1 and Hippo pathway fusions may play important roles in tumours without known driver mutations and that this prognostic factor may be associated with poor survival [73]. Several different gene fusions, viz. NF1-GOSR1, NF1-PSMD11, NF1-NLK, NF1-DRG2 and NF1-MYO15A, were also detected by transcriptome sequencing of lung cancers [73]. Interestingly, both lung ADC and SqCC DNA displayed a significantly increased frequency of guanine (cytosine) to thymine (adenine) mutations, a type of mutation associated with exposure to tobacco smoke [68]. Lung ADC genomes also manifest regional heterogeneity in terms of the distribution of mutations with sequencing data from lung cancer studies clearly indicating that lung cancer, at the molecular level, is a highly heterogeneous disease. Indeed, the mutational landscape of lung ADC is substantially different from that of SqCC of the lung or SCLC [74], with frequent receptor tyrosine kinase mutations found in lung ADC, that are rarely encountered in either SqCC or SCLC [75].

Mutations in *TP53*, *KRAS*, *LKB1*, *NF1* and *RBM10* are enriched in transversion-high tumours, whilst mutations in *EGFR*, *RB1* and *PIK3CA* and in-frame insertions in the receptor tyrosine kinases *EGFR* and *ERBB2* are enriched in transversion-low tumours [75]. The transversion-high group was found to be strongly associated with past or present smoking ($P < 2.2 \times 10^{-16}$) [72, 74, 75].

To compare lung ADC and SqCC and to identify new drivers of lung carcinogenesis, Campbell and colleagues examined the exome sequences and copy number profiles of 660 lung ADC and 484 lung SqCC tumour normal pairs [74]. They observed median somatic mutation rates of 8.7 mutations/Mbp and 9.7 mutations/Mbp for lung ADC and SqCC, respectively. At least 38 genes were significantly mutated in lung ADC and 20 genes in SqCC; however, only six genes, *TP53*, *RB1*, *ARIDIA*, *CDKN2A*, *PIK3CA* and *NF1*, were significantly mutated in both tumour types, and of these, *TP53*, *CDKN2A* and *PIK3CA* mutations had a significantly higher frequency in lung SqCC. Recurrent alterations in lung SqCC were more similar to those of other squamous carcinomas than to alterations in lung ADCs, whilst the significantly mutated genes in lung ADC were most similar to those associated with glioblastoma and colorectal cancer.

Small cell lung cancer

Although there is a paucity of data for small cell lung cancer (SCLC), the frequency of *NF1* mutations in SCLC was found to be 2.4 and 6.9% in two independent studies [76, 77]. In a subsequent study of 98 SCLC, DNA was sequenced to a high, uniform coverage and analysed for all classes of genomic alterations [78]. Of the seven most commonly altered genes identified, only one (*RICTOR*) was considered to be actionable in terms of treatment. The most common non-actionable genomic alterations were found in *TP53* (86% of SCLC cases), *RB1* (54%) and *MLL2* (17%), with *NF1* mutations identified in only 3% of SCLC, consistent with the earlier studies.

Myeloid malignancies

Myeloid malignancies are clonal disorders characterized by acquired somatic mutations in various haematopoietic progenitors. Constitutional *NF1* mutations are known to predispose individuals to myeloid malignancies such as chronic myelomonocytic leukaemia (CMML), JMML and acute myeloid leukaemia (AML) [79]. Somatic 17q11 deletions encompassing *NF1* have been described in many adult myeloid malignancies [80]. More generally, the RAS signalling pathway has been found to be fundamental in the development of myeloid malignancies, with somatic activating mutations in *NRAS* and *KRAS* genes estimated to be present in 20 to 40% of diagnosed cases of AML, CMML and JMML [81]. Recent advances in understanding the genetic basis of myeloid malignancies have

provided important insights into the pathogenesis of AML. Whilst somatic *KRAS* and *NRAS* mutations are frequently found in AML, mutations in other RAS signalling pathway genes, including *NF1*, occur at lower frequencies, although the reported frequency for *NF1* somatic mutations ranges quite widely from 3.5 to 23.6% [79, 82–85].

Parkin and colleagues identified *NF1* mutations in 7% of cases with AML, with a further 12% displaying copy number alterations (CNAs) involving *NF1*, mainly heterozygous deletions [85]. The absence of *NF1* expression was observed in 7% of adult AML associated with an increased RAS-GTP level. In another study of AML with CBHB-MYHII rearrangements, 16% of the samples harboured *NF1* deletions [84]. However, high-resolution studies have failed to provide any evidence for frequent *NF1* alterations in de novo AML, although they suggested that *NF1* mutations may contribute to tumour progression [82]. In this study, the authors screened a total of 488 previously untreated de novo AML patients for the *NF1* deletion using either array comparative genomic hybridization (aCGH) or real-time quantitative PCR/fluorescence in situ hybridization approaches. Using aCGH, a small ~0.3 Mbp minimally deleted region involving *NF1* was defined; the overall frequency of *NF1* deletion was 3.5% (17/485). Furthermore, *NF1* deletion was significantly associated with abnormal cytogenetics and a monosomal karyotype, whilst only one of five *NF1*-deleted patients acquired a coding mutation in the remaining allele. This study indicates that *NF1* microlesions are infrequent in de novo AML and may be secondary events in leukemic progression.

Myelodysplastic syndrome

The frequency of *NF1* changes in myelodysplastic syndrome has been found to vary between 0 and 9% [86, 87].

T cell acute lymphoblastic leukaemia

T cell acute lymphoblastic leukaemia (T-ALL) is a variant of acute lymphoblastic leukaemia (ALL), with features similar to some types of lymphoma. It accounts for about 15 and 25% of ALL in paediatric and adult cohorts, respectively.

T-ALL is a highly aggressive malignancy, characterized by rapid progression and high relapse rates [79]. Somatic mutations in a number of established T-ALL drivers such as *KRAS*, *NRAS*, *PIK3CA*, *PTEN*, *NOTCH1*, *PHF6* and *NF1* have been identified in T-ALL cell lines and patient samples [88]. Somatic *NF1* mutations have been found in 27.3% (9/33) of the T-ALL cohort; however, only 12.1% (4/33) were non-synonymous mutations [88]. The type 1 *NF1* microdeletion (1.4 Mb) was reported in 2.9% (3/103) of T-ALL patients [79]. None of these three individuals with the microdeletion exhibited any clinical characteristics of NF1.

Juvenile myelomonocytic leukaemia

JMML is a myeloproliferative neoplasm (MPN) of childhood, occurring when too many immature white blood cells (myelocytes and monocytes) are made in the bone marrow. In 1997, Side and colleagues reported constitutional *NF1* mutations in 15% of JMML patients [89]. JMML generally carries a very poor prognosis, with the only curative treatment being haematopoietic stem cell transplantation.

JMML was once considered a unique example of RAS-driven oncogenesis because it was thought to be initiated by mutually exclusive mutations in the RAS genes (*NRAS* or *KRAS*) or in several RAS pathway regulators (*PTPN11*, *NF1* or *CBL*) [90].

In an exploration of the somatic mutation landscape of 30 patients with syndromic (*n* = 8) or sporadic (*n* = 22) JMML, a combination of genome-wide DNA array analysis, whole-exome sequencing and targeted sequencing was used in paired germline and tumour samples [90]. In total, 85 somatically acquired genetic alterations were found in 83% (25/30) of patients in this sub-cohort. Genes containing somatic variants detected by whole-exome sequencing, or previously reported to be mutated in JMML, were then sequenced in the full cohort of 118 JMML cases. A total of 122 secondary clonal abnormalities, in addition to initiating RAS pathway mutations, were identified in 49% (58/118) of patients [90]. In addition, sequencing of isolated myeloid colonies demonstrated the coexistence of multiple RAS hits in the same myeloid progenitors in three of the JMML cases tested, challenging the concept of mutually exclusive RAS pathway mutations.

The polycomb recessive complex 2 (PRC2) is involved in cellular differentiation, maintenance of cell identity and proliferation as well as stem cell plasticity [91] and also drives myeloid malignancies. *Nf1/Kras* double-mutant mice have been shown to develop myeloid malignancies with reduced latency and increased severity in comparison to mice with only one of the two defects because copy number variations (CNVs) in *Nf1/Kras* mutant mice frequently resulted in haploinsufficiency for PRC2 core subunits (*SUZ12* or *EZH2*) or PRC2-associated factors necessary for optimal PRC2 activity (*AEBP2*, *CDYL* or *JARID2*) [92]. In addition, haploinsufficiency for multiple genes that regulate PRC2 function can cooperate in myeloid transformation, and other mutations in JMML target a small number of pathways specifically, including components of the RAS and PRC2 networks [93, 94]. Thus, RAS activation is a major player, and other pathways such as PRC2 are also important. Notably, PRC2 also plays a role in the development of MPNSTs. Loss of function of PRC2 (due to

mutations in *EED* or *SUZ12*) is also found in the vast majority of sporadic, NF1-associated, and radiotherapy-associated MPNSTs (where PRC2 loss amplifies Ras-driven transcription) [95, 96].

In a recent study focussing on characterization of serial samples from JMML patients at diagnosis and then beyond through relapse and transformation to AML, mutations were found in *NF1*, *NRAS*, *KRAS*, *PTPN11* or *CBL* in 85% of patients, as well as recurrent mutations in other genes involved in signal transduction, splicing, PRC2 and transcription. The number of somatic alterations present at diagnosis appeared to be important for the outcome of JMML [97].

Breast cancer

The *NF1* gene is reported to be frequently mutated in sporadic breast cancers, although in only a few studies has mutation frequency been published. NF1 patients have an increased risk of developing breast cancer as compared to the general population [8, 98]. In particular, women under the age of 50 with NF1 have an increased (4–5-fold) risk of developing breast cancer (standardized incidence ratio for women under 50) and also a 3.5-fold increased fatality risk (proportionate mortality ratio) [98–100]. A predisposition to breast cancer in NF1 patients has led researchers to postulate the potential involvement of somatic *NF1* mutations in initiating and driving the malignant transformation and progression of sporadic breast cancer. A number of breast cancer genome sequencing studies have identified *NF1* as one of a number of novel, recurrently mutated genes in sporadic tumours which could potentially be targeted in a therapeutic context [101, 102].

It was Ogata and colleagues, working with established breast cancer cell lines in 2001, who first identified a role for *NF1* in the malignant transformation of mammary cells [103]. Further analysis of the *NF1* deletion-bearing tumours revealed significantly higher levels of active RAS, indicating that RAS signal transduction pathway dysregulation, through *NF1* loss, may be responsible for driving malignancy in these cells. Neurofibromin was found to be below detectable levels in the highly malignant and treatment-resistant MB-231 breast cancer cell line as compared with four other less aggressive cell lines. Additionally, the MB-231 cells exhibited a 10-fold increase in pMAPK levels as a result of activated Ras, despite there being no changes in p120^{GAP}. Hence, this study suggested that under-expression of *NF1* and reduced neurofibromin activity may have a direct influence on malignant transformation and resistance to anti-cancer agents [103]. This is consistent with other studies and goes some way towards accounting for the presence of the somatic *NF1* mutations found in sporadic breast tumours.

The mouse model *Chaos3* is characterized by the spontaneous development of mammary tumours, due to a mutation in *Mcm4* leading to chromosomal instability through disruption of the MCM2-7 complex [104, 105]. Somatic *NF1* deletions were found in almost all (59/60) of the mammary tumours studied in this mouse model, and upon subsequent examination of TCGA data, it was noted that *NF1* is somatically mutated or deleted in 27.7% of human breast cancers [105, 106].

Large-scale NGS to compare primary and recurrent breast cancer has found mutations in recurrent tumours which were not present in matched primary tissue [107]. However, the difficulties inherent in studying recurrent tumours mean that the sample size was necessarily small in this study, with only 74 matched tumours from 43 patients across the various breast cancer subtypes. So, the precise role for *NF1* in breast cancer is still unclear and further studies are required.

CNAs dominate the breast cancer genome, with *NF1* gene amplification being a particular feature not seen in the other tumour types in which *NF1* mutations are observed (Fig. 1), suggesting that gain of neurofibromin function is especially important in breast cancer biology. In contrast, genes generally mutated in breast cancers are subject to a low frequency of somatic mutations, including single nucleotide mutations and indels in driver genes [105, 106].

Large-scale efforts by the TCGA and ICGC have contributed greatly towards determining the identity of genes mutated in breast cancer, but analysis of clinical associations in these data sets is limited by the scarcity of long-term patient follow-up data and the stringent criteria used for sample selection (e.g. tumour size, malignant cellularity) [41, 42].

In a recent study based on 2433 molecular profiles of breast cancer, it was noted that high levels of intra-tumour heterogeneity was generally associated with a worse clinical outcome, with one exception: highly aggressive breast tumours with 11q13–14 amplification had low levels of intra-tumour heterogeneity [108, 109]. Inactivating *NF1* mutations were also found to be associated with breast cancer severity score in oestrogen receptor-negative tumours.

As with melanoma and neuroblastoma, inactivation of *NF1* in breast cancer is associated with resistance to drug therapy. A potential mechanism for *NF1* and drug resistance in breast adenocarcinoma has been suggested following analysis of the MCF-7 breast cancer cell line [110]. Silencing of *NF1*, amongst several other genes, has been shown to confer a tamoxifen-resistant phenotype, although it was noted that resistance- or sensitivity-specific gene expression patterns may give a better prediction of treatment outcome as compared to single genes [111]. This is potentially of great clinical importance, of course, as, although tamoxifen is one of the most widely used anti-breast cancer agents, it is now apparent that up to ~40% of early-stage breast cancer patients who receive tamoxifen as an adjuvant therapy will ultimately develop tamoxifen resistance and relapse [111, 112].

Ovarian cancer

High-grade serous ovarian carcinoma (HGOSC) is the most common and malignant form of ovarian tumours accounting for up to 70% of all ovarian cancer cases. Some serous cancers may initiate in cells at the distal end of the fallopian tube, then spread to the ovary. There are different subtypes of epithelial ovarian cancer including mucinous, endometrioid, clear cell, undifferentiated or unclassifiable; therefore, HGOSC is a molecularly and clinically heterogeneous disease which accounts for the majority of ovarian cancer deaths.

More than a third of all ovarian serous carcinomas (OSCs) harbour somatic *NF1* mutations, identifying an alternative target for treatment and an additional prognostic marker. This is of particular importance when considering the disease heterogeneity, high relapse and fatality rates [113, 114].

A role for *NF1* in ovarian serous carcinoma (OSC) was first proposed by Sangha et al. in 2008 [113]. Genome-wide microarray analysis of 36 primary OSC identified homozygous *NF1* deletions in two tumours. This group subsequently screened 18 ovarian carcinoma-derived cell lines and 41 primary OSC for additional *NF1* alterations, with 8/18 cell lines exhibiting marked reduction or no expression of *NF1*. Homozygous *NF1* gene deletions and *NF1* splicing mutations were identified in 9/41 primary OSC. Additionally, tumours and cell lines with *NF1* lesions were found to lack *KRAS* and *BRAF* mutations, whilst exhibiting Ras pathway activation [113].

The Cancer Genome Atlas project analysed the expression of mRNA and microRNA, promoter methylation and DNA copy number in 489 HGOSC and performed genomic DNA analysis in 316 tumours. Loss of *NF1* function was identified in 12% (37/316) of samples, and of these, 24 had deletions, one had a duplication and the remaining (12) samples harboured other somatic mutations. The Australian Ovarian Cancer Study (AOCS) specifically examined CNAs and reported regions of copy number loss at the *NF1* locus in 34% (137/398) of ovarian cancer samples, comprising 157 serous adenocarcinomas from the TCGA cohort and a further 241 samples, of both endometrioid and serous subtypes [115].

HGOSC shows a simple mutational profile, with *TP53* nearly always mutated, but with other genes, including *NF1*, mutated at a low frequency [116]. Approximately 50% of all HGSOCs exhibit homologous recombination

(HR) deficiency, with such tumours being highly sensitive to PARP inhibitors [117]. However, *NF1* mutations identified in advanced HGOSC are associated with resistance to treatment because of the acquisition of different new mutations within the gene [116–118].

Paragangliomas and phaeochromocytomas

Phaeochromocytomas are rare tumours (annual incidence of 1–6 million per year) that develop from neural crest-derived chromaffin cells and produce excess catecholamine, resulting in hypertension and flushing. Despite being rare in the general population, the frequency of occurrence amongst NF1 patients is much higher, with 0.1–6% developing a phaeochromocytoma [119, 120].

NF1 is one of a number of known paraganglioma and phaeochromocytoma susceptibility genes, constitutional mutations in which are responsible for inherited tumour syndromes. Somatic *NF1* mutations occurred in 35/161 (21.7%) of sporadic phaeochromocytomas, with the majority exhibiting LOH and low *NF1* mRNA expression [121–123], whilst somatic mutations in the susceptibility genes *NF1*, *MAX*, *RET*, *VHL*, *SDHA*, *SDHB*, *SDHC*, *SDHD*, *SDHAF2*, *KIF1Bβ* and *TMEM127* are present in 11–19% of sporadic cases [124–126]. It has also been demonstrated that the majority (83%, 35/42) of sporadic phaeochromocytomas harbour a CNA in at least one of these susceptibility genes, thereby altering respective protein expression levels [123]. This is in addition to the 26% (11/42) of sporadic paragangliomas and phaeochromocytomas that have lost one *NF1* allele, associated with a reduction in *NF1* mRNA level. Furthermore, 10 of 11 tumours were also observed to harbour a somatic protein-truncating *NF1* mutation in the second allele [121]. This study also identified a correlation between *NF1* mutations and a biochemical phenotype: paragangliomas and phaeochromocytomas harbouring a somatic *NF1* mutation were found to display higher plasma levels of normetanephrine ($P = 0.005$) and metanephrine ($P = 0.0025$), markers for catecholamine-secreting tumours [121]. This could be of significance as plasma catecholamine levels are used in the diagnosis of phaeochromocytoma and paraganglioma; however, these findings were reported in only a small sample group and the biochemical data was non-centralized and incomplete, limiting their overall significance [123].

A large-scale analysis of a cohort of 202 paragangliomas and phaeochromocytomas, collected by the *Cortico et Médullosurrénale: les Tumeurs Endocrines* (COMETE) network, examined CNAs, somatic and constitutional mutations in known susceptibility genes [124]. Almost a quarter (25/119) of the sporadic phaeochromocytomas/paragangliomas carried an inactivating *NF1* mutation, of which 21/25 were associated with the loss of the wild-type allele. Of all the somatic mutations identified in the study, 56% were located in *NF1*, showing that *NF1* is frequently mutated in phaeochromocytomas/paragangliomas [124].

Neuroblastoma

Neuroblastoma is a neuroendocrine tumour that originates from neural crest cells of the sympathetic nervous system, with most tumours developing in the abdomen. Neuroblastoma is the second most common solid tumour in childhood and accounts for 8% of all childhood cancers. The treatment for neuroblastoma includes surgery, chemotherapy, radiation and bone marrow transplantation. Familial neuroblastoma cases comprise only a small fraction (~1–2%) of all neuroblastoma cases, and their genetic aetiology is relatively well understood [127, 128]. In contrast, far less is known of the genetic aetiology of sporadic neuroblastomas, despite their accounting for the majority of cases.

It was a quarter of a century ago when *NF1* was first reported to play a role in the development of neuroblastoma. In this study, 4/10 neuroblastoma cell lines were observed to express either a reduced level or a complete absence of neurofibromin, with *NF1* mutations being identified in two of these cell lines [129]. Furthermore, it was demonstrated that the introduction of a normal human chromosome 17 into a neuroblastoma cell line suppressed its tumorigenicity. Several *NF1*-deficient neuroblastoma cell lines exhibited only moderately elevated *Ras*–GTP levels, in contrast to *NF1* tumour cells, indicating that neurofibromin can contribute differently to the negative regulation of RAS in different cell types [130, 131].

Somatic *NF1* mutations in neuroblastomas have been correlated with reduced expression of neurofibromin and poor patient prognosis, whilst higher levels of expression are associated with longer progression-free survival [130, 131]. Hölzel and colleagues also reported a loss of neurofibromin expression in 8/25 neuroblastoma cell lines and that a further SNP analysis of 20 neuroblastoma cell lines detected 50% (10/20) with abnormal *NF1* alleles [130]. Genomic aberrations in *NF1* were also found in primary neuroblastomas but at a lower frequency of 6% (5/83).

A large-scale RNAi screen revealed an association of *NF1* loss in neuroblastoma cell lines with resistance to retinoic acid (RA) treatment which is used as targeted therapy in the treatment of neuroblastomas. Loss of *NF1* activates RAS-MEK signalling, which in turn represses *ZNF423*, a critical transcriptional coactivator of the retinoic acid receptors; neuroblastomas with low levels of both *NF1* and *ZNF423* have an extremely poor outcome. However, inhibition of MEK signalling downstream of *NF1* restores responsiveness to RA, suggesting a potential therapeutic strategy to overcome RA resistance in *NF1*-deficient neuroblastomas [130].

Glioblastoma

Glioblastomas are tumours that arise from astrocytes that comprise the supportive tissue of the brain. These tumours are usually aggressive as the cells divide rapidly and are also supported by a large network of blood vessels. The most aggressive subtype is glioblastoma multiforme (GBM) which is the most frequent form of brain cancer in adults, renowned for its lethality and poor prognosis and is thus an important target of study [132, 133].

Glioblastoma-associated *NF1* somatic mutations are well described [132, 134, 135], with recurrent driver mutations being identified in *NF1* and a number of other candidate genes (*IDH1*, *TP53*, *CDK4*, *EGFR*, *PI3KR1*, *PIK3CA*, *PTEN*, *RB1* and *CDNK2A*) in GBM [132]. *NF1* mutations were identified in at least 15% (16/105) of all GBM by Parsons and colleagues, although chromosomal translocations or epigenetic changes were not tested in this cohort [132].

A TCGA analysis assessed levels of gene expression, CNAs and DNA methylation in a cohort of 206 glioblastoma tumour samples, with recurrent mutations in *NF1*, *AKT3*, *PRK3R1* and *PARK2* being identified, and with 14% (13/91) of samples found to contain at least one somatic *NF1* mutation. Verhaak and colleagues subsequently performed large-scale genomic analysis of these TCGA data, dividing glioblastoma cases into four subtypes: proneural, neural, classical and mesenchymal [136]. They found that GBM with *NF1* and *PTEN* alterations had a distinct mesenchymal-like expression profile, with 53% of mesenchymal cases having an *NF1* mutation. The mutual exclusivity of *NF1* and *BRAF* mutations in GBM has also been reported [134].

In animal models, inactivation of *TP53* and *PTEN* may cooperate with *NF1* loss in the development of glioblastoma [137]. Haploinsufficiency of *NF1* is also reported to increase astrocyte proliferation and enhancement of angiogenesis in $Nf1^{+/-}$ heterozygous mouse models [138, 139].

Colorectal cancer

Colorectal cancer (CRC) is one of the leading causes of cancer-related deaths in the western world, with at least 50% of CRCs exhibiting dysregulation of the RAS/MAPK pathway. Reports of the type of *NF1* mutations in CRC vary widely, with *NF1* LOH first reported in 14–57%, and reported gains in part of, or even a complete duplication of, the *NF1* gene in 17% of CRC [140–142]. The 2012 TCGA genome-scale analysis of 212 CRC found that 24 genes were predominantly mutated, including *NF1* in approximately 5.6% (11/212) of cases [143]. Subsequent studies have confirmed this, with *NF1* mutations being identified in 5.6% (4/72) and 5.8% of cases (39/619), respectively [144, 145].

Several critical genes and pathways, such as WNT, RAS/MAPK, PI3K, TGF-β, P53 and DNA mismatch repair, are recognized in the initiation and progression of CRC [146, 147]. Although genetic alterations in the PI3K and RAS/MAPK pathways are common in CRC and *NF1* alterations have been detected in 5–6% of cases, it remains unclear as to whether *NF1* mutations in CRC are related to chemotherapeutic effect.

Urinary tract transitional cell carcinoma

The best documented molecular factors involved in urothelial transitional cell carcinoma (TCC) are the *RAS* proto-oncogene activation and *TP53* mutations. Alterations in *NF1* gene expression in TCC were first reported in 1999 [148], where decreased *NF1* gene expression was observed in 83% (23/29) of TCC specimens (as estimated by immunohistochemistry), whilst *NF1* mRNA levels were markedly lower in TCC tissue as compared with those in adjacent non-neoplastic urothelium. Neurofibromin levels were also decreased in high-grade TCC, suggesting that alterations of *NF1* gene expression might be involved in urinary TCC carcinogenesis. Whole genomic analysis performed on 35 stage IV urothelial cancers that had relapsed and progressed after primary surgery and conventional chemotherapy revealed *NF1* mutations in two cases (6%) [149]. Integrated analysis of 131 urothelial carcinomas showed recurrent mutations in 32 genes, with 14% of tumours having *NF1* mutations.

Other malignant tumours

There are a number of other malignant tumour types that have been found to harbour *NF1* alterations including neuroendocrine prostate cancer (24%), myxofibrosarcomas (10.5%) and pleomorphic liposarcomas (8%), pancreatic cancer (11%), gastric adenocarcinoma (10%) and rhabdomyosarcoma (7%) [44, 45]. Somatic *NF1* mutations have also been detected in 41–72% of sporadic MPNSTs, showing that *NF1* inactivation plays a major role in the development of this tumour type [96].

General discussion

Neurofibromatosis type 1, caused by constitutional inactivating mutations in the tumour suppressor gene *NF1*, is a neurodegenerative disorder predisposing individuals to both benign and malignant tumours [150–152]. Additionally, somatic mutations of *NF1* are also frequent in desmoplastic, cutaneous and mucosal melanoma, high-grade serous ovarian cancer, breast cancer, phaeochromocytomas and paragangliomas, glioblastoma multiforme, myeloid malignancies, neuroblastoma, and colorectal and urinary bladder transitional cell carcinoma (Table 1). Aberrations in neurofibromin result in the dysregulation of the RAS/MAPK pathway leading to unregulated cell growth and proliferation. The related mTOR pathway and other downstream activators and effectors of RAS including PI3K are also involved in cancer [17, 153].

Mutations (chromosomal aberrations, nucleotide substitutions and epigenetic aberrations) in a subset of candidate genes are likely to confer a growth advantage resulting in the development of cancer. Cancer encompasses more than 100 different diseases, the study of which provides insight into both the commonalities and differences between and amongst various types and subtypes of cancer [147]. In order to understand this complex disease and to develop novel targeted therapeutics, it is essential to characterize the somatic mutational spectra in each cancer genome in order to facilitate our understanding of the biological processes underlying the cancer as well as the pathways of evolutionary progression. The availability of the human genome reference sequence enabled the rapid resequencing of cancer genomes, leading to the discovery of many additional cancer genes, revealing for the first time the molecular heterogeneity of cancer genomes and identifying therapeutic targets. To improve the diagnosis and treatment of cancer patients, several large-scale cancer genomics projects, e.g. the TCGA, ICGC, cBioPortal and COSMIC, have been undertaken in recent years [41–44]. These pan-cancer projects have generated high-throughput data which provide valuable opportunities to understand the biology, initiation and progression of human cancers. One caveat, however, is distinguishing artefactual DNA damage from the bona fide mutations that actually occurred in the tumour, given that it has been reported that mutagenic damage accounts for the majority of the erroneous identification of variants with low to moderate (1 to 5%) frequency in whole (cancer) genome sequencing studies [154].

Generally, a large number of mutations occur in cancer genomes, such as somatic mutations, CNAs, methylation aberrations and histone modifications. It is critical to distinguish driver mutations and driver genes (which contribute to the progression of cancer from normal to malignant states) from passenger mutations and passenger genes (which accumulate in cells but do not contribute to cancer development). There is a subtle difference between a driver gene and a driver gene mutation. A driver gene harbours driver gene mutations but may also harbour passenger gene mutations. A driver mutation typically confers upon a tumour only a very small growth advantage, which may be as low as a 0.4% increase in the difference between cell birth and death rates [155]. More recently, Bozic and colleagues have shown that the first, and hence most abundant, passenger mutations are influenced both by the mutation rate and by the death-birth ratio of the cancer cells [156]. It should be appreciated that whilst passenger mutations do not, by definition, exert a strong selective growth advantage, they are not entirely neutral. Indeed, many are deleterious in terms of their effect on cellular

proliferation and cancer progression [157, 158]. It should also be appreciated that whilst the damaging effect of a non-synonymous passenger mutation is on average 100 times smaller than the effect of a driver mutation, passengers are 100 times more numerous than drivers [158]. The paucity of drivers in a sea of passenger mutations represents a challenge to identifying the former. This task is made all the more daunting by the possibility that drivers and passengers are not discrete entities but rather lie along a continuum which includes latent driver mutations which 'behave as passengers but coupled with other emerging mutations, drive cancer development and drug resistance' [159].

In 2004, Futreal and colleagues published a 'Census of human cancer genes' which aimed to list all genes that are causally implicated in tumorigenesis. This census has been kept up to date and currently includes 602 entries [43, 160]. This implies that more than 2% of all human genes are implicated in cancer. Of these, approximately 90% have somatic mutations in cancer; 20% have germline mutations that predispose to cancer; and 10% harbour both somatic and germline mutations. A second resource, the Network of Cancer Genes (NCG) contains a total of 1053 'cancer genes' whose possible involvement in cancer has been inferred by statistical means [161]. The number of genes recognized as being cancer-associated is likely to increase as new techniques are devised to identify the function of the associated proteins [162, 163].

Cooperativity and exclusivity of *NF1* somatic mutations

Mitogen-activated protein kinases (MAPK) and phosphoinositide-3 kinase (PI3K) pathways are key cellular growth regulators. In a normal cell, these control cell growth and survival but are often disrupted in a malignant cell with a deregulated MAPK or PI3K pathway. It is now well recognized that the focus should be upon cellular pathways rather than on individual genes to achieve a full understanding of cancer biology. Therefore, defining driver pathways is an important step to understanding the molecular mechanisms underlying cancer. Previous studies have focussed mainly on identifying the alterations in cancer genomes at the individual gene or single pathway level. However, a great deal of evidence indicates that multiple pathways often function cooperatively in carcinogenesis and other key biological processes. A common and restricted number of driver genes and pathways are probably responsible for most common forms of cancer [40, 147].

In general, mutations of the genes in one pathway usually exhibit mutual exclusivity, because a single mutation is usually enough to disturb one pathway and any further hits in other components of that pathway confer no added selectable advantage. Thus, sporadic tumours with *NF1* mutations are mutually exclusive for mutations in

MAPK kinase 1 (*MAP2K1*) or *NRAS*. Strongly activating 'canonical' mutations in oncogenes (for example G12D or G12V mutations in KRAS) can drive cancer formation on their own and are known to be epistatic in relation to other canonical mutations within the same pathway [164]. However, whether there are, for example, 'non-canonical' mutations that weakly activate oncogenes or only partially inactivate tumour suppressor activity and yet can drive cancer formation is less clear. Examination of genomic data from the Cancer Cell Line Encyclopedia (CCLE) and TCGA has indicated that whilst canonical *KRAS* mutations do not occur with increased frequency in the context of *NF1* mutations, non-canonical *KRAS* mutations certainly do, suggesting that such pairs of mutations might act together to confer a selective advantage in human tumours [164]. Activation of RAS guanine nucleotide exchange factors (RAS-GEFs) was predicted to have similar effects to neurofibromin loss and that non-canonical *KRAS* mutations co-occur with RAS-GEF mutations in TCGA and CCLE data [164]. Furthermore, increased frequencies of mutations in both *NF1* and other RAS pathway activators or effectors have been found which suggests that this principle could apply more broadly to other genes in the RAS network and possibly to other oncogenic signalling pathways [58]. Subsequently, *NF1* loss has been described as a key mediator of acquired and intrinsic *BRAF* inhibitor resistance following a high-throughput short hairpin RNA screening approach [53]. Furthermore, on the basis of analyses of somatic co-mutation patterns in the TCGA data sets (cBio Portal for Cancer Genomics), 9.6% of melanomas with *NF1* mutations also have mutations in *BRAF*, *NRAS* or *RAF1* [47]. But, whilst mutant *NF1* is known to cooperate with RASo-pathy genes (*RASA2*, *PTPN11*, *SOS1*, *RAF1* and *SPRED1*) in melanoma and although *NF1* is found to be frequently mutated (25–30%) in melanomas harbouring wild-type *BRAF* and *NRAS*, it is curious that melanoma is not a tumour type associated with NF1 [8, 49–51].

The capacity of *NF1* mutations to act both cooperatively and exclusively without *BRAF* and *NRAS* mutations in melanoma may be mediated through pathways other than the MAPK pathway. Maertens and colleagues have identified increased activation of the PI3K/AKT/mTOR pathway in *BRAF/NF1* double mutants, and a combinatorial MEK marker and mTOR inhibitor treatment has proven effective in many MEK inhibitor-resistant neoplasms [58]. In a glioblastoma animal model, *NF1* cooperates with both *TP53* and *PTEN*, but no co-occurrence of *NF1* and *BRAF* mutations is seen [137]. Moreover, whilst simultaneous inactivation of *Nf1* and expression of K-Ras^{G12D} in mouse haematopoietic cells results in AML that was fatal in primary mice within 4 weeks, in ovarian serous carcinomas, cooperation between mutant *TP53* and *NF1* results in a poor prognosis

[92, 117]. In addition, an association between inactivated *NF1* and *ZNF423* levels in neuroblastomas has been identified as a putative prognostic marker [130].

It should be appreciated that the same gene can function in completely opposite ways in different cell types. In melanomas harbouring *BRAF* V600E mutations, a BRAF inhibitor induces remission of the tumour; however, the same drug is ineffective in colorectal cancer cells harbouring identical mutations. This has been attributed to the expression of EGFR which occurs in some colorectal cancers, but not in melanomas [165].

Despite all the cancer genome information available regarding *NF1*, it remains unclear why NF1 patients are predisposed only to certain types of tumours. Why, for example, are NF1 patients not predisposed to lung tumours given that at least 10% of all sporadic lung cancers have *NF1* mutations [8, 65, 72, 166]?

NF1 and drug resistance

The RAS/MAPK pathway, with an important role in cancer biology, is a prime target for anti-cancer agents; however, the presence of an *NF1* mutation, resulting in reduced expression of neurofibromin, confers resistance to several therapeutic drugs. Furthermore, *NF1*-associated drug resistance to RAF and EGFR inhibitors, tamoxifen and retinoic acid, has been observed in melanoma, lung cancers, breast cancers and neuroblastoma, respectively, and melanoma cells with *BRAF/NF1* mutations develop resistance to BRAF inhibitors [58, 111, 130, 167]. It is not clear whether the specific nature of the mutations could have exerted an influence on the sensitivity of the drug, as complete inactivation of *NF1* has been noted to confer sensitivity to rapamycin in AML [85].

Mutational spectrum

Large constitutional *NF1* deletions, encompassing the *NF1* gene and many adjacent genes, occur in 5–10% of NF1 cases and are often associated with a more severe phenotype including learning disabilities and increased susceptibility to MPNSTs [168, 169]. Intriguingly, such mutations resulting in heterozygous or homozygous loss of *NF1* expression are found to occur more often as sporadic events in AML and ovarian carcinoma, based on cBioPortal data [45]. An *NF1* microdeletion in combination with an abnormal karyotype is an indicator of poor prognosis in AML; 7.6% of ovarian serous cystadeno-carcinomas, 2.8% of lung squamous cell carcinomas, 3.3% of glioblastomas and 1.9% of phaeochromocytomas/para-gangliomas harboured deletions [45, 82, 84].

NF1 amplification, and presumably increased neurofibromin expression and hence activity, has been identified in many cancers, including breast (17%), pancreatic (21.5%), uterine endometrial (1.8%) and neuroendocrine prostate cancer (21.5%) [45].

The pathological significance of sporadic *NF1* point mutations, especially putative missense mutations that have been identified in many sporadic tumours, is often unclear. Constitutional *NF1* missense mutations represent about 15% of all *NF1* mutations, but their frequency in sporadic tumours ranges widely from 15 to 71% [24, 25, 45, 72, 106, 143, 167, 170–172]. The characterization of such missense mutations has yielded new insights into the structure and function of neurofibromin. For example, through analysis of missense mutations, the arginine finger loop of the neurofibromin GRD has been found to be crucial for stabilizing the transition state of the GTPase reaction, and many missense mutations in the GRD have been found to exert a significant, pathological effect on Ras activity levels [36, 173, 174].

Conclusion

Somatic *NF1* mutations are present in tumours associated with NF1 and in a range of sporadic tumours, in different cell types and at various frequencies (Table 1). The frequency and temporal occurrence of somatic mutations and the range of histological types in which they occur therefore imply an important role for neurofibromin function in cancer development and progression. Whilst it is unclear whether the biallelic loss of *NF1* is common or if only heterozygous mutations of *NF1* contribute to tumour progression in sporadic tumours, mouse cells heterozygous for *Nf1* mutations show abnormal growth and invasion [138, 175].

Somatic *NF1* mutations may be critical drivers in multiple cancers as well as contributing to resistance to therapy. The mutational landscape of somatic *NF1* mutation should provide new insights into our understanding of the pathophysiology of cancer.

The introduction of a molecular genomics approach to cancer biology represents a major shift in our approach to the diagnosis and treatment of malignancy. The vast amount of genomic data generated over the last 10 years, which continues to be generated, is providing invaluable insights into the complexities of cancer genome structure, function and evolution. With recent advances in sequencing technology and high-throughput drug discovery, the increasing availability of more sophisticated animal models and the application of the state-of-the-art tumour imaging techniques and the diagnosis and treatment of cancer can only improve. The identification of somatic *NF1* mutations in such a wide spectrum of tumours, including types not associated with NF1, indicates that neurofibromin is likely to play a key role in cancer, far beyond that evident in the tumour predisposition syndrome NF1.

Abbreviations

ADC: Adenocarcinoma; AML: Acute myeloid leukaemia; AOCS: The Australian Ovarian Cancer Study; CCLE: Cancer Cell Line Encyclopedia; CMML: Chronic myelomonocytic leukaemia; CNS: Central nervous system; COSMIC: Catalogue of Somatic Mutations in Cancer; HGOSC: High-grade serous ovarian carcinoma; HR: Homologous recombination; ICGC: International Cancer Genome Consortium; JMML: Juvenile myelomonocytic leukaemia; MAPK: Mitogen-activated protein kinases; MPNST: Malignant peripheral nerve sheath tumour; NF1: Neurofibromatosis type 1; NSCLC: Non-small cell lung cancer; OSC: Ovarian serous carcinoma; PI3K: Phosphoinositide-3 kinase; RAS-GEFs: RAS guanine nucleotide exchange factors; SCLC: Small cell lung cancer; SqCC: Squamous cell lung cancer; T-ALL: T cell acute lymphoblastic Leukaemia; TCC: Urothelial transitional cell carcinoma; TCGA: The Cancer Genome Atlas

Acknowledgements
Not applicable.

Funding
We thank Sheila and Clive Owen for the financial support.

Authors' contributions
MU initiated the study, supported by CP, HT, IMF and DNC. All authors contributed to the writing and review of the manuscript. All authors read and approved the final manuscript.

Competing interests
The authors declare that they have no competing interests.

References

1. Bennett E, Thomas N, Upadhyaya M. Neurofibromatosis type 1: its association with the Ras/MAPK pathway syndromes. J Pediatr Neurol. 2009; 7(2):105–15.
2. Cooper DN, Upadhyaya M. The germline mutational spectrum in neurofibromatosis type 1 and genotype-phenotype correlations, Chapter 10. In: Upadhyaya M, Cooper DN, editors. Neurofibromatosis Type 1, vol. Chapter 10. Berlin: Springer Verlag; 2012. p. 115–34.
3. Huson SM, Compston DA, Clark P, Harper PS. A genetic study of von Recklinghausen neurofibromatosis in south east Wales. I. Prevalence, fitness, mutation rate, and effect of parental transmission on severity. J Med Genet. 1989;26(11):704–11.
4. Lammert M, Friedman JM, Kluwe L, Mautner VF. Prevalence of neurofibromatosis 1 in German children at elementary school enrollment. Arch Dermatol. 2005;141(1):71–4.
5. Upadhyaya M, Huson SM, Davies M, Thomas N, Chuzhanova N, Giovannini S, Evans DG, Howard E, Kerr B, Griffiths S, et al. An absence of cutaneous neurofibromas associated with a 3-bp inframe deletion in exon 17 of the NF1 gene (c.2970-2972 delAAT): evidence of a clinically significant NF1 genotype-phenotype correlation. Am J Hum Genet. 2007;80(1):140–51.
6. Upadhyaya M. Genetic basis of tumorigenesis in NF1 malignant peripheral nerve sheath tumors. Front Biosci (Landmark Ed). 2011;16:937–51.
7. Upadhyaya M, Kluwe L, Spurlock G, Monem B, Majounie E, Mantripragada K, Ruggieri M, Chuzhanova N, Evans DG, Ferner R, Thomas N, Guha A, Mautner V. Germline and somatic NF1 gene mutation spectrum in NF1-associated malignant peripheral nerve sheath tumors (MPNSTs). Hum Mutat. 2008;29(1):74–82.

8. Walker L, Thompson D, Easton D, Ponder B, Ponder M, Frayling I, Baralle D. A prospective study of neurofibromatosis type 1 cancer incidence in the UK. Br J Cancer. 2006;95(2):233–8.

9. Brems H, Beert E, de Ravel T, Legius E. Mechanisms in the pathogenesis of malignant tumours in neurofibromatosis type 1. Lancet Oncol. 2009;10(5):508–15.

10. Knudson Jr AG. Mutation and cancer: statistical study of retinoblastoma. Proc Natl Acad Sci U S A. 1971;68(4):820–3.

11. Viskochil D, Buchberg AM, Xu G, Cawthon RM, Stevens J, Wolff RK, Culver M, Carey JC, Copeland NG, Jenkins NA, et al. Deletions and a translocation interrupt a cloned gene at the neurofibromatosis type 1 locus. Cell. 1990;62(1):187–92.

12. Cichowski K, Jacks T. NF1 tumor suppressor gene function: narrowing the GAP. Cell. 2001;104(4):593–604.

13. McClatchey AI. Neurofibromatosis. Annu Rev Pathol. 2007;2:191–216.

14. Welti S, D'Angelo I, Scheffzek K. Structure and function of neurofibromin. In: Neurofibromatoses. Basel: Karger; 2008:113–28.

15. Scheffzek K, Welti S. Pleckstrin homology (PH) like domains—versatile modules in protein-protein interaction platforms. FEBS Lett. 2012;586(17):2662–73.

16. Scheffzek K, Welti S. Neurofibromin: protein domains and functional characteristics. In: Upadhyaya M, Cooper DN, editors. Neurofibromatosis Type 1. Berlin Heidelberg: Springer; 2012. p. 305–26.

17. Johannessen CM, Reczek EE, James MF, Brems H, Legius E, Cichowski K. The NF1 tumor suppressor critically regulates TSC2 and mTOR. Proc Natl Acad Sci U S A. 2005;102(24):8573–8.

18. Shilyansky C, Lee YS, Silva AJ. Molecular and cellular mechanisms of learning disabilities: a focus on NF1. Annu Rev Neurosci. 2010;33:221–43.

19. Hollstein PE, Cichowski K. Identifying the ubiquitin ligase complex that regulates the NF1 tumor suppressor and Ras. Cancer Discov. 2013;3(8):880–93.

20. Peltonen S, Kallionpaa RA, Peltonen J. Neurofibromatosis type 1 (NF1) gene: beyond cafe au lait spots and dermal neurofibromas. Exp Dermatol. 2016. doi:10.1111/exd.13212.

21. Gutmann DH, Parada LF, Silva AJ, Ratner N. Neurofibromatosis type 1: modeling CNS dysfunction. J Neurosci. 2012;32(41):14087–93.

22. Neurofibromin (NF1). https://grenada.lumc.nl/LOVD2/mendelian_genes/home.php?select_db=NF1. Accessed Mar 2017.

23. Griffiths S, Thompson P, Frayling I, Upadhyaya M. Molecular diagnosis of neurofibromatosis type 1: 2 years experience. Fam Cancer. 2007;6(1):21–34.

24. Messiaen LM, Callens T, Mortier G, Beysen D, Vandenbroucke I, Van Roy N, Speleman F, Paepe AD. Exhaustive mutation analysis of the NF1 gene allows identification of 95% of mutations and reveals a high frequency of unusual splicing defects. Hum Mutat. 2000;15(6):541–55.

25. Messiaen LM, Wimmer K. NF1 Mutational spectrum. In: neurofibromatoses. Kaufmann D, editor. Basel: Karger; 2008:63–77.

26. van Minkelen R, van Bever Y, Kromosoeto JN, Withagen-Hermans CJ, Nieuwlaat A, Halley DJ, van den Ouweland AM. A clinical and genetic overview of 18 years neurofibromatosis type 1 molecular diagnostics in the Netherlands. Clin Genet. 2014;85(4):318–27.

27. Stenson PD, Mort M, Ball EV, Evans K, Hayden M, Heywood S, Hussain M, Phillips AD, Cooper DN. The Human Gene Mutation Database: towards a comprehensive repository of inherited mutation data for medical research, genetic diagnosis and next-generation sequencing studies. Hum Genet. 2017. doi:10.1007/s00439-017-1779-6 [Epub ahead of print].

28. Evans DG, Bowers N, Burkitt-Wright E, Miles E, Garg S, Scott-Kitching V, Penman-Splitt M, Dobbie A, Howard E, Ealing J, et al. Comprehensive RNA analysis of the NF1 gene in classically affected NF1 affected individuals meeting NIH criteria has high sensitivity and mutation negative testing is reassuring in isolated cases with pigmentary features only. EBioMedicine. 2016;7:212–20.

29. Mautner VF, Kluwe L, Friedrich RE, Roehl AC, Bammert S, Hogel J, Spori H, Cooper DN, Kehrer-Sawatzki H. Clinical characterisation of 29 neurofibromatosis type-1 patients with molecularly ascertained 1.4 Mb type-1 NF1 deletions. J Med Genet. 2010;47(9):623–30.

30. Pros E, Gomez C, Martin T, Fabregas P, Serra E, Lazaro C. Nature and mRNA effect of 282 different NF1 point mutations: focus on splicing alterations. Hum Mutat. 2008;29(9):E173–193.

31. Bottillo I, Torrente I, Lanari V, Pinna V, Giustini S, Divona L, De Luca A, Dallapiccola B. Germline mosaicism in neurofibromatosis type 1 due to a paternally derived multi-exon deletion. Am J Med Genet A. 2010;152A(6):1467–73.

32. Colman SD, Rasmussen SA, Ho VT, Abernathy CR, Wallace MR. Somatic mosaicism in a patient with neurofibromatosis type 1. Am J Hum Genet. 1996;58(3):484–90.

33. Lazaro C, Ravella A, Gaona A, Volpini V, Estivill X. Neurofibromatosis type 1 due to germ-line mosaicism in a clinically normal father. N Engl J Med. 1994;331(21):1403–7.

34. Messiaen L, Vogt J, Bengesser K, Fu C, Mikhail F, Serra E, Garcia-Linares C, Cooper DN, Lazaro C, Kehrer-Sawatzki H. Mosaic type-1 NF1 microdeletions as a cause of both generalized and segmental neurofibromatosis type-1 (NF1). Hum Mutat. 2011;32(2):213–9.

35. Wimmer K, Yao S, Claes K, Kehrer-Sawatzki H, Tinschert S, De Raedt T, Legius E, Callens T, Beiglbock H, Maertens O, et al. Spectrum of single- and multiexon NF1 copy number changes in a cohort of 1,100 unselected NF1 patients. Genes Chromosomes Cancer. 2006;45(3):265–76.

36. Thomas L, Richards M, Mort M, Dunlop E, Cooper DN, Upadhyaya M. Assessment of the potential pathogenicity of missense mutations identified in the GTPase-activating protein (GAP)-related domain of the neurofibromatosis type-1 (NF1) gene. Hum Mutat. 2012;33(12):1687–96.

37. Kehrer-Sawatzki H, Vogt J, Mussotter T, Kluwe L, Cooper DN, Mautner VF. Dissecting the clinical phenotype associated with mosaic type-2 NF1 microdeletions. Neurogenetics. 2012;13(3):229–36.

38. Upadhyaya M. Neurofibromatosis type 1: diagnosis and recent advances. Expert Opin Med Diagn. 2010;4(4):307–22.

39. Tidyman WE, Rauen KA. Pathogenetics of the RASopathies. Hum Mol Genet. 2016;25(R2):R123–32.

40. Stratton MR, Campbell PJ, Futreal PA. The cancer genome. Nature. 2009; 458(7239):719–24.

41. The Cancer Genome Atlas (TCGA). http://cancergenome.nih.gov/. Accessed Sept 2016.

42. International Cancer Genome Consortium (ICGC). http://icgc.org/. Accessed Sept 2016.

43. Catalogue of Somatic Mutations in Cancer (COSMIC). http://cancer.sanger.ac.uk/cosmic. Accessed Sept 2016.

44. cBioPortal for Cancer Genomics. http://www.cbioportal.org/. Accessed Sept 2016.

45. Cerami E, Gao J, Dogrusoz U, Gross BE, Sumer SO, Aksoy BA, Jacobsen A, Byrne CJ, Heuer ML, Larsson E, et al. The cBio cancer genomics portal: an open platform for exploring multidimensional cancer genomics data. Cancer Discov. 2012;2(5):401–4.

46. Gao J, Aksoy BA, Dogrusoz U, Dresdner G, Gross B, Sumer SO, Sun Y, Jacobsen A, Sinha R, Larsson E, et al. Integrative analysis of complex cancer genomics and clinical profiles using the cBioPortal. Sci Signal. 2013;6(269):l1.

47. Ratner N, Miller SJ. A RASopathy gene commonly mutated in cancer: the neurofibromatosis type 1 tumour suppressor. Nat Rev Cancer. 2015;15(5): 290–301.

48. Andersen LB, Fountain JW, Gutmann DH, Tarle SA, Glover TW, Dracopoli NC, Housman DE, Collins FS. Mutations in the neurofibromatosis 1 gene in sporadic malignant melanoma cell lines. Nat Genet. 1993;3(2):118–21.

49. Krauthammer M, Kong Y, Bacchiocchi A, Evans P, Pornputtapong N, Wu C, McCusker JP, Ma S, Cheng E, Straub R, et al. Exome sequencing identifies recurrent mutations in NF1 and RASopathy genes in sun-exposed melanomas. Nat Genet. 2015;47(9):996–1002.

50. Krauthammer M, Kong Y, Ha BH, Evans P, Bacchiocchi A, McCusker JP, Cheng E, Davis MJ, Goh G, Choi M, et al. Exome sequencing identifies recurrent somatic RAC1 mutations in melanoma. Nat Genet. 2012;44(9):1006–14.

51. Hodis E, Watson IR, Kryukov GV, Arold ST, Imielinski M, Theurillat JP, Nickerson E, Auclair D, Li L, Place C, et al. A landscape of driver mutations in melanoma. Cell. 2012;150(2):251–63.

52. Nissan MH, Pratilas CA, Jones AM, Ramirez R, Won H, Liu C, Tiwari S, Kong L, Hanrahan AJ, Yao Z, et al. Loss of NF1 in cutaneous melanoma is associated with RAS activation and MEK dependence. Cancer Res. 2014;74(8):2340–50.

53. Whittaker SR, Theurillat JP, Van Allen E, Wagle N, Hsiao J, Cowley GS, Schadendorf D, Root DE, Garraway LA. A genome-scale RNA interference screen implicates NF1 loss in resistance to RAF inhibition. Cancer Discov. 2013;3(3):350–62.

54. Akbani R, Ng PK, Werner HM, Shahmoradgoli M, Zhang F, Ju Z, Liu W, Yang JY, Yoshihara K, Li J, et al. Corrigendum: a pan-cancer proteomic perspective on The Cancer Genome Atlas. Nat Commun. 2015;6:4852.

55. Akbani R, Ng PK, Werner HM, Shahmoradgoli M, Zhang F, Ju Z, Liu W, Yang JY, Yoshihara K, Li J, et al. A pan-cancer proteomic perspective on The Cancer Genome Atlas. Nat Commun. 2014;5:3887.

56. Hill VK, Gartner JJ, Samuels Y, Goldstein AM. The genetics of melanoma: recent advances. Annu Rev Genomics Hum Genet. 2013;14:257–79.

57. Garnett MJ, Marais R. Guilty as charged: B-RAF is a human oncogene. Cancer Cell. 2004;6(4):313–9.

58. Maertens O, Johnson B, Hollstein P, Frederick DT, Cooper ZA, Messiaen L, Bronson RT, McMahon M, Granter S, Flaherty K, et al. Elucidating distinct roles for NF1 in melanomagenesis. Cancer Discov. 2013;3(3):338–49.

59. Mar VJ, Wong SQ, Li J, Scolyer RA, McLean C, Papenfuss AT, Tothill RW, Kakavand H, Mann GJ, Thompson JF, et al. BRAF/NRAS wild-type melanomas have a high mutation load correlating with histologic and molecular signatures of UV damage. Clin Cancer Res. 2013;19(17):4589–98.

60. Wiesner T, Kiuru M, Scott SN, Arcila M, Halpern AC, Hollmann T, Berger MF, Busam KJ. NF1 mutations are common in desmoplastic melanoma. Am J Surg Pathol. 2015;39(10):1357–62.

61. Shain AH, Yeh I, Kovalyshyn I, Sriharan A, Talevich E, Gagnon A, Dummer R, North J, Pincus L, Ruben B, et al. The genetic evolution of melanoma from precursor lesions. N Engl J Med. 2015;373(20):1926–36.

62. Foster WJ, Fuller CE, Perry A, Harbour JW. Status of the NF1 tumor suppressor locus in uveal melanoma. Arch Ophthalmol. 2003;121(9):1311–5.

63. Cosgarea I, Ugurel S, Sucker A, Livingstone E, Zimmer L, Ziemer M, Utikal J, Mohr P, Pfeiffer C, Pfohler C, et al. Targeted next generation sequencing of mucosal melanomas identifies frequent NF1 and RAS mutations. Oncotarget. 2017.

64. Stewart B, Wild CP. World Cancer Report 2014. International Agency for Research on Cancer. Lyons: WHO Press; 2014.

65. Ding L, Getz G, Wheeler DA, Mardis ER, McLellan MD, Cibulskis K, Sougnez C, Greulich H, Muzny DM, Morgan MB, et al. Somatic mutations affect key pathways in lung adenocarcinoma. Nature. 2008;455(7216):1069–75.

66. Imielinski M, Berger AH, Hammerman PS, Hernandez B, Pugh TJ, Hodis E, Cho J, Suh J, Capelletti M, Sivachenko A, et al. Mapping the hallmarks of lung adenocarcinoma with massively parallel sequencing. Cell. 2012;150(6):1107–20.

67. Cancer Genome Atlas Research N. Comprehensive molecular profiling of lung adenocarcinoma. Nature. 2014;511(7511):543–50.

68. Redig AJ, Capelletti M, Dahlberg SE, Sholl LM, Mach S, Fontes C, Shi Y, Chalasani P, Janne PA. Clinical and molecular characteristics of NF1-mutant lung cancer. Clin Cancer Res. 2016;22(13):3148–56.

69. Jemal A, Bray F, Center MM, Ferlay J, Ward E, Forman D. Global cancer statistics. CA Cancer J Clin. 2011;61(2):69–90.

70. Lipson D, Capelletti M, Yelensky R, Otto G, Parker A, Jarosz M, Curran JA, Balasubramanian S, Bloom T, Brennan KW, et al. Identification of new ALK and RET gene fusions from colorectal and lung cancer biopsies. Nat Med. 2012;18(3):382–4.

71. de Bruin EC, Cowell C, Warne PH, Jiang M, Saunders RE, Melnick MA, Gettinger S, Walther Z, Wurtz A, Heynen GJ, et al. Reduced NF1 expression confers resistance to EGFR inhibition in lung cancer. Cancer Discov. 2014;4(5):606–19.

72. Cancer Genome Atlas Research N. Comprehensive genomic characterization of squamous cell lung cancers. Nature. 2012;489(7417):519–25.

73. Dhanasekaran SM, Balbin OA, Chen G, Nadal E, Kalyana-Sundaram S, Pan J, Veeneman B, Cao X, Malik R, Vats P, et al. Transcriptome meta-analysis of lung cancer reveals recurrent aberrations in NRG1 and Hippo pathway genes. Nat Commun. 2014;5:5893.

74. Campbell JD, Alexandrov A, Kim J, Wala J, Berger AH, Pedamallu CS, Shukla SA, Guo G, Brooks AN, Murray BA, et al. Distinct patterns of somatic genome alterations in lung adenocarcinomas and squamous cell carcinomas. Nat Genet. 2016;48(6):607–16.

75. Devarakonda S, Morgensztern D, Govindan R. Genomic alterations in lung adenocarcinoma. Lancet Oncol. 2015;16(7):e342–351.

76. Rudin CM, Durinck S, Stawiski EW, Poirier JT, Modrusan Z, Shames DS, Bergbower EA, Guan Y, Shin J, Guillory J, et al. Comprehensive genomic analysis identifies SOX2 as a frequently amplified gene in small-cell lung cancer. Nat Genet. 2012;44(10):1111–6.

77. Peifer M, Fernandez-Cuesta L, Sos ML, George J, Seidel D, Kasper LH, Plenker D, Leenders F, Sun R, Zander T, et al. Integrative genome analyses identify key somatic driver mutations of small-cell lung cancer. Nat Genet. 2012; 44(10):1104–10.

78. Ross JS, Wang K, Elkadi OR, Tarasen A, Foulke L, Sheehan CE, Otto GA, Palmer G, Yelensky R, Lipson D, et al. Next-generation sequencing reveals frequent consistent genomic alterations in small cell undifferentiated lung cancer. J Clin Pathol. 2014;67(9):772–6.

79. Balgobind BV, Van Vlierberghe P, van den Ouweland AM, Beverloo HB, Terlouw-Kromosoeto JN, van Wering ER, Reinhardt D, Horstmann M, Kaspers GJ, Pieters R, et al. Leukemia-associated NF1 inactivation in patients with pediatric T-ALL and AML lacking evidence of neurofibromatosis. Blood. 2008;111(8):4322–8.

80. Fioretos T, Strombeck B, Sandberg T, Johansson B, Billstrom R, Borg A, Nilsson PG, Van Den Berghe H, Hagemeijer A, Mitelman F, et al. Isochromosome 17q in blast crisis of chronic myeloid leukemia and in other hematologic malignancies is the result of clustered breakpoints in 17p11 and is not associated with coding TP53 mutations. Blood. 1999;94(1):225–32.

81. Braun BS, Shannon K. Targeting Ras in myeloid leukemias. Clin Cancer Res. 2008;14(8):2249–52.

82. Boudry-Labis E, Roche-Lestienne C, Nibourel O, Boissel N, Terre C, Perot C, Eclache V, Gachard N, Tigaud I, Plessis G, et al. Neurofibromatosis-1 gene deletions and mutations in de novo adult acute myeloid leukemia. Am J Hematol. 2013;88(4):306–11.

83. Garcia-Orti L, Cristobal I, Cirauqui C, Guruceaga E, Marcotegui N, Calasanz MJ, Castello-Cros R, Odero MD. Integration of SNP and mRNA arrays with microRNA profiling reveals that MiR-370 is upregulated and targets NF1 in acute myeloid leukemia. PLoS One. 2012;7(10):e47717.

84. Haferlach C, Grossmann V, Kohlmann A, Schindela S, Kern W, Schnittger S, Haferlach T. Deletion of the tumor-suppressor gene NF1 occurs in 5% of myeloid malignancies and is accompanied by a mutation in the remaining allele in half of the cases. Leukemia. 2012;26(4):834–9.

85. Parkin B, Ouillette P, Wang Y, Liu Y, Wright W, Roulston D, Purkayastha A, Dressel A, Karp J, Bockenstedt P, et al. NF1 inactivation in adult acute myelogenous leukemia. Clin Cancer Res. 2010;16(16):4135–47.

86. Misawa S, Horiike S, Kaneko H, Kashima K. Genetic aberrations in the development and subsequent progression of myelodysplastic syndrome. Leukemia. 1997;11 Suppl 3:533–5.

87. Kolquist KA, Schultz RA, Furrow A, Brown TC, Han JY, Campbell LJ, Wall M, Slovak ML, Shaffer LG, Ballif BC. Microarray-based comparative genomic hybridization of cancer targets reveals novel, recurrent genetic aberrations in the myelodysplastic syndromes. Cancer Genet. 2011;204(11):603–28.

88. Kalender Atak Z, De Keersmaecker K, Gianfelici V, Geerdens E, Vandepoel R, Pauwels D, Porcu M, Lahortiga I, Brys V, Dirks WG, et al. High accuracy mutation detection in leukemia on a selected panel of cancer genes. PLoS One. 2012;7(6):e38463.

89. Side L, Taylor B, Cayouette M, Conner E, Thompson P, Luce M, Shannon K. Homozygous inactivation of the NF1 gene in bone marrow cells from children with neurofibromatosis type 1 and malignant myeloid disorders. N Engl J Med. 1997;336(24):1713–20.

90. Caye A, Strullu M, Guidez F, Cassinat B, Gazal S, Fenneteau O, Lainey E, Nouri K, Nakhaei-Rad S, Dvorsky R, et al. Juvenile myelomonocytic leukemia displays mutations in components of the RAS pathway and the PRC2 network. Nat Genet. 2015;47(11):1334–40.

91. Margueron R, Reinberg D. The Polycomb complex PRC2 and its mark in life. Nature. 2011;469(7330):343–9.

92. Cutts BA, Sjogren AK, Andersson KM, Wahlstrom AM, Karlsson C, Swolin B, Bergo MO. Nf1 deficiency cooperates with oncogenic K-RAS to induce acute myeloid leukemia in mice. Blood. 2009;114(17):3629–32.

93. Abdel-Wahab O, Tefferi A, Levine RL. Role of TET2 and ASXL1 mutations in the pathogenesis of myeloproliferative neoplasms. Hematol Oncol Clin North Am. 2012;26(5):1053–64.

94. Abdel-Wahab O, Dey A. The ASXL-BAP1 axis: new factors in myelopoiesis, cancer and epigenetics. Leukemia. 2013;27(1):10–5.

95. De Raedt T, Beert E, Pasmant E, Luscan A, Brems H, Ortonne N, Helin K, Hornick JL, Mautner V, Kehrer-Sawatzki H, et al. PRC2 loss amplifies Ras-driven transcription and confers sensitivity to BRD4-based therapies. Nature. 2014;514(7521):247–51.

96. Lee W, Teckie S, Wiesner T, Ran L, Prieto Granada CN, Lin M, Zhu S, Cao Z, Liang Y, Sboner A, et al. PRC2 is recurrently inactivated through EED or SUZ12 loss in malignant peripheral nerve sheath tumors. Nat Genet. 2014; 46(11):1227–32.

97. Stieglitz E, Taylor-Weiner AN, Chang TY, Gelston LC, Wang YD, Mazor T, Esquivel E, Yu A, Seepo S, Olsen SR, et al. The genomic landscape of juvenile myelomonocytic leukemia. Nat Genet. 2015;47(11):1326–33.

98. Sharif S, Moran A, Huson SM, Iddenden R, Shenton A, Howard E, Evans DG. Women with neurofibromatosis 1 are at a moderately increased risk of developing breast cancer and should be considered for early screening. J Med Genet. 2007;44(8):481–4.

99. Evans DG, O'Hara C, Wilding A, Ingham SL, Howard E, Dawson J, Moran A, Scott-Kitching V, Holt F, Huson SM. Mortality in neurofibromatosis 1: in North West England: an assessment of actuarial survival in a region of the UK since 1989. Eur J Hum Genet. 2011;19(11):1187–91.

100. Madanikia SA, Bergner A, Ye X, Blakeley JO. Increased risk of breast cancer in women with NF1. Am J Med Genet A. 2012;158A(12):3056–60.

101. Sjoblom T, Jones S, Wood LD, Parsons DW, Lin J, Barber TD, Mandelker D, Leary RJ, Ptak J, Silliman N, et al. The consensus coding sequences of human breast and colorectal cancers. Science. 2006;314(5797):268–74.

102. Stephens PJ, Tarpey PS, Davies H, Van Loo P, Greenman C, Wedge DC, Nik-Zainal S, Martin S, Varela I, Bignell GR, et al. The landscape of cancer genes and mutational processes in breast cancer. Nature. 2012;486(7403):400–4.

103. Ogata H, Sato H, Takatsuka J, De Luca LM. Human breast cancer MDA-MB-231 cells fail to express the neurofibromin protein, lack its type I mRNA isoform and show accumulation of P-MAPK and activated Ras. Cancer Lett. 2001;172(2):159–64.

104. Shima N, Alcaraz A, Liachko I, Buske TR, Andrews CA, Munroe RJ, Hartford SA, Tye BK, Schimenti JC. A viable allele of Mcm4 causes chromosome instability and mammary adenocarcinomas in mice. Nat Genet. 2007;39(1):93–8.

105. Wallace MD, Pfefferle AD, Shen L, McNairn AJ, Cerami EG, Fallon BL, Rinaldi VD, Southard TL, Perou CM, Schimenti JC. Comparative oncogenomics implicates the neurofibromin 1 gene (NF1) as a breast cancer driver. Genetics. 2012;192(2):385–96.

106. Cancer Genome Atlas N. Comprehensive molecular portraits of human breast tumours. Nature. 2012;490(7418):61–70.

107. Meric-Bernstam F, Frampton GM, Ferrer-Lozano J, Yelensky R, Perez-Fidalgo JA, Wang Y, Palmer GA, Ross JS, Miller VA, Su X, et al. Concordance of genomic alterations between primary and recurrent breast cancer. Mol Cancer Ther. 2014;13(5):1382–9.

108. Pereira B, Chin SF, Rueda OM, Vollan HK, Provenzano E, Bardwell HA, Pugh M, Jones L, Russell R, Sammut SJ, et al. Erratum: the somatic mutation profiles of 2,433 breast cancers refine their genomic and transcriptomic landscapes. Nat Commun. 2016;7:11908.

109. Pereira B, Chin SF, Rueda OM, Vollan HK, Provenzano E, Bardwell HA, Pugh M, Jones L, Russell R, Sammut SJ, et al. The somatic mutation profiles of 2,433 breast cancers refines their genomic and transcriptomic landscapes. Nat Commun. 2016;7:11479.

110. Cui XY, Guo YJ, Yao HR. Analysis of microRNA in drug-resistant breast cancer cell line MCF-7/ADR. Nan Fang Yi Ke Da Xue Xue Bao. 2008;28(10):1813–5.

111. Mendes-Pereira AM, Sims D, Dexter T, Fenwick K, Assiotis I, Kozarewa I, Mitsopoulos C, Hakas J, Zvelebil M, Lord CJ, et al. Genome-wide functional screen identifies a compendium of genes affecting sensitivity to tamoxifen. Proc Natl Acad Sci U S A. 2012;109(8):2730–5.

112. Ring A, Dowsett M. Mechanisms of tamoxifen resistance. Endocr Relat Cancer. 2004;11(4):643–58.

113. Sangha N, Wu R, Kuick R, Powers S, Mu D, Fiander D, Yuen K, Katabuchi H, Tashiro H, Fearon ER, et al. Neurofibromin 1 (NF1) defects are common in human ovarian serous carcinomas and co-occur with TP53 mutations. Neoplasia. 2008;10(12):1362–72. following 1372.

114. Heintz AP, Odicino F, Maisonneuve P, Quinn MA, Benedet JL, Creasman WT, Ngan HY, Pecorelli S, Beller U. Carcinoma of the ovary. FIGO 26th Annual Report on the Results of Treatment in Gynecological Cancer. Int J Gynaecol Obstet. 2006;95 Suppl 1:S161–192.

115. Gorringe KL, George J, Anglesio MS, Ramakrishna M, Etemadmoghadam D, Cowin P, Sridhar A, Williams LH, Boyle SE, Yanaihara N, et al. Copy number analysis identifies novel interactions between genomic loci in ovarian cancer. PLoS One. 2010;5(9):e11408.

116. Cooke SL, Ng CK, Melnyk N, Garcia MJ, Hardcastle T, Temple J, Langdon S, Huntsman D, Brenton JD. Genomic analysis of genetic heterogeneity and evolution in high-grade serous ovarian carcinoma. Oncogene. 2010;29(35):4905–13.

117. Mittempergher L. Genomic characterization of high-grade serous ovarian cancer: dissecting its molecular heterogeneity as a road towards effective therapeutic strategies. Curr Oncol Rep. 2016;18(7):44.

118. Kulkarni-Datar K, Orsulic S, Foster R, Rueda BR. Ovarian tumor initiating cell populations persist following paclitaxel and carboplatin chemotherapy treatment in vivo. Cancer Lett. 2013;339(2):237–46.

119. Koch CA, Vortmeyer AO, Huang SC, Alesci S, Zhuang Z, Pacak K. Genetic aspects of pheochromocytoma. Endocr Regul. 2001;35(1):43–52.

120. Walther MM, Herring J, Enquist E, Keiser HR, Linehan WM. von Recklinghausen's disease and pheochromocytomas. J Urol. 1999;162(5):1582–6.

121. Welander J, Larsson C, Backdahl M, Hareni N, Sivler T, Brauckhoff M, Soderkvist P, Gimm O. Integrative genomics reveals frequent somatic NF1 mutations in sporadic pheochromocytomas. Hum Mol Genet. 2012;21(26):5406–16.

122. Opocher G, Schiavi F. Genetics of pheochromocytomas and paragangliomas. Best Pract Res Clin Endocrinol Metab. 2010;24(6):943–56.

123. Welander J, Soderkvist P, Gimm O. The NF1 gene: a frequent mutational target in sporadic pheochromocytomas and beyond. Endocr Relat Cancer. 2013;20(4):C13–17.

124. Burnichon N, Buffet A, Parfait B, Letouze E, Laurendeau I, Loriot C, Pasmant E, Abermil N, Valeyrie-Allanore L, Bertherat J, et al. Somatic NF1 inactivation is a frequent event in sporadic pheochromocytoma. Hum Mol Genet. 2012;21(26):5397–405.

125. Fishbein L, Nathanson KL. Pheochromocytoma and paraganglioma: understanding the complexities of the genetic background. Cancer Genet. 2012;205(1-2):1–11.

126. Galan SR, Kann PH. Genetics and molecular pathogenesis of pheochromocytoma and paraganglioma. Clin Endocrinol (Oxf). 2013;78(2):165–75.

127. Deyell RJ, Attiyeh EF. Advances in the understanding of constitutional and somatic genomic alterations in neuroblastoma. Cancer Genet. 2011;204(3):113–21.

128. Shojaei-Brosseau T, Chompret A, Abel A, de Vathaire F, Raquin MA, Brugieres L, Feunteun J, Hartmann O, Bonaiti-Pellie C. Genetic epidemiology of neuroblastoma: a study of 426 cases at the Institut Gustave-Roussy in France. Pediatr Blood Cancer. 2004;42(1):99–105.

129. The I, Murthy AE, Hannigan GE, Jacoby LB, Menon AG, Gusella JF, Bernards A. Neurofibromatosis type 1 gene mutations in neuroblastoma. Nat Genet. 1993;3(1):62–6.

130. Holzel M, Huang S, Koster J, Ora I, Lakeman A, Caron H, Nijkamp W, Xie J, Callens T, Asgharzadeh S, et al. NF1 is a tumor suppressor in neuroblastoma that determines retinoic acid response and disease outcome. Cell. 2010;142(2):218–29.

131. Han D, Spengler BA, Ross RA. Increased wild-type N-ras activation by neurofibromin down-regulation increases human neuroblastoma stem cell malignancy. Genes Cancer. 2011;2(11):1034–43.

132. Parsons DW, Jones S, Zhang X, Lin JC, Leary RJ, Angenendt P, Mankoo P, Carter H, Siu IM, Gallia GL, et al. An integrated genomic analysis of human glioblastoma multiforme. Science. 2008;321(5897):1807–12.

133. Louis DN. Molecular pathology of malignant gliomas. Annu Rev Pathol. 2006;1:97–117.

134. Brennan CW, Verhaak RG, McKenna A, Campos B, Noushmehr H, Salama SR, Zheng S, Chakravarty D, Sanborn JZ, Berman SH, et al. The somatic genomic landscape of glioblastoma. Cell. 2013;155(2):462–77.

135. Jones DT, Hutter B, Jager N, Korshunov A, Kool M, Warnatz HJ, Zichner T, Lambert SR, Ryzhova M, Quang DA, et al. Recurrent somatic alterations of FGFR1 and NTRK2 in pilocytic astrocytoma. Nat Genet. 2013;45(8):927–32.

136. Verhaak RG, Hoadley KA, Purdom E, Wang V, Qi Y, Wilkerson MD, Miller CR, Ding L, Golub T, Mesirov JP, et al. Integrated genomic analysis identifies clinically relevant subtypes of glioblastoma characterized by abnormalities in PDGFRA, IDH1, EGFR, and NF1. Cancer Cell. 2010;17(1):98–110.

137. Zhu Y, Guignard F, Zhao D, Liu L, Burns DK, Mason RP, Messing A, Parada LF. Early inactivation of p53 tumor suppressor gene cooperating with NF1 loss induces malignant astrocytoma. Cancer Cell. 2005;8(2):119–30.

138. Gutmann DH, Loehr A, Zhang Y, Kim J, Henkemeyer M, Cashen A. Haploinsufficiency for the neurofibromatosis 1 (NF1) tumor suppressor results in increased astrocyte proliferation. Oncogene. 1999;18(31):4450–9.

139. Wu M, Wallace MR, Muir D. Nf1 haploinsufficiency augments angiogenesis. Oncogene. 2006;25(16):2297–303.

140. Ahlquist T, Bottillo I, Danielsen SA, Meling GI, Rognum TO, Lind GE, Dallapiccola B, Lothe RA. RAS signaling in colorectal carcinomas through alteration of RAS, RAF, NF1, and/or RASSF1A. Neoplasia. 2008;10(7):680–6. 682 p following 686.

141. Cawkwell L, Lewis FA, Quirke P. Frequency of allele loss of DCC, p53, RB1, WT1, NF1, NM23 and APC/MCC in colorectal cancer assayed by fluorescent multiplex polymerase chain reaction. Br J Cancer. 1994;70(5):813–8.

142. Leggett B, Young J, Buttenshaw R, Thomas L, Young B, Chenevix-Trench G, Searle J, Ward M. Colorectal carcinomas show frequent allelic loss on the long arm of chromosome 17 with evidence for a specific target region. Br J Cancer. 1995;71(5):1070–3.

143. Cancer Genome Atlas N. Comprehensive molecular characterization of human colon and rectal cancer. Nature. 2012;487(7407):330–7.

144. Giannakis M, Mu XJ, Shukla SA, Qian ZR, Cohen O, Nishihara R, Bahl S, Cao Y, Amin-Mansour A, Yamauchi M, et al. Genomic correlates of immune-cell infiltrates in colorectal carcinoma. Cell Rep. 2016;17(4):1206.

145. Seshagiri S, Stawiski EW, Durinck S, Modrusan Z, Storm EE, Conboy CB, Chaudhuri S, Guan Y, Janakiraman V, Jaiswal BS, et al. Recurrent R-spondin fusions in colon cancer. Nature. 2012;488(7413):660–4.

146. Fearon ER. Molecular genetics of colorectal cancer. Annu Rev Pathol. 2011;6:479–507.

147. Vogelstein B, Papadopoulos N, Velculescu VE, Zhou S, Diaz Jr LA, Kinzler KW. Cancer genome landscapes. Science. 2013;339(6127):1546–58.

148. Aaltonen V, Bostrom PJ, Soderstrom KO, Hirvonen O, Tuukkanen J, Nurmi M, Laato M, Peltonen J. Urinary bladder transitional cell carcinogenesis is associated with down-regulation of NF1 tumor suppressor gene in vivo and in vitro. Am J Pathol. 1999;154(3):755–65.

149. Ross JS, Wang K, Al-Rohil RN, Nazeer T, Sheehan CE, Otto GA, He J, Palmer G, Yelensky R, Lipson D, et al. Advanced urothelial carcinoma: next-generation sequencing reveals diverse genomic alterations and targets of therapy. Mod Pathol. 2014;27(2):271–80.

150. Bader JL. Neurofibromatosis and cancer. Ann N Y Acad Sci. 1986;486:57–65.

151. Knudson AG. Antioncogenes and human cancer. Proc Natl Acad Sci U S A. 1993;90(23):10914–21.

152. Matsui I, Tanimura M, Kobayashi N, Sawada T, Nagahara N, Akatsuka J. Neurofibromatosis type 1 and childhood cancer. Cancer. 1993;72(9):2746–54.

153. Wullschleger S, Loewith R, Hall MN. TOR signaling in growth and metabolism. Cell. 2006;124(3):471–84.

154. Chen L, Liu P, Evans Jr TC, Ettwiller LM. DNA damage is a pervasive cause of sequencing errors, directly confounding variant identification. Science. 2017; 355(6326):752–6.

155. Bozic I, Antal T, Ohtsuki H, Carter H, Kim D, Chen S, Karchin R, Kinzler KW, Vogelstein B, Nowak MA. Accumulation of driver and passenger mutations during tumor progression. Proc Natl Acad Sci U S A. 2010;107(43):18545–50.

156. Bozic I, Gerold JM, Nowak MA. Quantifying clonal and subclonal passenger mutations in cancer evolution. PLoS Comput Biol. 2016;12(2):e1004731.

157. McFarland CD, Korolev KS, Kryukov GV, Sunyaev SR, Mirny LA. Impact of deleterious passenger mutations on cancer progression. Proc Natl Acad Sci U S A. 2013;110(8):2910–5.

158. McFarland CD, Mirny LA, Korolev KS. Tug-of-war between driver and passenger mutations in cancer and other adaptive processes. Proc Natl Acad Sci U S A. 2014;111(42):15138–43.

159. Nussinov R, Tsai CJ. 'Latent drivers' expand the cancer mutational landscape. Curr Opin Struct Biol. 2015;32:25–32.

160. Futreal PA, Coin L, Marshall M, Down T, Hubbard T, Wooster R, Rahman N, Stratton MR. A census of human cancer genes. Nat Rev Cancer. 2004;4(3): 177–83.

161. Network of Cancer Genes (NCG). http://ncg.kcl.ac.uk/. Accessed Sept 2016.

162. Lawrence MS, Stojanov P, Mermel CH, Robinson JT, Garraway LA, Golub TR, Meyerson M, Gabriel SB, Lander ES, Getz G. Discovery and saturation analysis of cancer genes across 21 tumour types. Nature. 2014;505(7484):495–501.

163. Lawrence MS, Stojanov P, Polak P, Kryukov GV, Cibulskis K, Sivachenko A, Carter SL, Stewart C, Mermel CH, Roberts SA, et al. Mutational heterogeneity in cancer and the search for new cancer-associated genes. Nature. 2013; 499(7457):214–8. doi:10.1038/nature12213.

164. Seton-Rogers S. Oncogenes: one of these things is not like the others. Nat Rev Cancer. 2016;16(1):5.

165. Prahallad A, Sun C, Huang S, Di Nicolantonio F, Salazar R, Zecchin D, Beijersbergen RL, Bardelli A, Bernards R. Unresponsiveness of colon cancer to BRAF(V600E) inhibition through feedback activation of EGFR. Nature. 2012;483(7387):100–3.

166. Furukawa K, Yanai N, Fujita M, Harada Y. Novel mutations of neurofibromatosis type 1 gene in small cell lung cancers. Surg Today. 2003;33(5):323–7.

167. Cancer Genome Atlas Research N. Comprehensive molecular characterization of urothelial bladder carcinoma. Nature. 2014;507(7492):315–22.

168. De Raedt T, Brems H, Wolkenstein P, Vidaud D, Pilotti S, Perrone F, Mautner V, Frahm S, Sciot R, Legius E. Elevated risk for MPNST in NF1 microdeletion patients. Am J Hum Genet. 2003;72(5):1288–92.

169. Pasmant E, Sabbagh A, Spurlock G, Laurendeau I, Grillo E, Hamel MJ, Martin L, Barbarot S, Leheup B, Rodriguez D, et al. NF1 microdeletions in neurofibromatosis type 1: from genotype to phenotype. Hum Mutat. 2010; 31(6):E1506–1518.

170. Cancer Genome Atlas Research N. Integrated genomic analyses of ovarian carcinoma. Nature. 2011;474(7353):609–15.

171. Cancer Genome Atlas Research N. Comprehensive genomic characterization defines human glioblastoma genes and core pathways. Nature. 2008; 455(7216):1061–8.

172. Messiaen L, Yao S, Brems H, Callens T, Sathienkijkanchai A, Denayer E, Spencer E, Arn P, Babovic-Vuksanovic D, Bay C, et al. Clinical and mutational spectrum of neurofibromatosis type 1-like syndrome. JAMA. 2009;302(19):2111–8.

173. Ahmadian MR, Kiel C, Stege P, Scheffzek K. Structural fingerprints of the Ras-GTPase activating proteins neurofibromin and p120GAP. J Mol Biol. 2003; 329(4):699–710.

174. Ahmadian MR, Wiesmuller L, Lautwein A, Bischoff FR, Wittinghofer A. Structural differences in the minimal catalytic domains of the GTPase-activating proteins p120GAP and neurofibromin. J Biol Chem. 1996;271(27):16409–15.

175. Ding H, Shannon P, Lau N, Wu X, Roncari L, Baldwin RL, Takebayashi H, Nagy A, Gutmann DH, Guha A. Oligodendrogliomas result from the expression of an activated mutant epidermal growth factor receptor in a RAS transgenic mouse astrocytoma model. Cancer Res. 2003;63(5):1106–13.

176. Kan Z, Jaiswal BS, Stinson J, Janakiraman V, Bhatt D, Stern HM, Yue P, Haverty PM, Bourgon R, Zheng J, et al. Diverse somatic mutation patterns and pathway alterations in human cancers. Nature. 2010;466(7308):869–73.

177. Kandoth C, McLellan MD, Vandin F, Ye K, Niu B, Lu C, Xie M, Zhang Q, McMichael JF, Wyczalkowski MA, et al. Mutational landscape and significance across 12 major cancer types. Nature. 2013;502(7471):333–9.

178. Bashashati A, Ha G, Tone A, Ding J, Prentice LM, Roth A, Rosner J, Shumansky K, Kalloger S, Senz J, et al. Distinct evolutionary trajectories of primary high-grade serous ovarian cancers revealed through spatial mutational profiling. J Pathol. 2013;231(1):21–34.

179. Kanchi KL, Johnson KJ, Lu C, McLellan MD, Leiserson MD, Wendl MC, Zhang Q, Koboldt DC, Xie M, Kandoth C, et al. Integrated analysis of germline and somatic variants in ovarian cancer. Nat Commun. 2014;5:3156.

180. Ross JS, Ali SM, Wang K, Palmer G, Yelensky R, Lipson D, Miller VA, Zajchowski D, Shawver LK, Stephens PJ. Comprehensive genomic profiling of epithelial ovarian cancer by next generation sequencing-based diagnostic assay reveals new routes to targeted therapies. Gynecol Oncol. 2013;130(3):554–9.

5

Identification of functional single nucleotide polymorphisms in the branchpoint site

Hung-Lun Chiang[1,2], Jer-Yuarn Wu[2,3] and Yuan-Tsong Chen[1,2,4*]

Abstract

Background: The human genome contains millions of single nucleotide polymorphisms (SNPs); many of these SNPs are intronic and have unknown functional significance. SNPs occurring within intron branchpoint sites, especially at the adenine (A), would presumably affect splicing; however, this has not been systematically studied. We employed a splicing prediction tool to identify human intron branchpoint sites and screened dbSNP for identifying SNPs located in the predicted sites to generate a genome-wide branchpoint site SNP database.

Results: We identified 600 SNPs located within branchpoint sites; among which, 216 showed a change in A. After scoring the SNPs by counting the As in the ± 10 nucleotide region, only four SNPs were identified without additional As (rs13296170, rs12769205, rs75434223, and rs67785924). Using minigene constructs, we examined the effects of these SNPs on splicing. The three SNPs (rs13296170, rs12769205, and rs75434223) with nucleotide substitution at the A position resulted in abnormal splicing (exon skipping and/or intron inclusion). However, rs67785924, a 5-bp deletion that abolished the branchpoint A nucleotide, exhibited normal RNA splicing pattern, presumably using two of the downstream As as alternative branchpoints. The influence of additional As on splicing was further confirmed by studying rs2733532, which contains three additional As in the ± 10 nucleotide region.

Conclusions: We generated a high-confidence genome-wide branchpoint site SNP database, experimentally verified the importance of A in the branchpoint, and suggested that other nearby As can protect branchpoint A substitution from abnormal splicing.

Keywords: RNA splicing, Single nucleotide polymorphism, Branchpoint site, Minigene

Background

Precursor messenger RNA (pre-mRNA) splicing is essential for gene expression in eukaryotes [1–3]. Splicing comprises a two-step trans-esterification reaction of intron removal and exon ligation. Splicing depends on the spliceosome, which is a large complex of small nuclear ribonucleoproteins (snRNPs; U1, U2, U4/U6, and U5) and non-snRNPs; these components recognize the target sequence and assemble on the pre-mRNA [4]. The intronic target sequences include a 5′ donor site, a 3′ acceptor site, a polypyrimidine tract (PPT) upstream of the 3′ acceptor, and a branchpoint site upstream of the PPT. The branchpoint contains a conserved splicing signal important for spliceosome assembly and lariat intron formation, with a consensus sequence (YNCTRAY, which differs slightly between species; Y is pyrimidine, N is any nucleotide, and R is purine) [5]. Tools to predict branchpoint sites based on the consensus sequence have been developed [6–10]; more recently, an NGS-based genome-wide study of splicing branchpoints was published [11–13].

Within the consensus branchpoint site sequence YNCTRAY, the well conserved A appears to be the most important one. A previous report showed that IVS4,-22A>G in the *LCAT* gene, which is an A to G change at the splicing branchpoint, resulted in intron inclusion and exon skipping of the mRNA and caused the Fish-eye disease [14]. There is also a report suggesting that mutations in the branchpoint sequence, especially the adenine (A) may result in aberrant pre-mRNA splicing and give rise to human genetic disorders [15].

* Correspondence: chen0010@ibms.sinica.edu.tw
[1]Institute of Clinical Medicine, National Yang-Ming University, Taipei, Taiwan
[2]Institute of Biomedical Sciences, Academia Sinica, Taipei, Taiwan
Full list of author information is available at the end of the article

There are millions of SNPs in the human genome; many are intronic, and have unknown functional significance. SNPs at the intron branchpoint sites, especially the adenine (A) nucleotide, would presumably affect splicing; however, this has not been systematically studied. It is therefore desirable to create a genome-wide branchpoint site SNP database, and perform functional analysis.

In the present study, we used an in silico splicing prediction program for branchpoint site prediction and combined its predictions with dbSNP data, to create a genome-wide branchpoint site SNP dataset. We experimentally verified the importance of A in the branchpoint, and further suggested that other nearby As may also influence RNA splicing.

Methods

Creating a dataset of SNPs located within branchpoint sites

All exon (n = 404,454) and intron (n = 363,190) sequences of the human genes were collected (human 1000genome v37), and the SROOGLE tool, which is based on two different algorithms, was used to predict branchpoint sites [8]. We were able to predict 338,787 (93.3%) branchpoint sites as output. Next, we screened NCBI's dbSNP for candidate SNPs located within the set of predicted branchpoint sites. Because adenine is the most important nucleotide at the branchpoint site, and 90% of branchpoint sites are upstream 19–37 bp from the 3′ acceptor [12, 13], we scored each SNP by the number of adenines found in the ± 10 nucleotide region (20 nucleotides total) surrounding the SNP. The SNPs identified in the predicted branchpoint sites and reported lariat sequences associated with these SNPs [12] are tabulated in Additional file 1.

Cell lines and genotyping

293T cells were obtained from The Bioresource Collection and Research Center (Hsinchu, Taiwan). Randomly selected EBV-transformed normal control B cell lines (n = 96) were obtained from the Taiwan Han Chinese Cell and Genome Bank [16]. Genomic DNA was extracted from the cell lines using the Gentra Puregene® Blood Kit (Gentra Systems, MN, USA) and genotyped for the SNPs of interest (*XPC* rs2733532, *PIP5KL1* rs13296170, *CYP2C19* rs12769205, *MYH11* rs75434223, and *KLC3* rs67785924), to identify cell lines carrying different branchpoint site SNP alleles (Table 1). The primer sequences are provided in Additional file 2.

Minigene constructs

Minigene constructs (Fig. 1) encompassing exons/introns of interest were prepared by amplifying introns and exons from genomic DNA; the amplified regions comprised *PIP5KL1* (chr9:130688147-130689612; 1466 bp), *CYP2C19* (chr10:96534815-96535296; 482 bp), *MYH11* (chr16:15833924-15835748; 1825 bp), and *KLC3* (chr19:45853898-45854704; 807 bp). The amplified minigenes were cloned into pJET1.2/blunt cloning vector (Thermo Scientific, Waltham, MA, USA), and subsequently sub-cloned into pEGFP-C1 vector (Additional file 2 indicates each restriction enzyme site). *PIP5KL1* and *MYH11*'s SNPs and *KLC3*'s seventh and eighth adenine substitution were used the GeneArt™ Site-Directed Mutagenesis System (Thermo Scientific, Waltham, MA, USA) with mutagenesis primers (Additional file 2). The complete sequences of the minigene constructs were confirmed by Sanger sequencing. Transient transfections of minigene constructs in 293T cells were performed using TransIT®-2020 transfection reagent (Mirus Bio, Inc., Madison, WI, USA). To isolate total RNA, the cells were harvested in TRIzol® reagent 24 h later, following the manufacturer's instructions to isolate total RNA.

Reverse transcription-PCR (RT-PCR)

Each cDNA was prepared from 2 μg total RNA, which was extracted from different minigenes of transfected cells and EVB-transformed B cells, using SuperScript®III reverse transcriptase, with oligo(dT)12–18 as primer, following the manufacturer's protocol (Invitrogen, CA, USA). All RT-PCR products were gel extracted and sequenced to confirm normal splicing, intron inclusion, and exon skipping forms.

Results

We identified 600 SNPs at the branchpoint sites; among these SNPs, 216 showed a change in adenine. After scoring the SNPs by counting the As in the ± 10 nucleotide region, only four SNPs were identified without any additional As; 17 SNPs had one additional A, and 29 SNPs had two additional As (Additional file 1).

The four SNPs identified without any additional As in the ± 10 nucleotide region were rs13296170, rs12769205, rs75434223, and rs67785924; these SNPs were the candidates most likely to affect RNA splicing (Table 1).

Table 1 Selected splice-site SNPs for functional studies

Chromosome	Position	Position	Gene name	SNP ID	Alleles	SNP ± 10 nucleotides sequence	Allele frequency
3	14187698	14187699	*XPC*	rs2733532	A/G	TCTGATTACT*A*ACCCTCGCCT	A = 0.363 G = 0.637
9	130689507	130689508	*PIP5KL1*	rs13296170	A/C	GGCCTCCCTC*A*CTCCCTGTCC	A = 1 C = 0
10	96535124	96535125	*CYP2C19*	rs12769205	A/G	TCTCCCTCCT*A*GTTTCGTTTC	A = 0.670 G = 0.330
16	15835555	15835556	*MYH11*	rs75434223	A/C	CGTGGGGCTC*A*CCCGCCTCCT	A = 1 C = 0
19	45854507	45854508	*KLC3*	rs67785924	–/ACCTC	CTTGCCCCTC*A*CCTCCCCTCC	– = 0.079 ACCTC = 0.921

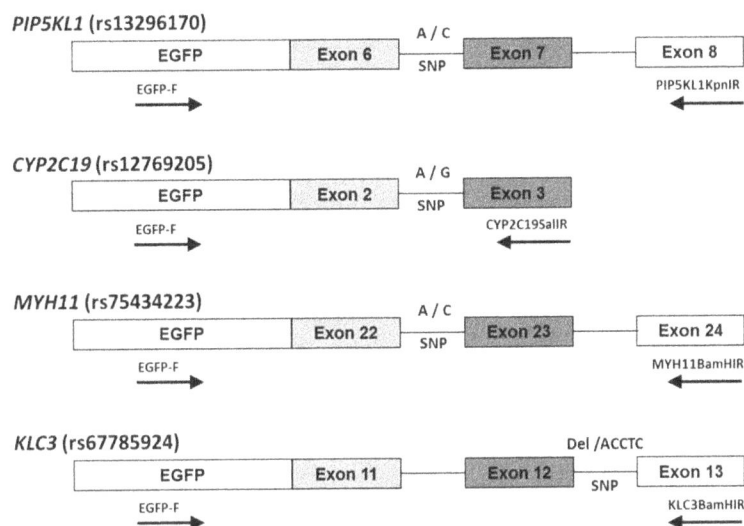

Fig. 1 Schematic representation of minigene constructs. SNPs in the branching point sites are indicated. Locations and orientations of RT-PCR primers (arrows) are shown. See Additional file 2: Table S2 for primer sequences

rs13296170, rs12769205, rs75434223, and rs67785924 are located on *PIP5KL1* intron6, *CYP2C19* intron2, *MYH11* intron22, and *KLC3* intron12, respectively (Fig. 1). These SNPs were further investigated for their functional significance. Minigenes containing the SNPs of interest were built using 3 exons and 2 introns, except for the *CYP2C19* SNP, for which two exons and one intron were used, because intron 3 of *CYP2C19* is large in size (4.9 kb).

RT-PCR of cDNAs prepared from 293T cells transfected with different minigene constructs showed that the rs12769205 A allele produced three bands (normal spliced, intron inclusion, and hybrid forms) when A was substituted with guanine (G) in *CYP2C19*, which spliced majorly in the intron inclusion form with lesser normal form (Fig. 2a). Since this construct comprised two exons and one intron, to make sure there was no exon skipping, we examined mRNA from EBV-transformed B cells carrying different genotypes for the spliced forms. The results showed that B cells had genotype AA spliced in the normal form, AG spliced equally in the normal and intron inclusion forms, and GG spliced mostly in the intron inclusion form (Fig. 2b). The results were further confirmed by using another set of primers such that the forward primer was located on intron 2, and it was noted that AG and GG genotypes spliced in the intron inclusion form (Fig. 2c).

We also studied the minigene constructs for the other three SNPs. When A was substituted with cytosine (C) in rs13296170, *PIP5KL1* spliced mostly into the exon skipping form and somewhat into the intron inclusion form, but not into the normal-spliced RNA form (Fig. 3a, lanes 5 and 6). While rs75434223 substituted A with C, *MYH11* spliced into the intron inclusion form, and not into the normal spliced form (Fig. 3b, lanes 8 and 9).

The SNP rs67785924 in *KLC3* has a normal (wild type) allele containing A and a deletion allele with five missing nucleotides, ACCTC. Both alleles produced normal spliced form, and some intron inclusion form. The level of intron inclusion form in the deletion allele was actually less than that in the normal A allele (Fig. 3b, lanes 2 and 3).

To understand why the deletion allele that did not contain branchpoint A still produces the normally spliced form, we checked the nearby intron sequence and found two other As located at the seventh and eighth nucleotides from the branchpoint A (Fig. 4a). We performed the branchpoint site prediction analysis using SROOGLE and Human Splicing Finder [9]; both tools predicted that these two nearby As also lie within the potential consensus branchpoint site sequence and can be used as alternative branchpoints in the deletion allele. We then tested the influence of these two nearby As on splicing using minigene constructs (Fig.4). In the wild-type allele, when the two nearby AA were changed to AG or GA, RNA spliced majorly in the normal form; when changed to GG, there was a decrease in the normal form and an increase in the intron inclusion form. In the deletion allele, when both AA were changed to GG, there was a further decrease in the normal form accompanied with a further increase in the intron inclusion form (Fig.4b). These results suggested other As nearby may serve as alternative branchpoints.

The influence of additional As on splicing was further examined for the branchpoint site SNP rs2733532 A/G, which contains three additional As in the ±10 nucleotide (Fig. 5a). This SNP is located in *XPC* and is reportedly associated with susceptibility to air pollution and childhood bronchitis [17]. In this case, EBV-transformed B cell lines from subjects carrying different genotypes at

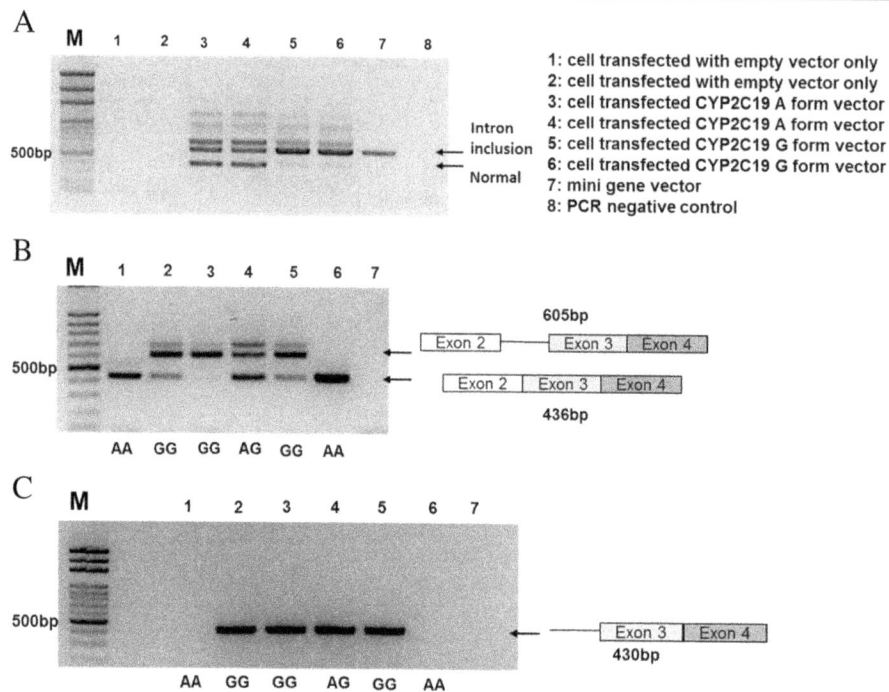

Fig. 2 *CYP2C19* alternative splicing forms in minigene-transfected 293T and in EBV-transformed B cells carrying different genotypes at SNP rs12769205. *CYP2C19* RT-PCR was performed with **a** 293T cells transfected with minigene of rs12769205, genotype A or G, using EGFP-F and *CYP2C19* SalIR primers, and **b** cDNA from B cells carrying different genotypes AA, AG, and GG at rs12769205 position using *CYP2C19* ex2F and *CYP2C19* ex4R primers or **c** cDNA from B cells using *CYP2C19* in2F and *CYP2C19* ex4R as primer set. Marker represents the 100-bp DNA ladder and indicated 500-bp site. See Additional file 2: Table S2 for primer sequences

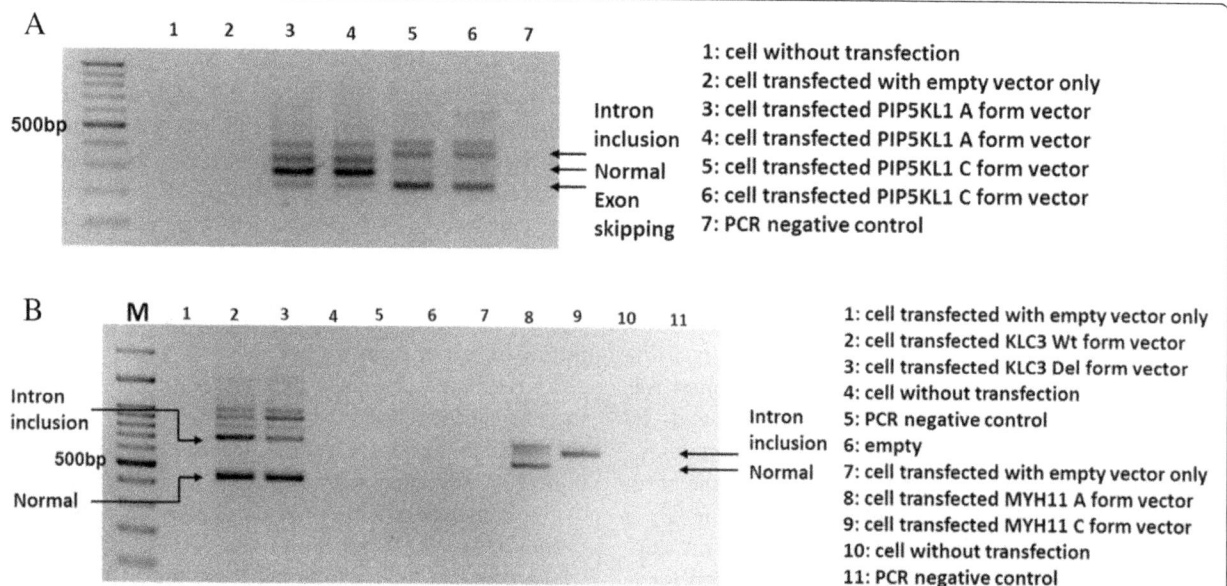

Fig. 3 *PIP5KL1*, *KLC3*, and *MYH11* alternative splicing in minigene-transected 293T cell. RT-PCR was performed in minigene-transfected 293T cells. **a** *PIP5KL1*; rs13296170, genotype A or C, was using EGFP-F and *PIP5KL1* KpnIR primers. **b** *KLC3* (land 1~5); rs67785924, genotype ACCTC (Wt) or deletion (Del), with EGFP-F and *KLC3* BamHIR primers, and *MYH11* (land 7~11); rs75434223, genotype A or C, was using EGFP-F and *MYH11* BamHIR primers. Marker represents the 100-bp DNA ladder and indicated 500-bp site. See Additional file 2: Table S2 for primer sequences

A

-gagctggagggtggatgtaacacttgcccctcAcctcccctccAAccatcccctgtgcctgtctccag [Exon 13]

↓

cttgcccctc*ccctccAAcc   **KLC3 Del form**

cttgcccctcAcctcccctccAGcc   **KLC3 AG form**

cttgcccctcAcctcccctccGAcc   **KLC3 GA form**

cttgcccctcAcctcccctccGGcc   **KLC3 GG form**

cttgcccctc*ccctccGGcc   **KLC3 Del with GG form**

B

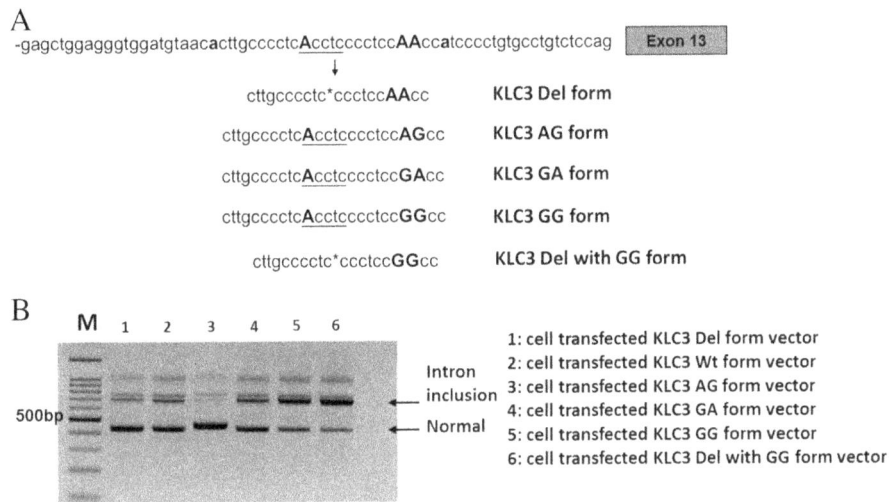

1: cell transfected KLC3 Del form vector
2: cell transfected KLC3 Wt form vector
3: cell transfected KLC3 AG form vector
4: cell transfected KLC3 GA form vector
5: cell transfected KLC3 GG form vector
6: cell transfected KLC3 Del with GG form vector

Fig. 4 Nucleotide sequences of *KLC3* intron 12 and alternative splicing forms in minigene-transected 293T cell. **a** Nucleotide sequences at 3'part of the *KLC3* intron 12. Possible splicing branchpoint adenine is indicated by bold and uppercase, SNP rs67785924 is underlined, and asterisk shown after deletion sequence. The following shown each A substituted minigene. **b** RT-PCR was performed in 293T cells transfected with different *KLC3* adenine substitution minigene constructs: ACCTC (Wt); ACCTC deletion (Del); Wt with AG (AG form); Wt with GA (GA form); Wt with GG (GG form) and Del with GG form. Marker represents the 100-bp DNA ladder and indicated 500-bp site. See Additional file 2: Table S2 for primer sequences

the branchpoint site, regardless of genotype (AA, AG, or GG), showed only the normally spliced form (Fig. 5b), suggesting that other As can serve as a branchpoint site.

Discussion

In the present study, we used SROOGLE to predict splice branchpoints and screened dbSNP for SNPs located within the branchpoint sites. Using minigene constructs and, when available, EBV-transformed cell lines carrying different SNP alleles, we experimentally verified that SNPs comprising a change to branchpoint A resulted in abnormal splicing, suggesting that the predicted sites are indeed involved in pre-mRNA splicing, and further confirming the functional importance of A. However, only 20% of the branchpoint sites that we identified had a reported corresponding lariat sequence

[12](see Additional file 1). This observation may be understandable given that the number of reported lariat sequences based on next generation sequencing represents only 28% of all introns in the genome [12].

We found only three branchpoint site SNPs that have a single A at the branchpoint site, without additional As nearby. It is possible that organisms evolved to have additional As in the branchpoint site to ensure proper splicing. Additional As in the ±10 nucleotide region may protect SNPs at the branchpoint A from abnormal splicing, by serving as alternative branchpoints. This mechanism has been demonstrated in the present study for SNP rs67785924 and SNP rs2733532 (Figs. 4 and 5). The latter SNP is located on *XPC* on chromosome 3, and has been reported to be associated with diseases related to air pollution and childhood bronchitis [17].

A

-ggggcttcctggtatctgAttActAAccctcgcctgtgtcctcccaccactgccacctgtccag [Exon 16]

B

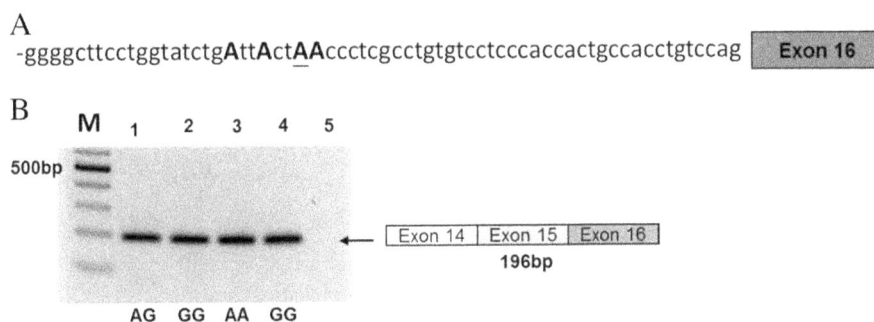

Exon 14 | Exon 15 | Exon 16
196bp

AG   GG   AA   GG

Fig. 5 *XPC* alternative splicing in different genotypes of EBV-transformed B cells. **a** Graphic representation 3'part of the *XPC* intron 15 sequences, possible splicing branchpoint adenine is indicated by bold and uppercase, underlining is rs2733532. **b** cDNA from normal control B cells of different genotypes AA, AG, and GG at rs2733532 using *XPC* ex14F and *XPC* ex16R primers. Marker represents the 100-bp DNA ladder and indicated 500-bp site. See Additional file 2: Table S2 for primer sequences

The risk allele G of the branchpoint SNP A/G resides in the population at a frequency of ~ 0.637. Both the lariat sequence database and our prediction algorithms classified it as a branchpoint site. However, our experiments demonstrated that this branchpoint A to G SNP did not influence splicing; this observation presumably results from the presence of additional nearby As, which serve as alternative splicing sites; this explanation implies that other mechanisms may be involved in this disease association.

Several algorithms and tools have been used to predict branchpoints [6–10], and surprisingly, no branchpoint site SNP database has been reported. Because minigene constructs are time-consuming and not all SNPs in the branchpoint sites have cell lines available for study, in the present study we have tested only five SNPs, and verified their significance. More functional studies are needed to examine the functional significance of other SNPs, especially those SNPs that do not involve A changes at branchpoints.

In conclusion, we have generated a high-confidence genome-wide branchpoint site SNP database, experimentally verified the importance of A in the branchpoint, and suggested that other nearby As may serve as alternative branchpoints and ensure proper pre-mRNA splicing. These results improve upon the prediction of functional SNPs at branchpoint sites, and inform the study of the SNPs at intron branchpoint sites.

Abbreviations
A: Adenine; C: Cytosine; G: Guanine; PPT: Polypyrimidine tract; pre-mRNA: Precursor messenger RNA; SNP: Single nucleotide polymorphism; snRNPs: Small nuclear ribonucleoproteins

Acknowledgements
Not applicable.

Funding
This work was supported by Academia Sinica Genomic Medicine Multicenter Study, Taiwan [40-05-GMM] and National Resource Center for Genomic Medicine MOST 105-2319-B-001-001]. The funding organization had no role in the design or conduct of this research. The authors alone are responsible for the content and writing of the paper.

Authors' contributions
HLC, JYW, and YTC conceived and designed the experiments. HLC performed the experiments and wrote the paper. All authors analyzed the data and approved the final manuscript.

Competing interests
The authors are no competing of interest to declare.

Author details
[1]Institute of Clinical Medicine, National Yang-Ming University, Taipei, Taiwan. [2]Institute of Biomedical Sciences, Academia Sinica, Taipei, Taiwan. [3]Graduate Institute of Chinese Medical Science, China Medical University, Taichung, Taiwan. [4]Department of Pediatrics, Duke University Medical Center, Durham, USA.

References
1. Berget SM, Moore C, Sharp PA. Spliced segments at the 5' terminus of adenovirus 2 late mRNA. Proc Natl Acad Sci U S A. 1977;74(8):3171–5.
2. Chow LT, Gelinas RE, Broker TR, Roberts RJ. An amazing sequence arrangement at the 5' ends of adenovirus 2 messenger RNA. Cell. 1977; 12(1):1–8.
3. Gilbert W. Why genes in pieces? Nature. 1978;271(5645):501.
4. Will CL, Luhrmann R. Spliceosome structure and function. Cold Spring Harb Perspect Biol. 2011;3(7). doi:10.1101/cshperspect.a003707.
5. Kramer A. The structure and function of proteins involved in mammalian pre-mRNA splicing. Annu Rev Biochem. 1996;65:367–409.
6. Kol G, Lev-Maor G, Ast G. Human-mouse comparative analysis reveals that branch-site plasticity contributes to splicing regulation. Hum Mol Genet. 2005;14(11):1559–68.
7. Schwartz SH, Silva J, Burstein D, Pupko T, Eyras E, Ast G. Large-scale comparative analysis of splicing signals and their corresponding splicing factors in eukaryotes. Genome Res. 2008;18(1):88–103.
8. Schwartz S, Hall E, Ast G. SROOGLE: webserver for integrative, user-friendly visualization of splicing signals. Nucleic Acids Res. 2009;37(Web Server issue): W189–92.
9. Desmet FO, Hamroun D, Lalande M, Collod-Beroud G, Claustres M, Beroud C. Human Splicing Finder: an online bioinformatics tool to predict splicing signals. Nucleic Acids Res. 2009;37(9):e67.
10. Faber K, Glatting KH, Mueller PJ, Risch A, Hotz-Wagenblatt A. Genome-wide prediction of splice-modifying SNPs in human genes using a new analysis pipeline called AAS sites. BMC bioinformatics. 2011;12(Suppl 4):S2.
11. Taggart AJ, DeSimone AM, Shih JS, Filloux ME, Fairbrother WG. Large-scale mapping of branchpoints in human pre-mRNA transcripts in vivo. Nat Struct Mol Biol. 2012;19(7):719–21.
12. Mercer TR, Clark MB, Andersen SB, Brunck ME, Haerty W, Crawford J, Taft RJ, Nielsen LK, Dinger ME, Mattick JS. Genome-wide discovery of human splicing branchpoints. Genome Res. 2015;25(2):290–303.
13. Taggart AJ, Lin CL, Shrestha B, Heintzelman C, Kim S, Fairbrother WG. Large-scale analysis of branchpoint usage across species and cell lines. Genome Res. 2017;27(4):639–49.
14. Kuivenhoven JA, Weibusch H, Pritchard PH, Funke H, Benne R, Assmann G, Kastelein JJ. An intronic mutation in a lariat branchpoint sequence is a direct cause of an inherited human disorder (fish-eye disease). J Clin Invest. 1996;98(2):358–64.
15. Kralovicova J, Lei H, Vorechovsky I. Phenotypic consequences of branch point substitutions. Hum Mutat. 2006;27(8):803–13.
16. Pan WH, Fann CS, Wu JY, Hung YT, Ho MS, Tai TH, Chen YJ, Liao CJ, Yang ML, Cheng AT, et al. Han Chinese cell and genome bank in Taiwan: purpose, design and ethical considerations. Hum Hered. 2006;61(1):27–30.
17. Ghosh R, Rossner P, Honkova K, Dostal M, Sram RJ, Hertz-Picciotto I. Air pollution and childhood bronchitis: interaction with xenobiotic, immune regulatory and DNA repair genes. Environ Int. 2016;87:94–100.

6

Identification of protein complexes from multi-relationship protein interaction networks

Xueyong Li[1,2], Jianxin Wang[1]*, Bihai Zhao[2]*, Fang-Xiang Wu[3] and Yi Pan[4]

Abstract

Background: Protein complexes play an important role in biological processes. Recent developments in experiments have resulted in the publication of many high-quality, large-scale protein-protein interaction (PPI) datasets, which provide abundant data for computational approaches to the prediction of protein complexes. However, the precision of protein complex prediction still needs to be improved due to the incompletion and noise in PPI networks.

Results: There exist complex and diverse relationships among proteins after integrating multiple sources of biological information. Considering that the influences of different types of interactions are not the same weight for protein complex prediction, we construct a multi-relationship protein interaction network (MPIN) by integrating PPI network topology with gene ontology annotation information. Then, we design a novel algorithm named MINE (identifying protein complexes based on Multi-relationship protein Interaction NEtwork) to predict protein complexes with high cohesion and low coupling from MPIN.

Conclusions: The experiments on yeast data show that MINE outperforms the current methods in terms of both accuracy and statistical significance.

Background

With the completion of the sequencing of the human genome, proteomic research becomes one of the most important areas in the life science. One important task in proteomics is to detect protein complexes based on protein-protein interaction (PPI) data generated by various experimental technologies, e.g., yeast-two-hybrid [1], tandem affinity purification [2], and mass spectrometry [3]. Protein complexes are molecular aggregations of proteins assembled by PPIs, which play critical roles in biological processes. Many proteins are functional only when they are assembled into a protein complex and interact with other proteins in this complex. Protein complexes are key molecular entities to perform cellular functions. Even in the relatively simple model organism *Saccharomyces cerevisiae*, these complexes are comprised of many subunits that work

in a coherent fashion. Besides applications of PPI networks, such as protein function predictions [4] and essential protein discoveries [5–11], prediction of protein complexes is another active topic. Actually, protein complexes are of great importance for understanding the principles of cellular organization and function.

Many computational methods for predicting protein complexes from PPI networks have been developed. Pairwise protein interactions can be modelled as a graph or network, where vertices are proteins and edges are PPIs. Since proteins in the same complex are highly interactive with each other, protein complexes generally correspond to dense subgraphs in the PPI network and many previous studies have been proposed based on this observation, such as MCODE (Molecular Complex detection) [12], MCL (Markov Cluster algorithm) [13], R-MCL (Regularized MCL) [14], CMC (Maximal Clique algorithm) [15], RRW (Repeated Random Walks) [16], SPICi (Speed and Performance in Clustering algorithm) [17], HC-PIN (Hierarchical Clustering based on Protein-Protein Interaction Network) [18], IPC-MCE (Identifying Protein

* Correspondence: jxwang@mail.csu.edu.cn; bihaizhao@163.com
[1]School of Information Science and Engineering, Central South University, Changsha 410083, China
[2]Department of Information and Computing Science, Changsha University, Changsha 410003, China
Full list of author information is available at the end of the article

Complexes based on Maximal Clique Extension) [19], and IPCA (Identification of Protein Complexes Algorithm) [20]. Nepusz et al. [21] proposed an algorithm to find overlapping protein complexes from PPI networks, named ClusterONE (Clustering with Overlapping Neighborhood Expansion). For the convenience of researchers, MCODE, ClusterONE, etc. have been designed as plus-in for protein complex prediction and biological network analysis. ClusterViz [22] is such a Cytoscape APP to complete this work.

However, these abovementioned approaches for extracting dense subgraphs fail to take into account the inherent organization. Recent analysis of experimentally detected protein complexes [23] has revealed that a complex consists of a core component and attachments. Core proteins are highly co-expressed and share high functional similarity, and each attachment protein binds to a subset of core proteins to form a biological complex. Based on the core-attachment concept, some algorithms have been proposed, including COACH (Core-Attachment-based method) [24], CORE [25], MCL-Caw [26], DCU (Detecting Complex based on Uncertain graph model) [27], and WPNCA (a Weighted PageRank-Nibble algorithm with Core-Attachment structure) [28].

In spite of the advances in computational approaches and related fields, accurate identification protein complexes are still a bottleneck. One of the most important reasons is that the PPI network contains a lot of false positives which greatly reduce the complex detection accuracy. To address this problem, biological information other than PPIs has been integrated with network topology to improve the precision of protein complex detection methods. Wu et al. proposed a method called CACHET to discover protein complexes with core-attachment structures from tandem affinity purification (TAP) data [29]. Tang et al. [30] constructed time course PPI networks by incorporating gene expression into PPI networks and applied it successfully to the identification of function modules. Wang et al. [31] proposed a three-sigma method to identify active time points of each protein in a cellular cycle, where three-sigma principle is used to compute an active threshold for each gene according to the characteristics of its expression curve. A dynamic PPI network (DPIN) is constructed for the detection of protein complexes. Li et al. proposed novel algorithms, such as TSN-PCD [32] and DPC [33], to identify dynamic protein complexes by integrating PPI data and dynamic gene expression profiles. Zhao et al. [34] reconstructed a weighted PPI network by using dynamic gene expression data and developed a novel protein complex identification algorithm, named PCIA-GeCo.

There exist complex and diverse relationships among proteins after integrating multiple sources of biological information. However, comparing PPI data is difficult because they are often diverse and play different roles under different conditions. Current existing approaches failed to take into account and combined the interactions with different natures into one interaction effectively. Taking into account the influences of different types of interactions are not the same weight for protein complex prediction, we construct a multi-relationship protein interaction network (MPIN) by integrating PPI network topology with gene ontology (GO) annotation information. Then, a new method named MINE (identify protein complexes based on Multi-relationship protein Interaction NEtwork) is proposed. We have conducted an experiment on yeast data. Experimental results show that MINE outperforms the existing methods in terms of both accuracy and p value.

Methods
Multi-relationship protein interaction network

Complex networks have now been a new research focus because of surging networks in various fields such as engineering, social science, and life science. In reality, connections among nodes in complex networks are diversified. Multi-relationship means that there is more than one connection between two nodes and each of them has its own property. For instance, in social networks [35], persons contact with each other via emails, telephones, MSN, etc. and hence make up a complex multi-relationship network. Similarly, in biological networks, there are diverse links among proteins like physical interaction, co-expression, and co-annotation. However, multi-relationship networks are much more difficult to analyze than single-relationship networks. Multi-relationship networks are also essential in better reflecting the real world.

Definition 1 Multi-relationship network
Consider a PPI network $G = (V, E)$, where $V = \{v_1, v_2,..., v_n\}$ represents a set of proteins and $E = \{e_1, e_2,..., e_m\}$ represents a set of interactions. A multi-relationship network is defined as MG $= (V, E \cup E', T)$, where $T(e_i) = t_i$ ($i = 1, 2...m$) is the interaction type of e_i. E' is the set of new generated interactions.

In a multi-relationship network, a pair of proteins may be connected by more than one type of links. If there are two or more links between a pair of proteins, they are called parallel interactions. Figure 1 illustrates a typical multi-relationship network. From Fig. 1, we can see that proteins A and B have physical interaction in the PPI network and at the same time, A and B are also co-expression based on gene expression profiles and co-annotations based on gene ontology annotation information. In the multi-relationship network, multiple connections between A and B are kept.

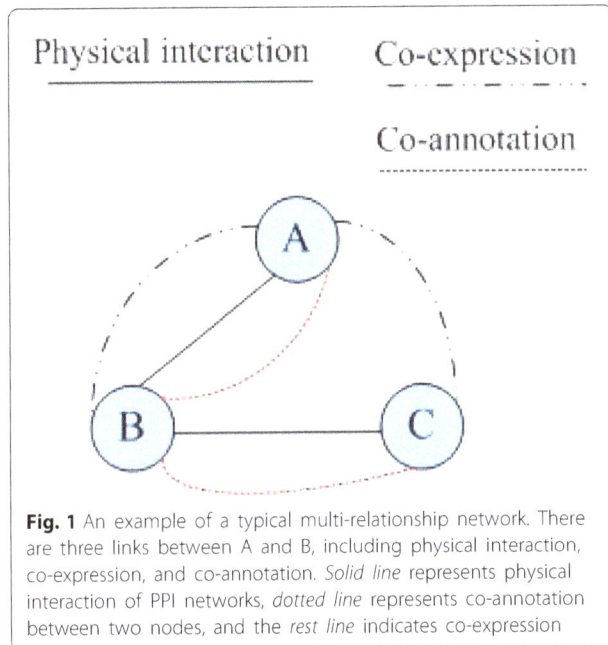

Fig. 1 An example of a typical multi-relationship network. There are three links between A and B, including physical interaction, co-expression, and co-annotation. *Solid line* represents physical interaction of PPI networks, *dotted line* represents co-annotation between two nodes, and the *rest line* indicates co-expression

Researches [27, 36] show that PPI data obtained through high-throughput biological experiments contains relatively high rates of false positives and false negatives. False positives become obstacle to the precision of prediction algorithm. False negatives lead to the loss of interaction data and continue to inhibit the increase of the number of protein complexes correctly matched. To overcome these problems, researches have begun to integrate the PPI network and other biological information, such as gene expression profiles, essential proteins, and GO annotation information. Due to the similar biological properties of protein complexes, GO annotation is a valuable addition to PPI data for protein complex prediction. Therefore, in this study we construct a multi-relationship protein interaction network by integrating PPI network topology and GO annotation information.

The GO database consists of three separate categories of annotations, namely molecular function (MF), biological process (BP), and cellular component (CC). MF describes activities, such as catalytic or binding activities, at the molecular level. BP describes biological goals accomplished by one or more ordered assemblies of molecular functions. CC describes locations, at the levels of subcellular structures and macromolecular complexes. In this study we integrate the PPI network and three categories of GO annotations to construct a multi-relationship protein interaction network. In our constructed multi-relationship network, four kinds of interactions at most can be considered between two proteins, namely the interactions of the PPI network and the interactions of sharing molecular functions,

sharing biological processes, and sharing cellular components. Figure 2 describes the process of a multi-relationship network construction.

In the constructed multi-relationship protein interaction network, two proteins are connected if they interact with each other in the PPI network or have common functions, including biological processes, molecular functions, and cellular components. After constructing a multi-relationship protein interaction network, we do some further processing, such as weighting and filtering. Studies [9, 10, 36] show that the performance of prediction algorithms based on weighted networks is generally superior to that based on unweighted networks. The reason is simple: weight stands for the relative reliability/importance of interactions; thus, weighted networks can be more valuable than unweighted networks in the representative of PPI networks. For the first type of interaction in our constructed multi-relationship network, interacting with each other in the PPI network, we weight these interactions through the analysis of topological features of PPI networks. Generally speaking, for a pair of interacting proteins, the strength of an interaction can be reflected by the number of its common neighbors. This study uses ECC to calculate the weight of protein pairs, which is defined as

$$
\text{ECC}(v_i, v_j) = \begin{cases} \dfrac{|N_i \cap N_j|^2}{(|N_i|-1) * (|N_j|-1)} & , \quad |N_i| > 1 \text{ and } |N_j| > 1 \\ 0 & , \quad |N_i| = 1 \text{ or } |N_j| = 1 \end{cases},
$$

(1)

where N_i and N_j are the neighborhood sets of v_i and v_j, respectively. To reduce the negative effect of false positive on the protein complex prediction, we remove interactions whose ECC values are zero.

For the rest three types of interaction, we weight interactions according to the number of common functions (including BP, MF, and CC) between two proteins. For a pair of proteins v_i and v_j, BP_i and BP_j are sets of biological processes of v_i and v_j, respectively. W_BP (v_i, v_j) represents the strength of sharing biological processes, which is calculated as follows:

$$
\text{W\_BP}(v_i, v_j) = \begin{cases} \dfrac{|BP_i \cap BP_j|^2}{|BP_i| * |BP_j|} & , \quad |BP_i| * |BP_j| > 0 \\ 0 & , \quad |BP_i| * |BP_j| = 0 \end{cases}
$$

(2)

In Eq. (2), $BP_i \cap BP_j$ denotes the set of common biological processes of v_i and v_j. In a similar way, W_MF (v_i, v_j) and W_CC (v_i, v_j) denote the strengths of sharing molecular functions and cellular components of v_i and v_j, respectively. They can be calculated as follows:

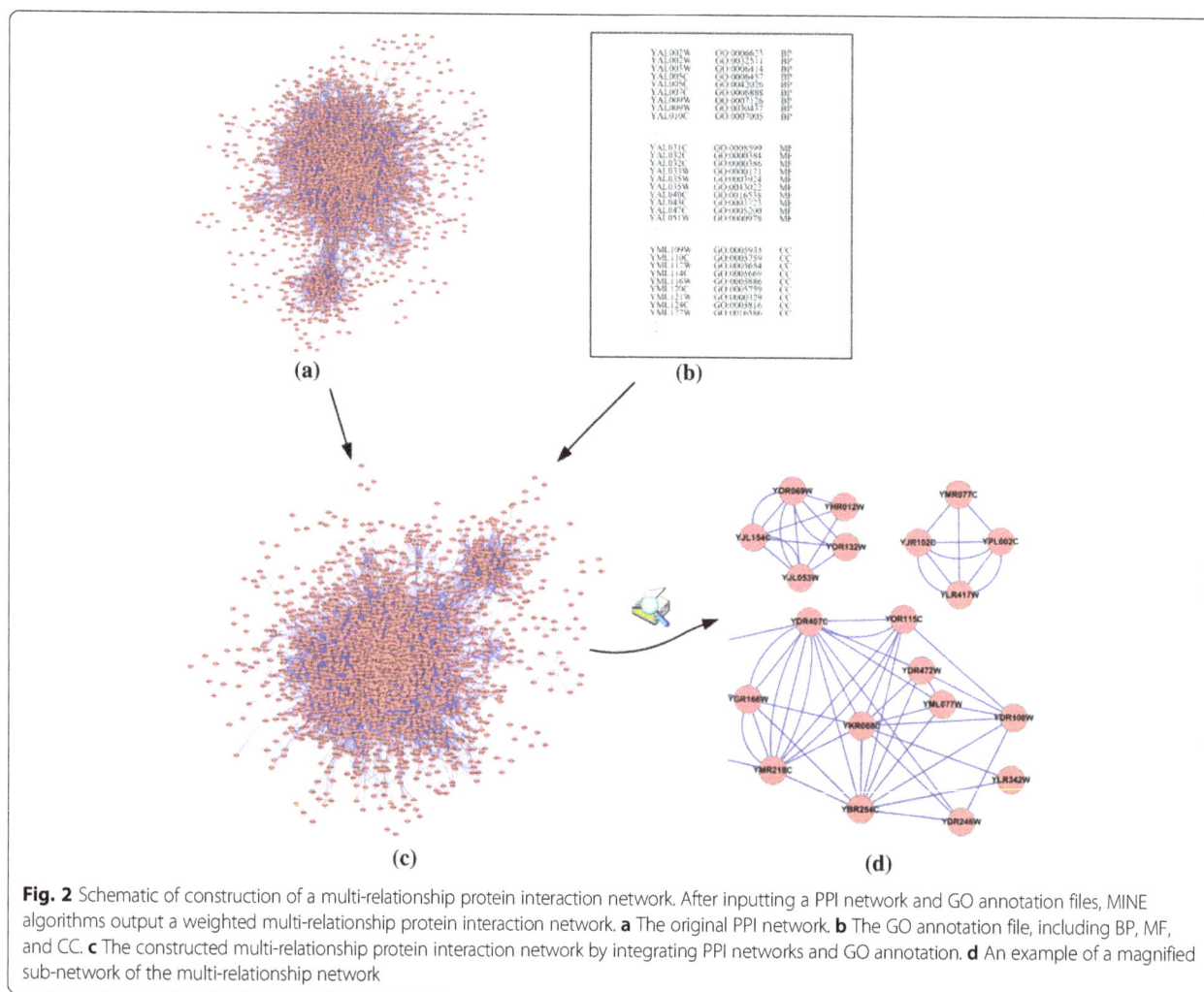

Fig. 2 Schematic of construction of a multi-relationship protein interaction network. After inputting a PPI network and GO annotation files, MINE algorithms output a weighted multi-relationship protein interaction network. **a** The original PPI network. **b** The GO annotation file, including BP, MF, and CC. **c** The constructed multi-relationship protein interaction network by integrating PPI networks and GO annotation. **d** An example of a magnified sub-network of the multi-relationship network

$$
\text{W\_MF}(v_i, v_j) = \begin{cases} \dfrac{|MF_i \cap MF_j|^2}{|MF_i| * |MF_j|} & , \quad |MF_i| * |MF_j| > 0 \\ 0 & , \quad |MF_i| * |MF_j| = 0 \end{cases} \tag{3}
$$

$$
\text{W\_CC}(v_i, v_j) = \begin{cases} \dfrac{|CC_i \cap CC_j|^2}{|CC_i| * |CC_j|} & , \quad |CC_i| * |CC_j| > 0 \\ 0 & , \quad |CC_i| * |CC_j| = 0 \end{cases} \tag{4}
$$

For the three types of interactions, we perform more stringent filter operations than the first type because they are newly generated interactions. For a pair of function-shared proteins, if they have only one common function or no common neighbors in the PPI network, interactions between them are removed. After performing the above operations, a weighted multi-relationship protein interaction network is constructed.

MINE algorithm
Considering the influences of different types of interactions in protein complex prediction are not the same, we construct a multi-relationship protein interaction network by integrating PPI networks and GO annotation information. To test the effectiveness of the multi-relationship network, we design a new method for predicting protein complexes, named MINE (based on Multi-relationship protein Interaction NEtwork). Multi-relationship networks have more complex attributes than single networks. Current protein complex prediction methods are mainly based on single networks. So, converting a multi-relationship network into single networks is key to design the MINE algorithm. A simple way for addressing this problem is to combine interactions with different natures to one interaction effectively. In reality, it is inappropriate for us to combine multiple interactions between two proteins because they are often derived under different conditions and play different roles in protein complex prediction. Considering that different types of interactions play different roles in detecting protein complexes, we decompose the multi-relationship network into several single networks,

including the PPI network, BPN (sharing biological processes), MFN (sharing molecular functions) and CCN (sharing cellular components). Figure 3 displays the framework of multi-relationship decomposition.

And then, we identify protein complexes through mining density subgraphs from the four networks. Intuitively, a subgraph representing a protein complex should satisfy two simple structural properties: it should contain many reliable interactions between its subunits, and it should be well-separated from the rest of the network [21]. Inspired by the notion, we take into account the density of a subgraph and connections between nodes of the subgraph and nodes out of the subgraph. To describe MINE simply and clearly, we provide the following definitions, firstly.

Definition 2 Weighted Density [27]

Given a weighted network $G = (V, E, W)$. $V = \{v_1, v_2, ..., v_n\}$, $E = \{e_1, e_2, ..., e_m\}$, $W = \{w(e_1), w(e_2), ..., w(e_m)\}$, $w(e_i)$ is the weight of an edge e_i. WD (G) denotes the weighted density of G and is defined as

$$\mathrm{WD}(G) = \frac{\sum_{i=1}^{m} p(e_i) \times 2}{\max_{1 \leq i \leq |m|} (p(e_i)) \times (|V| \times (|V|-1))} \quad (5)$$

Definition 3 Sub-network Weighted Degree [36]

Given a weighted sub-network $G = (V, E, W)$ and a vertex u, u V. $V = \{v_1, v_2, ..., v_n\}$, $E = \{e_1, e_2, ..., e_m\}$, $W = \{w(e_1), w(e_2), ..., w(e_m)\}$, $w(e_i)$ is the weight of an edge e_i. SWD (u, G) denotes the weighted degree of u within G and is defined as

$$\mathrm{SWD}(u, G) = \sum_{i=1}^{n} w(u, v_i), (u, v_i) \in E \quad (6)$$

Based on these definitions, we are now ready to describe our proposed MINE algorithm to detect protein complexes. Our method visits the four single networks, respectively, to discover density subgraphs as protein complexes. For a selected network, MINE starts from a randomly chosen protein vertex and add protein vertices via a greedy procedure to form a candidate complex

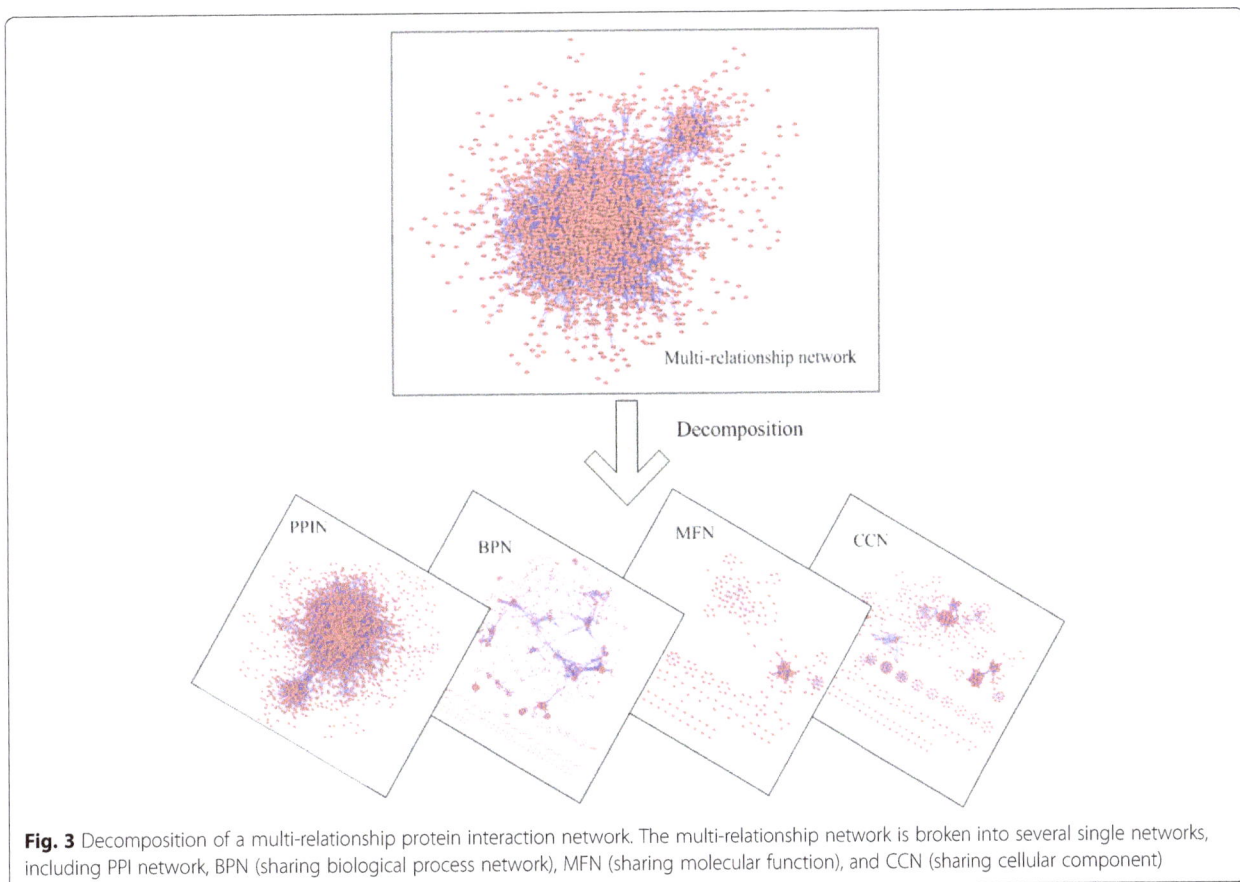

Fig. 3 Decomposition of a multi-relationship protein interaction network. The multi-relationship network is broken into several single networks, including PPI network, BPN (sharing biological process network), MFN (sharing molecular function), and CCN (sharing cellular component)

with high cohesion and low coupling. The growth process is repeated from all vertices to form non-redundant complex sets. Since some vertices have similar neighborhood graphs, the candidate complexes detected from their neighborhood graphs may have large overlaps, which result in high redundancy. Hence, a redundancy-filtering procedure is applied to quantify the extent overlap between each pair of complexes and discard the complexes with low density or small size.

MINE algorithm (Algorithm 1) describes the overall procedure to identify protein complexes. MINE algorithm processes four single networks according to the multi-relationship network, such as PPIN, BPN, MFN, and CCN, in line 1. For a selected network G_k, we first generate candidate complexes according to neighbors of all proteins in the network, in lines 3–8. The seed is inserted into the candidate set CCS, and then all neighbors of the seed are put into CCS one by one. If the weighted density of CCS is less than the threshold WDT, the new added neighbor node is removed from CCS. After this process, a candidate complex with high cohesion is formed. Then, we remove some nodes highly connected with the neighbor subgraph to form a candidate complex with low coupling, in lines 9–12. Figure 4 illustrates an example of removing high-coupling proteins. In Fig. 4, SWD(D, CCS) = 0.2, SWD(D, NS) = 0.3 + 0.4 = 0.7, D is removed from CCS.

Finally, if CCS is not a subset of complex in the set of protein complex SC, CCS is inserted into SC.

The second stage of our method is redundancy-filtering, in lines 15–20. Complexes overlapping to a very high extent should be discarded. With quantifying the extent of overlap between each pair of complexes, a complex with small weighted density or a small number of proteins is discarded for which overlap score of the pair is above the threshold. In our method, the overlap threshold is typically set as 0.8 [21, 27], where the matching score of two complexes A and B is defined as follows [15, 24]:

$$MS(A, B) = \frac{|A \cap B|^2}{|A| \times |B|} \tag{7}$$

Algorithm 1: Protein complexes identification

Input: multi-relationship network MG= (V, E, W, T);

weighted density threshold WDT; the threshold for overlap T;

Output: SC: the set of protein complexes;

1. GS= {G_1, G_2, G_3, G_4} is a network set generated from MG;

2. for each network $G_k \in GS$ (k=1, 2, 3, 4)

3.   for each vertex $v \in V_k$

4.   Insert v into CCS;// Candidate complex set

5.   for each neighbor q of v

6.   insert q into CCS;

7.   If WD (CCS)< WDT

8.   remove q from CCS

9.   NS is a neighbor subgraph of nodes in CCS

10.   for each vertex $u \in CS$

11.   if SWD(u , CCS) <= SWD (u , NS)

12.   remove u from CCS;

13.   if CCS is not a subset of element in SC

14.   insert CCS into SC;

15.   for each element $A \in SC$

16.   for each element $B \in SC$ and A≠B

17:      if NA(A,B)>T

18.   if WD(A)≥WD(B) or Size(A)≥Size(B)

19.   remove B from SC ;

20.   else remove A from SC ;

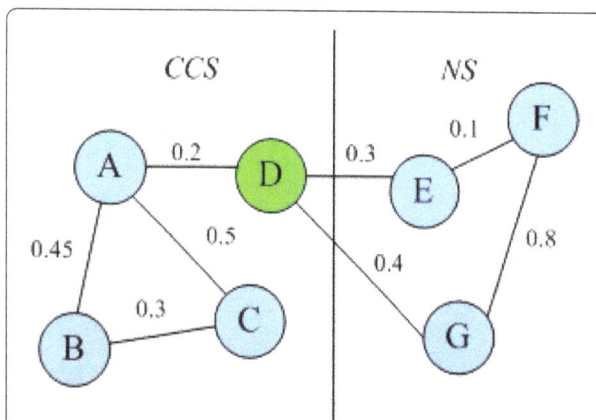

Fig. 4 An example of removing high-coupling proteins. The sum of weighted degree in CCS is 0.2, while that value in NS is 0.7, so D is removed from CCS, due to high coupling with neighbor set NS

Results and discussion

In order to evaluate the performance of our proposed algorithm, we compare it with other five competing algorithms, including CMC [15], RRW [16], COACH [24], SPICi [17], and ClusterONE [21]. For all those competing algorithms, the parameters are set as recommended by their authors. We have applied our MINE method and other methods on two yeast PPI networks, including DIP [37] and Krogan [38]. These PPI datasets are available online, which varied from each other a lot. In this section, we will first present in details the results on DIP data. The results using Krogan data will also be briefly presented to demonstrate the effectiveness of our proposed method.

The DIP dataset consists of 5023 proteins and 22,570 interactions. The Krogan dataset contains 3672 proteins and 14,317 interactions. Self-interactions and repeated interactions are filtered out in the three PPI networks. To evaluate the protein complexes predicted by our method, a benchmark set is obtained from the reference [39], which consists of 408 complexes.

To assess the quality of predicted complexes, we employed several evaluation measures, including precision, recall, F-measure, and functional enrichment of GO terms.

Precision, recall, and F-measure

We describe how well the predicted protein complexes match with the benchmark complex set, firstly. A predicted protein complex is considered to match with a benchmark complex, if its matching score MS (see Eq. (7)) is no less than a threshold. Typically, the threshold is set as 0.2 [24, 27]. Precision and recall are the commonly used measures to evaluate the performance of protein complex prediction algorithms. Precision measures the percentage of predicted protein complexes that match benchmark complexes in all the predicted protein complexes. Recall is the fraction of benchmark complexes that are retrieved. Mathematically, precision and recall are defined as follows:

$$\text{Precision} = \frac{N_{cp}}{|P|} \quad (8)$$

$$\text{Recall} = \frac{N_{cb}}{|B|} \quad (9)$$

where N_{cp} is the number of predicted complexes matched by benchmark complexes, N_{cb} is the number of benchmark complexes that are matched by predicted complexes, P is the set of predicted protein complexes and B is the benchmark complex set.

F-measure, as the harmonic mean of precision and recall, can be used to evaluate the overall performance of the different techniques [21, 24]. Table 1 shows the basic information about predicted complexes by various methods on DIP data, where the best values are italized.

In Table 1, PC represents the total number of predicted complexes, while N_{pcp} is the number of complexes perfectly matching the benchmark complexes. In other words, the matching score between a predicted complex and a benchmark complex is 1. From Table 1, we can see that MINE produces the largest number of correctly predicted complexes and the second-largest number

Table 1 The matching results of various algorithms

Algorithms	PC	N_{cp}	N_{cb}	N_{pcp}
MINE	*606*	*345*	*218*	*19*
CMC	235	119	124	8
COACH	902	319	219	15
RRW	250	118	136	4
SPICi	574	118	143	7
ClusterONE	371	155	136	6

of benchmark complexes after COACH, respectively, while PC of our method (606) is far less than COACH's (902). The fifth column of Table 1 shows that MINE has the absolute advantage to obtain the largest number of perfectly matched complexes. N_{pcp} of MINE is 137.5, 26.67, 375, 171.43, and 216.67 % higher than that of CMC, COACH, RRW, SPICi, and ClusterONE, respectively. Figure 5 shows the overall comparison in terms of precision, recall, and F-measure.

On DIP data, F-measure of MINE is 0.551, which is 45.05, 29.23, 41.02, 112.62, and 48.59 % higher than that of CMC, COACH, RRW, SPICi, and ClusterONE, respectively. Our MINE method can achieve the highest F-measure by providing the highest precision and the same highest recall as COACH, which shows that our method can predict protein complexes very good.

Functional enrichment analysis

Another evaluation measure is the function enrichment which measures the biological significance of predicted protein complexes by various algorithms. To substantiate the biological significance of our predicted complexes, we calculate their p values, which represent the probability of co-occurrence of proteins with common functions [27]. In this wok, we employ the tool BiNGO

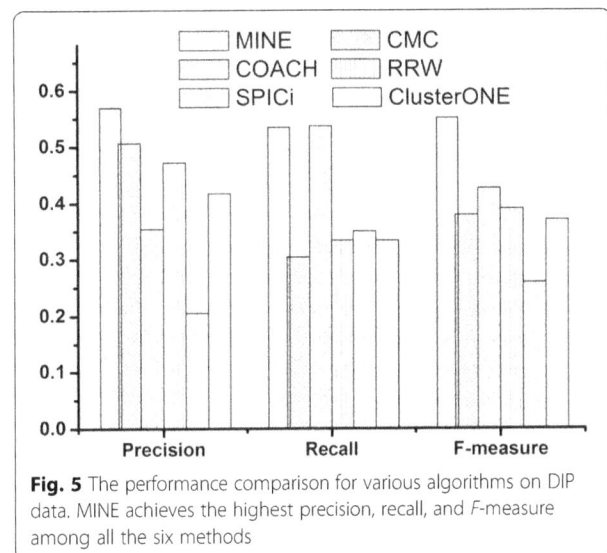

Fig. 5 The performance comparison for various algorithms on DIP data. MINE achieves the highest precision, recall, and F-measure among all the six methods

[40] to calculate p values for predicted complexes. BiNGO is a Java-based tool to determine which GO categories are statistically overrepresented in a set of genes or a subgraph of a biological network. BiNGO is implemented as a plug-in for Cytoscape [41], which is an open-source bioinformatics software platform for visualizing and integrating molecular interaction networks. A low p value of a predicted complex indicates that those proteins in the complex do not happen merely by chance, so the complex has high statistical significance. Generally, a complex is considered to be significant with p value <0.01. In addition, the p-score is also used as an effective evaluation measure, which is defined as

$$p\text{-score} = \frac{1}{n}\sum_{i=1}^{n} -\lg(p\ \text{value}_i)|p\ \text{value}_i < 0.01 \quad (10)$$

Table 2 lists comparative results of various algorithms based on GO annotation, where the best values are italized. In Table 2, SC is the number of significant predicted complexes. That is, their p values are less than 0.01. Our MINE method achieves the highest proportion of significantly predicted complexes and p-score values among all algorithms. The p-score of MINE is 12.16, 18.41, 32.08, 48.38, and 20.20 % higher than that of CMC, COACH, RRW, SPICi, and ClusterONE, respectively. In addition, Table 2 indicates that RRW gets the highest proportion of significant complexes, while achieves a lower p-score values than ClusterONE because the p value of significant complexes predicted by ClusterONE are lower than RRW's. These results suggest that the complexes predicted by MINE had the most biological significance.

Effect of parameters on prediction performance

In MINE, we introduce a user-defined parameter WDT (weighted density threshold) to discover density subgraphs with high cohesion to form candidate complexes. To investigate the effect of parameter WDT on performance of MINE, we evaluate the prediction accuracy in terms of precision, recall, and F-measure by setting different values of WDT, ranging from 0 to 1. Figure 6 shows that the performance of our method fluctuates

Table 2 The comparison of various methods in terms of function enrichment

Algorithms	PC	SC	Proportion (%)	p-score
MINE	*606*	*499*	*82.34*	*11.9*
CMC	235	187	79.57	10.61
COACH	902	676	74.94	10.05
RRW	250	191	76.40	9.01
SPICi	574	262	45.64	8.02
ClusterONE	371	235	63.34	9.9

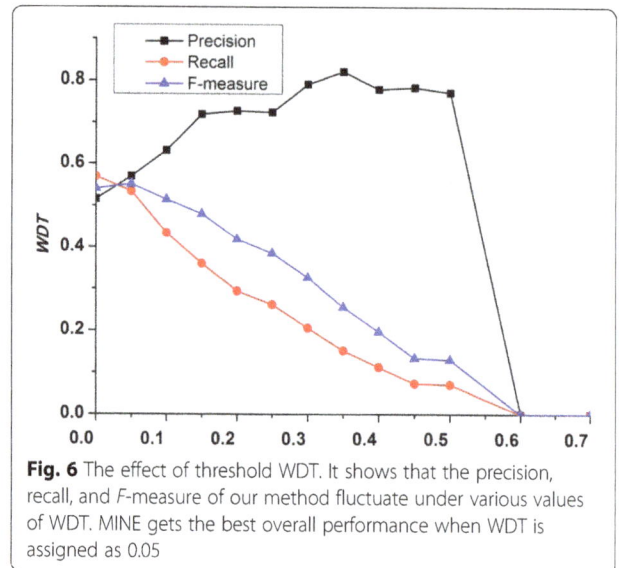

Fig. 6 The effect of threshold WDT. It shows that the precision, recall, and *F*-measure of our method fluctuate under various values of WDT. MINE gets the best overall performance when WDT is assigned as 0.05

under various values of WDT. Figure 6 clearly indicates that MINE gets the best performance when WDT is assigned as 0.05.

Results using Krogan data

We also performed MINE method on the Krogan PPI network. The precision, recall, and F-measure of each algorithm based on Krogan data are shown in Fig. 7.

Figure 7 indicates that our method gets the best performance among all these methods in terms of precision, recall, and F-measure. The F-measure of our method is 0.5, which is 68.63, 33.52, 45.53, 69.71, and 47.73 % higher than that of CMC, COACH, RRW, SPICi, and ClusterONE, respectively.

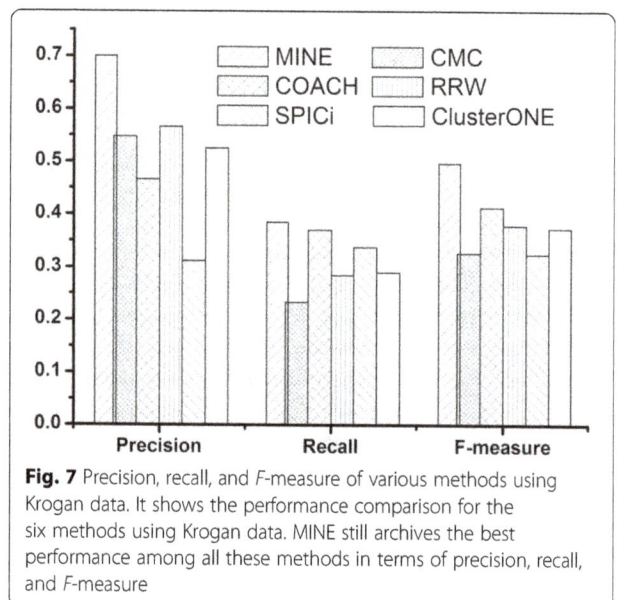

Fig. 7 Precision, recall, and *F*-measure of various methods using Krogan data. It shows the performance comparison for the six methods using Krogan data. MINE still archives the best performance among all these methods in terms of precision, recall, and *F*-measure

Conclusions

In this paper, we have constructed a multi-relationship protein interaction network (MPIN) by integrating PPI network topology with GO annotation information. For a pair of proteins in the MPIN, there exists more than one kind of interactions between them. To test the effectiveness of the MPIN, we have developed a novel method named MINE to predict protein complexes. MINE first decomposes the MPIN into four single relationship networks. Then, MINE visits four networks in turn for predicting protein complexes with high cohesion and low coupling. The results of experiments based on yeast PPI networks show that not only MINE achieves higher prediction accuracy than other existing methods but also majority of complexes predicted by MINE possess high biological significance. All results have proved that the constructed MPIN is useful for predicting protein complexes.

Competing interests
The authors declare that they have no competing interests.

Authors' contributions
XYL and BHZ obtained the protein-protein interaction data, gene ontology annotation data, and protein complex data. XYL and BHZ designed the new method MINE and analyzed the results. XYL and BHZ drafted the manuscript together. JW, FXW, and YP participated in revising the draft. All authors have read and approved the manuscript.

Acknowledgements
This work is supported in part by the National Natural Science Foundation of China under Grant No. 61472133, No. 31560317, and No. 61428209 and the Program for New Century Excellent Talents in University under Grant NCET-12-0547.

Declarations
Publication of this article has been funded by the National Natural Science Foundation of China (No. 61472133).
This article has been published as part of *Human Genomics* Volume 10 Supplement 2, 2016: From genes to systems genomics: human genomics. The full contents of the supplement are available online at http://humgenomics.biomedcentral.com/articles/supplements/volume-10-supplement-2.

Author details
[1]School of Information Science and Engineering, Central South University, Changsha 410083, China. [2]Department of Information and Computing Science, Changsha University, Changsha 410003, China. [3]Department of Mechanical Engineering and Division of Biomedical Engineering, University of Saskatchewan, Saskatoon, SK S7N 5A9, Canada. [4]Department of Computer Science, Georgia State University, Atlanta, GA 30302-4110, USA.

References
1. Ito T, Chiba T, Ozawa R, Yoshida M, Hattori M, Sakaki Y. A comprehensive two-hybrid analysis to explore the yeast protein interactome. Proc Natl Acad Sci. 2001;98:4569–74.
2. Rigaut G, Shevchenko A, Rutz B, Wilm M, Mann M, Séraphin B. A generic protein purification method for protein complex characterization and proteome exploration. Nat Biotechnol. 1999;17:1030–2.
3. Ho Y, Gruhler A, Heilbut A, et al. Systematic identification of protein complexes in Saccharomyces cerevisiae by mass spectrometry. Nature. 2002;415:180–3.
4. Peng W, Li M, Chen L, and Wang L S. Predicting protein functions by using unbalanced random walk algorithm on three biological networks. IEEE/ACM Transactions on Computational Biology and Bioinformatics. doi 10.1109/TCBB.2015.2394314.
5. Li M, Lu Y, Niu Z B, Wu F X. United complex centrality for identification of essential proteins from PPI networks. IEEE/ACM Transactions on Computational Biology and Bioinformatics. doi: 10.1109/TCBB.2015.2394487.
6. Li M, Lu Y, Wang JX, Wu FX, Pan Y. A topology potential-based method for identifying essential proteins from PPI networks. IEEE/ACM Trans Comput Biol Bioinform. 2015;12(2):372–83.
7. Ren J, Wang JX, Li M, Wu FX. Discovering essential proteins based on PPI network and protein complex. Int J Data Min Bioinform. 2015;12(1):24–43.
8. Li M, Zheng RQ, Zhang HH, Wang JX, Pan Y. Effective identification of essential proteins based on priori knowledge, network topology and gene expressions. Methods. 2014;67(3):325–33.
9. Li M, Wang JX, Wang H, Pan Y. Identification of essential proteins from weighted protein interaction networks. J Bioinform Comput Biol. 2013;11(3):1341002.
10. Wang JX, Li M, Wang H, Pan Y. Identification of essential proteins based on edge clustering coefficient. IEEE/ACM Trans Comput Biol Bioinform. 2012;9(4):1070–80.
11. Tang Y, Li M, Wang JX, Pan Y, Wu FX. CytoNCA: a cytoscape plugin for centrality analysis and evaluation of biological networks. BioSystems. 2015;127:67–72.
12. Bader G, Hogue C. An automated method for finding molecular complexes in large protein interaction networks. BMC Bioinformatics. 2003;4:2.
13. Enright AJ, Dongen SV, Ouzounis CA. An efficient algorithm for large-scale detection of protein families. Nucleic Acids Res. 2002;30:1575–84.
14. Shih YK, Parthasarathy S. Identifying functional modules in interaction networks through overlapping Markov clustering. Bioinformatics. 2012;28:i473–9.
15. Liu G, Wong L, Chua HN. Complex discovery from weighted PPI networks. Bioinformatics. 2009;25:1891–7.
16. Macropol K, Can T, Singh AK. RRW: repeated random walks on genome-scale protein networks for local cluster discovery. BMC Bioinformatics. 2009;10:283.
17. Jiang P, Singh M. SPICi: a fast clustering algorithm for large biological networks. Bioinformatics. 2010;26:1105–11.
18. Wang JX, Li M, Chen JE, Pan Y. A fast hierarchical clustering algorithm for functional modules discovery in protein interaction networks. IEEE/ACM Trans Comput Biol Bioinform. 2011;8(3):607–20.
19. Li M, Wang JX, Chen JE, Cai Z, Chen G. Identifying the overlapping complexes in protein interaction networks. Int J Data Min Bioinform (IJDMB). 2010;4(1):91–108.
20. Li M, Chen J, Wang J, et al. Modifying the DPClus algorithm for identifying protein complexes based on new topological structures. BMC Bioinformatics. 2008;9(1):398.
21. Nepusz T, Yu H, Paccanaro A. Detecting overlapping protein complexes in protein-protein interaction networks. Nature Methods. 2012;9:471–5.
22. Wang JX, Zhong JC, Chen G, et al. ClusterViz: a Cytoscape APP for clustering analysis of biological network. IEEE/ACM Trans Comput Biol Bioinform. 2015;12(4):815–22.
23. Gavin A, Aloy P, Grandi P, et al. Proteome survey reveals modularity of the yeast cell machinery. Nature. 2006;440:631–6.
24. Wu M, Li X, Kwoh CK, Ng S. A core-attachment based method to detect protein complexes in PPI networks. BMC Bioinformatics. 2009;10:169.
25. Leung HC, Xiang Q, Yiu SM, Y CF. Predicting protein complexes from PPI data: a core-attachment approach. J Comput Biol. 2009;16:133–44.
26. Srihari S, Ning K, Leong HW. MCL-CAw: a refinement of MCL for detecting yeast complexes from weighted PPI networks by incorporating core-attachment structure. BMC Bioinformatics. 2010;11:504.
27. Zhao B, Wang J, Li M, et al. Detecting protein complexes based on uncertain graph model. IEEE/ACM Trans Comput Biol Bioinform. 2014;11:486–97.
28. Peng W, Wang J, Zhao B, et al. Identification of protein complexes using weighted PageRank-Nibble algorithm and core-attachment structure. IEEE/ACM Trans Comput Biol Bioinform. 2014;12:179–92.
29. Wu M, Li X, Kwoh C, et al. Discovery of protein complexes with core-attachment structures from Tandem Affinity Purification (TAP) data. J Comput Biol. 2012;19:1027–42.

30. Tang X, Wang J, Liu B, et al. A comparison of the functional modules identified from time course and static PPI network data. BMC Bioinformatics. 2011;12(1):339.

31. Wang J, Peng X, Li M, et al. Construction and application of dynamic protein interaction network based on time course gene expression data. Proteomics. 2013;13:301–12.

32. Li M, Wu X, Wang J, et al. Towards the identification of protein complexes and functional modules by integrating PPI network and gene expression data. BMC Bioinformatics. 2012;13:109.

33. Li M, Chen W, Wang J, et al. Identifying dynamic protein complexes based on gene expression profiles and PPI networks. BioMed Res Int. 2014;2014 (375262):10.

34. Zhao J, Hu X, He T, et al. An edge-based protein complex identification algorithm with gene co-expression data. IEEE Trans Nanobioscience. 2014; 13:80–8.

35. Fan W, Yeung KH. Similarity between community structures of different online social networks and its impact on underlying community detection. Commun Nonlinear Sci Numer Simul. 2015;20:1015–25.

36. Zhao BH, Wang JX, Li M, et al. Prediction of essential proteins based on overlapping essential modules. IEEE Transactions on NanoBioscience. 2014;13:415–24.

37. Xenarios X et al. DIP: the database of interacting proteins. Nucleic Acids Res. 2000;28:289–91.

38. Krogan N et al. Global landscape of protein complexes in the yeast Saccharomyces cerevisiae. Nature. 2006;440:637–43.

39. Pu S, Wong J, Turner B, et al. Up-to-date catalogues of yeast protein complexes. Nucleic Acids Res. 2009;37:825–31.

40. Maere S, Heymans K, Kuiper M. BiNGO: a Cytoscape plugin to assess overrepresentation ontology categories in biological network. Bioinformatics. 2005;21:3448–9.

41. Shannon P et al. Cytoscape: a software environment for integrated models of biomolecular interaction networks. Genome Res. 2003;13:2498–504.

The genetic structure of the Belgian population

Jimmy Van den Eynden[1,2]* (iD), Tine Descamps[1], Els Delporte[1], Nancy H. C. Roosens[1], Sigrid C. J. De Keersmaecker[1],
Vanessa De Wit[1], Joris Robert Vermeesch[3], Els Goetghebeur[4], Jean Tafforeau[1], Stefaan Demarest[1],
Marc Van den Bulcke[1] and Herman Van Oyen[1,5]*

Abstract

Background: National and international efforts like the 1000 Genomes Project are leading to increasing insights in the genetic structure of populations worldwide. Variation between different populations necessitates access to population-based genetic reference datasets. These data, which are important not only in clinical settings but also to potentiate future transitions towards a more personalized public health approach, are currently not available for the Belgian population.

Results: To obtain a representative genetic dataset of the Belgian population, participants in the 2013 National Health Interview Survey (NHIS) were invited to donate saliva samples for DNA analysis. DNA was isolated and single nucleotide polymorphisms (SNPs) were determined using a genome-wide SNP array of around 300,000 sites, resulting in a high-quality dataset of 189 samples that was used for further analysis. A principal component analysis demonstrated the typical European genetic constitution of the Belgian population, as compared to other continents. Within Europe, the Belgian population could be clearly distinguished from other European populations. Furthermore, obvious signs from recent migration were found, mainly from Southern Europe and Africa, corresponding with migration trends from the past decades. Within Belgium, a small north-west to south-east gradient in genetic variability was noted, with differences between Flanders and Wallonia.

Conclusions: This is the first study on the genetic structure of the Belgian population and its regional variation. The Belgian genetic structure mirrors its geographic location in Europe with regional differences and clear signs of recent migration.

Keywords: Genetic variability, Population genomics, Public health genomics

Background

After the completion of the Human Genome Project in 2003, international efforts were initiated to map human genetic variation between populations. This variation has been described for 26 populations worldwide via the 1000 Genomes Project [1, 2]. While this is a valuable resource for studying global genetic variation, both the number of samples per population and the total number of populations studied are relatively low. To gain sufficient statistical power and avoid false positives/negatives due to unmatched control populations in genotype-phenotype association

studies, population-based genetic reference data are required from more specific and extended populations [3]. To address this, population-based whole genome sequencing initiatives have been performed at the national level throughout Europe [4–7]. From these genetic population studies, it has become clear that there is a strong correlation between the geographical location and the genetic structure of different populations [8, 9], also at the more regional level (e.g., along a north-south axis in the Netherlands) [6, 7, 9, 10]. Currently, this genetic information is not available for the Belgian population.

Therefore, a population-based cross-sectional study, called BelPHG-21 (Belgian Public Health Genomics in the twenty-first century), was organized that aims at describing the genetic variability in the Belgian population and relating

* Correspondence:
jimmy.van.den.eynden@gu.se; herman.vanoyen@wiv-isp.be
[1]Scientific Institute of Public Health, Brussels, Belgium
Full list of author information is available at the end of the article

this variability to several indicators of health and disease to anticipate a future transition towards precision public health. To accomplish this, the BelPHG-21 study was organized in the context of the 2013 Belgian National Health Interview Survey (NHIS). The NHIS is a population-based survey that has been periodically organized since 1997. It has the purpose to assess the health status and its distribution in the population and to describe the association of this health status with its main determinants [11].

Here, we report on the BelPHG-21 results related to the genetic structure of the Belgian population. By incorporating NHIS information about the study subject's residence and parental country of birth, we demonstrate small but clear genetic differences between different regions and illustrate how the population's genetic structure is shaped by recent migration waves.

Results

Factors determining consent for former NHIS participants to participate in the BelPHG-21 population genetic study

To study the genetic structure and variability in the Belgian population, a subset of participants from the most recent NHIS, conducted on 10,829 inhabitants in 2013 [12], was invited to donate saliva samples for DNA analysis (Fig. 1). From the invited subsample of 1468 individuals, 210 (14%) consented and submitted saliva samples for DNA analysis. Using the NHIS information related to demographics, education, employment, income, health behavior, lifestyle characteristics, physical and social environment, and wellbeing characteristics, we applied a predictive weighted binomial regression analysis to identify the factors that determined consent to participate in this study. This resulted in a model containing four variables (smoking behavior, education, age, and region of residence) (Table 1). The odds for consent were higher in non-smokers (and higher in former smokers than never smokers), higher age, and higher educational attainment. Furthermore, the likelihood for consent was also higher in the Flemish Region compared to the other regions.

DNA sampling from the Belgian population

DNA was extracted from saliva samples obtained from 210 consenting participants. Three of these samples contained insufficient saliva, while the DNA concentration of eight other samples was considered too low for downstream analysis (Fig. 1). From the remaining 199 samples, single nucleotide polymorphisms (SNPs) at ± 300,000 sites were measured using the whole genome scanning Illumina HumanCytoSNP-12 microarray. Microarray results from 10 samples were excluded due to insufficient call rates (i.e., lower than 0.6), resulting in 189 samples that were used for further analysis. These samples were genotyped using the hg19 human

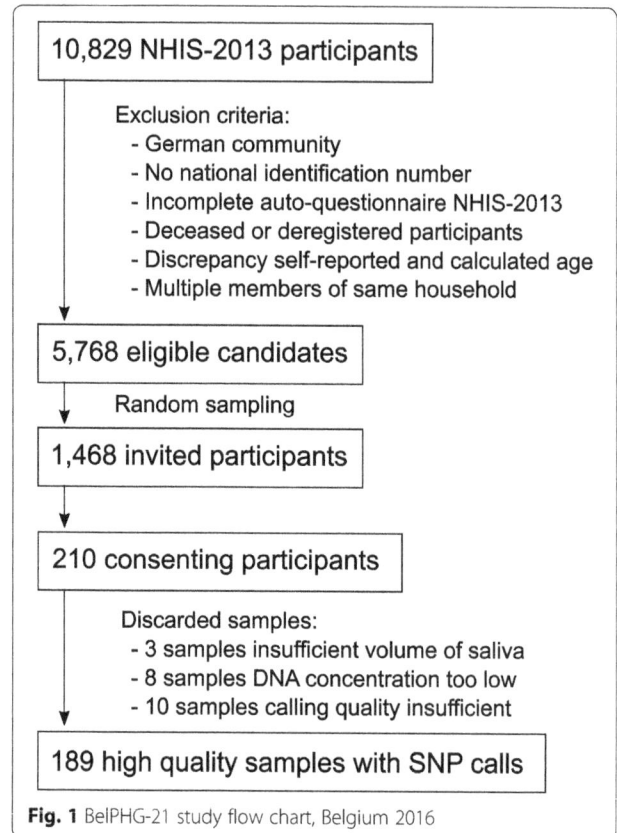

Fig. 1 BelPHG-21 study flow chart, Belgium 2016

genome build as a reference and variant allele frequencies were calculated for a total number of 261,079 SNPs for which genotyping information was available (Additional file 1: Table S1).

Belgium is composed of three different geographical regions: Flanders, Brussels, and Wallonia. The 189 samples that were used for analysis in this study were donated by volunteers in all three regions: 98 from Flanders, 62 from Wallonia, and 29 from Brussels

Table 1 Variables predicting consent, BelPHG-21 study, Belgium 2016

Variable	Parameter	OR	95% CI OR
Smoking habits (ref "Smoker")	Former smoker	2.21	[1.38, 3.62]
	Never smoker	1.38	[0.92, 2.15]
Age	Age (years)	1.02	[1.01, 1.02]
Residence (ref "Flanders")	Brussels' region	0.45	[0.24, 0.77]
	Walloon region	0.58	[0.41, 0.80]
Education (ref "No diploma")	Lower secondary	2.29	[1.38, 7.02]
	Higher secondary	4.13	[2.12, 9.50]
	Higher	6.66	[3.40, 15.44]
	Not applicable	5.31	[2.25, 14.06]

A weighted binomial regression analysis to predict consent contained four variables (smoking habits, age, residence, and education). For each parameter, the odds ratio (OR) and 95% CI interval are given

(Fig. 2). These numbers are proportional to the population size of the respective regions with an overrepresentation from the Brussels region (15.3, 17.3, and 24.7 samples per million inhabitants for Flanders, Wallonia, and Brussels respectively) (Additional file 2: Table S2). This oversampling of the Brussels region is related to the way the NHIS was constructed [11]. Similarly, the distribution of these samples was relatively proportional to the population size from each of 10 provinces in Belgium with a variation from 11.3 to 26.7 samples per million inhabitants (Fig. 2 and Additional file 2: Table S2).

From the samples used for analysis, 35 (18.5%) were donated by an individual with non-Belgian roots (here defined as an individual whose mother and/or father was born outside Belgium, as registered in NHIS). These individuals mainly originated from neighboring countries (16), Southern Europe (7), and Africa (6). Proportionally, the highest numbers of non-Belgian samples were obtained from individuals living in Brussels (11/29 samples; 37.9%), followed by Wallonia (18/62; 29.0%), and Flanders (6/98; 6.1%) (Fig. 2). These numbers are representative for the current structure of Belgian population, with important migration waves in the past 50 years, mainly from Southern Europe and Northern Africa, and with the highest immigration numbers found in the Brussels region [13].

The Belgian population is a typical European population with genetic signals of recent migration from the African continent

We first compared the genetic structure of the Belgian population with other populations worldwide. To restrict this analysis to the most informative and independent SNPs, only SNPs located on autosomes with a minor allele frequency of at least 5%, less than 2% missing values, and a linkage disequilibrium lower than 0.2 were used for structural comparison. These filtering criteria resulted in a selection of 47,802 SNPs. These SNPs were used for a principal component (PC) analysis using continental population data (i.e., African, American, South Asian, East Asian, and European populations) from the 1000 Genomes Project [1, 2, 14]. The main variance was captured by the first four PCs (10.4%, Additional file 3: Figure S1a). Using the first two PCs, which capture 5.2 and 3.2% of the total variance respectively, an expected and clear separation was observed between the different continental populations, with the largest differences between African, East Asian, and European populations (Fig. 3). By applying this PC model on the Belgian SNP genotype data, 184/189 samples were perfectly mapped on the European population. The remaining five samples were mapped towards or on the African population, and for four of these samples, an African origin was indeed confirmed in the NHIS data (Fig. 3 and Additional file 3: Figure S1b). These

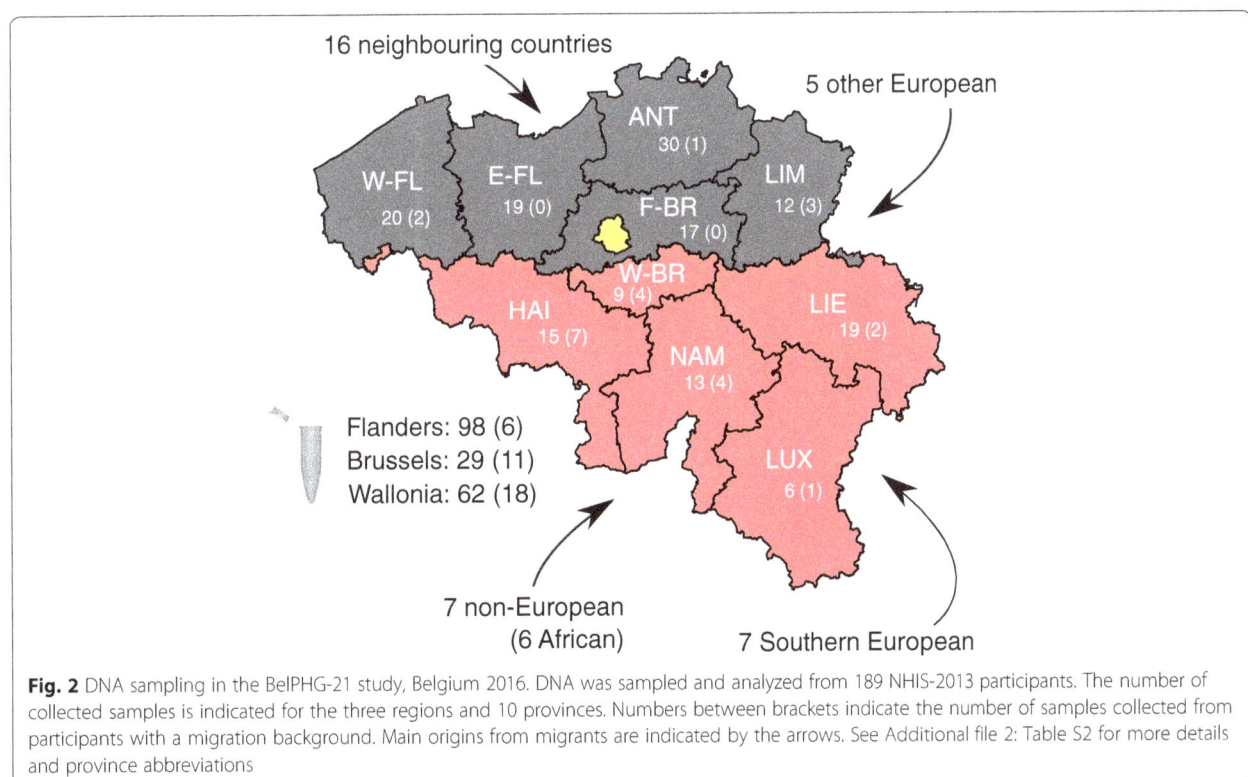

Fig. 2 DNA sampling in the BelPHG-21 study, Belgium 2016. DNA was sampled and analyzed from 189 NHIS-2013 participants. The number of collected samples is indicated for the three regions and 10 provinces. Numbers between brackets indicate the number of samples collected from participants with a migration background. Main origins from migrants are indicated by the arrows. See Additional file 2: Table S2 for more details and province abbreviations

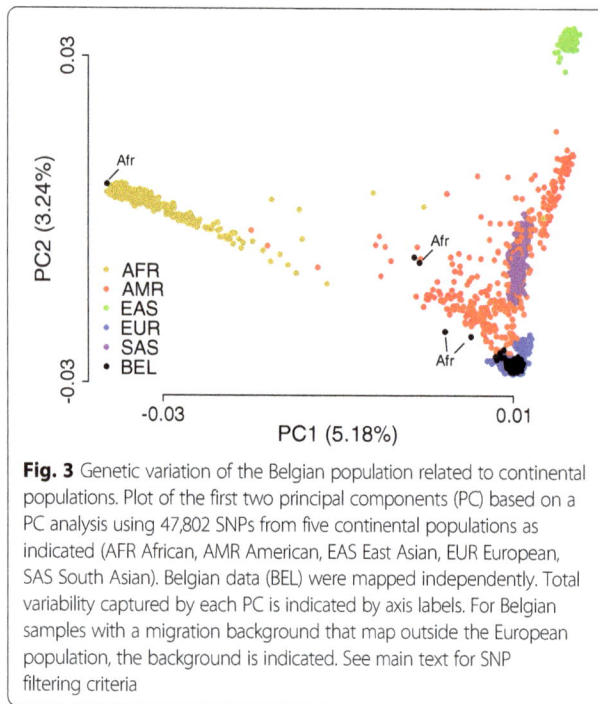

Fig. 3 Genetic variation of the Belgian population related to continental populations. Plot of the first two principal components (PC) based on a PC analysis using 47,802 SNPs from five continental populations as indicated (AFR African, AMR American, EAS East Asian, EUR European, SAS South Asian). Belgian data (BEL) were mapped independently. Total variability captured by each PC is indicated by axis labels. For Belgian samples with a migration background that map outside the European population, the background is indicated. See main text for SNP filtering criteria

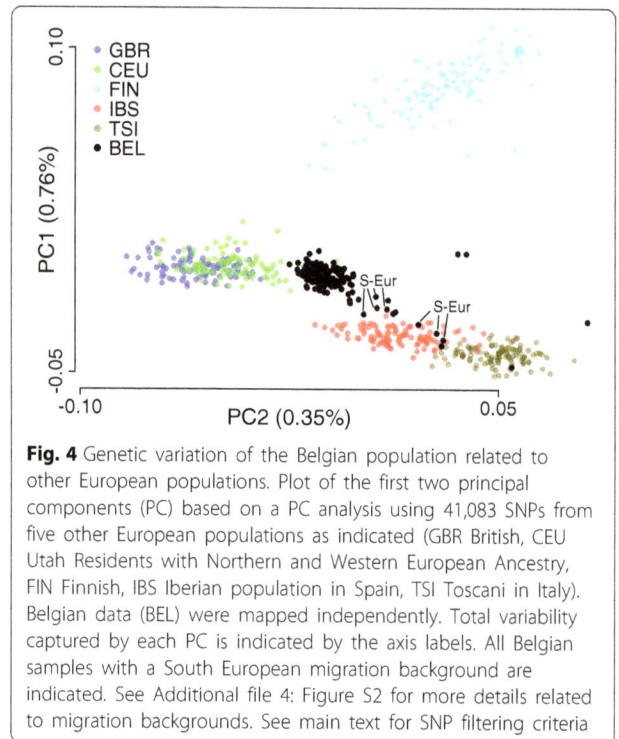

Fig. 4 Genetic variation of the Belgian population related to other European populations. Plot of the first two principal components (PC) based on a PC analysis using 41,083 SNPs from five other European populations as indicated (GBR British, CEU Utah Residents with Northern and Western European Ancestry, FIN Finnish, IBS Iberian population in Spain, TSI Toscani in Italy). Belgian data (BEL) were mapped independently. Total variability captured by each PC is indicated by the axis labels. All Belgian samples with a South European migration background are indicated. See Additional file 4: Figure S2 for more details related to migration backgrounds. See main text for SNP filtering criteria

findings show that the genetic structure of the Belgian population is a typical European population with signals of recent migration from the African continent.

The genetic structure of the Belgian population mirrors its geographical location in Europe

Our next goal was to examine how the Belgian population differs from other European populations. After a similar SNP filtering strategy as described above, the PC analysis was repeated using the European populations from the 1000 Genomes Project. Only the first two PCs were informative for a rather small variance of 0.76 and 0.35% respectively (Additional file 4: Figure S2a). As expected, the PC plot mimics European geography with a clear separation between Finnish, British, and South European populations. In agreement with this geographical orientation, most of the Belgian population mapped between the British and Southern European populations. Few samples mapped closer or within the South European populations, and for seven of these, a South European origin could indeed be confirmed (Fig. 4 and Additional file 4: Figure S2b). These data show the uniqueness of the Belgian genetic structure in Europe with geographically related differences with the other European populations.

Minor genetic differences between Flanders and Wallonia

To examine potential differences between the three main geographic regions in Belgium, we excluded the 35 samples with non-Belgian origins and indicated regional information on the European PC model (Fig. 5). This PC analysis demonstrates a minor but clear genetic substructure in the

Belgian population along a north-west to south-east geographic gradient, with Flemish inhabitants mapping in the north-west, Walloon inhabitants mapping in the south-east, and individuals from Brussels in between. A similar analysis based on sample origin information from the 10 different provinces confirmed these geographic-related genetic differences (Additional file 5: Figure S3).

To quantify the genetic differences between the three Belgian regions and compare them with other European

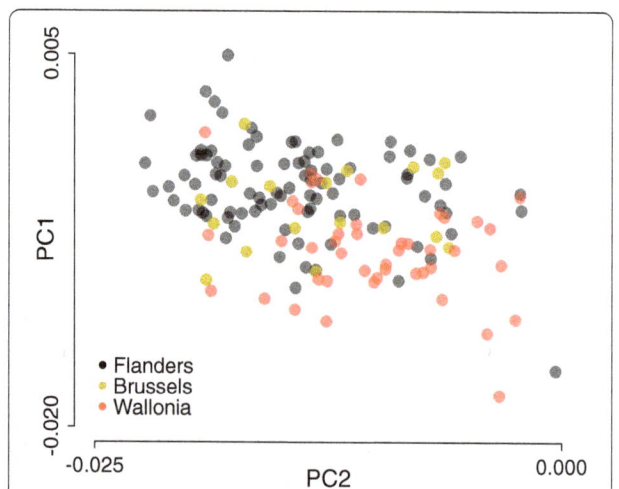

Fig. 5 Regional genetic variation within the Belgian population. Belgian samples were mapped on the European PC model (41,083 SNPs) and colored based on the region of inhabitance as indicated

populations, we calculated fixation indices (i.e., Fst values). Fst is a metric with values between 0 and 1 that is used to measure genetic distance between populations, in which high pairwise values indicate large population differentiation and vice versa. Fst values between the three Belgian regions were very small (between 1.8 and 2.5e–04) and smaller than with any other European population (Fst 3.2e–04 or higher) (Table 2), confirming the results from the PC analyses.

Finally, we correlated the variant allele frequencies of the Belgian population with other European populations. This analysis also allowed us to compare the Belgian population to the geographically and linguistically related population of the Netherlands, for which allele frequency data, but no genotyping data, are publicly available (Genome of the Netherlands project, GoNl [6]). As expected, and similar to the PC and Fst analysis, extremely good correlations were found with all European populations (Pearson correlation coefficients of 0.972 and higher). The best correlation was found with the GoNl data (Pearson correlation coefficient of 0.992; Additional file 6: Figure S4).

In summary, these data show minor but clear genetic differences between the different regions in Belgium with a north-west to south-east geographical correlation. However, these differences were smaller than with any other European population.

Discussion

The BelPHG-21 study aims at developing an approach to estimate genetic variability at the level of the Belgian population and exploring how this genetic information can be associated with information collected via NHIS questionnaires. Here, we reported on the genetic structure of the Belgian population using ± 300,000 genome-wide SNPs, derived from saliva DNA sampled from 189 participants from the latest NHIS (2013). This is the first study on the genetic structure of the Belgian population and its regional differences. The Belgian population was found to be a typical European population with signals of recent migration from the African continent. Within Europe, the Belgian population has its unique properties,

which clearly mirrors the geographic orientation and again with signs of recent migration from Southern Europe. While minor genetic differences were observed between the different Belgian regions, these were smaller than with any other population studied.

The linkage possibilities to health, demographic, and related data from the NHIS provide a unique opportunity to study the different factors that determine participation in a genetic study and to better understand public willingness to participate in population genetic research. Consent rates to participate in this study were rather low (14%). Related studies that recruited people with previous participation in health research reported on variable consent rates between 21 and 85% [15–18]. The 3-year time gap between the NHIS and the second contact, inviting participation in the BelPHG-21 study, may be a reason for the relatively low participation rate. Furthermore, subjects were contacted only by an invitation letter (and reminder). We noted regional differences in the consent rate, a higher consent for non-smokers and a positive association with age and education level. The higher likelihood of educated people to give consent is in agreement with other studies [19–21]. The correlation with age is more ambiguous, with reports of both younger age as well as older age being associated with lower consent [15, 20, 22]. The observation of smokers to be less likely to provide consent is in contradiction to other studies [23]. However, in our study, the difference was attributed to a higher consent rate for former smokers than for current smokers, while no significant difference was observed between current smokers and never smokers, indicating a more complex association with smoking status.

The close mirroring of population genetic variation with geography is a well-known phenomenon that has been described at the European level previously [8, 9]. Novembre et al. described a geographical map of Europe that arose naturally as an efficient PCA-based two-dimensional summary of genetic variation in European individuals from different countries (including 43 Belgians) [8]. This has been shown not only on national, but also on regional levels,

Table 2 Fst pairwise genetic distances between Belgian regional and other European populations, BelPHG-21 study, Belgium 2016

	GBR	FIN	IBS	CEU	TSI	Flanders	Wallonia	Brussels
GBR	0							
FIN	6.7e–03	0						
IBS	2.4e–03	1.0e–02	0					
CEU	3.2e–04	6.2e–03	2.2e–03	0				
TSI	3.7e–03	1.1e–02	1.5e–03	3.3e–03	0			
Flanders	6.5e–04	6.7e–03	1.9e–03	3.2e–04	2.7e–03	0		
Wallonia	7.1e–04	7.1e–03	1.4e–03	4.1e–04	2.1e–03	2.5e–04	0	
Brussels	6.5e–04	7.0e–03	1.8e–03	4.3e–04	2.5e–03	1.8e–04	1.8e–04	0

as exemplified by genetic substructures that were observed in Sweden [10, 24], Finland [7, 25], the Netherlands [6], and several other European countries [9]. While this mirroring of the Belgian genetic structure with its geographical orientation in Europe was expected, it is quite remarkable to see the same phenomenon at regional and to a lesser extent even at provincial levels in a small country like Belgium.

Belgium is a country of immigration, with substantial labor-related migration waves after the Second World War [13]. This is reflected in this study, in which 18.5% of the samples originated from individuals with a migration background. Apart from the expected origin from neighboring countries, the most frequent migration backgrounds were South European and African, in agreement with migration data. This non-Belgian origin was clearly reflected in the genetic structure of the Belgian population. Information on migration background was derived from NHIS data and based on to the country of birth of the parents of the study participant. While this study demonstrated the usefulness of this type of NHIS-related information, there are some limitations. First, the information is limited to the first generation only (parents). This likely explains why one individual with a clear non-European genetic background was not found to have a migration background based on our criteria, which is unlikely. Secondly, there is also a risk of false positive migration findings as country of birth does not necessarily imply the individual (or his parents) originated in that country.

The NHIS contains information related to health, lifestyle, environment, etc. [11]. Therefore, linking genetic information to NHIS data has great potential for genome-wide association studies. While the current sample size (189) is rather limited, we will use the experience gathered in this study to set up a larger genetic study linked to the next NHIS (2018) where we aim to sequence the entire genome from a representative sample of ± 1000 individuals from the Belgian population using whole genome sequencing techniques. This genetic epidemiology study will also give a concrete idea about the expected number of harmful variants in the genome of a typical Belgian individual, including the prevalence of several genetic disease carriers. Results from these studies will be an invaluable resource in the transition towards precision public health, focusing on subsets of the population at increased risk, rather than on the entire population.

Conclusions

This is the first study on the genetic structure of the Belgian population and its regional variation. The Belgian population is a typical European population with minor but clear differences between the regions and clear signs of recent migration.

Methods
BelPHG-21 study design

The BelPHG-21 study is a cross-sectional population-based study, conducted in 2016. The study population was selected from the participants of the most recent (2013) NHIS. Persons from the German community or with a missing national identification number were excluded for logistic reasons. Only one member per household was included, and the participants that did not complete the auto-questionnaire part of the NHIS in 2013 (which contains information on health, lifestyle, and environment), that were deceased, deregistered or with a discrepancy between self-reported and calculated age were excluded. From the resulting 5768 eligible candidates, a random subsample of 1468 individuals was invited to participate in the BelPHG-21 study. Individuals were invited via postal mail. They received an invitation letter with all the information on the BelPHG-21 study as well as informed consent forms to return in case of participation. Individuals that consented to participate in the study were subsequently sent a saliva sample collection kit (Oragene® saliva collection device (OG-500, DNA Genotek Inc. Ottawa, Canada)) accompanied by an information letter, a user manual for sample collection, a safety bag, and a pre-paid and UN3373-labeled bubble. Each package complied with the guidance on regulations for the transport of infectious substances. All communication with study participants (consent, sampling kits) was performed by a trusted third party (Belgian Federal Service of Internal Affairs) that was not involved in the downstream research in any way. They submitted the received samples to the BelPHG-21 research team and provided linking information to the NHIS database.

Sample preparation and SNP array

Upon receipt of saliva samples by the BelPHG-21 research team, DNA was manually extracted from the total sample following the manufacturer's instructions (DNA Genotek, PD-PR-015 Issue 10/2015-01). DNA samples were quantified using UV absorbance, and SNPs at ± 300,000 sites were determined using the whole genome scanning 12-sample Illumina HumanCytoSNP-12v2.1 BeadChip according to the manufacturer's instructions. Images were captured on Cytoscan (Illumina), and data were primarily analyzed using Illumina's GenomeStudio software.

NHIS data

Information related to the study participants' residence (region and province), migration background, and a set of variables that could influence the consent rate was obtained from the NHIS-2013 database. A subject was considered to have a migration background when at least one of its parents was born outside of Belgium. The variables that were considered to potentially influence consent rates were the background characteristics (demographic information, education, employment, income), health behavior and lifestyle characteristics (substance abuse, nutritional status, physical activity), physical and social environment characteristics (housing, passive smoking), and health and wellbeing characteristics (chronic diseases, mental health, perceived health). Selection of the variables for the predictive model was conducted by stepwise-weighted binomial regression analysis. Survey weights were calculated based on age, gender, and region of residence.

Demographic and geographic data

Demographic data from the 2013 Belgian population were downloaded from Eurostat (http://ec.europa.eu/eurostat). Belgian geographic data were obtained using the BelgiumMaps.Statbel R package (available at http://www.datatailor.be/rcube/).

SNP data processing

Genotype calls were imported in R and converted in a *sample x SNP* matrix. Samples with genotyping call rates lower than 0.6 were excluded from further analysis. All genotypes were converted so that the reference allele always referred to the positive strand of the human genome build hg19. Genomic coordinates for all SNPs were retrieved from dbSNP Build 144 [26]. SNPs not present in dbSNP were excluded from further analysis. The R SNPRelate package [27] was used for downstream analysis (calculation of allele frequencies, principal component analysis, ...). Therefore, genotyping data were first converted in genomic data structure (gds) format.

Principal component analysis

A principal component (PC) analysis was performed using phase 3 data from 1000 genomes [2]. VCF and sample information data were downloaded from the 1000 genomes ftp site (ftp://ftp.1000genomes.ebi.ac.uk/vol1/ftp/release/20130502/), and genotype information from all SNPs overlapping with the BelPHG-21 study was extracted using the R VariantAnnotation package [28]. Belgian data were mapped independently on the PC model. The PC analysis was performed using the most informative SNPs by applying the following filtering criteria: (1) SNPs measured in all datasets, (2) lower than 2% missing values in both the 1000 genome dataset that was used to perform the PC analysis and the Belgian data, (3) only autosomes, (4) minor allele frequency higher than 5%, and (5) linkage disequilibrium lower than 0.2.

Variant allele frequency correlations

Correlations between variant allele frequencies (VAF) were determined using Pearson's correlation. Correlations were determined for SNPs after filtering using the higher mentioned criteria. Variant allele frequencies from the Genome of the Netherlands (GoNl) project were derived from the release 5 vcf files downloaded at https://molgenis26.target.rug.nl/downloads/gonl_public/variants/release5/.

Additional files

Additional file 1: Table S1. SNP variant allele frequencies of the Belgian population, BelPHG-21 study, Belgium 2016. Variant allele frequencies (VAF) for all SNPs were calculated with reference to the human genome build hg19 on all samples or after exclusion of samples with a foreign origin (indicated by tab names). Columns indicate SNP ids, chromosome, position, reference allele, variant allele, VAF, and frequencies of homozygous reference (AA), heterozygous (AB), and homozygous variant (BB) alleles respectively.

Additional file 2: Table S2. Population details of the samples analyzed in the BelPHG-21 study, Belgium 2016. Indication of the number of samples taken from NHIS-2013 participants in each region and province, total number of inhabitants in 2013, number of samples taken per million inhabitants,

Additional file 3: Figure S1. Genetic variation of the Belgian population related to continental populations. Principal component (PC) analysis using 47,802 SNPs from five continental populations with mapping of the Belgian population. (a) Screeplot showing the variability captured by the first 10 PCs. (b) Pairwise plots of the first four PCs. Populations are indicated below the plot (AFR: African; AMR: American;

Additional file 4: Figure S2. Genetic variation of the Belgian population related to other European populations. Principal component (PC) analysis based on 41,083 SNPs from five different European populations (see Fig. 4 for details). (a) Screeplot showing the variability captured by the first 10 PCs. (b) PC plot of five European populations with mapping of the Belgian population and indication of their migration backgrounds. For visualization purposes, the other European populations

Additional file 5: Figure S3. Provincial genetic variation within the Belgian population. Belgian data were mapped on the European PC model (41,083 SNPs). Panels show plots of the first two PCs with indication of the province of inhabitance as indicated. The central map of Belgium shows the geographical location of each province. Panels with Flemish provinces are shown on top while Walloon province panels are

Additional file 6: Figure S4. Variant allele frequency correlations between Belgian and other populations. Variant allele frequencies (VAF) for all SNPs were calculated with reference to the human genome build hg19. Plots show the VAF of Belgian versus other continental (a) and European (b) populations. Pearson correlation coefficients are shown on top of each plot. For visualization purposes, only 1000 random points are

Abbreviations

PC: Principal component; SNP: Single nucleotide polymorphism; VAF: Variant allele frequency

Acknowledgements

We wish to thank all colleagues at the WIV-ISP that contributed to the accomplishment of the BelPHG-21 project. We acknowledge the support of the Platform Biotechnology and Bioinformatics, the ICT team, the dispatch center, and the communication team of the WIV-ISP as well as the Federal Service of Internal Affairs for the sample coding. Finally, we acknowledge all study subjects for their participation.

Funding

The BelPHG-21 study is funded by the Belgian Science Policy via the BRAIN.be (Belgian Research Action through Interdisciplinary Network) research program (BR/121/PI/BELPHG-21).

Authors' contributions

MVDB, JT, HVO, and VDW designed the BelPHG-21 study. JVdE analyzed the genomic data and wrote the manuscript. TD and EG did the statistical analysis related to factors determining consent rates. SDK and NR were responsible for the sample preparations and DNA extractions. JRV was responsible for the micro-array analysis. SD and JT performed the NHIS 2013 correlations. ED and VDW prepared the BelPHG-21 applications to ethical and privacy committees. All authors read and approved the final manuscript.

Competing interests

The authors declare that they have no competing interests.

Author details

[1]Scientific Institute of Public Health, Brussels, Belgium. [2]Department of Medical Biochemistry and Cell Biology, Institute of Biomedicine, The Sahlgrenska Academy, University of Gothenburg, Gothenburg, Sweden. [3]Laboratory of Cytogenetics and Genome Research, Department of Human Genetics, KU Leuven, Leuven, Belgium. [4]Department of Applied Mathematics, Computer Science and Statistics, Ghent University, Ghent, Belgium. [5]Department of Public Health, Ghent University, Ghent, Belgium.

References

1. Abecasis GR, Auton A, Brooks LD, MA DP, Durbin RM, Handsaker RE, Kang HM, Marth GT, McVean GA. An integrated map of genetic variation from 1,092 human genomes. Nature. 2012;491:56–65.
2. Auton A, Abecasis GR, Altshuler DM, Durbin RM, Abecasis GR, Bentley DR, Chakravarti A, Clark AG, Donnelly P, Eichler EE, Flicek P, Gabriel SB, Gibbs RA, Green ED, Hurles ME, Knoppers BM, Korbel JO, Lander ES, Lee C, Lehrach H, Mardis ER, Marth GT, McVean GA, Nickerson DA, Schmidt JP, Sherry ST, Wang J, Wilson RK, Gibbs RA, Boerwinkle E, et al. A global reference for human genetic variation. Nature. 2015;526:68–74.
3. Jiang Y, Epstein MP, Conneely KN. Assessing the impact of population stratification on association studies of rare variation. Hum Hered. 2013;76:28–35.
4. Ameur A, Dahlberg J, Olason P, Vezzi F, Karlsson R, Lundin P, Che H, Thutkawkorapin J, Kusalananda Kahari A, Dahlberg M, Viklund J, Hagberg J, Jareborg N, Jonasson I, Johansson A, Lundin S, Nilsson D, Nystedt B, Magnusson P, Gyllensten U. SweGen: a whole-genome map of genetic variability in a cross-section of the Swedish population. bioRxiv. 2016;
5. Gudbjartsson DF, Helgason H, Gudjonsson SA, Zink F, Oddson A, Gylfason A, Besenbacher S, Magnusson G, Halldorsson BV, Hjartarson E, Sigurdsson GT, Stacey SN, Frigge ML, Holm H, Saemundsdottir J, Helgadottir HT, Johannsdottir H, Sigfusson G, Thorgeirsson G, Sverrisson JT, Gretarsdottir S, Walters GB, Rafnar T, Thjodleifsson B, Bjornsson ES, Olafsson S, Thorarinsdottir H, Steingrimsdottir T, Gudmundsdottir TS, Theodors A, et al. Large-scale whole-genome sequencing of the Icelandic population. Nat Genet. 2015;47:435–44.
6. Genome of the Netherlands Consortium LC, Menelaou A, Pulit SL, van Dijk F, Palamara PF, Elbers CC, PBT N, Ye K, Guryev V, Kloosterman WP, Deelen P, Abdellaoui A, van Leeuwen EM, van Oven M, Vermaat M, Li M, JFJ L, Karssen LC, Kanterakis A, Amin N, Hottenga JJ, Lameijer E-W, Kattenberg M, Dijkstra M, Byelas H, van Setten J, van Schaik BDC, Bot J, Nijman IJ, Renkens I, et al. Whole-genome sequence variation, population structure and demographic history of the Dutch population. Nat Genet. 2014;46:818–25.
7. Jakkula E, Rehnström K, Varilo T, Pietiläinen OPH, Paunio T, Pedersen NL, de Faire U, Järvelin M-R, Saharinen J, Freimer N, Ripatti S, Purcell S, Collins A, Daly MJ, Palotie A, Peltonen L. The genome-wide patterns of variation expose significant substructure in a founder population. Am J Hum Genet. 2008;83:787–94.
8. Novembre J, Johnson T, Bryc K, Kutalik Z, Boyko AR, Auton A, Indap A, King KS, Bergmann S, Nelson MR, Stephens M, Bustamante CD. Genes mirror geography within Europe. Nature. 2008;456:98–101.
9. Nelis M, Esko T, Mägi R, Zimprich F, Zimprich A, Toncheva D, Karachanak S, Piskáčková T, Balaščák I, Peltonen L, Jakkula E, Rehnström K, Lathrop M, Heath S, Galan P, Schreiber S, Meitinger T, Pfeufer A, Wichmann H-E, Melegh B, Polgár N, Toniolo D, Gasparini P, D'Adamo P, Klovins J, Nikitina-Zake L, Kučinskas V, Kasnauskienė J, Lubinski J, Debniak T, et al. Genetic structure of Europeans: a view from the north–east. PLoS One. 2009;4:e5472.
10. Humphreys K, Grankvist A, Leu M, Hall P, Liu J, Ripatti S, Rehnström K, Groop L, Klareskog L, Ding B, Grönberg H, Xu J, Pedersen NL, Lichtenstein P, Mattingsdal M, Andreassen OA, O'Dushlaine C, Purcell SM, Sklar P, Sullivan PF, Hultman CM, Palmgren J, Magnusson PKE. The genetic structure of the Swedish population. PLoS One. 2011;6:e22547.
11. Demarest S, Van der Heyden J, Charafeddine R, Drieskens S, Gisle L, Tafforeau J. Methodological basics and evolution of the Belgian health interview survey 1997–2008. Arch Public Heal. 2013;71:24.
12. Drieskens S, Demarest S, D'Hoker N, Ortiz B, Tafforeau J. Is a Health Interview Survey an appropriate tool to assess domestic violence? Eur J Pub Health. 2017;27:903–9.
13. Martiniello M. Belgium, migration, 1946 to present. In: The encyclopedia of global human migration. Oxford: Blackwell Publishing Ltd; 2013.
14. Durbin RM, Altshuler DL, Durbin RM, Abecasis GR, Bentley DR, Chakravarti A, Clark AG, Collins FS, De La Vega FM, Donnelly P, Egholm M, Flicek P, Gabriel SB, Gibbs RA, Knoppers BM, Lander ES, Lehrach H, Mardis ER, McVean GA, Nickerson DA, Peltonen L, Schafer AJ, Sherry ST, Wang J, Wilson RK, Gibbs RA, Deiros D, Metzker M, Muzny D, Reid J, et al. A map of human genome variation from population-scale sequencing. Nature. 2010;467:1061–73.
15. Bogner HR, Wittink MN, Merz JF, Straton JB, Cronholm PF, Rabins PV, Gallo JJ. Personal characteristics of older primary care patients who provide a buccal swab for apolipoprotein E testing and banking of genetic material: the spectrum study. Community Genet. 2005;7:202–10.
16. Le Marchand L, Lum-jones A, Saltzman B, Marchand L, Visaya V, AMY N, Kolonel LN. Feasibility of collecting buccal cell DNA by mail in a cohort study feasibility of collecting buccal cell DNA by mail in a cohort study 1. Cancer Epidemiol Biomark Prev. 2001;10:701–3.
17. Cozier YC, Palmer JR, Rosenberg L. Comparison of methods for collection of DNA samples by mail in the Black Women's Health Study. Ann Epidemiol. 2004;14:117–22.
18. Moorman PG, Skinner CS, Evans JP, Newman B, Sorenson JR, Calingaert B, Susswein L, Crankshaw TS, Hoyo C, Schildkraut JM. Racial differences in enrolment in a cancer genetics registry. Cancer Epidemiol Biomark Prev. 2004;13:1349–54.
19. Audrain J, Tercyak KP, Goldman P, Bush A. Recruiting adolescents into genetic studies of smoking behavior recruiting adolescents into genetic studies of smoking behavior 1. Cancer Epidemiol Biomark Prev. 2002;11:249–52.
20. Sterling R, Henderson GE, Corbie-Smith G. Public willingness to participate in and public opinions about genetic variation research: a review of the literature. Am J Public Health. 2006;96:1971–8.
21. Royal C, Baffoe-Bonnie A, Kittles R, Powell I, Bennett J, Hoke G, Pettaway C, Weinrich S, Vijayakumar S, Ahagotu C, Mason T, Johnson E, Obeikwe M, Simpson C, Mejia R, Boykin W, Roberson P, Frost J, Faison-Smith L, Meegan C, Foster N, Furbert-Harris P, Carpten J, Bailey-Wilson J, Trent J, Berg K, Dunston G, Collins F. Recruitment experience in the first phase of the African American Hereditary Prostate Cancer (AAHPC) study. Ann Epidemiol. 2000;10(8 Suppl):S68–77.
22. Oliver JM, Slashinski MJ, Wang T, Kelly PA, Hilsenbeck SG, McGuire AL. Balancing the risks and benefits of genomic data sharing: genome research participants' perspectives. Public Health Genomics. 2012;15:106–14.
23. Audrain J, Tercyak KP, Goldman P, Bush A. Recruiting adolescents into genetic studies of smoking behavior. Cancer Epidemiol Biomark Prev. 2002;11:249–52.
24. Ameur A, Dahlberg J, Olason P, Vezzi F, Karlsson R, Martin M, Viklund J, Kähäri AK, Lundin P, Che H, Thutkawkorapin J, Eisfeldt J, Lampa S, Dahlberg M, Hagberg J, Jareborg N, Liljedahl U, Jonasson I, Johansson Å, Feuk L, Lundeberg J, Syvänen A-C, Lundin S, Nilsson D, Nystedt B, Magnusson PK, Gyllensten U. SweGen: a whole-genome data resource of genetic variability in a cross-section of the Swedish population. Eur J Hum Genet. 2017;25:1253–60.
25. McEvoy BP, Montgomery GW, McRae AF, Ripatti S, Perola M, Spector TD, Cherkas L, Ahmadi KR, Boomsma D, Willemsen G, Hottenga JJ, Pedersen NL, Magnusson PKE, Kyvik KO, Christensen K, Kaprio J, Heikkilä K, Palotie A, Widen E, Muilu J, Syvänen A-C, Liljedahl U, Hardiman O, Cronin S, Peltonen L, Martin NG, Visscher PM. Geographical structure and differential natural selection among North European populations. Genome Res. 2009;19:804–14.

26. Sherry ST, Ward MH, Kholodov M, Baker J, Phan L, Smigielski EM, Sirotkin K. dbSNP: the NCBI database of genetic variation. Nucleic Acids Res. 2001;29:308–11.

27. Zheng X, Levine D, Shen J, Gogarten SM, Laurie C, Weir BS. A high-performance computing toolset for relatedness and principal component analysis of SNP data. Bioinformatics. 2012;28:3326–8.

28. Obenchain V, Lawrence M, Carey V, Gogarten S, Shannon P, Morgan M. VariantAnnotation: a Bioconductor package for exploration and annotation of genetic variants. Bioinformatics. 2014;30:2076–8.

Single nucleotide polymorphisms in the angiogenic and lymphangiogenic pathways are associated with lymphedema caused by *Wuchereria bancrofti*

Linda Batsa Debrah[1,2†], Anna Albers[3†], Alexander Yaw Debrah[4], Felix F. Brockschmidt[5,6], Tim Becker[7], Christine Herold[7], Andrea Hofmann[3], Jubin Osei-Mensah[1], Yusif Mubarik[1], Holger Fröhlich[8], Achim Hoerauf[3*] and Kenneth Pfarr[3*]

Abstract

Background: Lymphedema (LE) is a chronic clinical manifestation of filarial nematode infections characterized by lymphatic dysfunction and subsequent accumulation of protein-rich fluid in the interstitial space—lymphatic filariasis. A number of studies have identified single nucleotide polymorphisms (SNPs) associated with primary and secondary LE. To assess SNPs associated with LE caused by lymphatic filariasis, a cross-sectional study of unrelated Ghanaian volunteers was designed to genotype SNPs in 285 LE patients as cases and 682 infected patients without pathology as controls. One hundred thirty-one SNPs in 64 genes were genotyped. The genes were selected based on their roles in inflammatory processes, angiogenesis/lymphangiogenesis, and cell differentiation during tumorigenesis.

Results: Genetic associations with nominal significance were identified for five SNPs in three genes: vascular endothelial growth factor receptor-3 (VEGFR-3) rs75614493, two SNPs in matrix metalloprotease-2 (MMP-2) rs1030868 and rs2241145, and two SNPs in carcinoembryonic antigen-related cell adhesion molecule-1 (CEACAM-1) rs8110904 and rs8111171. Pathway analysis revealed an interplay of genes in the angiogenic/lymphangiogenic pathways. Plasma levels of both MMP-2 and CEACAM-1 were significantly higher in LE cases compared to controls. Functional characterization of the associated SNPs identified genotype GG of CEACAM-1 as the variant influencing the expression of plasma concentration, a novel finding observed in this study.

Conclusion: The SNP associations found in the MMP-2, CEACAM-1, and VEGFR-3 genes indicate that angiogenic/lymphangiogenic pathways are important in LE clinical development.

Keywords: Lymphatic filariasis, Angiogenesis, Lymphangiogenesis, Single nucleotide polymorphisms, Genotypes

Background

Worldwide, more than 850,000 people live in areas endemic for *Wuchereria bancrofti*, *Brugia malayi*, and *Brugia timori* filial nematodes that cause lymphatic filariasis, a disease of severe morbidity [1]. Lymphatic disease symptoms are characterized by a cascade of events that leads to lymphatic dysfunction with associated fibrosis

[2]. Lymphedema (LE) and hydrocele are pathologies that can develop in *Wuchereria bancrofti* infected individuals. These clinical symptoms are usually preceded by dilated and tortious lymphatic vessels and scrotal lymphangiectasia [3, 4]. Of these two pathologies, LE is the most debilitating, affecting about 7% of the population in a lymphatic filariasis (LF) endemic community even though all individuals in the endemic area may be inoculated with the parasite and the majority (80%) may be infected [5, 6].

LE is a condition caused by the leakage of plasma from the arterial blood capillaries that is then trapped in the

* Correspondence: achim.hoeraruf@ukbonn.de; kenneth.pfarr@ukbonn.de
†Equal contributors
[3]Institute for Medical Microbiology, Immunology and Parasitology, University Hospital Bonn, Sigmund-Freud-Str. 25, 53127 Bonn, Germany
Full list of author information is available at the end of the article

soft tissues as a result of the dysfunction of the lymphatic vessel that originates from the infection with the filarial parasites *Wuchereria bancrofti* or *Brugia* spp. [7]. The global burden of LE in 2000 was 14.84 million [8]. After 13 years of treatment with ivermectin and albendazole or diethylcarbamazine, to eliminate the infection [1], and morbidity management procedures, there still remained 14.41 million LE cases [8], although an estimated 116–250 million DALYS have been averted within that period. This highlights the need for alternative strategies to current morbidity management procedures to help prevent or even ameliorate LE in the affected persons.

Individuals infected with lymphatic filariasis parasites do not show recognizable clinical symptoms. However, a third of those infected developed a clinical disease. What causes the expression of clinical disease is not well understood. Several reasons have been given to explain the differences in the cause(s) of heterogeneity in infection and disease of filarial infection. These include the immune interaction between the human host and the parasite [9–12], transmission potential of the mosquito vector [13], in utero exposure to parasite antigens [14, 15], and secondary bacterial/fungal infections superimposed on the lymphatic dysfunction [16].

The contribution of host immunogenetics to this heterogeneity has also been investigated, leading to the finding that susceptibility to infection, parasite load and pathology cluster in families [17–21], indicating an underlying genetic component is involved in the disease. Gene polymorphisms such as the variant Leu10Pro of transforming growth factor-β-1 (TGFβ-1) was found to be associated with both lack of microfilariae and differential microfilarial loads [22]. In that study, it was shown that the differential microfilaria loads and the lack of circulating microfilariae (Mf) in the blood exhibited by people in endemic areas have genetic propensity. Hence, some people in endemic areas may be infected with the adult worm but would have no Mf in the peripheral blood. Also, polymorphisms in TLR-2 (+ 597 > C, 1450T > C and –96 to –173 deletion) were found to be associated with higher asymptomatic bancroftian filariasis [23]. Association has also been found in the HH variant of Chitinase-1 (CHIT-1) that correlated with decreased activity as well as levels of chitotriosidase and susceptibility of filarial infection. The XX genotype in the mannose-binding lectin-2 (MBL-2) genes has been associated with susceptibility to bancroftian infection [24]. Positive association was reported for all variants of rs733618 of cytotoxic T-lymphocyte-associated protein 4 (CTLA-4) gene among asymptomatic amicrofilaremic cases [25]. IL-10 promoter haplotypes and *IL-10 RA* S138G polymorphisms have also been identified as possible genetic determinants of susceptibility to lymphatic filariasis [26]. All the above SNPs that

have been found to be associated with filarial infections were the basis for our study.

We were among the first to show that angiogenic/lymphangiogenic molecules such as vascular endothelial growth factors (VEGFs) may be involved in the development of LE and hydrocele in humans [27, 28]. In these studies, we showed that VEGF-C and its receptor VEGFR-3 are elevated in the plasma of LE patients and treating them with antiangiogenic drugs such as doxycycline reduced the factors prior to ameliorating early stages of pathology [27]. We went further to show that another angiogenic molecule, VEGF-A, is genetically associated with hydrocele caused by bancroftian infections. Treatment with doxycycline again reversed the pathology in men with early stages of hydrocele [28]. Other authors have also shown the involvement of angiogenic/lymphangiogenic molecules in the clinical manifestations of LF [29, 30].

SNPs in FOXC-2 and FLT-4 genes have been identified to be involved in lymphedema progression [31].

While LE is clinically well described, there have been few investigations of host genetic contributions to filarial LE. In this study, we have further shown an association of SNPs in genes of the angiogenic/lymphangiogenic pathways with LE. Identified SNPs could contribute to the search of biomarkers for diagnosis of LE and potential methods to ameliorate LE symptoms.

Results

Demographic and pathology information of study participants

The mean age of study participants was not statistically different between cases and controls (Table 1). Predominantly, 71% of them were females and 29% were males. In the control group, the majority were males (57%). The volunteers had stayed in the study community from a year to over 50 years. In the cases group, 171 people (60%) had been a resident for more than 40 years. A greater number of cases had stages 2 and 3 (32 and 37%, respectively) pathology according to Dreyer et al. [32, 33], while stages 4 and 7 (2% each) were the least frequent stage of pathology among the cases (Table 1).

Single marker analysis

One hundred and forty-seven (147) single nucleotide polymorphisms (SNPs) were initially selected for genotyping (Additional file 1). Sixteen (16) were rejected during the assay design because the primer sequences produced were prone to primer dimerization or the masses of the sequences were too similar to be distinguished by mass spectrometry. Eight out of the 16 rejected SNPs are in the coding region resulting in

Table 1 Demographic and pathology profile of study participants

Variable	Cases N = 285	Controls N = 682
Mean age/years (range)	44.4 (16–73)	40.8 (16–93)
Gender		
Male % (N)	29.5 (84)	57 (389)[a]
Female % (N)	70.5 (201)	43 (293)
Duration in community/years		
1–10	2	55
11–20	10	90
21–30	42	178
31–40	57	132
41–50	79	109
> 50	92	118
Stages of lymphedema		
Stage 1	11	–
Stage 2	90	–
Stage 3	106	–
Stage 4	5	–
Stage 5	20	–
Stage 6	49	–
Stage 7	4	–

[a]Fisher's exact test, $P \leq 0.05$ controls compared to cases

amino acid changes, three were in the promoter region with no amino acid change, and six were in non-coding regions (Additional file 1). With the exception of tumor necrosis factor-α (TNF-α), CTLA-4, and interleukin-4 (IL-4), all the rejected genes were represented by at least one other SNP in the Sequenom data. Thus, 131 SNPs in 64 genes were genotyped.

The single marker analysis compared 285 LE patients (cases) and 682 infected patients without LE pathology (controls). Of the 131 SNPs genotyped, 5 SNPs in three genes were associated with LE with nominal significance (Table 2): 2 SNPs in matrix metalloprotease-2 (MMP-2 rs1030868, $P = 0.0094$; rs2241145, $P = 0.0116$), 2 SNPs in carcinoembryonic antigen-related cell adhesion molecule-1 (CEACAM-1 rs8110904, $P = 0.024$; rs8111171, $P = 0.026$), and 1 SNP in vascular endothelial growth factor receptor-3 (VEGFR-3 rs75614493, $P = 0.034$). None of the nominally associated SNPs withstood correction for multiple testing (Benjamini-Hochberg). All the associated SNPs were in Hardy-Weinberg equilibrium (HWE, $P > 0.05$) with the exception of CEACAM-1 rs8110904 (controls $P = 2.93E{-}10$).

The risk alleles for MMP-2 SNPs rs1030868 and rs2241145 were A and C, respectively, each conferring a 1.3-fold risk to LE development (Table 2). Both alleles fit in a recessive model of association (Additional file 2: Table S1).

No individual in the cohort was homozygous for the T allele in VEGFR-3 SNP rs75614493, and only three people were heterozygous (Table 2). The participants with the C allele of the VEGFR-3 SNP had a 3.4-fold risk of LE development. Due to the lack of homozygosity for the T allele in the cohort, no model of association, whether dominant or recessive, could be assigned (Additional file 2: Table S1). The risk alleles for CEACAM-1 SNPs rs8110904 and rs8111171 were A and T and confer a 1.2- and 1.3-fold risk, respectively, of LE development (Table 2). Both alleles fit a dominant model of association (Additional file 2: Table S1).

Haplotype analysis

Two or more SNPs in a gene or on the same chromosome can form haplotypes that are inherited together [34]. Analysis of haplotype association with LE was done using the FamHap software package [35]. A likelihood ratio test with one degree of freedom was used to assess the significance of haplotype frequencies among SNPs on the same gene. Only haplotypes that were significantly associated at one degree of freedom were reported (Table 3).

Two CEACAM-1 SNPs, rs8110904 and rs8111171, were associated with LE in a single marker analysis with nominal significance. From these SNPs, three haplotypes were generated. The frequency of haplotype GG was significantly higher in the controls than the cases ($P = 0.026$); there was a trend in haplotype AT ($P = 0.055$) but there was no difference in haplotype GT between cases and controls (Table 3).

Six different haplotypes comprising SNPs rs11643630, rs1030868, rs2241145, and rs1992116 in the MMP-2 gene (GACG, GGCA, GGGG, TACG, TGCG, and TGGG) were predicted by the FamHap analysis. Haplotype TACG was significantly higher in cases than controls ($P = 0.046$), and this significance was even strengthened after multiple testing with 200,000 simulations, ($P = 0.03$, Table 3). The remaining haplotypes were not significant in either cases or controls.

The VEGFR-3 SNPs rs75614493 and rs3587489 formed three haplotypes (CC, CT, and TT). The TT haplotype was rare in this population and was significantly associated with controls ($P = 0.023$), but was lost after correcting for multiple testing ($P = 0.08$, Table 3).

Plasma levels of angiogenic/lymphangiogenic molecules

Plasma concentrations of the proteins encoded by the genes associated with LE development were measured to evaluate the functional phenotypes. CEACAM-1 and MMP-2 were measured using commercially available kits to compare the plasma levels between LE patients and infected controls. The plasma levels of CEACAM-1 were significantly elevated in LE patients ($P < 0.02$, Fig. 1a).

Table 2 Genotype frequencies and odds ratio of SNPs associated with lymphedema patients and infected controls

Gene (dbSNP rs#)	Functional category of SNP	Genotypes	Cases (%)	Controls (%)	P value P_{ATT} [a]	Adjusted[b]	OR[c] (95% CI)
CEACAM-1 (rs8110904)	Missense	AA	26 (9)	57 (9)	0.024	0.370	(A) 1.2 (0.99–1.49)
		AG	182 (67)	385 (59)			
		GG	65 (24)	213 (32)			
CEACAM-1 (rs8111171)	Missense	GG	61 (22)	205 (31)	0.026	0.370	(T) 1.3 (1.03–1.56)
		GT	145 (52)	311 (46)			
		TT	73 (26)	157 (23)			
FLT-4/VEGFR-3 (rs75614493)	Missense	CC	282 (99)	658 (96)	0.034	0.232	(C) 3.4 (1.02–11.29)
		CT	3 (1)	24 (4)			
		TT	0 (0)	0 (0)			
MMP-2 (rs1030868)	Intron	AA	69 (24)	113 (17)	0.0094	0.232	(A) 1.3 (1.07–1.58)
		AG	134 (47)	337 (49)			
		GG	82 (29)	232 (34)			
MMP-2 (rs2241145)	Intron	CC	86 (30)	158 (23)	0.0116	0.232	(C) 1.3 (1.06–1.57)
		CG	136 (48)	334 (49)			
		GG	63 (22)	190 (28)			

[a]Cochrane-Armitage test for trend
[b]Adjusted P values according to Benjamini-Hochberg
[c]Odds ratio with 95% confidence intervals for the risk allele

MMP-2 protein concentration was also significantly higher in the LE patients ($P = 0.025$, Fig. 1b).

To functionally characterize the genotypes, plasma levels of CEACAM-1 and MMP-2 were correlated with the respective genotypes. CEACAM-1 plasma level was higher in people with the GG genotype in both rs8110904 and rs8111171 SNPs (Fig. 2). Plasma levels of MMP-2 did not correlate with any of the SNP genotypes in this population.

Pathway interaction of lymphedema associated genes

The MetaCore™ software package was used to analyze the genotyped genes for pathways of protein interaction.

Table 3 SNP haplotypes in genes associated with lymphedema

Gene	dbSNPrs#	Allele	Distribution cases (%)	Distribution controls (%)	P value (1df)	Global P value[a]
CEACAM-1	rs8110904	G	48.3	54.0	*0.026*	0.092
	rs8111171	G				
	rs8110904	A	48.0	39	*0.046*	0.092
	rs8111171	T				
VEGFR-3	rs75614493	T	0.5	1.8	*0.023*	0.080
	rs3587489	T				
MMP-2	rs2241145	T	33.1	28.3	*0.046*	*0.030*
	rs1030868	A				
	rs11643630	C				
	rs1992116	G				

Italic text indicates a significant association
[a]Calculated by an omnibus statistic with 200,000 simulations in FamHap version 19

Because of the candidate gene approach of this case-control study, it is not surprising that the associated genes are in the angiogenesis pathway. Nevertheless, candidates for further study for their role in LE development are identified by this analysis. The three genes (gray circles) with SNPs associated with filarial LE interact with each other (CEACAM-1 and VEGFR-3) and 11 proteins in the angiogenesis pathway (Fig. 3). CEACAM-1 is predicted to up-regulate VEGFR-3 expression directly and up-regulates PROX-1, VEGF-C, and VEGF-D, which also up-regulate VEGFR-3. CEACAM-1 can also up-regulate MMP-2 via the up-regulation of TALIN. It down-regulates beta-catenin, a protein that up-regulates MMP-2 directly and also indirectly via up-regulation of VEFG-A, and up-regulates VEGFR-3 indirectly via PROX-1. MMP-2 is predicted to up-regulate TGF-β1, MMP-9, and VEGFR-1.

Discussion

Pathological effects of lymphatic filariasis such as LE and hydrocele are observed in a fraction of the individuals in endemic areas even though up to 80% may be infected with *W. bancrofti* [5, 36]. LE, the most debilitating pathology, occurs in ~ 7% of the endemic population [6, 8].

Different studies have been undertaken to unravel the genetic basis of this heterogeneity, but they concentrated on infection and hydrocele development [24, 28]. Filarial LE is the single largest cause of secondary lymphedema

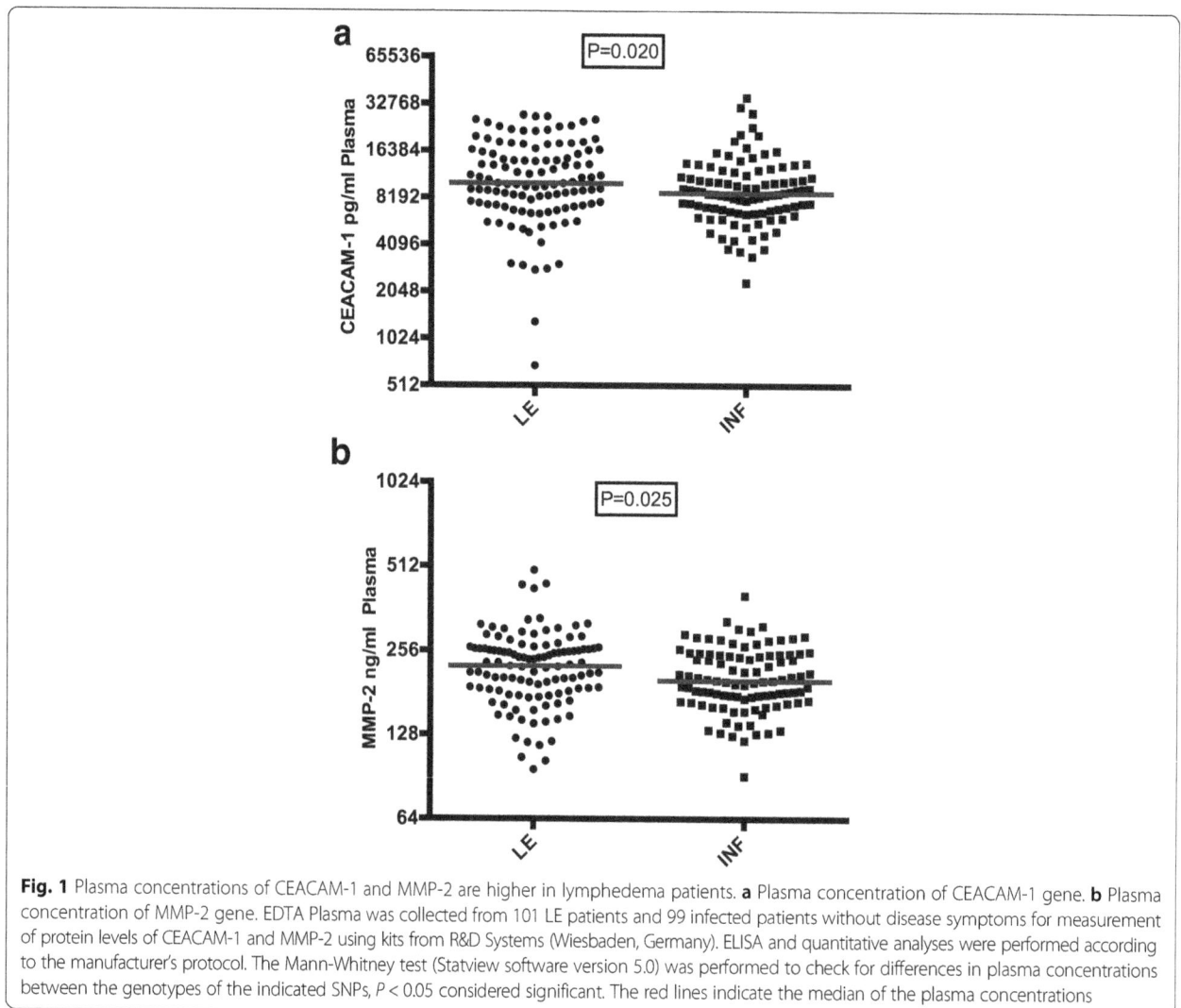

Fig. 1 Plasma concentrations of CEACAM-1 and MMP-2 are higher in lymphedema patients. **a** Plasma concentration of CEACAM-1 gene. **b** Plasma concentration of MMP-2 gene. EDTA Plasma was collected from 101 LE patients and 99 infected patients without disease symptoms for measurement of protein levels of CEACAM-1 and MMP-2 using kits from R&D Systems (Wiesbaden, Germany). ELISA and quantitative analyses were performed according to the manufacturer's protocol. The Mann-Whitney test (Statview software version 5.0) was performed to check for differences in plasma concentrations between the genotypes of the indicated SNPs, $P < 0.05$ considered significant. The red lines indicate the median of the plasma concentrations

[37], an inflammatory disease resulting from the destruction of the lymphatic vessel with associated fibrosis as a result of the presence and death of the adult filarial worms, larval death, and the release of *Wolbachia* endosymbionts [38]. Since the immune response of the host plays an integral role in disease etiology by inducing the expression of particular genes [38], host immunogenetics was exploited in this study to answer the question as to which SNPs could be causative variants in filarial LE development.

Five SNPs in three genes were identified to be associated with LE. The associations did not withstand correction for multiple testing, which is probably attributable to the low sample size and/or the small contributing effects of the SNPs on the disease.

Carcinoembryonic antigen-related cell adhesion molecule 1 (CEACAM-1) is a type 1 transmembrane protein involved in cell-to-cell adhesion [39]. It has been shown to be a potent stimulator of vascular endothelial growth

factor (VEGF) mediated angiogenesis [40, 41]. It also stimulates microvascular endothelial cell growth in the presence of VEGF [40]. However, the overexpression of CEACAM-1 is associated with cancers such as thyroid cancer, gastric cancer, and metastasizing malignant melanomas [42].

Two SNPs in the CEACAM-1 gene (rs8110904 and rs8111171) were associated with LE development. The frequencies for the minor alleles A and T are consistent with the values reported for rs8111171 and rs8110904 from the Yorubian population (rs8110904 G = 57% A = 43%, rs8111171 G = 56% T = 44%) using 120 and 48 participants, respectively [43]. The minor allele A in rs8110904 was higher in the cases than in the controls, and patients with the A allele had an odds ratio of 1.2 (CI 0.99–1.49). The minor T allele frequency in rs8111171 was also higher in the cases than in the controls with a 1.3-fold risk (CI 1.03–1.56) of developing LE. The significant haplotype association of the

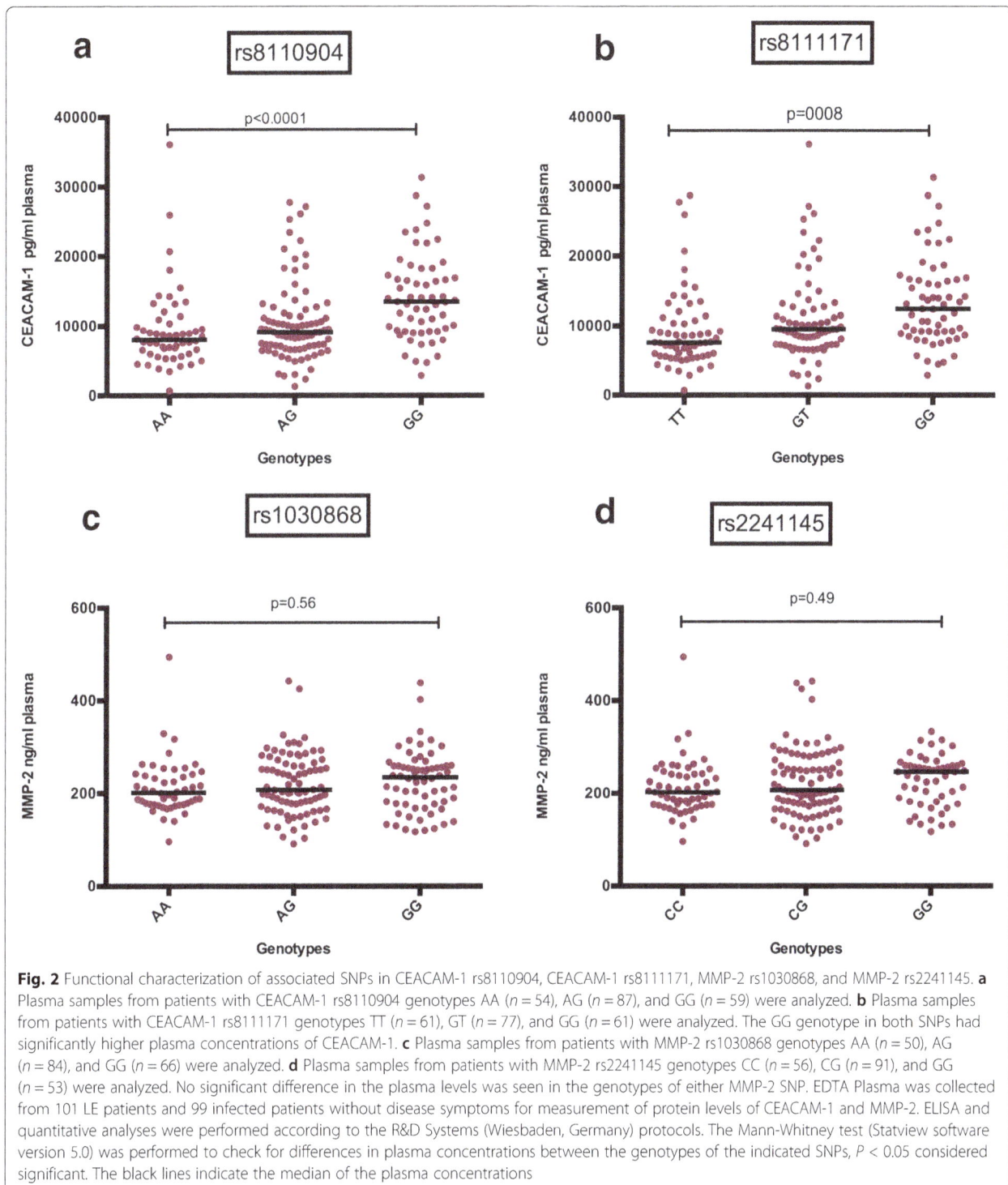

Fig. 2 Functional characterization of associated SNPs in CEACAM-1 rs8110904, CEACAM-1 rs8111171, MMP-2 rs1030868, and MMP-2 rs2241145. **a** Plasma samples from patients with CEACAM-1 rs8110904 genotypes AA ($n = 54$), AG ($n = 87$), and GG ($n = 59$) were analyzed. **b** Plasma samples from patients with CEACAM-1 rs8111171 genotypes TT ($n = 61$), GT ($n = 77$), and GG ($n = 61$) were analyzed. The GG genotype in both SNPs had significantly higher plasma concentrations of CEACAM-1. **c** Plasma samples from patients with MMP-2 rs1030868 genotypes AA ($n = 50$), AG ($n = 84$), and GG ($n = 66$) were analyzed. **d** Plasma samples from patients with MMP-2 rs2241145 genotypes CC ($n = 56$), CG ($n = 91$), and GG ($n = 53$) were analyzed. No significant difference in the plasma levels was seen in the genotypes of either MMP-2 SNP. EDTA Plasma was collected from 101 LE patients and 99 infected patients without disease symptoms for measurement of protein levels of CEACAM-1 and MMP-2. ELISA and quantitative analyses were performed according to the R&D Systems (Wiesbaden, Germany) protocols. The Mann-Whitney test (Statview software version 5.0) was performed to check for differences in plasma concentrations between the genotypes of the indicated SNPs, $P < 0.05$ considered significant. The black lines indicate the median of the plasma concentrations

"protective" haplotype GG ($P = 0.0256$) and haplotype of the case-associated alleles AT ($P = 0.046$) supports a role for this gene in disease development.

CEACAM-1 is up-regulated in some cancers such as thyroid and gastric cancers. The initial metastasis of these cancers is through the lymphatic vessels to the regional lymph nodes similar to the pathogenesis of LE

which mainly occurs after dilation of the lymphatic vessel with associated fibrosis [44]. Multicellular activities such as angiogenesis have been attributed to encoded proteins of CEACAM-1. The serum of CEACAM-1 served as a useful indicator for the presence of pancreatic cancer [45]. CEACAM-1 is a potent inducer of VEGFs. The receptor 3 of VEGF-C and D has been

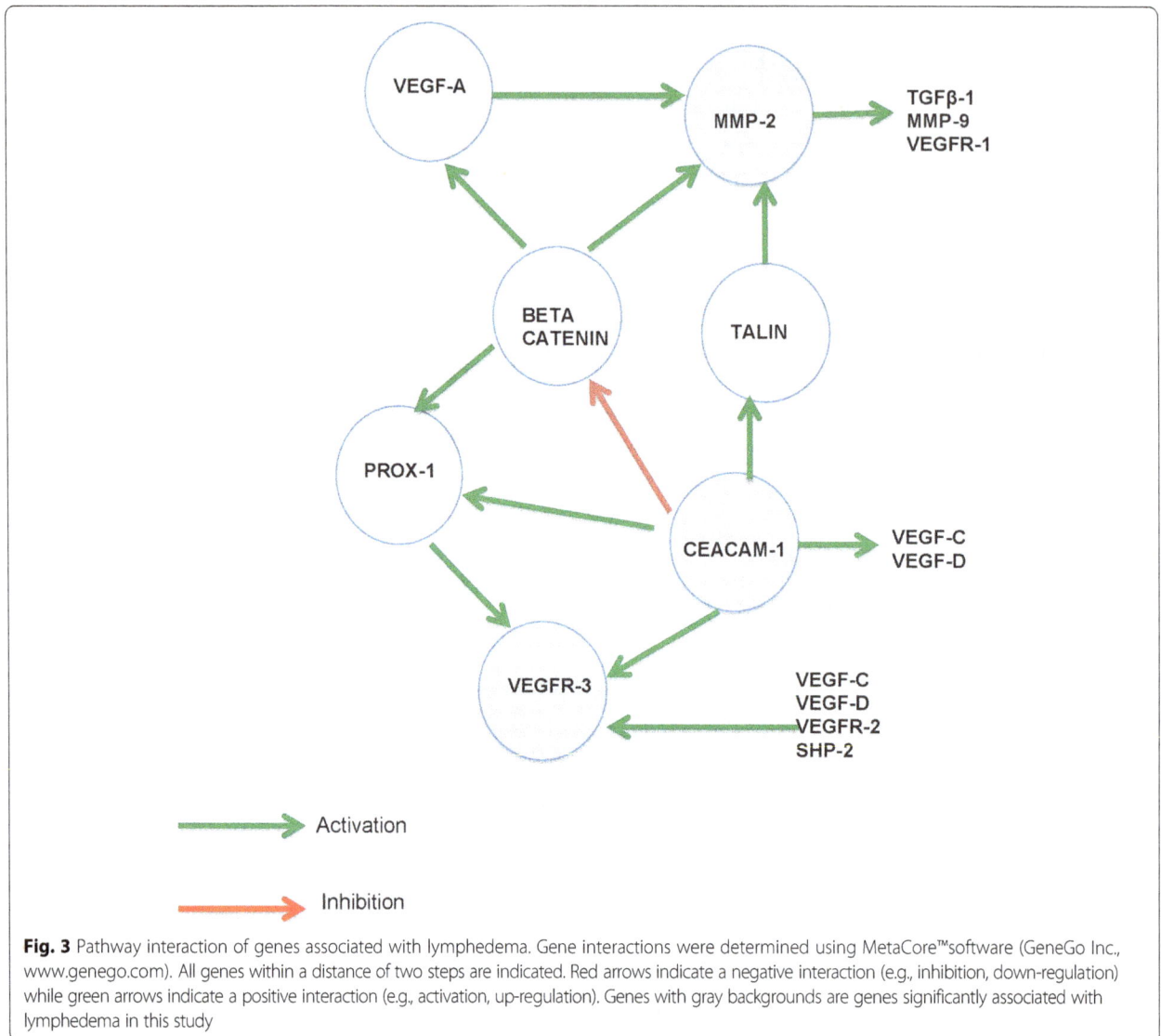

Fig. 3 Pathway interaction of genes associated with lymphedema. Gene interactions were determined using MetaCore™software (GeneGo Inc., www.genego.com). All genes within a distance of two steps are indicated. Red arrows indicate a negative interaction (e.g., inhibition, down-regulation) while green arrows indicate a positive interaction (e.g., activation, up-regulation). Genes with gray backgrounds are genes significantly associated with lymphedema in this study

associated with LE, and its plasma was found to be elevated in LE [27]. If CEACAM-1 stimulates VEGFs and the plasma levels of the receptors influence LE then higher plasma levels of CEACAM-1 in LE could play a role in the development of the disease. The significant increase in plasma protein concentration of CEACAM-1 gene in LE patients (Fig. 1a) correlates with the genotype and is an indication that CEACAM-1 might play a role in LE development. The plasma protein level was also observed to be higher with the GG genotype compared with the other genotypes indicating that the genotype GG directly or indirectly impacts the expression of CEACAM-1 plasma proteins and could be a variant for LE development.

Matrix metalloprotease-2 (MMP2) is a known angiogenic factor whose activity involves the breakdown of extracellular matrix in physiological processes such as embryonic development, reproduction, and tissue remodeling [46]. Mutations in the MMP-2 gene lead to a number of disease processes, such as arthritis and metastasis, tumor growth vascular aneurysmal disease development, Winchester syndrome, and nodulosis-arthropathy-osteolysis (NAO) syndrome [47–50].

The significant association of MMP-2 SNPs rs1030868 ($P = 0.0094$) and rs2241145 ($P = 0.0116$) is an indication that this gene might be involved in LE development. Patients with rs1030868 (minor allele A) and rs2241145 (minor allele C) SNPs have a 1.3-fold (CI 1.07–1.58 and CI 1.06–1.57, respectively) risk of developing LE than those who do not have these alleles (Table 2). In National Center for Biotechnology Information database of single nucleotide polymorphism (NCBI dbSNP), these minor alleles have a frequency of C = 52% (rs2241145) and A = 42% (rs1030868) in the Yorubian population ($n =$ 120) and are similar to the values calculated from our larger sample size [43]. These SNPs have also been found to

Single nucleotide polymorphisms in the angiogenic and lymphangiogenic pathways are associated...

83

be associated with development of lacunar stroke [51], and higher levels of MMP-2 protein and activity have been described. The authors hypothesize that more MMP-2 alters and remodels the extracellular matrix around the vessels that contribute to the development of edema [52, 53], a hypothesis supported by the finding that MMP-2 also disrupts tight junctions [54]. Thus, extravasation of fluid occurs and contributes to stroke. A similar phenomenon is seen in LE development in which the lymph vessels dilate, reducing lymph flow. With destruction/remodeling of the vessel architecture, here hypothesized to be in part caused by MMP-2, lymph fluid enters the surrounding tissue causing lymphedema. The affected limb then enlarges progressively due to fibroadipose deposition [7].

MMP-2 mRNA levels are known to be higher in lymphedematous specimens compared to non-lymphedematous specimens of progenitor cells [7], and a blockage or downregulation of this gene leads to reduced lymphangiogenesis [55]. Therefore, the significant increase in the plasma concentration of MMP-2 in LE patients (Fig. 1b) is an indication that this gene might have a role in the LE development. Even though the plasma concentration was evenly distributed among the genotypes (Fig. 2c, d), the identified associations of these intronic SNPs seem to account for another genetic effect which is independent of the plasma level. Thus, these intronic SNPs may act as proxy markers for another, yet to be identified, functional SNP in this chromosomal region.

Tetracycline and its derivatives have been shown to profoundly inhibit mammalian MMPs by a mechanism that is independent of their antimicrobial activity, thereby reducing excessive degradation or remodeling at the healing enthesis after rotator cuff repair [56, 57]. It has been shown by Debrah et al. [27, 58] that doxycycline improves the condition of disease symptoms of LF patients with early stages of LE. However, the mechanism of action was not clear. This study supports that the effect might be a direct effect on MMP-2 and explains why doxycycline is able to ameliorate LE pathology even though most LE patients do not have active infections. Additionally, pathway analysis with MetaCore shows that MMP-2 positively influences the expression of VEGFs, and therefore, inhibition of MMP-2 may result in additive or synergistic effects with other factors in this pathway.

VEGFR-3, a tyrosine-protein kinase, emerged as one of the genes associated with LE development in this study. A single marker association was found between the VEGFR-3 SNP (rs75614493) in the exon region of chromosome 5 and LE development (Table 2, $P = 0.034$). There was no patient homozygous TT in the study population even though 1 and 2% of patients carried the T allele in the cases and control groups, respectively. The allelic distribution from this study is consistent with earlier work done in sub-Saharan Africa

(Yorubian population) involving 118 patients (NCBI dbSNP). The allelic frequency of the study was 97.5% for the C allele and 2.5% for the T allele [59].

From this present study, the C allele was significantly more frequent in the cases compared to the controls with an odds ratio of 3.4 (CI 1.02–11.29). Even though the genotype frequencies are 99 and 96% in cases vs controls, a statistical difference was observed and a significant difference in haplotype frequencies between rs75614493 and rs3587489 was also observed in the TT haplotype with one degree of freedom.

VEGFR-3 is restricted largely to the lymphatic endothelium and acts as a cell surface receptor for VEGF-C and VEGF-D [60]. The other two receptors of VEGFs that have been identified, VEGFR-1 and VEGFR-2, are expressed mainly in the blood vascular endothelium [61]. Studies on the molecular mechanisms controlling the lymphatic vessels have shown that vascular endothelial growth factors C and D specifically control lymphangiogenesis in humans by activating the VEGF receptor-3 (VEGFR-3) [62, 63] [61, 64]. VEGFR-3 has also been linked to human hereditary LE [65].

VEGFs and VEGFR3 are needed for the development of lymphatic vessels. However, their overproduction leads to lymphatic dilation and LE development [66]. In animal models, overexpression of VEGF-C in the skin of transgenic mice resulted in lymphatic endothelial proliferation and dilation of lymph vessels [64] with a resemblance to lymphatics infected with filarial parasites. These transgenic mice then developed a lymphedema-like phenotype characterized by swelling of feet, edema, and dermal fibrosis [67], similar to what is observed in humans.

Several studies by Debrah et al. [27, 28, 58], involving our study participants, showed that plasma levels of VEGFs and a VEGF soluble receptor, sVEGFR-3, are significantly elevated in patients infected with filarial worms, and a correlation was found between sVEGFR-3, lymphatic dilation, and pathology development. Targeting the filarial worms by doxycycline reduced the levels of VEGFs/sVEGFR-3, with amelioration of dilated supratesticular lymphatic vessels and reduction in LE and hydrocele stages. A mechanism that could be due to the non-antimicrobial activity of tetracyclines. The fact that the VEGF and sVEGFR-3 reduction preceded the improvement of pathology indicates a possible causal interaction between lymphangiogenic factors and lymphatic pathology, rather than only a coincidence or an epiphenomenon.

Pathway interaction of associated genes was done using the MetaCore software package [68]. Genes in the angiogenic pathway were shown to be involved in a complex relationship (Fig. 3). Genes in gray background had SNPs that were directly associated with LE in this study (MMP-2, CEACAM-1, and VEGFR-3). However, during pathway analysis, other genes were found to either activate or inhibit those genes that were found to be directly associated with LE.

CEACAM-1, MMP-2, and VEGFR-3 genes are directly found to be involved in LE development. The pathway interaction of LE associated genes provides information on the involvement of other genes and probably other SNPs in the development of LE. CEACAM-1 is known to be involved in angiogenesis, and its overexpression in human dermal microvascular endothelial cells (HDMEC) leads to an up-regulation of VEGF-C, VEGF-D, and VEGFR-3 [39, 69]. The down-regulation of CEACAM-1 results in deregulation of beta-catenin, which is known to be associated with malignant transformation [70, 71]. TALIN interacts with CEACAM-1 and increases its activity [72].

Prospero homeobox protein-1 (PROX-1) activates VEGFR-3 with a subsequent increase in receptor expression [73]. Activation of PROX-1 is positively regulated by beta-catenin signaling [74]. VEGF-A is essential for cancer neovascularization and cancer invasion by promoting endothelial mitogenesis and permeability. However, the overexpression is known to increase MMP-2 levels in glioblastoma [75]. At the same time, MMP-2 up-regulates TGF beta-1, MMP-9, and VEGFR-1 (Fig. 3). The interaction of these genes can, therefore, be said to contribute to the disease.

This study is the first to determine the genotype frequencies of CEACAM-1 and MMP-2 in our study population. We have gone a further step to confirm the involvement of lymphangiogenic/angiogenic factors in the development of pathology of LF. Our pathway analysis also supports the assertion that LE due to *W. bancrofti* infection is a complex disease and not caused by a single genetic factor.

Conclusion

SNPs in the angiogenic and lymphangiogenic pathway contribute to the development of filarial LE. The genes whose SNPs were found to be associated with LE (CEACAM-1, MMP-2, and VEGFR-3) have an influence in the vascular endothelial growth factors either directly or indirectly, supporting the fact that VEGFs are major functional proteins in filarial LE development and that the identified angiogenic/lymphangiogenic factors function through influencing the VEGFs. The direct activity of MMP-2 on the extracellular matrix which results in the progressive damage of vascular walls in vascular diseases when elevated could also have direct influence in the development of LE. The outcomes of this study are important in the diagnosis of the disease as well as the development of future vaccine. Although the associations were not as strong as anticipated, they underscore

the fact that LE is a complex disease caused by multiple genetic markers. This complex interaction of genes therefore calls for a first-stage genome-wide association study (GWAS) to identify all genes associated with LE development that could serve as markers for diagnosis of the disease, and identify pathways that could be targeted by chemotherapeutics to prevent/reduce lymphedema, providing amelioration of disease to the thousands of people with LE.

The 1000 Genome haplotypes is a valuable resource to infer information on further SNPs via genotype imputation. Unfortunately, the number of SNPs per linkage disequilibrium/gene region available in our study was not sufficient to enable the application of the IMPUTE2 software. In our ongoing GWAS study with a larger sample size, we hope to be able to achieve denser genotyping to be able to make use of public resources like 1000 Genomes or the haplotype reference panel (http://www.haplotype-reference-consortium.org/).

Methods
Study design
The study participants were selected from the Nzema East and Ahanta West districts in the Western Region of Ghana, which are the LF endemic districts in Ghana.

Participants numbering 967—comprising 285 lymphedema patients (Cases) and 682 infected patients without pathology (controls) were enrolled into the study. All volunteers included in the study underwent finger prick blood collection at night for assessment and quantification of microfilariae (Mf) in the peripheral blood. Circulating filarial antigen (CFA) test to identify infected patients who did not have Mf was also done. The procedures for microfilaria and CFA determination were done as described [27, 76]. LE patients were examined separately by a clinician conversant with the symptoms of LF, and the staging was done according to Dreyer et al. [32].

Genotyping
DNA extraction
In the field lab, volunteer's blood was mixed with equal volumes of 8 M urea for preservation at ambient temperature. The Chemagen platform (Chemagen Biopolymer-Technologies AG, Baesweiler, Germany) in Bonn was used for the DNA extraction as per kit instructions. After the genomic DNA was isolated, a DNA stock concentration of 100 ng/ml was diluted to 15 ng/μl working concentration with Tris-EDTA buffer. Quality-checked DNA samples with an A260/A280 ratio between 1.7 and 2.0 were pipetted into aliquots of 2 μl (30 ng DNA) per well in a 384-well plate for genotyping.

SNP genotyping

To investigate several candidate genes conferring susceptibility or protection to LE, the SNP databases National Center for Biotechnology Information (NCBI) and Online Mendelian Inheritance in Man (OMIM) were used [77, 78]. These databases provide information on genetic variations. SNP Annotation and Proxy Search (SNAP) (http://www.broadinstitute.org) was also used to find proxy SNPs based on linkage disequilibrium, physical distance, and/or membership in selected commercial genotyping arrays. Pair-wise linkage disequilibrium was pre-calculated based on phased genotype data from the International HapMap Project (www.hapmap.org), which has since been replaced by the 1000 Genomes Project (www.1000genomes.org).

In all, 64 genes of interest known to have a role in inflammation, angiogenesis/lymphangiogenesis, extravasation of fluid, and also in other mechanisms, such as cell differentiation during tumorigenesis, were selected. A total of 131 functional variants from the 64 genes were successfully genotyped and analyzed (Additional file 2: Table S1). Genotyping was done in multiplex reactions using the MassARRAY (Sequenom Inc., San Diego, USA) platform. Identified monoallelic SNPs and SNPs with genotyping call rates of < 95% were excluded from the analysis.

Determination of plasma levels of angiogenic/ lymphangiogenic molecules

Plasma concentrations of the angiogenic/lymphangiogenic molecules associated SNPs were assessed as a measure of the functional phenotypes in the genotyped samples. Blood from cases and controls was taken with ethylenediaminetetraacetic acid (EDTA) tubes, and plasma was collected for measurement of protein levels of CEACAM-1 and MMP-2 using commercially available kits (R&D Systems, Wiesbaden, Germany) according to the manufacturer's protocol. ELISA plates were read with a Wallac VICTOR^2 1420 (PerkinElmer Inc., Waltham MA, USA) at 450 nm and corrected with a second read at 540 nm. A standard curve was created for each plate using a four-parameter logistic (4-PL) curve fit. Only plates with a standard curve $r^2 > 0.99$ were evaluated.

Statistical analyses

FamHap version 19 software was used for single marker analysis as well as haplotype analysis of association of the SNPs with cases or controls [79]. Genotype and haplotype frequencies were summarized as percentages. Statistical significance for the single marker SNP analysis was calculated using the Cochrane-Armitage test for trend with $P_{ATT} \leq 0.05$ considered significant. The Armitage test is less influenced by deviation from Hardy-Weinberg equilibrium (HWE), and the result obtained is valid and acceptable even when a group is not in HWE [35].

Genotype-specific risks were estimated as odds ratios (ORs) with 95% confidence intervals (CIs). Analysis of dominant or recessive association was done using the DeFinetti formula at ihg.gsf.de/cgi-bin/hw/hwa1.pl.

Haplotype analyses calculated an omnibus statistic using 200,000 simulations of the case-control data correcting for multiple testing (global P value). MetaCore™ software (GeneGo Inc., St. Joseph, MI, USA) was used to test for SNP interaction and network analysis [68]. Unpaired t test with GraphPad Prism version 6 (La Jolla, California, USA, www.graphpad.com) software was used for comparing the differences in the plasma concentration of the samples and for plotting the graphs from data generated. $P \leq 0.05$ were considered statistically significant.

Abbreviations

CEACAM-1: Carcinoembryonic antigen-related cell adhesion molecule-1; CHIT-1: Chitinase-1; CTLA-4: Cytotoxic T-lymphocyte-associated protein 4; EDTA: Ethylenediaminetetraacetic acid; ELISA: Enzyme-linked immunosorbent assay; IL-4: Interleukin-10; LE: Lymphedema; LF: Lymphatic filariasis; MBL-2: Mannose-binding lectin-2; MHC: Major histocompatibility complex; MMP-2: Matrix metalloprotease-2; PROX-1: Prospero homeobox protein-1; SNP: Single nucleotide polymorphism; TGFβ-1: Transforming growth factor-β-1; TNF-α: tumor necrosis factor-alpha; VEGFR-3: Vascular endothelial growth factor receptor-3

Acknowledgements

We thank all the volunteers in the study, as well as the Ahanta West and Nzema East District Health Directorates in the Western Region of Ghana for their cooperation. We are grateful to the staff of filariasis team at Kumasi Centre for Collaborative Research into Tropical Medicine for their support and cooperation. We are again grateful to the DFG, the Bill and Melinda Gates Foundation, the European Commission (No. 242121, EPIAF), and the European Foundation Initiative for African Research into Neglected Tropical Diseases for funding this work.
The technical assistance of Lydia Lust, Institute for Medical Microbiology, Immunology and Parasitology is gratefully appreciated.
We are also thankful for the helpful discussions of the results with Dr. Johannes Schumacher and Dr. Kerstin Ludwig of the Institute of Human Genetics, University of Bonn.

Funding

This work was funded through the Deutsche Forschungsgemeinschaft (DFG, German Research Foundation) within the German-African Cooperation Projects in Infectology (PF 673/2-1 and PF 673/4-1). Volunteers were recruited, and samples for genotyping were collected with support through grants to Achim Hoerauf from the Liverpool School of Tropical Medicine as part of the A-WOL (Anti-Wolbachia) Consortium funded by the Bill and Melinda Gates Foundation, the European Commission (No. 242121, EPIAF), and a grant to Alexander Yaw Debrah from the European Foundation Initiative for African Research into Neglected Tropical Diseases Grant (No. 1/81995 and 8652).

Authors' contributions

AYD, AH, and KP conceptualized the study and obtained funding. AYD, LBD, JOM, and YM performed the field work and obtained patient samples. LBD and AA organized patient samples. LBD, AA, and FFB performed the experiments. LBD, TB, CH, and JHF analyzed the data. LBD, AA, and KP wrote the manuscript. AH contributed critical suggestions for the manuscript. All authors read and approved the final manuscript.

Competing interests

The authors declare that they have no competing interests.

Author details

[1]Kumasi Centre for Collaborative Research in Tropical Medicine, Kumasi, Ghana. [2]Department of Clinical Microbiology, Kwame Nkrumah University of Science and Technology, Kumasi, Ghana. [3]Institute for Medical Microbiology, Immunology and Parasitology, University Hospital Bonn, Sigmund-Freud-Str. 25, 53127 Bonn, Germany. [4]Faculty of Allied Health Sciences of Kwame Nkrumah University of Science and Technology, Kumasi, Ghana. [5]Institute of Human Genetics, University of Bonn, Bonn, Germany. [6]Department of Genomics, Life and Brain Center, University of Bonn, Bonn, Germany. [7]Institute for Medical Biometry, Informatics and Epidemiology, University of Bonn, Bonn, Germany. [8]Bonn-Aachen International Center for Information Technology (B-IT), University of Bonn, Bonn, Germany.

References

1. WHO. Global programme to eliminate lymphatic filariasis: progress report, 2016. Wkly Epidemiol Rec. 2017;92(40):594–607.
2. Hoerauf A, Pfarr K, Mand S, Debrah AY, Specht S. Filariasis in Africa—treatment challenges and prospects. Clin Microbiol Infect. 2011; 17(7):977–85.
3. Noroes J, Addiss D, Santos A, Medeiros Z, Coutinho A, Dreyer G. Ultrasonographic evidence of abnormal lymphatic vessels in young men with adult Wuchereria bancrofti infection in the scrotal area. J Urol. 1996; 156(2 Pt 1):409–12.
4. Noroes J, Addiss D, Amaral F, Coutinho A, Medeiros Z, Dreyer G. Occurrence of living adult Wuchereria bancrofti in the scrotal area of men with microfilaraemia. Trans R Soc Trop Med Hyg. 1996;90(1):55–6.
5. Nutman TB, Kumaraswami V. Regulation of the immune response in lymphatic filariasis: perspectives on acute and chronic infection with Wuchereria bancrofti in South India. Parasite Immunol. 2001;23(7): 389–99.
6. Tisch DJ, Hazlett FE, Kastens W, Alpers MP, Bockarie MJ, Kazura JW. Ecologic and biologic determinants of filarial antigenemia in bancroftian filariasis in Papua New Guinea. J Infect Dis. 2001;184(7):898–904.
7. Couto RA, Kulungowski AM, Chawla AS, Fishman SJ, Greene AK. Expression of angiogenic and vasculogenic factors in human lymphedematous tissue. Lymphat Res Biol. 2011;9(3):143–9.
8. Ramaiah KD, Ottesen EA. Progress and impact of 13 years of the global programme to eliminate lymphatic filariasis on reducing the burden of filarial disease. PLoS Negl Trop Dis. 2014;8(11):e3319.
9. Steel C, Nutman TB. CTLA-4 in filarial infections: implications for a role in diminished T cell reactivity. J Immunol. 2003;170(4):1930–8.
10. Babu S, Blauvelt CP, Kumaraswami V, Nutman TB. Regulatory networks induced by live parasites impair both Th1 and Th2 pathways in patent lymphatic filariasis: implications for parasite persistence. J Immunol. 2006; 176(5):3248–56.
11. Taylor MJ, Cross HF, Bilo K. Inflammatory responses induced by the filarial nematode Brugia malayi are mediated by lipopolysaccharide-like activity from endosymbiotic Wolbachia bacteria. J Exp Med. 2000;191(8):1429–36.
12. Harnett W, Harnett MM, Leung BP, Gracie JA, McInnes IB. The anti-inflammatory potential of the filarial nematode secreted product, ES-62. Curr Top Med Chem. 2004;4(5):553–9.
13. King CL, Connelly M, Alpers MP, Bockarie M, Kazura JW. Transmission intensity determines lymphocyte responsiveness and cytokine bias in human lymphatic filariasis. J Immunol. 2001;166(12):7427–36.
14. Steel C, Guinea A, McCarthy JS, Ottesen EA. Long-term effect of prenatal exposure to maternal microfilaraemia on immune responsiveness to filarial parasite antigens. Lancet. 1994;343(8902):890–3.
15. Malhotra I, Ouma JH, Wamachi A, Kioko J, Mungai P, Njzovu M, Kazura JW, King CL. Influence of maternal filariasis on childhood infection and immunity to Wuchereria bancrofti in Kenya. Infect Immun. 2003;71(9):5231–7.
16. Mahanty S, Ravichandran M, Raman U, Jayaraman K, Kumaraswami V, Nutman TB. Regulation of parasite antigen-driven immune responses by interleukin-10 (IL-10) and IL-12 in lymphatic filariasis. Infect Immun. 1997; 65(5):1742–7.
17. Cuenco KT, Halloran ME, Louis-Charles J, Lammie PJ. A family study of lymphedema of the leg in a lymphatic filariasis-endemic area. Am J Trop Med Hyg. 2004;70(2):180–4.
18. Cuenco KT, Halloran ME, Lammie PJ. Assessment of families for excess risk of lymphedema of the leg in a lymphatic filariasis-endemic area. Am J Trop Med Hyg. 2004;70(2):185–90.
19. Terhell AJ, Price R, Koot JW, Abadi K, Yazdanbakhsh M. The development of specific IgG4 and IgE in a paediatric population is influenced by filarial endemicity and gender. Parasitology. 2000;121(5):535–43.
20. Wahyuni S, Houwing-Duistermaat JJ, Syafruddin ST, Yazdanbakhsh M, Sartono E. Clustering of filarial infection in an age-graded study: genetic, household and environmental influences. Parasitology. 2004;128(3):315–21.
21. Chesnais CB, Sabbagh A, Pion SD, Missamou F, Garcia A, Boussinesq M. Familial aggregation and heritability of Wuchereria bancrofti infection. J Infect Dis. 2016;
22. Debrah AY, Batsa L, Albers A, Mand S, Toliat MR, Nurnberg P, Adjei O, Hoerauf A, Pfarr K. Transforming growth factor-beta1 variant Leu10Pro is associated with both lack of microfilariae and differential microfilarial loads in the blood of persons infected with lymphatic filariasis. Hum Immunol. 2011;72(11):1143–8.
23. Junpee A, Tencomnao T, Sanprasert V, Nuchprayoon S. Association between toll-like receptor 2 (TLR2) polymorphisms and asymptomatic bancroftian filariasis. Parasitol Res. 2010;107(4):807–16.
24. Choi EH, Zimmerman PA, Foster CB, Zhu S, Kumaraswami V, Nutman TB, Chanock SJ. Genetic polymorphisms in molecules of innate immunity and susceptibility to infection with Wuchereria bancrofti in South India. Genes Immun. 2001;2(5):248–53.
25. Idris ZM, Miswan N, Muhi J, Mohd TA, Kun JF, Noordin R. Association of CTLA4 gene polymorphisms with lymphatic filariasis in an east Malaysian population. Hum Immunol. 2011;72(7):607–12.
26. Yasmeen Sheik1 SFQ, Ananthapur Venkateshwari SN, BMAP N. Association of IL-10 & IL-10RA polymorphisms with lymphatic Filariasis in south Indian population. Int J Trop Dis Health. 2012:2.
27. Debrah AY, Mand S, Specht S, Marfo-Debrekyei Y, Batsa L, Pfarr K, Larbi J, Lawson B, Taylor M, Adjei O, et al. Doxycycline reduces plasma VEGF-C/sVEGFR-3 and improves pathology in lymphatic filariasis. PLoS Pathog. 2006; 2(9):e92.
28. Debrah AY, Mand S, Toliat MR, Marfo-Debrekyei Y, Batsa L, Nurnberg P, Lawson B, Adjei O, Hoerauf A, Pfarr K. Plasma vascular endothelial growth factor-a (VEGF-A) and VEGF-A gene polymorphisms are associated with hydrocele development in lymphatic filariasis. Am J Trop Med Hyg. 2007;77(4):601–8.
29. Panda AK, Sahoo PK, Kerketta AS, Kar SK, Ravindran B, Satapathy AK. Human lymphatic filariasis: genetic polymorphism of endothelin-1 and tumor necrosis factor receptor II correlates with development of chronic disease. J Infect Dis. 2011;204(2):315–22.
30. Weinkopff T, Mackenzie C, Eversole R, Lammie PJ. Filarial excretory-secretory products induce human monocytes to produce lymphangiogenic mediators. PLoS Negl Trop Dis. 2014;8(7):e2893.
31. Sheik Y, Qureshi SF, Mohhammed B, Nallari P. FOXC2 and FLT4 gene variants in lymphatic Filariasis. Lymphat Res Biol. 2015;13(2):112–9.
32. Dreyer GDA, Dreyer P, Noroes J. Basic lymphoedema management: treatment and prevention of problems associated with lymphatic filariasis. London: Royal Free and University College Medical School; 2002.
33. Mand S, Debrah AY, Klarmann U, Batsa L, Marfo-Debrekyei Y, Kwarteng A, Specht S, Belda-Domene A, Fimmers R, Taylor M, et al. Doxycycline improves filarial lymphedema independent of active filarial infection: a randomized controlled trial. Clin Infect Dis. 2012;55(5):621–30.
34. Clark AG. The role of haplotypes in candidate gene studies. Genet Epidemiol. 2004;27(4):321–33.
35. Armittage P. Tests for linear trends in proportions and frequencies. Biometrics. 1995;11:375–86.
36. Kumaraswami V. The clinical manifestation of lymphatic filariasis. In: Lymphatic Filariasis. Volume 1, edn. Edited by Nutman T. London: Imperial College Press; 2000.
37. Karpanen T, Alitalo K. Molecular biology and pathology of lymphangiogenesis. Annu Rev Pathol. 2008;3:367–97.
38. Pfarr KM, Debrah AY, Specht S, Hoerauf A. Filariasis and lymphoedema. Parasite Immunol. 2009;31(11):664–72.
39. Gu A, Tsark W, Holmes KV, Shively JE. Role of Ceacam1 in VEGF induced vasculogenesis of murine embryonic stem cell-derived embryoid bodies in 3D culture. Exp Cell Res. 2009;315(10):1668–82.

40. Ergun S, Kilik N, Ziegeler G, Hansen A, Nollau P, Gotze J, Wurmbach JH, Horst A, Weil J, Fernando M, et al. CEA-related cell adhesion molecule 1: a potent angiogenic factor and a major effector of vascular endothelial growth factor. Mol Cell. 2000;5(2):311–20.

41. Oliveira-Ferrer L, Tilki D, Ziegeler G, Hauschild J, Loges S, Irmak S, Kilic E, Huland H, Friedrich M, Ergun S. Dual role of carcinoembryonic antigen-related cell adhesion molecule 1 in angiogenesis and invasion of human urinary bladder cancer. Cancer Res. 2004;64(24):8932–8.

42. Matsuda Y. CEACAM1 (carcinoembryonic antigen-related cell adhesion molecule 1 (biliary glycoprotein)). Atlas Database. 2009;14(4):4.

43. http://www.ncbi.nlm.nih.gov/snp. AA.

44. Bennuru S, Maldarelli G, Kumaraswami V, Klion AD, Nutman TB. Elevated levels of plasma angiogenic factors are associated with human lymphatic filarial infections. Am J Trop Med Hyg. 83(4):884–90.

45. Simeone DM, Ji B, Banerjee M, Arumugam T, Li D, Anderson MA, Bamberger AM, Greenson J, Brand RE, Ramachandran V, et al. CEACAM1, a novel serum biomarker for pancreatic cancer. Pancreas. 2007;34(4):436–43.

46. Bennuru S, Nutman TB. Lymphangiogenesis and lymphatic remodeling induced by filarial parasites: implications for pathogenesis. PLoS Pathog. 2009;5(12):e1000688.

47. Zankl A, Pachman L, Poznanski A, Bonafe L, Wang F, Shusterman Y, Fishman DA, Superti-Furga A. Torg syndrome is caused by inactivating mutations in MMP2 and is allelic to NAO and Winchester syndrome. J Bone Miner Res. 2007;22(2):329–33.

48. Bedi A, Fox AJ, Kovacevic D, Deng XH, Warren RF, Rodeo SA. Doxycycline-mediated inhibition of matrix metalloproteinases improves healing after rotator cuff repair. Am J Sports Med. 38(2):308–17.

49. Candelario-Jalil E, Thompson J, Taheri S, Grossetete M, Adair JC, Edmonds E, Prestopnik J, Wills J, Rosenberg GA. Matrix metalloproteinases are associated with increased blood-brain barrier opening in vascular cognitive impairment. Stroke. 2011;42(5):1345–50.

50. Peng ZH, Wan DS, Li LR, Chen G, ZH L, XJ W, Kong LH, Pan ZZ. Expression of COX-2, MMP-2 and VEGF in stage II and III colorectal cancer and the clinical significance. Hepato-Gastroenterology. 2011;58(106):369–76.

51. Fatar M, Stroick M, Steffens M, Senn E, Reuter B, Bukow S, Griebe M, Alonso A, Lichtner P, Bugert P, et al. Single-nucleotide polymorphisms of MMP-2 gene in stroke subtypes. Cerebrovasc Dis. 2008;26(2):113–9.

52. Shigemori Y, Katayama Y, Mori T, Maeda T, Kawamata T. Matrix metalloproteinase-9 is associated with blood-brain barrier opening and brain edema formation after cortical contusion in rats. Acta Neurochir Suppl. 2006;96:130–3.

53. Kelly MA, Shuaib A, Todd KG. Matrix metalloproteinase activation and blood-brain barrier breakdown following thrombolysis. Exp Neurol. 2006; 200(1):38–49.

54. Yang Y, Estrada EY, Thompson JF, Liu W, Rosenberg GA. Matrix metalloproteinase-mediated disruption of tight junction proteins in cerebral vessels is reversed by synthetic matrix metalloproteinase inhibitor in focal ischemia in rat. J Cereb Blood Flow Metab. 2007;27(4):697–709.

55. Detry B, Erpicum C, Paupert J, Blacher S, Maillard C, Bruyere F, Pendeville H, Remacle T, Lambert V, Balsat C, et al. Matrix metalloproteinase-2 governs lymphatic vessel formation as an interstitial collagenase. Blood. 2012;119(21):5048–56.

56. Pasternak B, Fellenius M, Aspenberg P. Doxycycline impairs tendon repair in rats. Acta Orthop Belg. 2006;72(6):756–60.

57. Lo IK, Marchuk LL, Hollinshead R, Hart DA, Frank CB. Matrix metalloproteinase and tissue inhibitor of matrix metalloproteinase mRNA levels are specifically altered in torn rotator cuff tendons. Am J Sports Med. 2004;32(5):1223–9.

58. Debrah AY, Mand S, Marfo-Debrekyei Y, Batsa L, Pfarr K, Lawson B, Taylor M, Adjei O, Hoerauf A. Reduction in levels of plasma vascular endothelial growth factor-a and improvement in hydrocele patients by targeting endosymbiotic Wolbachia sp. in Wuchereria bancrofti with doxycycline. Am J Trop Med Hyg. 2009;80(6):956–63.

59. http://www.ncbi.nlm.nih.gov/projects/SNP/snp_ref.cgi?rs=75614493#locus. Accessed 14 May 2010.

60. Spiegel R, Ghalamkarpour A, Daniel-Spiegel E, Vikkula M, Shalev SA. Wide clinical spectrum in a family with hereditary lymphedema type I due to a novel missense mutation in VEGFR3. J Hum Genet. 2006;51(10):846–50.

61. Veikkola T, Jussila L, Makinen T, Karpanen T, Jeltsch M, Petrova TV, Kubo H, Thurston G, McDonald DM, Achen MG, et al. Signalling via vascular endothelial growth factor receptor-3 is sufficient for lymphangiogenesis in transgenic mice. EMBO J. 2001;20(6):1223–31.

62. Korpelainen EI, Alitalo K. Signaling angiogenesis and lymphangiogenesis. Curr Opin Cell Biol. 1998;10(2):159–64.

63. Achen MG, Jeltsch M, Kukk E, Makinen T, Vitali A, Wilks AF, Alitalo K, Stacker SA. Vascular endothelial growth factor D (VEGF-D) is a ligand for the tyrosine kinases VEGF receptor 2 (Flk1) and VEGF receptor 3 (Flt4). Proc Natl Acad Sci USA. 1998;95(2):548–53.

64. Jeltsch M, Kaipainen A, Joukov V, Meng X, Lakso M, Rauvala H, Swartz M, Fukumura D, Jain RK, Alitalo K. Hyperplasia of lymphatic vessels in VEGF-C transgenic mice. Science. 1997;276(5317):1423–5.

65. Yu Z, Wang J, Peng S, Dong B, Li Y. Identification of a novel VEGFR-3 missense mutation in a Chinese family with hereditary lymphedema type I. J Genet Genomics. 2007;34(10):861–7.

66. Makinen T, Jussila L, Veikkola T, Karpanen T, Kettunen MI, Pulkkanen KJ, Kauppinen R, Jackson DG, Kubo H, Nishikawa S, et al. Inhibition of lymphangiogenesis with resulting lymphedema in transgenic mice expressing soluble VEGF receptor-3. Nat Med. 2001;7(2):199–205.

67. Kaipainen A, Korhonen J, Mustonen T, van Hinsbergh VW, Fang GH, Dumont D, Breitman M, Alitalo K. Expression of the fms-like tyrosine kinase 4 gene becomes restricted to lymphatic endothelium during development. Proc Natl Acad Sci USA. 1995;92(8):3566–70.

68. Froehlich H, Fellmann M, Sueltmann H, Poustka A, Beissbarth T. Large scale statistical inference of signaling pathways from RNAi and microarray data. BMC Bioinformatics. 2007;8:386.

69. Horst AK, Ito WD, Dabelstein J, Schumacher U, Sander H, Turbide C, Brummer J, Meinertz T, Beauchemin N, Wagener C. Carcinoembryonic antigen-related cell adhesion molecule 1 modulates vascular remodeling in vitro and in vivo. J Clin Invest. 2006;116(6):1596–605.

70. Jin L, Li Y, Chen CJ, Sherman MA, Le K, Shively JE. Direct interaction of tumor suppressor CEACAM1 with beta catenin: identification of key residues in the long cytoplasmic domain. Exp Biol Med. 2008;233(7):849–59.

71. Reyes M, Rojas-Alcayaga G, Maturana A, Aitken JP, Rojas C, Ortega AV. Increased nuclear beta-catenin expression in oral potentially malignant lesions: a marker of epithelial dysplasia. Med Oral Patol Oral Cir Bucal. 2015; 20(5):e540–6.

72. Muller MM, Singer BB, Klaile E, Obrink B, Lucka L. Transmembrane CEACAM1 affects integrin-dependent signaling and regulates extracellular matrix protein-specific morphology and migration of endothelial cells. Blood. 2005; 105(10):3925–34.

73. Kilic N, Oliveira-Ferrer L, Neshat-Vahid S, Irmak S, Obst-Pernberg K, Wurmbach JH, Loges S, Kilic E, Weil J, Lauke H, et al. Lymphatic reprogramming of microvascular endothelial cells by CEA-related cell adhesion molecule-1 via interaction with VEGFR-3 and Prox1. Blood. 2007; 110(13):4223–33.

74. Karalay O, Doberauer K, Vadodaria KC, Knobloch M, Berti L, Miquelajauregui A, Schwark M, Jagasia R, Taketo MM, Tarabykin V, et al. Prospero-related homeobox 1 gene (Prox1) is regulated by canonical Wnt signaling and has a stage-specific role in adult hippocampal neurogenesis. Proc Natl Acad Sci USA. 2011;108(14):5807–12.

75. Gong J, Zhu S, Zhang Y, Wang J. Interplay of VEGFa and MMP2 regulates invasion of glioblastoma. Tumour Biol. 2014;35(12):11879–85.

76. Debrah AY, Mand S, Marfo-Debrekyei Y, Batsa L, Albers A, Specht S, Klarmann U, Pfarr K, Adjei O, Hoerauf A. Macrofilaricidal activity in Wuchereria bancrofti after 2 weeks treatment with a combination of rifampicin plus doxycycline. J Parasitol Res. 2011;2011:201617.

77. http://www.ncbi.nlm.nih.gov/snp. Accessed 14 May 2010.

78. http://omim.org/entry/109770. Accessed 14 May 2010.

79. Herold C, Becker T. Genetic association analysis with FAMHAP: a major program update. Bioinformatics. 2009;25(1):134–6.

9

Attitudes of stakeholders in psychiatry towards the inclusion of children in genomic research

Anna Sundby[1,2]*, Merete Watt Boolsen[3], Kristoffer Sølvsten Burgdorf[4], Henrik Ullum[4], Thomas Folkmann Hansen[2,5,6] and Ole Mors[1,2]

Abstract

Background: Genomic sequencing of children in research raises complex ethical issues. This study aims to gain more knowledge on the attitudes towards the inclusion of children as research subjects in genomic research and towards the disclosure of pertinent and incidental findings to the parents and the child.

Methods: Qualitative data were collected from interviews with a wide range of informants: experts engaged in genomic research, clinical geneticists, persons with mental disorders, relatives, and blood donors. Quantitative data were collected from a cross-sectional web-based survey among 1227 parents and 1406 non-parents who were potential stakeholders in psychiatric genomic research.

Results: Participants generally expressed positive views on children's participation in genomic research. The informants in the qualitative interviews highlighted the age of the child as a critical aspect when disclosing genetic information. Other important aspects were the child's right to an autonomous choice, the emotional burden of knowing imposed on both the child and the parents, and the possibility of receiving beneficial clinical information regarding the future health of the child. Nevertheless, there was no consensus whether the parent or the child should receive the findings. A majority of survey stakeholders agreed that children should be able to participate in genomic research. The majority agreed that both pertinent and incidental findings should be returned to the parents and to the child when of legal age. Having children does not affect the stakeholder's attitudes towards the inclusion of children as research subjects in genomic research.

Conclusion: Our findings illustrate that both the child's right to autonomy and the parents' interest to be informed are important factors that are found valuable by the participants. In future guidelines governing children as subjects in genomic research, it would thus be essential to incorporate the child's right to an open future, including the right to receive information on adult-onset genetic disorders.

Keywords: Child, Minors, Attitude, Whole genome sequencing, Ethics research, Mental disorders

Background

Genome sequencing, i.e., whole genome and whole exome sequencing, has now become a widely used tool in research, for example, in psychiatric genetic research. However, genome sequencing generates huge amounts of genomic information, and some of the information is clinically useful. There is an ongoing debate regarding the return of individual genetic research findings unrelated to the condition under investigation [1–7]. The community of clinical genetics refers to these types of results as incidental findings [8]. Because incidental findings should be expected as a part of genomic sequencing, other terms as secondary findings, additional findings, and non-pertinent findings have been suggested [8, 9]. However, the increasing number of large-scale genomic research projects and the inclusion of children in genomic research

* Correspondence: anna.sundby@regionh.dk
[1]Department of Clinical Medicine, Psychosis Research Unit, Aarhus University Hospital, Skovagervej 2, 8240 Risskov, Denmark
[2]The Lundbeck Foundation Initiative for Integrative Psychiatric Research, iPSYCH, Copenhagen, Denmark
Full list of author information is available at the end of the article

have made it important to continue the debate regarding the return of individual genetic research findings.

Children are included in genomic research because some disorders are childhood-onset [10]. For example, to study genetic factors for attention deficit hyperactivity disorder (ADHD) or autism spectrum disorder, blood and buccal cell samples from children with ADHD and autism spectrum disorder are often taken in the clinical setting and used for research. Research on children can also be done using already existing biological samples stored in a biobank. For example, the Danish Neonatal Screening Biobank holds archived blood samples from all newborns in Denmark after screening for phenylketonuria (PKU) and several other congenital diseases [11, 12]. The dried blood spot samples from the neonates provide an opportunity to use DNA from children in research on a very large scale [13].

The ethical issues of including children in genomic research differ from those raised when including adults [10, 14, 15]. One of the biggest differences is that a third party (the parent) must mediate the relationship between the researcher and the research subject (the child) [10, 14, 16, 17]. Furthermore, young children do not have the same capacity to understand the research information or the implications of the findings. Common questions related to involvement of children in genomic research include the following: Should children be research subjects at all? Should the findings be returned to the child or to the parents? [5, 10, 14, 17–22].

If samples are to be collected and used for research purposes in Denmark, the research subject must be of legal age (18 years) to voluntarily consent to participate. If the research subject is not able to consent, for example, due to the age, such authority lies with the parents or the guardians [23]. If a research project obtains significant information about the health status of the research subject, the research subject should be informed, unless the subject has specifically expressed that s/he does not want the information [24]. The Danish National Committee on Health Research Ethics has developed a guideline on genomic research [25]. The guideline addresses inclusion of children in genomic research and return of incidental findings. It is emphasized that there must be a direct health benefit for the individual child to justify inclusion in whole genome research and that it is not sufficient to include children simply to study the genetics of a disease. Return of results to research subjects is only the norm for genetic variants with high penetrance that predispose to serious curable or treatable disease, whereas no return of results is usually provided for genetic variants with low or moderate penetrance and uncertain clinical significance [25]. The guideline furthermore addresses that exemptions from obtaining consent from parents can be given if the research project uses biological samples archived in a biobank [25].

The legal regulations in Denmark on the return of findings based on children's DNA are complex and unclear. This makes it difficult for researchers and research subjects to navigate the regulations governing the return of findings from children's DNA. We assume that the severity, treatability, and preventability of the disease; the age of the child; and the decision on whether to return incidental findings are discussed at the time of donation of the sample as all these issues are relevant in the decision-making. It is unclear whether the return of genetic risk variants with high penetrance that predispose to severe, curable, or treatable diseases encompasses all known genetic risk variants, including those for adult-onset disorders. Furthermore, it is unclear if results should be returned to the child or to the parents or whether results should be conveyed only when the child reaches legal age.

Previous studies have found that parents generally think that children should be involved in genomic research and that parents have a right to know about incidental findings concerning their child(ren) [26–28]. However, to our knowledge, no large studies have investigated the attitudes towards the involvement of children in genomic research among potential research subjects. Researching such attitudes is important to create policy strategies and to design future genomic research projects that meet the concerns and expectations of potential research subjects. We chose to study this topic in the context of mental disorders because they are some of the commonest disorders in the population and because large genome sequencing studies have been conducted in this area [13, 29, 30].

This study aims to explore attitudes among stakeholders in psychiatric genetic research towards (i) children as genomic research subjects, (ii) return of pertinent and incidental findings, and (iii) disclosure to participants (i.e., children) or their parents.

Methods

For the purpose of this study, we use pertinent findings for the results that are directly relevant to the condition under investigation and incidental findings for results that are not directly related to the research project but may have health importance for the individual research subject. We use a definition of childhood, starting from birth to 18 years of age, referring to the legal age of majority in Denmark. According to Statistics Denmark, individuals under age 26 living at home are defined as home-living children because the child has parental reference to at least one adult [31]. Therefore, we define a parent as a male or female with children under age 26 years living at home.

Mixed-methods

We used a mixed-methods design as we collected both qualitative and quantitative data [32]. This approach was taken to address the overall aim at different levels and to complement the strengths of a single-method design. The motivation for using a mixed-methods design was to use qualitative interviews to develop and modify the quantitative survey, but the qualitative interviews also helped to approach the field regarding inclusion of children in genomic research from a different angle.

The qualitative interviews

The interviews were conducted to explore the attitudes towards ethical issues regarding the use of genomic sequencing in psychiatric research among experts engaged in genomic research and among potential research participants in psychiatric genetic research. The interview guides were developed on the basis of relevant literature and the research questions of the overall study. The overall interview guides focused on attitudes towards (i) sharing findings, (ii) consenting procedures, (iii) duties of genomic researchers, (iv) including children in genomic research, and (v) misuse of knowledge in genetics. All interviews were conducted from 5 December 2012 to 11 December 2013, and each interview lasted between 30 and 90 min.

The informants

The informants in the interviews were experts (doctors and nurses), working with issues surrounding genomic research in Denmark, including the Faroe Islands, and persons with schizophrenia. The informants in the focus group interviews comprised persons with ADHD, parents to children with ADHD, clinical geneticists, and healthy controls (blood donors from the Danish Blood Donor Study (DBDS)). The persons with schizophrenia and ADHD were all diagnosed by psychiatrists and were stable in daily life. All blood donors who participated in the interview (and in the survey) are part of DBDS and have all given a broad informed consent to participate in a biobank for research and are potential healthy controls in genomic research. To be included in DBDS, the individual is not subjected to any medical treatment [33, 34]. Participants in the interview were all voluntary and informants were recruited through direct email contact, paper flyers at an activity center for mentally ill, invitations posted in an ADHD Facebook group, an ADHD clinic, a psychiatrist working in private practice, Copenhagen Hospital Biobank, and a blood donor Facebook group.

The data analysis

All interviews were audio-recorded, transcribed verbatim, coded, and analyzed using the software package NVivo 11 [35]. NVivo helped to organize and manage the data. We were based on Grounded Theory as a method to analyze the data because this analytical strategy suggests a systematic analysis and enabled us to explore and identify attitudes towards inclusion of children in genomic research [36]. All transcripts were analyzed after a three-step process: open coding, axial coding, and selective coding [36]. We examined the emerging core concepts overall and how they differed across informants. We used some of the core concepts to develop items for the survey. For this paper, we selected relevant and illustrative quotes regarding inclusion of children in genome research and return of results. All quotes were translated from Danish into English by a professional translator.

The cross-sectional survey

After the interviews, we conducted a cross-sectional web-based survey to explore specific attitudes towards the use of genomic research in Denmark. The survey was a translated and modified version of an English web-based survey developed at the Wellcome Trust Sanger Institute in Cambridge, UK [3, 37–40]. Details of the development of both the English and Danish survey versions have been presented elsewhere [39, 41]. On basis of the qualitative interviews, we modified the Danish version of the survey to also include items on informed consent, inclusion of children, and personal and familial experience with mental disorders. Items on children in genomic research were included because it was a key topic in the interviews and because the category of "age" came up in all the interviews. The survey also included self-reported sociodemographic information. Ten explanatory video films with subtitles and voice-over were used to illustrate the ethical issues raised in the survey (https://svaros.dk/holdning). The data collection began in August 2014 and ended April 2015. An average survey took approximately 23 min to complete.

The stakeholders

Potential stakeholders in psychiatric genomic research were recruited: (i) 241 persons with mental disorders (who are potential cases in genomic research), (ii) 671 relatives to individuals with mental disorders (who are potential controls in genomic research), (iii) 1623 blood donors from DBDS (who serve as healthy controls in genomic research) [33, 34], (iv) 28 clinical geneticists (who analyze, return, and explain genomic data to patients and relatives in their clinical work and who must validate sequencing findings obtained in research), and (v) 74 psychiatrists (who diagnose and treat people with mental disorders) ($N = 2637$). We recruited the stakeholders through email, paper flyers at psychiatric hospitals, invitations posted in an ADHD Facebook group, and links at the homepages of the Danish Psychiatric

Association, the Danish Society of Medical Genetics, and user groups of psychiatric patients and their relatives.

Statistical analysis

We expected parents to hold a different attitude from non-parents because of their parenthood and interest in the health of their child. For example, parents might be motivated to participate in genomic research with the hope of receiving crucial information about the health of their child. Therefore, we decided to divide the stakeholders into parents (persons with children under age 26 years living at home) or non-parents (persons without children).

Descriptive statistics were used to characterize the study sample. Unadjusted associations between items and stakeholders were estimated using χ^2 tests. Multivariable logistic regression with 95% confidence interval (CI) and a

p value of 0.05 was used to estimate the association between item and stakeholder adjusted for parenthood, gender, age, educational level, marital status, and stakeholder group. "Don't know" answers were omitted from the regression model but are a part of the analysis regarding the questions towards the return of pertinent and incidental finding in children (Figs. 1 and 2). The analysis of the data was carried out using SAS® 9.4 [42].

The two questions regarding return of pertinent and incidental findings from research could be answered in four different ways, and respondents were allowed to choose more than one answer. We analyzed all answers and identified six combinations for pertinent findings and the same six combinations for incidental findings: (i) The child should have the opportunity to get information about pertinent/incidental findings, (ii) The child should not have

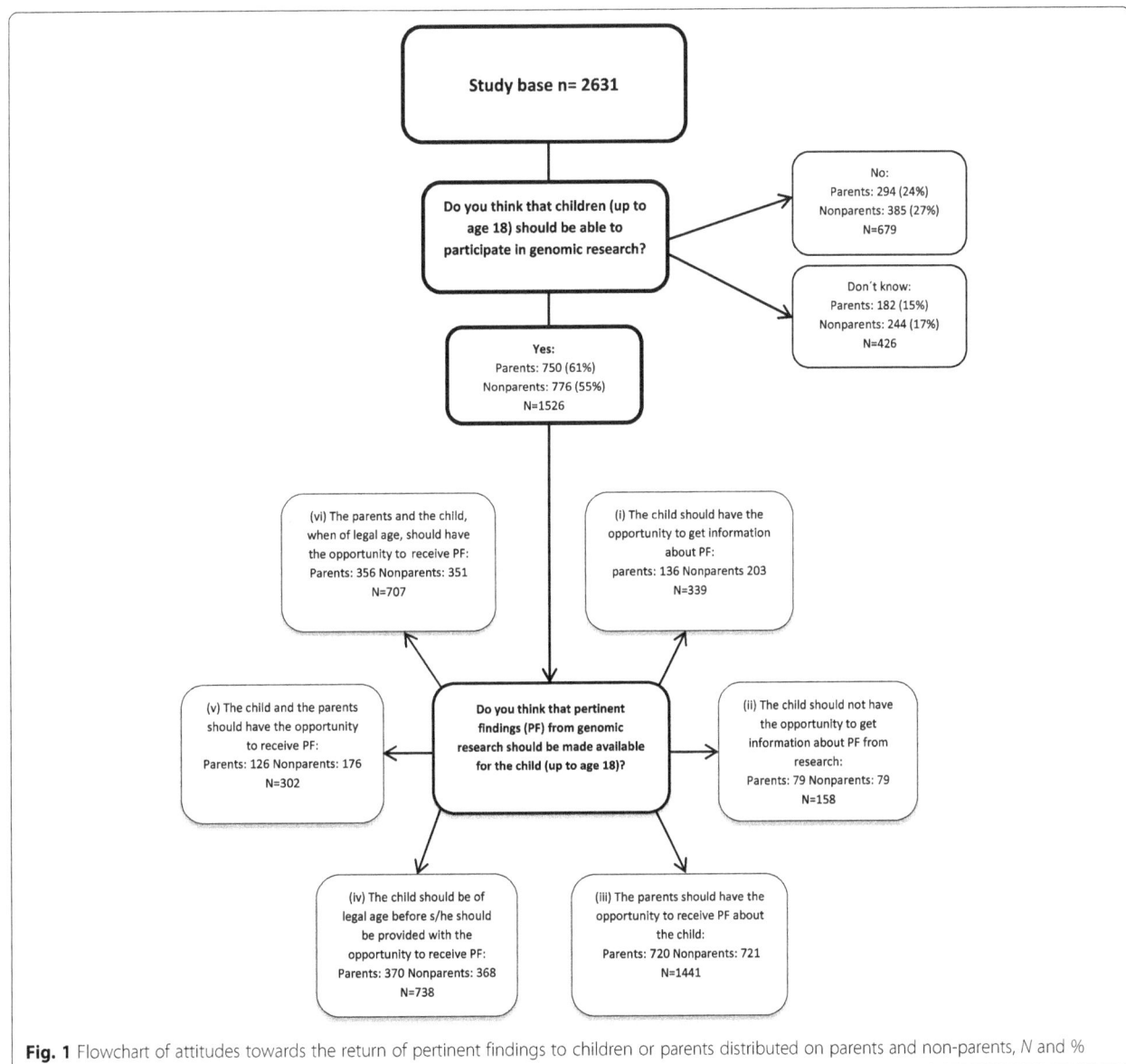

Fig. 1 Flowchart of attitudes towards the return of pertinent findings to children or parents distributed on parents and non-parents, N and %

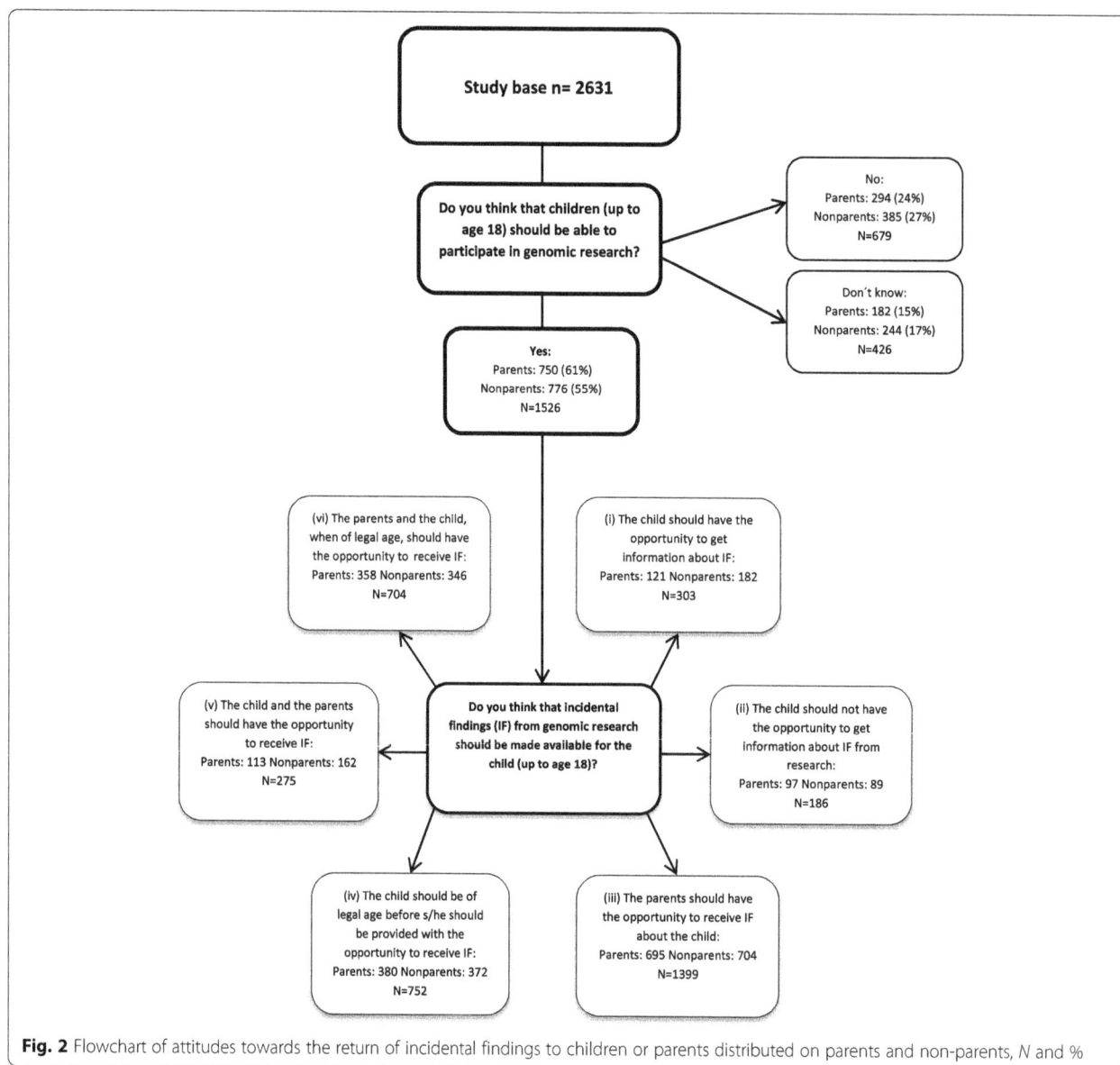

Fig. 2 Flowchart of attitudes towards the return of incidental findings to children or parents distributed on parents and non-parents, *N* and %

the opportunity to get information about pertinent/incidental findings from research, (iii) The parents should have the opportunity to receive pertinent findings about the child if they would like to receive such information, (iv) The child should be of legal age before getting the opportunity to receive pertinent/incidental findings, (v) The child and the parents should have the opportunity to receive pertinent/incidental findings, (vi) The parents and the child, when of legal age (18 years), should have the opportunity to receive pertinent/incidental findings (Figs. 1 and 2).

Results

The qualitative interviews

Sample characteristics

A total of 10 semi-structured qualitative interviews were conducted in this study: four focus-group interviews, one

group interview, and five individual interviews. The informants consisted of 12 males and 17 females (Table 1).

Attitudes towards using children as genomic research subjects

The attitudes towards children as genomic research subjects varied. Experts, persons with ADHD, and parents of children with ADHD generally had a positive view, whereas clinical geneticists, persons with schizophrenia, and blood donors tended to have more ambiguous views. As a person with schizophrenia expressed: "Children should not be part of a research project, really. That makes a mess."

The age of the child played a major role in the talks and discussions about children as research subjects. The overall attitudes were that parents should make the decision on whether their child should be included or not, that parents should give informed consent on behalf

Table 1 Overview of sample characteristics in the qualitative interviews

Interview	Informants	Supplementary information
Focus-group interview	Persons with ADHD ($n = 5$)	Male 4; female 1, Denmark
Focus-group interview	Parents to children with ADHD ($n = 6$)	Male 1; female 5, Denmark
Focus-group interview	Danish blood donors from DBDS ($n = 5$)	Male 3; female 2, Denmark
Focus-group interview	Clinical geneticists ($n = 6$)	Male 1; female 5, Denmark
Group interview	Experts ($n = 2$)	Females, Faroe Islands
Individual interview	Expert	Female, Faroe Islands
Individual interview	Expert	Male, Denmark
Individual interview	Person with schizophrenia	Female, Denmark
Individual interview	Person with schizophrenia	Male, Denmark
Individual interview	Person with schizophrenia	Male, Denmark

The table presents type of interview and background of informants, their gender, and country of origin

of their child, and that the child should be involved in the decisions depending on the age of the child: the older the child, the more the child should be involved in the decision-making.

The willingness to enroll children in genomic research was often associated with the dilemma of receiving the individual results:

Is it fair to deny the child the right to receive this knowledge [about genetic findings] from a research project – to say yes or no regarding information about himself or herself? [...] I don't think that we should cancel the research, but I think that the problem occurs when you start to involve the families in the return of individual results. (Clinical geneticist)

During the interview with the clinical geneticists, the discussion addressed the use of PKU samples in research and two informants discussed use of their own children's archived neonatal PKU samples:

Clinical geneticist A, "My children, they should no longer be registered in the Danish Neonatal Screening Biobank. I will make the call next week."

Clinical geneticist B, "What then if they become ill, and you could have known it?"

Clinical geneticist A, "Yes. I know that."

Clinical geneticist B concludes, "But it is exactly post-rationalization that is difficult. I mean, beforehand, we may say that we don't want to know, but what then if

we suddenly have a sick child; and we could have done something?"

The clinical geneticists discussed the return of individual research results in relation to a child's right to make an autonomous decision, but the discussion also touched on the possibility of using the research results as clinical information with potential health benefits for their child.

Several informants agreed that there is an emotional burden linked to the recipient's age at the time when information about such findings is received and that returning the findings too early in the child's life "could ruin the person's life." (blood donor)

There is great difference between a man of 51, such as myself, with certain life experience – both good and bad – and a young person with certain ideas about how hers life should be and who would be terribly disturbed by knowing of an 80 percent risk of getting, for example, breast cancer. So you have to consider when in life you should [return knowledge about findings], I think that is what I believe. (Other blood donor)

Some of the informants also expressed that there is an emotional burden associated with the return of findings to parents:

Well, I would say that neither I nor the children should know anything before they have turned 18. I really don't think that the children can handle knowledge about it at their age and I... I should obviously not have that knowledge about my children before they are 18. Because I cannot handle such knowledge either. (Mother of a child with ADHD)

Nevertheless, there was no consensus among the informants as to whether the parents or the child should receive the findings:

There is no doubt that I love him, my son. I love him more than anything, but I would still like to have that knowledge because it is a hard life. (Father of a child with ADHD)

The two parents of children with ADHD have different attitudes to the return of findings from research. The mother states that she should not receive the findings until her child is of legal age, whereas the father focuses on the opportunity to receive information that could help his son get a better life.

In short, the attitudes towards children as genomic research subjects varied among informants. There was no consensus whether children should be genomic research subjects and whether the child or the parents should receive the genomic findings. The attitudes of involving children in genomic research focused on the child's right to take an autonomic choice when of legal age, the emotional burden of knowing of both children and parents, and the possibility of receiving clinical information that could benefit the future health of the child.

The survey
Sample characteristics
A total of 1227 parents and 1406 non-parents completed the survey. Their characteristics are presented in Table 2. There was an almost equal distribution between males and females. Parents were significantly older than non-parents. The mean age was 45 years (standard deviation (SD) 8) for parents and 48 years (SD 15) for non-parents. A higher proportion of parents than non-parents had a

Table 2 Socioeconomic characteristics of survey respondents

	Parents (n = 1227) % (n*)	Non-parents (n = 1406) % (n*)	p value**
Sex			0.37
Female	52 (634)	53 (751)	
Male	48 (591)	47 (653)	
Age groups, years			< 0.0001
20–40	28 (347)	36 (504)	
41–60	70 (852)	37 (526)	
61–76	2 (25)	27 (373)	
Age, mean (SD)	45 (8)	48 (15)	
Level of high education***			< 0.0001
None higher education	2 (17)	3 (34)	
Short higher(< 3 years)	28 (348)	29 (409)	
Medium higher (3–4 years)	29 (356)	32 (449)	
Long higher (> 4 years)	38 (470)	31 (439)	
Other education	3 (35)	5 (74)	
Marital status			< 0.0001
Married/cohabiting	84 (1032)	52 (727)	
Partnership	6 (70)	17 (241)	
Single	10 (122)	31 (437)	
Stakeholder groups			0.23
Persons with mental disorders	8 (103)	10 (138)	
Relatives to persons with mental disorders	26 (322)	25 (348)	
Blood donors	61 (749)	62 (871)	
Clinical geneticists	2 (18)	1 (10)	
Psychiatrists	3 (35)	2 (39)	

Socio-economic characteristics of the sample; specified in percentage and number of participants divided by parents, non-parents, and total. Values that were significant at p < 0.05 are set in italics
*n varies because of missing data
**χ^2
***Children must receive 10 years of compulsory education in Denmark

long level of education and was married/cohabiting. The majority of persons with mental disorders were diagnosed with depression, anxiety, or obsessive compulsive disorder by a doctor. The majority of relatives was first or second degree relatives (data not shown). No statistically significant differences were found for gender and stakeholder group membership between parents and non-parents (Table 2). Thus, parents were older, better educated (due to their age), and—not surprisingly—married.

Attitudes towards children as research subjects
Table 3 shows the respondents' attitudes towards children as research subjects in genomic research and the association with parenthood, age, educational level, marital status, and stakeholder group.

Significantly more males (76%) than females (63%) and significantly less persons with short higher education (67%) and other education (61%) than persons with long higher education responded that children should be able to participate in genomic research.

A consistent finding was that parents were more positive towards this statement than non-parents. Persons in the young age group (20–40 years), the older age group (61–76 years), single persons, persons with mental disorders, psychiatrists, and clinical geneticists were more negative towards the statement than persons in the mid age group (41–60 years), persons in a partnership, and blood donors (Table 3).

Attitudes towards the return of pertinent and incidental findings in children
As shown in Table 3, a majority of parents and non-parents responded that children should be able to participate in genomic research. However, 24% parents and 27% non-parents responded that children should not be able to participate in genomic research, whereas 15% parents and 17% non-parents did not know (Figs. 1 and 2).

The parents and non-parents who responded in the survey that children should be able to participate in genomic research (N = 1526) were asked about their opinion on the return of pertinent and incidental findings (Figs. 1 and 2). Firstly, both for pertinent (N = 1441) and incidental findings (N = 1399), parents and non-parents agreed that the parents should have the opportunity to receive both types of findings. Secondly, the child should be of legal age before s/he should be provided with the opportunity to receive pertinent (N = 738) and incidental findings (N = 752).

Discussion
Main findings
Two main discussion points emerged from the study. These will be discussed below.

Table 3 Attitudes towards children as research subjects in genomic research

Do you think that children (up to age 18) should be able to participate in genomic research?

	N	Yes % (n)	OR $_{adj}$ (95% CI)*	p value
Parenthood	2205			
Non-parent		67 (776)	1.00	
Parent		72 (750)	1.19 (0.96–1.48)	0.12
Sex	2204			
Female		63 (714)	1.00	
Male		76 (813)	1.77 (1.46–2.14)	*< 0.0001*
Age groups, years	2202			
41–60		70 (806)	1.00	
20–40		69 (501)	0.95 (0.76–1.19)	0.67
61–76		68 (218)	0.92 (0.68–1.24)	0.58
Level of high education	2206			
Long higher (> 4 years)		73 (562)	1.00	
None higher education		60 (25)	0.54 (0.29–1.06)	0.07
Short higher (< 3 years)		67 (424)	0.75 (0.59–0.96)	*0.03*
Medium higher (3–4 years)		69 (456)	0.87 (0.68–1.11)	0.26
Other education		61 (60)	0.59 (0.38–0.93)	*0.02*
Marital status	2204			
Married/cohabiting		70 (1034)	1.00	
Partnership		70 (186)	1.09 (0.79–1.50)	0.62
Single		65 (305)	0.95 (0.75–1.22)	0.69
Stakeholder group	2207			
Blood donors		70 (956)	1.00	
Persons with mental disorder		66 (130)	1.00 (0.73–1.39)	0.99
Relatives		70 (386)	1.05 (0.84–1.31)	0.69
Clinical geneticists		67 (18)	0.88 (0.40–2.12)	0.77
Psychiatrists		69 (38)	0.84 (047–1.59)	0.59

Multivariable logistic regression was used to assess the attitudes towards children as research subjects in genomic research and the association with parenthood, stakeholder group, gender, age, educational level, and marital status, with 95% CI and p value of < 0.05. Values that were significant at p < 0.05 are set in italics
*Adjusted for parenthood, stakeholder group, gender, age, educational level, and marital status

Children as genomic research subjects

In a hypothetical scenario, participants are overall likely to hold positive views on the question whether a child should be able to participate in genomic research. Our findings are similar to Fernandez et al. [26], who found that the majority of participants reported that children should be able to take part in genomic research, whether the condition under study began in childhood or not and independent of the existence of effective treatment. We expected that parents in the survey would hold a more positive view and that non-parents would be more indifferent, but we found only slightly higher agreement among parents than among non-parents.

There was a significant higher agreement towards involving children in genomic research among males than females indicating that males have less protective or more chance-taking behaviors than females. Having short higher education and other education was significantly associated with less agreement toward the statement than persons with long higher education. Individuals with low level of education may have greater difficulties in understanding the consequences of genomic data and thus more worries of letting children participate in genomic research.

Return of results: the child's right to know

Participants expressed an attitude and also an expectation towards receiving research findings concerning children. In the interviews, there was no consensus whether the child or the parents should receive the findings. However, the return of findings were discussed in relation to the child's age, the child's right to an autonomous choice, the possibility of the emotional burden of knowing, and the possibility of receiving important clinical information. The majority in the survey agreed that both pertinent and incidental findings should be returned to the parents and to the child when of legal age. As parents might be more interested than non-parents in receiving clinical information, we expected that parents would take a more positive approach than non-parents. Nevertheless, we found that parents and non-parents had very similar attitudes. Thus, having children does not seem to affect stakeholder's attitudes towards return of findings in children.

Furthermore, there were no differences in participant's attitudes towards the return of pertinent or incidental findings, and they are interested in receiving both types of findings regarding the child. Our results illustrate that there are an interest in receiving information and that the child's right to an autonomous choice and the parent's interest to be informed are both important for the participants. The results in the survey study are consistent with those of Kleiderman et al. [28], who found that parents of children affected by a wide range of rare diseases expressed an interest in receiving their child's research results. However, our results further illustrate that the guideline on genomic research from The Danish National Committee on Health Research Ethics [25] is more restrictive than participants' attitudes toward the inclusion of children in genomic research. The participants accept inclusion of children in research without having direct health benefit for the child, including studies of the genetics of a disorder. Additionally, they are more positive towards the return of findings than the guideline.

Although the child does not have full autonomy when joining a genomic research project, the child will have autonomy in the future as an adult. As genomic research may provide clinical findings about both child-onset and adult-onset genetic diseases, it is important to consider the child's future and right to know and not to know. Respecting the right to an open future means that the child can make his or her own autonomous decisions when reaching adulthood [10, 14, 27, 43, 44]. Feinberg [45] holds that children have a right, while they still are children, to remain ignorant of disease predisposition until they reach adulthood, presumably capable of making a well-informed decision. While the child is still a child, these "future interests" include interests that the child will in fact come to have in the future, including future interests that might never happen [45]. The right to an open future protects the child against having important life choices determined by parents (and others) before having the ability to make them for themselves. The parents can disrupt the child's right to an open future if they act in a way that will cut off possibilities for the child in adulthood. For example, if the parents receive findings regarding breast cancer because of mutations in *BRCA1* or *BRCA2* genes, it can conflict with the child's right to an open future if knowledge is disclosed that the child would have wanted to live without as an adult. Nevertheless, withholding discoverable information from the child could also close a child's future if the child were interested in receiving the information as a child. The legal regulations in Denmark are unclear whether the return of genomic results encompasses adult-onset disorders and whether the results should be returned to the child or to the parents. Thus, it is uncertain whether parents have a right to be informed about all their child's genomic research findings, including adult-onset genetic diseases. The Clinical Sequencing Exploratory Research (CSER) Consortium and the Electronic Medical Records and Genomics (eMERGE) Network aim to develop practical strategies for addressing questions concerning the return of results in genomic research [44]. For example, CSER and eMERGE address whether adult-onset findings should be offered for pediatric research participants. They conclude that, during the consent process, the parents should be offered the choice of whether or not to have the adult-onset actionable incidental findings returned along with counseling [44]. In the Danish clinical setting, children are not being offered genetic testing for adult-onset conditions. However, the Danish legislation in this area is unclear concerning the research setting. The results of this study suggest that it is important to incorporate the child's right to an open future and to address the return of information of adult-onset genetic diseases in the (legal) discussion of children as research subjects.

Strengths and limitations

It is a strength of the study design that we used both interview and survey data because the two methods contribute different insights to the topic. The interviews provided an in-depth perspective concerning the attitudes and views of the informants, and the survey data provided a broader and more general attitudinal perspective. It is also a strength that the first part of our data collection was used to inform the second part as the qualitative interviews inspired us to include additional items in the questionnaire survey to focus its scope. In the survey, we were measuring genomic research broadly and not specific at psychiatric genomic research. However, no larger studies have investigated the attitudes of patients, relatives, and health professionals in psychiatry and genetics towards inclusion of children in genomic research. The results illustrate that persons with mental disorder and relatives do not differ in attitudes from blood donors or clinical geneticists. This study thus contributes with new original knowledge in relation to stakeholders in psychiatry in Denmark. Each mode of the data collection provided preferential access to certain parts of the population. It is a strength that we used web-based survey since this method is known to recruit hard-to-reach groups [46, 47]. At the same time, using a web-based survey requires the participants to be familiar and have access to smartphones, tables, laptops, or computers, and this may have excluded potential participants without these skills or without access to such technical equipment or to the internet. Therefore, it is likely that the included stakeholders comprise a more homogeneous group, more positive of genomic research than potential participants who did not participate.

The study had some further limitations. Firstly, the survey and interviews had the inherent weaknesses of measuring hypothetical scenarios as the participants did not have direct experience with genomic research. "Real" requests to use children in genomic research could produce different results. Responses to hypothetical scenarios often anticipate behaviors and future intentions rather than actual behavior [48]. Therefore, studies are needed to test actual behavior in a real-life situation. However, we still think hypothetical scenario methodology is an important tool for predicting interest in research and to understand attitudes. Secondly, participants were included on a voluntary basis, and we cannot assess the effects of non-response. Participants may be more favorably inclined towards genomic research than the general population since the participants must be willing to take part in this study and thereby have an influence on the generalizability of the study results. The survey might have been too difficult or too long to maintain the engagement of the participants. This potential selection bias could mean that the results do not represent all possible stakeholders in genomic research in Denmark. Thirdly, persons with schizophrenia are difficult to recruit into trials [49]. In this study, it was difficult to recruit persons with schizophrenia to a focus-group interview. As a result, we decided to conduct individual interviews in this group of informants. A focus-group interview allows for interaction between the informants and may have given some more knowledge about the mechanisms behind certain attitudes expressed by the informants. Furthermore, it is possible that other core concepts would have emerged including persons with different mental disorders and psychiatrists because it is not certain that the focus-group interview went to saturation with the included interviews. Fourthly, we used a broad age category of children in the survey. As the age of the child could influence the participant's attitudes, it is important to divide the children into several age categories in future studies. Fifthly, the participants were not specifically recruited because of their status as parents or non-parents. Instead, in consideration of the overall aim, we focused on recruiting a wide range of stakeholders in psychiatric genomic research: persons with mental disorders, relatives, blood donors, psychiatrists, and clinical geneticists. Finally, it could have been interesting to study the participants' attitudes towards the return of pertinent and incidental findings in children subdivided into childhood-onset and adult-onset diseases.

Conclusion

Participants generally reported positive views on the inclusion of children in genomic research. Additionally, our results illustrate that both the child's right to autonomy and the parent's interest in receiving information are important and valuable factors for the participants. They hold more positive and comprehensive views than the current Danish Guidelines on the inclusion of children and return of findings. However, having children does not affect the participant's attitudes towards the inclusion of children as research subjects in genomic research.

Genomic research on children raises complex ethical issues and it is important to consider the view of potential stakeholders who rarely get a voice. Despite the Danish Guidelines, the issue of when to include children as research subjects and how to deliver research findings is still unclear and subject to legal challenges. We hope that sharing their attitudes will help the mobilization of knowledge on children as genomic research subjects, the return of findings regarding adult-onset genetic diseases, and the children's right to an open future. Similarly, we think it is important to address these issues in the legal discussion of children as research subjects.

Acknowledgements
The authors would like to thank Professor Mette Hartlev for valuable constructive comments on an earlier draft of this article.

Funding
We would like to acknowledge the Deciphering Developmental Disorders (DDD) study for funding the films that were used in this research. The DDD study presents independent research commissioned by the Health Innovation Challenge Fund (grant number: HICF-1009-003), a parallel funding partnership between the Wellcome Trust and the Department of Health, UK. This study was supported financially by the Lundbeck Foundation Initiative for Integrative Psychiatric Research, iPSYCH, Denmark (grant number: R155-2014-1724) and Aarhus University. The funding sources were not involved in the study design, data collection and analysis, writing of the manuscript, or decision regarding publication.

Authors' contributions
AS, MWB, TFH, and OM conceived the study and its design. AS, KSB, and HU recruited participants from the Danish Blood Donor Study. AS recruited the participants for the interviews and survey, collected the data, and performed the data analyses and the statistical analyses. AS drafted the manuscript. All authors reviewed and commented on drafts of the manuscript, and all authors approved the final version of the manuscript.

Competing interests
The authors declare that they have no competing interests.

Author details
[1]Department of Clinical Medicine, Psychosis Research Unit, Aarhus University Hospital, Skovagervej 2, 8240 Risskov, Denmark. [2]The Lundbeck Foundation Initiative for Integrative Psychiatric Research, iPSYCH, Copenhagen, Denmark. [3]Department of Political Science, Copenhagen University, Copenhagen, Denmark. [4]Department of Clinical Immunology, Copenhagen University Hospital, Copenhagen, Denmark. [5]Institute for Biological Psychiatry, Mental Health Centre Sct. Hans, Copenhagen University Hospital, Copenhagen, Denmark. [6]Danish Headache Center, Department of Neurology, Rigshospitalet-Glostrup, Copenhagen, Denmark.

References
1. Christenhusz GM, Devriendt K, Dierickx K. To tell or not to tell? A systematic review of ethical reflections on incidental findings arising in genetics contexts. Eur J Hum Genet. 2013;21:248–55.
2. Klitzman R, Appelbaum PS, Fyer A, Martinez J, Buquez B, Wynn J, et al. Researchers' views on return of incidental genomic research results: qualitative and quantitative findings. Genet Med. 2013;15:888–95.
3. Middleton A, Morley KI, Bragin E, Firth HV, Hurles ME, Wright CF, et al. Attitudes of nearly 7000 health professionals, genomic researchers and publics toward the return of incidental results from sequencing research. Eur J Hum Genet. 2016;24:21–9.
4. Parens E, Appelbaum P, Chung W. Incidental findings in the era of whole genome sequencing? Hastings Cent Rep. 2013;43:16–9.
5. Ryan KA, De Vries RG, Uhlmann WR, Roberts JS, Gornick MC. Public's views toward return of secondary results in genomic sequencing: It's (almost) all about the choice. J Genet Couns. 2017;26:1197–212.
6. Solberg B, Steinsbekk KS. Managing incidental findings in population based biobank research. J Epidemiol. 2012;21:195–202.
7. Yu J-H, Harrell TM, Jamal SM, Tabor HK, Bamshad MJ. Attitudes of genetics professionals toward the return of incidental results from exome and whole-genome sequencing. Am J Hum Genet. 2014;95:77–84.
8. Tan N, Amendola LM, O'Daniel JM, Burt A, Horike-Pyne MJ, Boshe L, et al. Is "incidental finding" the best term? A study of patients' preferences. Genet Med. 2017;19:176–81.
9. Mitchell C, Ploem C, Chico V, Ormondroyd E, Hall A, Wallace S, et al. Exploring the potential duty of care in clinical genomics under UK law. Med Law Int. 2017;17:158–82.

10. Holm IA. Pediatric issues in return of results and incidental findings: Weighing autonomy and best Interests. Genet Test Mol Biomark. 2017;21: 155–8.

11. Nørgaard-Pedersen B, Hougaard DM. Storage policies and use of the Danish Newborn Screening Biobank. J Inherit Metab Dis. 2007;30:530–6.

12. Nørgaard-Pedersen B, Simonsen H. Biological specimen banks in neonatal screening. Acta Pædiatrica. 1999;88:106–9.

13. Pedersen CB, Bybjerg-Grauholm J, Pedersen MG, Grove J, Agerbo E, Bækvad-Hansen M, et al. The iPSYCH2012 case–cohort sample: new directions for unravelling genetic and environmental architectures of severe mental disorders. Mol Psychiatry. 2017; https://doi.org/10.1038/mp.2017.196.

14. Hens K. Whole genome sequencing of children's DNA for research: points to consider. J Clin Res Bioeth. 2011; https://doi.org/10.4172/2155-9627.1000106e.

15. Hens K, Van El CE, Borry P, Cambon-Thomsen A, Cornel MC, Forzano F, et al. Developing a policy for paediatric biobanks: principles for good practice. Eur J Hum Genet. 2013;21:2–7.

16. Hens K, Cassiman J-J, Nys H, Dierickx K. Children, biobanks and the scope of parental consent. Eur J Hum Genet. 2011;19:735–9.

17. Sénécal K, Thys K, Vears DF, Van Assche K, Knoppers BM, Borry P. Legal approaches regarding health-care decisions involving minors: implications for next-generation sequencing. Eur J Hum Genet. 2016;24:1559–64.

18. Zawati MH, Rioux A. Biobanks and the return of research results: Out with the old and in with the new? J Law Med Ethics. 2011;39:614–20.

19. Anderson JA, Meyn MS, Shuman C, Zlotnik Shaul R, Mantella LE, Szego MJ, et al. Parents perspectives on whole genome sequencing for their children: qualified enthusiasm? J Med Ethics. 2016; https://doi.org/10.1136/medethics-2016-103564.

20. Dodson DS, Goldenberg AJ, Davis MM, Singer DC, Tarini BA. Parent and public interest in whole-genome sequencing. Public Health Genomics. 2015;18:151–9.

21. Sabatello M, Appelbaum PS. Raising genomic citizens: Adolescents and the return of secondary genomic findings. J Law Med Ethics. 2016;44:292–308.

22. Newson AJ. Whole genome sequencing in children: ethics, choice and deliberation. J Med Ethics. 2017; https://doi.org/10.1136/medethics-2016-103943.

23. The Danish Ministry of Health. Bekendtgørelse af lov om videnskabsetisk behandling af sundhedsvidenskabelige forskningsprojekter (in Danish) [Danish Act on Research Ethics Review of Health Research Projects and later amendments]. (2017). https://www.retsinformation.dk/Forms/R0710.aspx?id=192671. Accessed 17 Sep 2017.

24. The Danish Ministry of Health. Bekendtgørelse om information og samtykke til deltagelse i sundhedsvidenskabelige forskningsprojekter samt om anmeldelse af og tilsyn med sundhedsvidenskabelige forskningsprojekter (in Danish) [Executive Order no. 1464 of 2 December 2016 on information and consent at inclusion of trial subjects in biomedical research projects and the notification and supervision of health research projects]. (2017).https://www.retsinformation.dk/Forms/R0710.aspx?id=185233. Accessed 12 Jun 2017.

25. The Danish National Committee on Health Research Ethics. Vejledning om genomer af 1. Februar 2017 (in Danish) [Guidelines on genomes of 1 February 2017]. (2017). http://www.nvk.dk/emner/genomer/vejledning-om-genomer. Accessed 16 Sep 2017.

26. Fernandez CV, Bouffet E, Malkin D, Jabado N, O'Connell C, Avard D, et al. Attitudes of parents toward the return of targeted and incidental genomic research findings in children. Genet Med. 2014;16:633–40.

27. Fernandez CV, O'Connell C, Ferguson M, Orr AC, Robitaille JM, Knoppers BM, et al. Stability of attitudes to the ethical issues raised by the return of incidental genomic research findings in children: a follow-up study. Public Health Genomics. 2015;18:299–308.

28. Kleiderman E, Knoppers BM, Fernandez CV, Boycott KM, Ouellette G, Wong-Rieger D, et al. Returning incidental findings from genetic research to children: views of parents of children affected by rare diseases. J Med Ethics. 2014;40:691–6.

29. Yu TW, Chahrour MH, Coulter ME, Jiralerspong S, Okamura-Ikeda K, Ataman B, et al. Using whole-exome sequencing to identify inherited causes of autism. Neuron. 2013;77:259–73.

30. Demontis D, Lescai F, Børglum A, Glerup S, Østergaard SD, Mors O, et al. Whole-exome sequencing reveals increased burden of rare functional and disruptive variants in candidate risk genes in individuals with persistent attention-deficit/hyperactivity disorder. J Am Acad Child Adolesc Psychiatry. 2016;55:521–3.

31. Statistics Denmark. Statistikdokumentation for Boligopgørelsen 2017 (in Danish) [Statistical documentation for the housing inentory]. (2017). www.dst.dk/Site/Dst/SingleFiles/kvaldeklbilag.aspx?filename=794ee8d0-1b80-4eb0-a077-1a0c22aca5ecBoligopg%C3%B8relsen. Accessed 7 Dec 2017

32. Johnson RB, Onwuegbuzie AJ. Mixed methods research: a research paradigm whose time has come. Educ Res. 2004;33:14–26.

33. Pedersen OB, Erikstrup C, Kotzé SR, Sørensen E, Petersen MS, Grau K, et al. The Danish Blood Donor Study: a large, prospective cohort and biobank for medical research. Vox Sang. 2012;102:271.

34. The Danish Blood Donor Study. The Danish Blood Donor Study. http://www.dbds.dk/defaultuk.htm (2016). Accessed 16 Sep 2017.

35. QSR International. Nvivo. Daresbury: Daresbury, Cheshire, WA4 4AB United Kingdom; 2017.

36. Strauss AL, Corbin JM. Basics of qualitative research: techniques and procedures for developing grounded theory. 2nd ed. Thousand Oaks: Sage Publications; 1998.

37. Middleton A, Wright CF, Morley KI, Bragin E, Firth HV, Hurles ME, et al. Potential research participants support the return of raw sequence data. J Med Genet. 2015;52:571–4.

38. Middleton A, Bragin E, Parker M. Finding people who will tell you their thoughts on genomics—recruitment strategies for social sciences research. J Community Genet. 2014:291–302.

39. Middleton A, Bragin E, Morley KI, Parker M. Online questionnaire development: using film to engage participants and then gather attitudes towards the sharing of genomic data. Soc Sci Res. 2013:211–23.

40. Middleton A, Parker M, Wright CF, Bragin E, Hurles ME, On behalf of the DDD Study. Empirical research on the ethics of genomic research. Am J Med Genet A. 2013;161:2099–101.

41. Sundby A, Boolsen MW, Burgdorf KS, Ullum H, Hansen TF, Middleton A, et al. Stakeholders in psychiatry and their attitudes toward receiving pertinent and incident findings in genomic research. Am J Med Genet A. 2017;173: 2649–58.

42. SAS Institute Inc. SAS® 9.4. Cary; 2017.

43. Davis DS. Genetic dilemmas and the child's right to an open future. Hastings Cent Rep. 1997;27:7.

44. Jarvik GP, Amendola LM, Berg JS, Brothers K, Clayton EW, Chung W, et al. Return of genomic results to research participants: The floor, the ceiling, and the choices in between. Am J Hum Genet. 2014;94:818–26.

45. Feinberg J. The child's right to an open future. In: Whose child? Children's right, parental authority, and state power. Auth. State Power. 1st ed. New Jersey: Littlefield, Adams & Co; 1980. p. 124–53.

46. Barratt MJ, Ferris JA, Lenton S. Hidden populations, online purposive sampling, and external validity: taking off the blindfold. Field Methods. 2015; 27:3–21.

47. Frippiat D, Marquis N, Wiles-Portier E. Web surveys in the social sciences: an overview. Population. 2010;65:285–311.

48. Persky S, Kaphingst KA, Condit CM, McBride CM. Assessing hypothetical scenario methodology in genetic susceptibility testing analog studies: a quantitative review. Genet Med. 2007;9:727–38.

49. Jørgensen R, Munk-Jørgensen P, Lysaker PH, Buck KD, Hansson L, Zoffmann V. Overcoming recruitment barriers revealed high readiness to participate and low dropout rate among people with schizophrenia in a randomized controlled trial testing the effect of a Guided Self-Determination intervention. BMC Psychiatry. 2014;14:28.

10

Variants in congenital hypogonadotrophic hypogonadism genes identified in an Indonesian cohort of 46,XY under-virilised boys

Katie L. Ayers[1,2], Aurore Bouty[1,3], Gorjana Robevska[1], Jocelyn A. van den Bergen[1], Achmad Zulfa Juniarto[4], Nurin Aisyiyah Listyasari[4], Andrew H. Sinclair[1,2†] and Sultana M. H. Faradz[4*†]

Abstract

Background: Congenital hypogonadotrophic hypogonadism (CHH) and Kallmann syndrome (KS) are caused by disruption to the hypothalamic-pituitary-gonadal (H-P-G) axis. In particular, reduced production, secretion or action of gonadotrophin-releasing hormone (GnRH) is often responsible. Various genes, many of which play a role in the development and function of the GnRH neurons, have been implicated in these disorders. Clinically, CHH and KS are heterogeneous; however, in 46,XY patients, they can be characterised by under-virilisation phenotypes such as cryptorchidism and micropenis or delayed puberty. In rare cases, hypospadias may also be present.

Results: Here, we describe genetic mutational analysis of CHH genes in Indonesian 46,XY disorder of sex development patients with under-virilisation. We present 11 male patients with varying degrees of under-virilisation who have rare variants in known CHH genes. Interestingly, many of these patients had hypospadias.

Conclusions: We postulate that variants in CHH genes, in particular *PROKR2*, *PROK2*, *WDR11* and *FGFR1* with *CHD7*, may contribute to under-virilisation phenotypes including hypospadias in Indonesia.

Keywords: Congenital hypogonadotrophic hypogonadism, Under-virilisation, Hypospadias, Targeted gene sequencing, Disorder of sex development

Background

Proper function of the hypothalamic-pituitary-gonadal (H-P-G) axis is essential for the development of the reproductive system. Gonadotrophin-releasing hormone (GnRH), secreted by the hypothalamus, stimulates the biosynthesis and the release of gonadotrophins from the anterior pituitary gland. These gonadotrophins (luteinising hormone (LH) and follicle-stimulating hormone (FSH)) both play distinct roles in the gonads during embryonic development. In males, FSH stimulates the proliferation of immature Sertoli cells and spermatogonia [1]. FSH also stimulates the secretion of inhibin, which acts in a negative feedback loop directly to the anterior pituitary. LH stimulates the production and secretion of testosterone from the Leydig cells, which is thought to occur through the LH receptor after 10 weeks post conception [2]. Disruption to the H-P-G axis (through deficient production, secretion or action of the gonadotrophins) can result in hypogonadotrophic hypogonadism (HH). While this can be associated with additional anomalies or syndromes such as Dandy-Walker syndrome, Gorden Holmes syndrome and CHARGE [3], when observed alone, it is termed congenital or idiopathic HH (CHH) (OMIM 146110). CHH can be coupled with a decreased or absent sense of smell due to the abnormal migration of the GnRH neurons [4, 5]. The co-occurrence of CHH with anosmia is termed Kallmann syndrome (KS (OMIM 308700, 147950, 244200, 610628, 612370 and 612702)).

* Correspondence: sultanafaradz@gmail.com
†Equal contributors
4Division of Human Genetics, Centre for Biomedical Research, Faculty of Medicine, Diponegoro University (FMDU), JL. Prof. H. Soedarto, SH, Tembalang, Semarang 50275, Central Java, Indonesia
Full list of author information is available at the end of the article

Estimates of the prevalence of CHH range between 1 and 10 in 100,000 live births, with approximately two thirds of cases arising from KS [6]. CHH in 46,XY males can cause a reduced level of circulating androgens due to hypogonadism. Isolated or apparently isolated CHH (i.e. in a patient with KS who does not complain of an absent or diminished sense of smell) is most commonly diagnosed in teenagers or young men who present with pubertal failure. During foetal development, testosterone is responsible for virilisation of the reproductive tract and dihydrotestosterone (DHT), a highly potent derivative of testosterone, drives differentiation of the external genitalia. The appearance of clinical characteristics depends on when HH begins. When GnRH deficiency occurs in the late foetal or early neonatal periods, a significant decrease in androgens can lead to some CHH patients being diagnosed postnatally with under-virilisation phenotypes such as cryptorchidism, micropenis [7] and, in some rare cases, hypospadias [8]. Patients also typically showed delayed or absent puberty including minimal virilisation, low libido, lack of sexual function and a reduced or absent growth spurt [3]. In addition to the physical anomalies, physiological impairments have also been reported such as low self-esteem, distorted body image and, in some cases, problems in sexual identity [9, 10]. Finally, CHH may be diagnosed following adolescence, later in life when infertility is a concern. Given these complex and significant physical and psychological implications, early diagnosis and treatment of CHH is essential. Clinically, CHH can phenocopy partial androgen insensitivity syndrome (PAIS) or other disorders of sex development (DSDs) in which a reduction of testosterone during development can cause reduced virilisation. If blood hormone testing is not routinely carried out, these patients may be misdiagnosed and clinical management may differ.

Genetically, CHH is highly complex. More than 30 genes have been implicated in CHH and/or KS including nine genes that cause an overlapping syndrome [3]. To complicate matters, a large degree of variability in inheritance, penetrance and expressivity is seen in CHH and an increasing body of evidence suggests that this disorder can be caused by variants in more than one gene (oligogenicity) [11, 12]. Variants in known CHH genes currently account for only 50% of CHH cases [13] meaning that more genes are yet to be found. Here, we present genetic mutational analysis of CHH genes in Indonesian 46,XY patients presenting with under-virilisation phenotypes.

Materials and methods
Clinical data
Patients with 46,XY DSD were referred to the Center for Biomedical Research, Faculty of Medicine, Diponegoro University (FMDU), Semarang, Indonesia. The medical ethics committee of the Dr. Kariadi Hospital/FMDU approved this study, and informed consent was obtained from all participants, as well as their parents or guardians, prior to their participation in this study. Following informed consent, a detailed interview was performed at recruitment and data concerning medical history, age of initial presentation, sex of rearing, family history (relatives with a genital disorder) and consanguinity were collected. Patients were clinically evaluated by a trained andrologist; a detailed description of the external genitalia was obtained and, in many cases, images taken. A blood sample was obtained for karyotyping, hormonal analysis and DNA extraction. Referral and data collection took place between 2004 and 2010. Eighty-eight of these patients have been described previously [14]. A total of 47 males with 46,XY under-virilisation phenotypes (including uni- or bilateral cryptorchidism, hypospadias, bifid scrotum, micropenis and, in some cases, severe hypospadias) were included in this study. Hormone analysis was carried out for some patients including base level LH and FSH and testosterone (T). Reference levels for FSH and LH are based on paediatric measurements depending on age [15]. In some cases, T levels were also measured following Leydig cell stimulation by human chorionic gonadotrophin (hCG). For more details on blood hormone analysis, see [14].

Gene panel sequencing
Genomic DNA was obtained from peripheral EDTA-blood samples using the salting out method [16]. The DNA underwent quality control at the Murdoch Childrens Research Institute (MCRI), Melbourne, Australia. Total genomic DNA was sequenced using a targeted panel (Haloplex, Agilent) that covers 64 diagnostic DSD genes [17]. This included 19 genes implicated in CHH (*CHD7, GNRH1, GNRHR, HESX1, LEP, PROKR2, PROP1, TAC3, FGFR1, KAL1, LHX3, FGF8, PROK2, KISS1R, WDR11, SPRY4, FSHB, CGA, SOX10*). Library preparation and sequencing were carried out as detailed in [17]. Raw data was analysed using a modified pipeline created at MCRI—C-pipe, which calls variants and provides data on frequency and pathogenicity [18].

Following C-pipe analysis, variants were checked for quality and depth and were filtered for those less than 1% minor allele frequency (MAF) in both the ESP6500 and 1000 genome project. As non-affected controls from Indonesia were not included, variants that were found very frequently in our screen (greater than 5% of total samples run) were also discounted. We manually check variant frequency in EVS and extracted ExAC data on frequency in Asia (South Asia and East Asia). Variants were checked for previous implication in human disease via ClinVAR and HMGD. Predicted pathogenicity of each variant was analysed using a range of up-to-date in silico prediction tools (SIFT, PolyPhen-2, LRT and

MutationTaster). Effects on protein structure and function were predicted using the HOPE tool [19].

Results

Patient cohort

All forty-seven 46,XY DSD patients from Indonesia were first analysed for mutations in DSD genes that cause androgen insensitivity or reduced testosterone production (e.g. *androgen receptor* (*AR*), *SRD5A2*, *HSD17B3*). Rare and damaging mutations in these genes were found in 19 patients [17] of the 47. The other 28 did not have a causative variant identified. These patients ranged in age from newborn to 14 years old, with a variety of 46,XY DSD phenotypes including hypospadias, bifid scrotum, cryptorchidism/undescended testis, microtestis and micropenis. All patients identify as male. Many have undergone hypospadias repair. The phenotypes of the eleven patients with a CHH variant are shown in Table 1, and representative images are shown in Fig. 1.

The hallmarks of CHH can include low levels of testosterone (due to hypogonadism), which can often be increased by hCG stimulation. Indeed, we found that all of the patients tested showed moderate to high increases in testosterone after hCG stimulation (Table 1). In addition, low levels of LH and FSH are often indicative of CHH; however, the natural levels of these hormones are low during childhood. Indeed, most patients were between mini-puberty and puberty when FSH/LH levels are expected to be low (<0.1–4 IU/l for LH and <0.1–8 IU/l for FSH). For all patients of this age, assayed LH and FSH levels were within the normal range. Patient 169, who was 14 at the time, had an LH measurement of 2.7 IU/l, which is within normal range, but an FSH of 9.24 IU/l, which is considered slightly elevated. Patient 147 was within mini-puberty at the time of measurement and subsequently had an elevated LH level of 10.8 and FSH of 6.23. This may suggest that secretion of these gonadotrophins is not inhibited in this patient. Patient 143 did not have hormonal analysis.

CHH genetic variants

The remaining 28 patients were then analysed for mutations in the exonic regions of CHH genes as previously detailed in [17]. Eleven patients had one or more rare variants (<1% MAF in g1000 and ESP6500) in a CHH gene (Table 2). In total, we found 14 variants in CHH genes in these patients. The variants are described below.

PROKR2

Four patients had variants in the *PROKR2* gene. Two patients (173 and 143) had the same variant—*PROKR2*:c.C563T:pS188L (Table 2). This variant has not been found in our DSD panel previously (in over 300

DSD patients; see [17]) but has a total allele frequency of 1.65e–05 in ExAC (although it has not been recorded in SA or EA). This change has been recorded to be likely pathogenic (ClinVar) [20, 21] (Table 2). Previous functional analysis has shown this variant has a strong defect in G-protein coupling [21]. The two patients with this variant (patients 173, 143) had under-virilisation phenotypes including micropenis, scrotal hypospadias and cryptorchidism (Fig. 1, Table 1). Interestingly, one of these patients also had additional anomalies. Patient 173 had spina bifida, incontinence and suspected intellectual disability—suggesting additional genetic or environmental contributors (Table 1). Indeed, the mother of this patient had a suspected folic acid deficiency during pregnancy.

Two other patients had heterozygous missense variants in the *PROKR2* gene (Table 2). c.G991A:p.V331M was found in patient 159 who has perineal hypospadias and unilateral cryptorchidism (Fig. 1, Table 1). This variant (rs117106081) has a total frequency in ExAC of 0.0065 (and was greater than 0.01 in both SA and EA). It is not predicted to be damaging in any of the in silico prediction tools and was not highly conserved. Nevertheless, this variant has been previously reported in CHH/KS patients, and functional analysis in both publications suggested a reduction in function (in particular a mild G-protein coupling defect) [21–23]. In contrast, another variant c.T1054G:p.W352G was not found in ExAC or EVS and was predicted to be damaging and highly conserved among different species (Table 2 and Fig. 2a). This was found in a patient 171, who has bilateral cryptorchidism and scrotal hypospadias (Fig. 1 and Table 1). In this case, the mutated residue is located on the surface of a domain with unknown function (Fig. 2b). The mutant residue (glycine) is smaller than the wild-type residue and differs in hydrophobicity to the wild-type residue (tryptophan). This may cause a loss of external interactions in particular a loss of hydrophobic interactions with other molecules on the surface of the protein.

From this, we hypothesise that *PROKR2* variants, in particular the variant p.S188L, represent a significant cause of under-virilisation including cryptorchidism, micropenis and, in some cases, hypospadias in Indonesian 46,XY DSD patients.

PROK2

One patient (47) was found to harbour a variant in this gene (*PROK2*:c.G68A:p.R23H). This missense heterozygous variant was not found in any of the online databases; however, it was not predicted to be pathogenic (Table 2). This patient has a micropenis, scrotal hypospadias and unilateral cryptorchidism (Table 1). The first 27 amino acids of PROK2 are a signal peptide, important

Table 1 Patient clinical details

Patient ID	Age at initial appointment	Gender		Clinical description				Associated malformations	Anosmia reported?	hCG stimulation test	Image provided?
		Genetic	Sex of rearing	Testes	Scrotum	Micropenis	Urethral meatus (type of hypospadias)			Increased T?	
173	12	46,XY	Male	Bilaterally non palpable	Bifid	Yes	Scrotal	Spina bifida	Unknown	Moderate	
143	6	46,XY	Male	R, not palpable L, 1 ml, scrotal	Bifid	Yes	Scrotal		No		Figure 1b
159	2	46,XY	Male	R, 1 ml, scrotal L, fetractile	Bifid	No	Perineal		Unknown		
171	4	46,XY	Male	R, 1–2 ml, scrotal L, 2 ml, scrotal	Bifid	Yes	Scrotal		No	Yes	Figure 1a
47	3	46,XY	Female, changed to male at 3 years	R, 2 ml, scrotal L, not palpable	Bifid	Yes	Scrotal		No	Yes	
174	3	46,XY	Male	R, not palpable L, 1 ml, scrotal	Fused	Yes	Penoscrotal		No	Yes	
164	3	46,XY	Male	Bilaterally 2 ml, scrotal	Bifid	No	Penoscrotal		No	Yes	
163	10	46,XY	Male	Bilaterally 3 ml, scrotal	Bifid	Yes	Penile		No	Yes	Figure 1c
147	1 m	46,XY	Male	R, inguinal L, not palpable	Bifid	No	Scrotal		No	Yes	
101	3	46,XY	Male	Bilaterally 2 ml, scrotal	Bifid	Yes	Scrotal		Unknown	Yes	Figure 1d
169	14	46,XY	Male	R, 4 ml, scrotal L, 6 ml, scrotal	Bifid	no	Penoscrotal		No	Yes	

Patient identification number and age at first consultation are shown, as well as sex chromosome complement and gender. A description of anomalies is also included. Response to hCG stimulation is shown. Testosterone reference levels were considered as 0.3–0.5 nmol/l except for patients 169, 163 and 8 (where reference was considered 3–6.5 nmol/l)

for its secretion. The affected amino acid (arginine at position 23) lies within this region.

WDR11

Three patients had heterozygous missense variants in *WDR11* (Table 2, patients 174, 164, 163). The first of these was one of a pair of twins, who have concordant phenotypes (patient 174, twin not analysed). This variant, *WDR11*:c.G2409T:p.W803C, was not found in online databases and is predicted to be pathogenic with strong conservation—even down to zebrafish (Table 2,

Fig. 2c). Patient 174 has a micropenis with penoscrotal hypospadias and chordee (Fig. 1, Table 1). The second variant found was *WDR11*:c.A1352G:p.H451R (Table 2). This variant (rs199920020) has a total frequency of 0.0001 in ExAC but is rare in Asia and was found in a patient with penoscrotal hypospadias and bifid scrotum but no micropenis or cryptorchidism (patient 164, Fig. 1, Table 1). Like the previous variant, this amino acid is highly conserved (Fig. 2c). The third variant (*WDR11*:c.T1279A:p.L427I) was not previously found in any online databases and was predicted to be

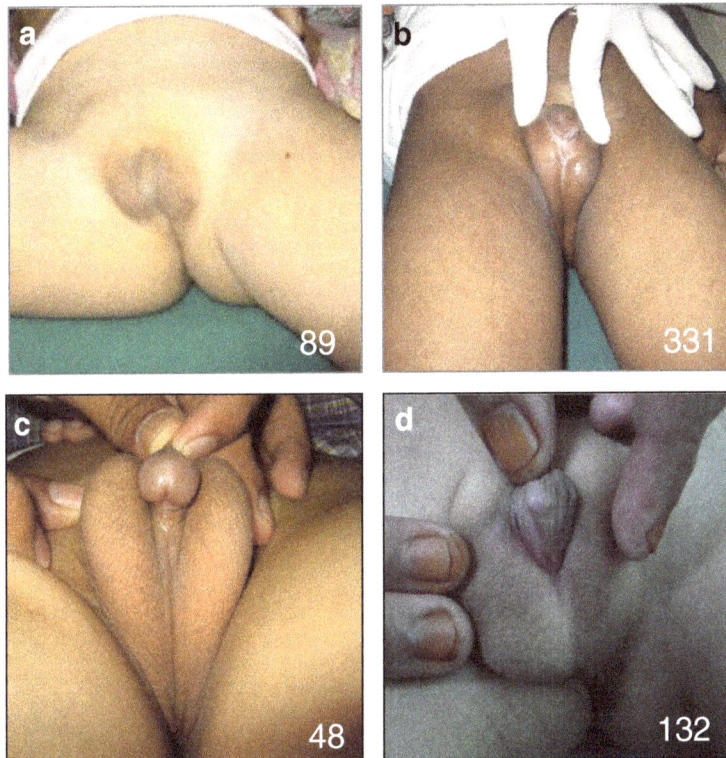

Fig. 1 Under-virilisation in patients with CHH gene variants. **a–d** Representative images of external genitalia for four patients presenting with 46,XY DSD (see Table 1 for details)

damaging and highly conserved (Fig. 2c). This was found in patient 163, who has a micropenis and penile hypospadias (Fig. 1, Table 1).

FGFR1
Three patients had the *FGFR1* variant rs140382957 (*FGFR1*:c.C320T:p.S107L) (Table 2). This variant has a MAF in EVS of 0.0077 and in ExAC of 0.0023 (and while it is predicted to be pathogenic in two prediction tools, one record in ClinVar has it logged as being benign [24].)

CHD7
Curiously, two of the three patients who had a *FGFR1* variant also had a variant in *CHD7*. One of these, *CHD7*: c.G1565T:p.G522V has an ExAC MAF of 0.002318 and was predicted damaging (Table 2); however, it has been reported as benign for CHARGE on ClinVar. This was found in patient 101. Another novel variant was rare (ExAC MAF = 9.2e–05) (*CHD7*:c.C2347T:p.P783S). No other *CHD7* variants were found.

Discussion
In this study, we have investigated variants in CHH-related genes in a cohort of Indonesian 46,XY DSD patients who had an under-virilisation phenotype. After

excluding patients with mutations in known DSD genes, we found rare and damaging variants in CHH genes in 11 of the remaining 28 patients. CHH and KS can present at birth with under-virilisation phenotypes in males such as micropenis and cryptorchidism [25]. Our study suggests that CHH may be a cause of under-virilisation in Indonesia. While forty-seven 46,XY DSD patients were initially recruited, 19 of these were found to harbour mutation in a known DSD genes such as *AR* (data not shown). Of the remaining 28, we found a likely CHH variant(s) in 11 patients, making this a total of 25% of the total original cohort. In addition, while our targeted DSD panel has a comprehensive list of diagnostic DSD genes, it only covers 19 of approximately 24 genes that cause CHH/KS without an associated syndrome. Sequencing of the entire list of known CHH genes, including those that cause CHH in association with additional anomalies, may increase the diagnostic yield of a genetic screen like this. This will be important for future studies of this cohort.

Penile and urethral morphology is established before 14 weeks gestation meaning that the foetal pituitary-hypothalamic axis is typically thought to be unnecessary for normal penile development (instead relying on maternal hCG). However, after week 14, continued increase in penile length is dependent upon the hypothalamic-

Table 2 Rare variants found in CHH genes in 46,XY DSD patients

Patient ID	CHH gene	Variant location	Change	Variant details	dbSNP	EVS MAF	ExAC total freq.	ExAC SA/EA	ClinVar/HGMD	In silico predictions	GERP+ + RS score	Previous functional studies
173	PROKR2	chr20:5283278-5283279	G/A	PROKR2:NM_144773:c.C563T:p.S188L	rs376239580	0.0077	0.00002	0/0	Yes—likely pathogenic for CHH	3 of 4	5.31	Cole et al. (2008); Zhu et al. (2015)
143	PROKR2	chr20:5283278-5283279	G/A	PROKR2:NM_144773:c.C563T:p.S188L	rs376239580	0.0077	0.00002	0/0	Yes—likely pathogenic for CHH	3 of 4	5.31	Cole et al. (2008); Zhu et al. (2015)
159	PROKR2	chr20:5282850-5282851	C/T	PROKR2:NM_144773:c.G991A:p.V331M	rs117106081	0.0154	0.00652	0.03119/0.02901	Yes—CHH	0 of 4	2.01	Dodé (2006); Monnier et al. (2009); Cole et al. (2008)
171	PROKR2	chr20:5282787-5282788	A/C	PROKR2:NM_144773:c.T1054G:p.W352G	Not found	0	0.00000	0.00	Not found	4 of 4	5.05	
47	PROK2	chr3:71834136-71834137	C/T	PROK2:NM_001126128:c.G68A:p.R23H	Not found	0	0.00000	0/0	Not found	0 of 4	2.47	
174	WDR11	chr10:122650293-122650294	G/T	WDR11:NM_018117:c.G2409T:p.W803C	Not found	0	0.00000	0/0	Not found	4 of 4	5.79	
164	WDR11	chr10:122630739-122630740	A/G	WDR11:NM_018117:c.A1352G:p.H451R	rs199920020	0	0.00007	0/0.00104	Not found	2 of 4	3.575	
163	WDR11	chr10:122626666-122626667	T/A	WDR11:NM_018117:c.T1279A:p.L427I	Not found	0	0.00000	0/0	Not found	3 of 4	3.11	
147	FGFR1	chr8:38287238-38287239	G/A	FGFR1:NM_001174063:c.C320T:p.S107L	rs140382957	0.0077	0.00253	0.0002393/0.0454	1 record—benign	2 of 4	3.6	Sato (2004); Sykiotis (2010); Fukami et al. (2013)
101	CHD7	chr8:61655556-61655557	G/T	CHD7: NM_017780:c.G1565T:p.G522V	rs142962579	0	0.00232	0.0003717/0.03098	Not found	3 of 4	5.67	
	FGFR1	chr8:38287238-38287239	G/A	FGFR1:NM_001174063:c.C320T:p.S107L	rs140382957	0.0077	0.00253	0.0002393/0.0454	1 record—benign	2 of 4	3.6	Sato (2004); Sykiotis (2010); Fukami et al (2013)
169	FGFR1	chr8:38287238-38287239	G/A	FGFR1:NM_001174063:c.C320T:p.S107L	rs140382957	0.0077	0.00253	0.0002393/0.0454	1 record—benign	2 of 4	3.6	Sato (2004); Sykiotis (2010); Fukami et al. (2013)
	CHD7	chr8:61713055-61713056	C/T	CHD7:NM_017780:c.C234T:p.P783S	rs373873996	0	0.00009	6.152e-05/0.00117	1 record—benign for CHARGE	2 of 4	5.81	
	LEP	chr7:127892124-127892125	A/G	LEP:NM_000230:c.A53G:p.Y18C	rs148407750	0.0461	0.00041	6.056e-05/0.003004	Not found	0 of 4	1.13	

Patient number is shown and the gene, variant location and DNA change. The allele frequency (from ExAC) is shown for all populations (MAF) and also specifically for both South Asia (AS) and East Asia (EA). Details are shown in the variant in found in Clinvar or in HMGD, and if reported previously, the reference is shown. Four in silico prediction programs were used for each variant, and the number of these showing a likely pathogenic/damaging score is shown. GERP++ scores are also shown

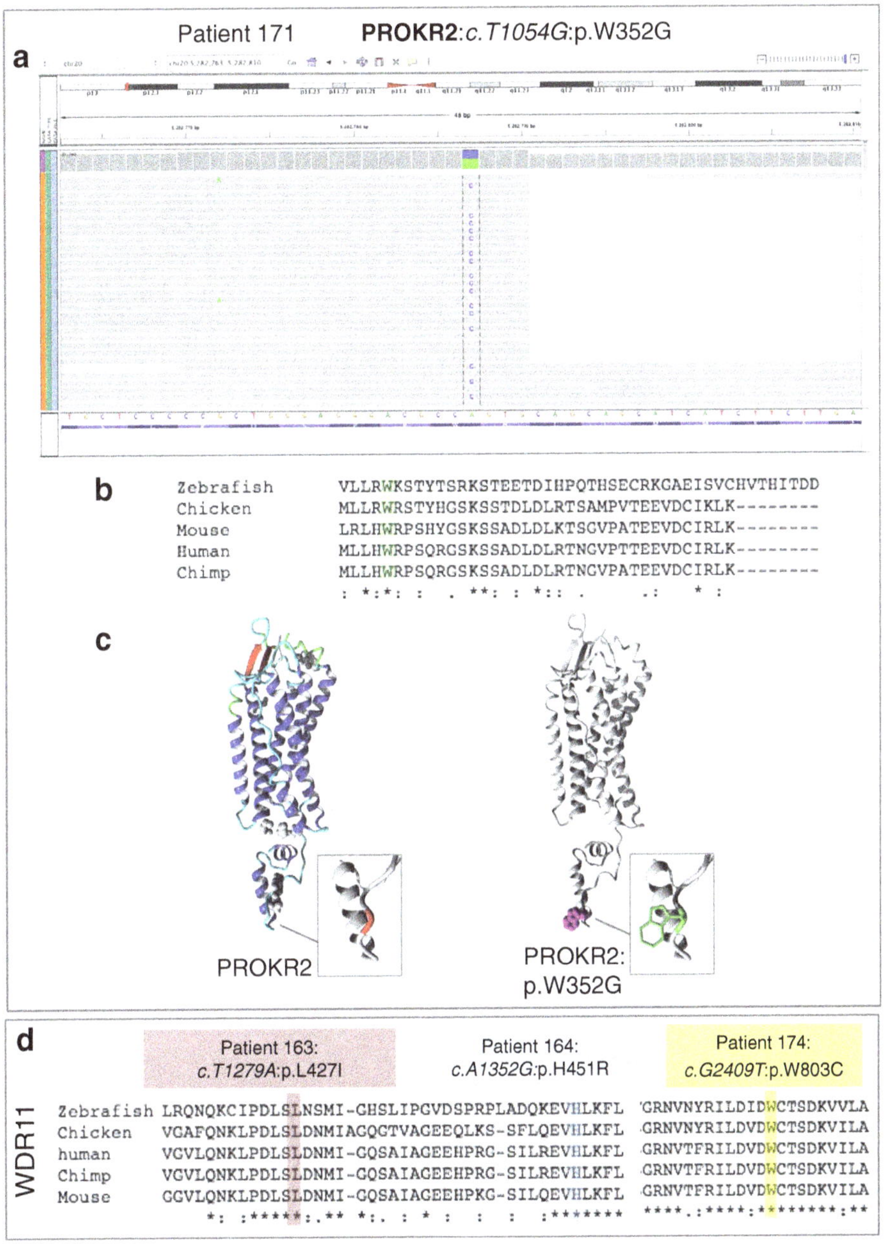

Fig. 2 Novel variants in CHH genes. Just one novel variant in *PROKR2* was found (p.W352G). This change found in patient 171, *c.T1054G*:p.W352G, is heterozygous and has good quality and depth (**a**). This change falls on a highly conserved residue (**b**) and lies within the cytoplasmic tail of this transmembrane receptor (**c**). Three novel variants in WDR11 were found in our cohort—all of which affect a highly conserved residue (**d**)

pituitary axis. Therefore, boys with hypogonadism will often have micropenis but normal phallic morphology. However, we found that many of individuals in our cohort had varying degrees of hypospadias. Given this, it is interesting to note that while rare, hypospadias in patients with CHH or KS has been described. A large study found two patients with CHH and hypospadias [26], and several other studies have described patients with KS or CHH and hypospadias of varying degrees [8, 27–29]. Nevertheless, hypospadias in CHH is a rare combination, and it is interesting to speculate why our cohort has an over-representation of variants in CHH genes in patients with hypospadias. It is possible that in our cohort of Indonesian patients, CHH and KS manifest in a unique way, as we have not found this association in patients with 46,XY DSD of other nationalities (data not shown). Or, it may be that these variants simply contribute to a phenotype in these patients that could involve additional undetected variants in genes controlling either gonadal or penile development. It is also possible that these genes/variants have an interaction with environmental cues in this population, resulting in more common under-virilisation in CHH than in other populations. Indeed, many of the described patients come from low socio-economic communities, and many of them are involved in agriculture. Both genetic and environmental factors are thought to contribute to isolated hypospadias (reviewed in [30]), and numerous studies in different populations have shown agriculture and pesticides to be a risk factor for reproductive development and health, e.g. [31–34]. Finally, it is possible that these variants detected in CHH genes are non-damaging variants over-represented in the Indonesian population. However, three patients had a *PROKR2* variant previously shown to be deleterious in functional studies, and we have sequenced more than 100 individuals from Indonesia (include severe DSD patients, parents and siblings) who were not enriched for these or other rare variants in CHH genes (data not shown).

Mutations in *PROK2* and *PROKR2* are thought to contribute to around 9% of patients with KS [23]. In our cohort, a total of four patients had a variant in *PROKR2* and one with *PROK2*. We also had three patients with *WDR11* variants, meaning this gene may also play a significant role in Indonesian 46,XY DSD patients. Overall, we have found eight variants in CHH genes that have not been previously described in this disorder. Of these, four are not present in online variant databases ExAC or EVS. The PROKR2 variant p.W352G lies within the cytoplasmic tail of this transmembrane receptor. Other variants have been described in this region (such as p.V331M—which we also found, and p.R357W) [21]. In this case, the mutant residue (glycine) is smaller than the wild-type residue and differs in hydrophobicity to the wild-type residue (tryptophan). This may cause a loss of external interactions in particular a loss of hydrophobic interactions with other molecules on the surface of the protein. One patient had a variant in *PROK2* (p.R23H) that has not been previously described. The affected amino acid lies within the signal peptide region, and the mutant residue (histidine) is smaller than the wild-type residue and has a different charge (neutral rather than positive). This may change the activity of the signal peptide, and a patient with a variant affecting the neighboring amino acid (p.A24P) has been described previously in CHH [21].

The PROKR2 p.V331M variant that we and others have found has been shown to have reduced functional activity (albeit weaker than other variants) [21–23]; however, it is not predicted to be damaging by any of the four prediction tools used. This is likely due to the fact that several orthologous proteins in other species have a methionine in this protein position. It has been suggested that filtering variants based on currently available pathogenicity tools may lead to under-reporting of such compensated variants [35]. Therefore, while we have included the *in silico* predictions of pathogenicity in our pipeline, we have chosen to report all rare variants in this manuscript regardless of these predictions.

Finally, two novel *WDR11* variants were found in our screen. WDR11 is predicted to exhibit two β propellers made up of WD domains. Protein structure modelling has predicted that WDR11 has 12 WD domains and that nine of them (second through tenth) participate in the genesis of two consecutive β propellers [36]. The p.W803C variant in which a tryptophan is replaced by a cysteine at position 803 falls within the 12th WD domain and is a highly conserved amino acid [36]. Cysteine is a smaller residue than the wild-type residue, which could interrupt with the WD function. The p.L427I change is predicted to fall adjacent to WD domain 6, where at least two other human variants have been described [36].

Interestingly, we also found two patients with both *FGFR1* and *CHD7* variants. Indeed, oligogenicity has been described to be a feature of CHH (for a summary, see [3]). Specifically, oligogenic inheritance has been previously reported for *FGFR1*, while no reports for *CHD7* oligogenicity have yet been published. While *CHD7* has most frequently been associated with CHARGE syndrome, of which hypospadias can be a feature, a recent paper has detailed patients in which *CHD7* single-nucleotide variants (SNVs) were not associated with classical CHARGE syndromic features. Indeed, they show that rare deleterious SNVs in this gene contribute to the mutational burden of patients with both KS and CHH in the absence of full CHARGE syndromic features [37]. It may be that a combination of variant alleles in *FGFR1* and *CHD7* can cause hypospadias and under-virilisation. However, several of the *FGFR1* and *CHD7* variants had a total MAF of around 0.2%, with a prevalence of 0.3 or 0.4% in East Asia indicating that they may be over-represented in the Indonesian population. Further studies to address the pathogenicity of these variants and the interaction between *FGFR1* and *CHD7* are required and are beyond the scope of this study.

Hormonal analysis at the right age can be highly informative in a clinical diagnosis of CHH. This includes assays of the levels of the gonadotrophins FSH and LH, as well as testosterone levels before and after hCG stimulation. Diagnosis of KS and CHH in many of these patients has been limited by access to detailed blood hormone analysis (in particular as many are pre-pubescent children meaning that measuring LH and FSH is not informative). Most of our patients showed low levels of testosterone (consistent with their age), but these levels were stimulated by hCG. Nevertheless, the genetic results of this study suggest that boys presenting with under-virilisation phenotypes in Indonesian clinics should be tested for CHH or KS. The patients presented here will be monitored as they develop, and we recommend they have their gonadotrophin levels retested at a later date when reduced levels can be detected.

A genetic diagnosis can inform family planning and fertility investigations, as well as direct clinical management. Treatments exist for many of the features of CHH. In early life, this can include low-dose testosterone or gonadotrophins for micropenis and stimulation of gonadal development. Later, during adolescence or adulthood, testosterone therapy can also induce puberty including psychosocial development [3]. CHH-associated infertility can also be treated, for example, by administering GnRH or gonadotrophins [3]. Thus, given the therapeutic options, having a genetic diagnosis may allow earlier or tailored intervention. Gene panel testing is a viable option to deliver this genetic diagnosis.

Conclusion

We conclude that variants in CHH genes, in particular *PROKR2*, *PROK2*, *WDR11* and *FGFR1* with *CHD7*, may contribute to under-virilisation phenotypes including hypospadias in Indonesian boys. We suggest that in this population, 46,XY DSD patients should be monitored for signs of CHH including hormonal and genetic analysis.

Abbreviations

CHH: Congenital hypogonadotrophic hypogonadism; DHT: Dihydrotestosterone; DSD: Disorder of sex development; FSH: Follicle-stimulating hormone; GnRH: Gonadotrophin-releasing hormone; hCG: Human chorionic gonadotrophin; KS: Kallmann syndrome; LH: Luteinising hormone

Acknowledgements
The authors would like to thank the patients who kindly consented to be part of this study.

Funding
KA, GR and JvdB are funded by a National Health and Medical Research Council (NHMRC) program grant (number APP1074258). AS is funded by a NHMRC research fellowship.

Authors' contributions
KLA analysed and interpreted the data and wrote the manuscript. AB interpreted the data and critically revised the manuscript. GR and JvdB handled the DNA, carried out sequencing, and analysed data. NAL and AZJ collected and analysed the patient clinical data. AHS and SMHF supervised the work, contributed to the study design and interpretation, and critically reviewed the manuscript. All authors have read and approved the manuscript for publication.

Competing interests
The authors declare that they have no competing interests.

Author details
[1]Murdoch Childrens Research Institute, Melbourne, Victoria, Australia. [2]Department of Paediatrics, University of Melbourne, Melbourne, Victoria, Australia. [3]The Royal Children's Hospital, Melbourne, Victoria, Australia. [4]Division of Human Genetics, Centre for Biomedical Research, Faculty of Medicine, Diponegoro University (FMDU), JL. Prof. H. Soedarto, SH, Tembalang, Semarang 50275, Central Java, Indonesia.

References
1. Walker WH, Cheng J. FSH and testosterone signaling in Sertoli cells. Reproduction. 2005;130:15–28. Society for Reproduction and Fertility.
2. Svechnikov K, Landreh L, Weisser J, Izzo G, Colón E, Svechnikova I, et al. Origin, development and regulation of human Leydig cells. Horm Res Paediatr. 2010;73:93–101.
3. Boehm U, Bouloux P-M, Dattani MT, de Roux N, Dodé C, Dunkel L, et al. Expert consensus document: European Consensus Statement on congenital hypogonadotropic hypogonadism—pathogenesis, diagnosis and treatment. Nat Rev Endocrinol. 2015;11:547–64. Nature Publishing Group.
4. Teixeira L, Guimiot F, Dodé C, Fallet-Bianco C, Millar RP, Delezoide A-L, et al. Defective migration of neuroendocrine GnRH cells in human arrhinencephalic conditions. The Journal of clinical investigation. Am Soc Clin Invest. 2010;120:3668–72.
5. Schwanzel-Fukuda M, Pfaff DW. Origin of luteinizing hormone-releasing hormone neurons. Nature. 1989;338:161–4. Nature Publishing Group.
6. Bianco SDC, Kaiser UB. The genetic and molecular basis of idiopathic hypogonadotropic hypogonadism. Nat Rev Endocrinol. 2009;5:569–76. Nature Publishing Group.
7. Fraietta R, Zylberstejn DS, Esteves SC. Hypogonadotropic hypogonadism revisited. Clinics (Sao Paulo). 2013;68 Suppl 1:81–8. Hospital das Clinicas da Faculdade de Medicina da Universidade de Sao Paulo.
8. Moriya K, Mitsui T, Tanaka H, Nakamura M, Nonomura K. Long-term outcome of pituitary-gonadal axis and gonadal growth in patients with hypospadias at puberty. J Urol. 2010;184:1610–4.
9. Ediati A, Juniarto AZ, Birnie E, Drop SLS, Faradz SMH, Dessens AB. Body image and sexuality in Indonesian adults with a disorder of sex development (DSD). J Sex Res. 2013;52:15–29.
10. Ediati A, Faradz SMH, Juniarto AZ, van der Ende J, Drop SLS, Dessens AB. Emotional and behavioral problems in late-identified Indonesian patients with disorders of sex development. J Psychosom Res. 2015;79:76–84. Elsevier Inc.
11. Izumi Y, Suzuki E, Kanzaki S, Yatsuga S, Kinjo S, Igarashi M, et al. Genome-wide copy number analysis and systematic mutation screening in 58 patients with hypogonadotropic hypogonadism. Fertil Steril. 2014;102:1130–3.
12. Raivio T, Sidis Y, Plummer L, Chen H, Ma J, Mukherjee A, et al. Impaired fibroblast growth factor receptor 1 signaling as a cause of normosmic idiopathic hypogonadotropic hypogonadism. J Clin Endocrinol Metab. 2009;94:4380–90.
13. Miraoui H, Dwyer AA, Sykiotis GP, Plummer L, Chung W, Feng B, et al. Mutations in FGF17, IL17RD, DUSP6, SPRY4, and FLRT3 are identified in individuals with congenital hypogonadotropic hypogonadism. Am J Hum Genet. 2013;92:725–43.
14. Juniarto Z, van der Zwan YG, Santosa A, Ariani MD, Eggers S, Hersmus R, et al. Hormonal evaluation in relation to phenotype and genotype in 286 patients with a disorder of sex development from Indonesia. Clin Endocrinol (Oxf). 2016;n/a–n/a.
15. Soldin OP, Hoffman EG, Waring MA, Soldin SJ. Pediatric reference intervals for FSH, LH, estradiol, T3, free T3, cortisol, and growth hormone on the DPC IMMULITE 1000. Clin Chim Acta. 2005;355:205–10.
16. Miller SA, Dykes DD, Polesky HF. A simple salting out procedure for extracting DNA from human nucleated cells. Nucleic Acids Res. 1988;16:1215. Oxford University Press.
17. Eggers S, Sadedin S, van den Bergen JA, Robevska G, Ohnesorg T, Hewitt J, et al. Disorders of sex development: insights from targeted gene sequencing of a large international patient cohort. Genome Biol. 2016;17:243. BioMed Central.
18. Sadedin SP, Dashnow H, James PA, Bahlo M, Bauer DC, Lonie A, et al. Cpipe: a shared variant detection pipeline designed for diagnostic settings. Genome Med. 2015;7:68.

19. Venselaar H, Beek Te TAH, Kuipers RKP, Hekkelman ML, Vriend G. Protein structure analysis of mutations causing inheritable diseases. An e-Science approach with life scientist friendly interfaces. BMC Bioinformatics. 2010;11: 548. BioMed Central.

20. Zhu J, Choa RE-Y, Guo MH, Plummer L, Buck C, Palmert MR, et al. A shared genetic basis for self-limited delayed puberty and idiopathic hypogonadotropic hypogonadism. J Clin Endocrinol Metab. 2015;100: E646–54. Endocrine Society Chevy Chase.

21. Cole LW, Sidis Y, Zhang C, Quinton R, Plummer L, Pignatelli D, et al. Mutations in prokineticin 2 and prokineticin receptor 2 genes in human gonadotrophin-releasing hormone deficiency: molecular genetics and clinical spectrum. J Clin Endocrinol Metab. 2008;93:3551–9.

22. Monnier C, Dodé C, Fabre L, Teixeira L, Labesse G, Pin J-P, et al. PROKR2 missense mutations associated with Kallmann syndrome impair receptor signalling activity. Hum Mol Genet. 2009;18:75–81. Oxford University Press.

23. Dodé C, Rondard P. PROK2/PROKR2 signaling and Kallmann syndrome. Front Endocrinol (Lausanne). 2013;4:19. Frontiers.

24. Fukami M, Iso M, Sato N, Igarashi M, Seo M, Kazukawa I, et al. Submicroscopic deletion involving the fibroblast growth factor receptor 1 gene in a patient with combined pituitary hormone deficiency. Endocr J. 2013;60:1013–20.

25. Costa-Barbosa FA, Balasubramanian R, Keefe KW, Shaw ND, Tassan Al N, Plummer L, et al. Prioritizing genetic testing in patients with Kallmann syndrome using clinical phenotypes. J Clin Endocrinol Metab. 2013;98:E943–53.

26. Vizeneux A, Hilfiger A, Bouligand J, Pouillot M, Brailly-Tabard S, Bashamboo A, et al. Congenital hypogonadotropic hypogonadism during childhood: presentation and genetic analyses in 46 boys. Veitia RA, editor. PLoS ONE. 2013;8:e77827. Public Library of Science.

27. Kurzrock EA, Delair S. Hypospadias and Kallmann's syndrome: distinction between morphogenesis and growth of the male phallus. J Pediatr Urol. 2006;2:515–7.

28. Knorr JR, Ragland RL, Brown RS, Gelber N. Kallmann syndrome: MR findings. AJNR Am J Neuroradiol. 1993;14:845–51.

29. Ponticelli C, Frosini P, Masi L. Kallmann's syndrome. Apropos of 2 personal cases. Acta Otorhinolaryngol Ital. 1991;11:603–8.

30. Bouty A, Ayers KL, Pask A, Heloury Y, Sinclair AH. The genetic and environmental factors underlying hypospadias. Sex Dev. 2015;9:239–59. Karger Publishers.

31. Strazzullo M, Matarazzo MR. Epigenetic effects of environmental chemicals on reproductive biology. Curr Drug Targets. 2016.

32. Bianca S, Li Volti G, Caruso-Nicoletti M, Ettore G, Barone P, Lupo L, et al. Elevated incidence of hypospadias in two sicilian towns where exposure to industrial and agricultural pollutants is high. Reprod Toxicol. 2003;17:539–45.

33. Xu L-F, Liang C-Z, Lipianskaya J, Chen X-G, Fan S, Zhang L, et al. Risk factors for hypospadias in China. Asian J Androl. 2014;16:778–81.

34. Kristensen P, Irgens LM, Andersen A, Bye AS, Sundheim L. Birth defects among offspring of Norwegian farmers, 1967-1991. Epidemiology. 1997;8:537–44.

35. Azevedo L, Mort M, Costa AC, Silva RM, Quelhas D, Amorim A, et al. Improving the in silico assessment of pathogenicity for compensated variants. Eur J Hum Genet. 2016;25:2–7.

36. Kim H-G, Ahn J-W, Kurth I, Ullmann R, Kim H-T, Kulharya A, et al. WDR11, a WD protein that interacts with transcription factor EMX1, is mutated in idiopathic hypogonadotropic hypogonadism and Kallmann syndrome. Am J Hum Genet. 2010;87:465–79.

37. Balasubramanian R, Choi J-H, Francescatto L, Willer J, Horton ER, Asimacopoulos EP, et al. Functionally compromised CHD7 alleles in patients with isolated GnRH deficiency. Proceedings of the National Academy of Sciences. National Acad Sci. 2014;111:17953–8.

Ensemble genomic analysis in human lung tissue identifies novel genes for chronic obstructive pulmonary disease

Jarrett D. Morrow[1*], Michael H. Cho[1,2], John Platig[3], Xiaobo Zhou[1], Dawn L. DeMeo[1,2], Weiliang Qiu[1], Bartholome Celli[2], Nathaniel Marchetti[4], Gerard J. Criner[4], Raphael Bueno[5], George R. Washko[2], Kimberly Glass[1], John Quackenbush[3], Edwin K. Silverman[1,2] and Craig P. Hersh[1,2]

Abstract

Background: Genome-wide association studies (GWAS) have identified single nucleotide polymorphisms (SNPs) significantly associated with chronic obstructive pulmonary disease (COPD). However, many genetic variants show suggestive evidence for association but do not meet the strict threshold for genome-wide significance. Integrative analysis of multiple omics datasets has the potential to identify novel genes involved in disease pathogenesis by leveraging these variants in a functional, regulatory context.

Results: We performed expression quantitative trait locus (eQTL) analysis using genome-wide SNP genotyping and gene expression profiling of lung tissue samples from 86 COPD cases and 31 controls, testing for SNPs associated with gene expression levels. These results were integrated with a prior COPD GWAS using an ensemble statistical and network methods approach to identify relevant genes and observe them in the context of overall genetic control of gene expression to highlight co-regulated genes and disease pathways. We identified 250,312 unique SNPs and 4997 genes in the cis(local)-eQTL analysis (5% false discovery rate). The top gene from the integrative analysis was *MAPT*, a gene recently identified in an independent GWAS of lung function. The genes *HNRNPAB* and *PCBP2* with RNA binding activity and the gene *ACVR1B* were identified in network communities with validated disease relevance.

Conclusions: The integration of lung tissue gene expression with genome-wide SNP genotyping and subsequent intersection with prior GWAS and omics studies highlighted candidate genes within COPD loci and in communities harboring known COPD genes. This integration also identified novel disease genes in sub-threshold regions that would otherwise have been missed through GWAS.

Keywords: eQTL, Expression QTL, Integrative genomics, Network medicine, Ensemble methods, Bayesian methods

Background

Chronic obstructive pulmonary disease (COPD) is characterized by progressive airflow obstruction accompanied by chronic inflammation. It is a major cause of morbidity and mortality worldwide [1]. Although environmental exposures such as cigarette smoking are risk factors, a genetic component to susceptibility has been observed [2–5]. Multiple genome-wide association studies (GWAS) have identified loci associated with COPD susceptibility across various populations [6–9]. However, most of these associations have small effect sizes, so there are likely additional COPD genes to be discovered. Understanding the gene regulatory implications of the significant and sub-genome-wide significant (sub-threshold) GWAS variants in lung tissue may identify genes and loci relevant to COPD for future validation experiments.

Prioritization of previously identified genomic loci enhances the molecular understanding of complex disease [10, 11]. Additionally, sub-threshold genetic loci may play a role in complex diseases [12] such as COPD, as

---

* Correspondence: jarrett.morrow@channing.harvard.edu
[1]Channing Division of Network Medicine, Brigham and Women's Hospital, 181 Longwood Avenue, Boston, MA 02115, USA
Full list of author information is available at the end of the article

they likely carry a significant biological signal and may reach significance in later higher powered studies. Increasing the power to identify additional associations often requires a much larger sample size [13], which greatly increases study expense. Integration with omics data can provide insight into the regulatory effects of these variants [12, 14, 15], without increasing sample size. Expression quantitative trait locus (eQTL) analysis tests the association between genetic variants and gene expression and can point to relevant single nucleotide polymorphisms (SNPs) and genes within GWAS loci [15–17] using the observation that trait-associated SNPs are likely to be eQTLs/eSNPs [17] and/or have gene regulatory implications [18].

In this study of genetic control of gene expression, we performed eQTL analysis in lung tissue samples from severe COPD cases and ex-smoker controls and integrated the findings with results from a prior GWAS [8]. We used the Bayesian method Sherlock [19] to identify genes having collective associations within the significant and sub-threshold GWAS SNPs. To observe these genes in the overall context of genetic control of gene expression, we constructed a bipartite network and identified communities [20] harboring the Sherlock-derived genes. We observed that some of these communities contained differentially expressed genes and genes with CpG sites differentially methylated by COPD status. This integration of previous omics studies hones in on the communities demonstrating greater relevance to COPD.

The central hypothesis of this study is that sub-threshold GWAS SNPs, in addition to genome-wide significant SNPs, both influence gene expression and confer disease susceptibility through effects better observed using network and integrative statistical methods. The foundation of this study is the aggregation of the gene expression signals from SNPs identified in prior GWAS, both significant and sub-threshold, using regulatory evidence via an ensemble Bayesian and network approach. This integrative method extracts the additional genetic and genomic signals contained in the sub-threshold SNPs by combining evidence across genotyping, gene expression and DNA methylation datasets and highlights novel genes and loci within regions that may not have been identified through GWAS. This motivates hypotheses regarding the biological role of these findings in disease and informs selection of targets for further functional investigations.

Results

Gene expression data were available for lung tissue samples from 86 severe COPD cases (mean FEV_1 26.4% predicted) and 31 controls with normal spirometry, all Caucasians (Additional file 1: Table S1). There were no significant differences between cases and controls by sex or age. The cases had higher lifetime smoking intensity in pack-years and quit smoking on average 8.7 fewer years in the past ($p = 0.0006$). We identified eQTLs using the gene expression and imputed genotyping data and integrated them with prior GWAS and omics studies using an ensemble approach of statistical and network methods (Fig. 1).

Using the lung tissue gene expression profiling and imputed genotyping data from the cases and controls, we performed cis- and trans-eQTL analysis (see the "Methods" section). We identified 347,251 significant cis-eQTL results (FDR < 5%) out of 55,550,191 total tests. Within these results, there were 250,312 unique cis-eQTL SNPs (eSNPs) and 5878 unique eQTL genes (eGenes, 4997 gene symbols) (Additional file 1: Table S2). This represents 4.2% of the SNPs and 24% of the expression probes tested. The trans results contain 8519 significant results (FDR < 5%), out of 146,665,850,054 total tests, with 6930 unique eSNPs and 451 unique eGenes (434 gene symbols) (Additional file 1: Table S3).

We intersected the significant cis-eQTL results with the GWAS at a suggestive level of significance ($p < 10^{-4}$) [8] and observed that 292 of these 1847 significant and sub-threshold GWAS SNPs were eSNPs (4.3 fold enrichment, hypergeometric p value < 0.00001). The top intersection results are shown in (Additional file 1: Table S4). Regional genomic plots of significant cis-eQTLs (FDR < 5%) for 5 of these 13 loci highlight the regulatory information for the top eSNPs and SNPs in linkage disequilibrium (LD) (Additional file 1: Figures S1–S5). Two of the eSNPs from (Additional file 1: Table S4) are located within the

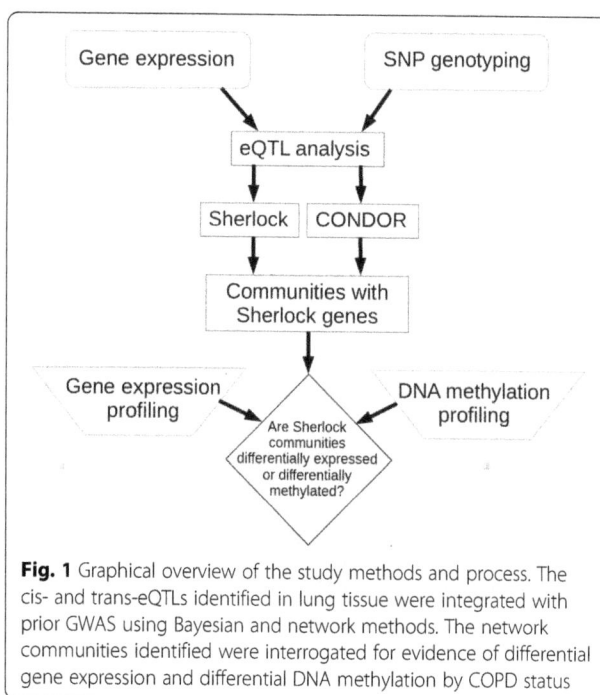

Fig. 1 Graphical overview of the study methods and process. The cis- and trans-eQTLs identified in lung tissue were integrated with prior GWAS using Bayesian and network methods. The network communities identified were interrogated for evidence of differential gene expression and differential DNA methylation by COPD status

associated eGene (rs1504550-*IREB2* and rs2252518-*ACVR1B*; Additional file 1: Figures S1 and S2). Two others (rs12461383-*C19orf54* and rs11852372-*CHRNA5*; Additional file 1: Figures S3 and S4) are in promoter flanking and transcription factor binding regions within DNase hypersensitivity (DHS) sites. The last eSNP (rs151321-*SULT1A2*; Additional file 1: Figure S5) is in LD (shaded in red) with several SNPs located in regulatory regions. To observe overall genetic control of gene expression in a disease context, we intersected all cis-eQTL results with the nominally significant GWAS SNPs ($p < 0.05$) [8] and plotted the p values from the two sets (Fig. 2). Each point in the plot represents an eQTL result (eSNP-eGene pair); prior COPD gene expression profiling results [21] are overlaid in color. We observed that eQTLs with COPD GWAS associations are generally not enriched for differentially expressed genes; regions with sub-threshold GWAS p values ($p < 10^{-4}$) and significant eQTL p values lack differentially expressed genes (FDR < 5%). Therefore, we used additional statistical and network methods to extract the signal in these results, given this complex relationship between the disease and the genetic control of gene expression.

We integrated the nominally significant cis-eQTLs ($p < 10^{-3}$) and trans-eQTLs ($p < 10^{-6}$) with prior GWAS using the Bayesian method Sherlock [19], seeking genes with collective associations across the significant and sub-threshold GWAS results. The 438,536 SNPs common to the eQTL, GWAS, and GWAS permutation data were the basis for this integrative analysis. A total of 50 Sherlock results had p values < 10^{-3} (Table 1, Additional file 2: Table S5). This p value threshold corresponds to a LBF

(logarithm of Bayes factor) sum of 1.94. Of the 50 genes identified, 13 were previously found in the intersection between cis-eQTLs and GWAS ($p < 10^{-4}$) results. Several genes have been identified in previous COPD GWAS studies. We repeated the Sherlock analysis using the eQTL results from GTEx V7 (using the same p value thresholds) and observed the results for these top 50 genes (Table 1). We further sought to place our 50 Sherlock-derived genes in the context of overall genetic control of gene expression using network methods, since co-regulated genes may have shared function. This process has the potential to reveal additional COPD genes of interest.

We constructed a bipartite network using the cis- and trans-eQTLs with p value thresholds identical to those for Sherlock (cis: $p < 10^{-3}$ and trans: $p < 10^{-6}$). After all filtering steps (see the "Methods" section), 171,490 eSNPs and 11,348 eGenes were used in the construction of the network. The power-law nature of the degree distribution for this network is heavy-tailed (Additional file 1: Figure. S6) and similar to that seen in other bipartite eQTL networks [20], suggesting a scale-free structure characterized by the presence of hubs. We identified 250 communities within this network and focused on the 14 that contain Sherlock-derived genes (Table 2, Additional file 1: Table S6). We also examined two communities that contained putative interactors (*HMGB1* and *CD79A*) of genes near GWAS loci from our previous study [21]. These differentially expressed interactors were identified using gene expression profiling in lung tissue and in vitro, in vivo, and in silico datasets that identified genes with evidence of

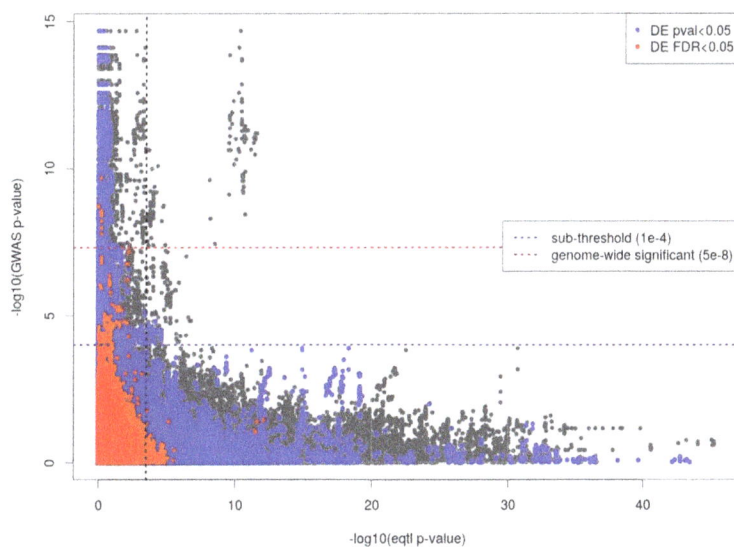

Fig. 2 Plot of COPD GWAS *p* values vs. the cis-eQTL *p* values. Each point in the plot represents a cis-eQTL result with an rsID found in the prior GWAS. GWAS *p* values (*y* axis) are plotted against the expression QTL *p* values (*x* axis). A vertical dotted line indicates the threshold of significance (FDR < 5%) for the eQTL. Horizontal lines delineate genome-wide significant (red) and sub-threshold (blue) GWAS *p* values. The significant (red; FDR < 5%) and nominally significant (blue; *p* < 0.05) eGenes from gene expression profiling in COPD lung tissue are highlighted

Table 1 COPD genes identified in the Sherlock analysis

Gene symbol	Total LBF score	Sherlock p value	Differentially expressed probe ($p < 0.05$)	Differentially methylated site ($p < 0.05$, effect > 5%)	GTEx V7 (cis-only, LBF score)	GTEx V7 (cis-only, p value)
MAPT	7.65	6.91E-07	Yes	No	7.31	6.41E-07
LRRC37A4	7.46	6.91E-07	No	No	2.13	1.8E-3
C17orf69	7.38	6.91E-07	Yes	No	2.39	1.3E-3
IREB2 *	6.40	6.91E-07	No	No	4.37	5.89E-05
C19orf54 *	5.45	5.53E-06	No	No	5.01	1.79E-05
ACVR1B *	5.40	5.53E-06	No	Yes	4.77	2.82E-05
EIF3CL *	4.45	1.94E-05	No	No	N/A	N/A
TUFM *	4.29	2.49E-05	Yes	No	5.31	8.97E-06
FAM13A	4.09	3.60E-05	No	No	5.69	3.84E-06
PCBP2	3.97	4.43E-05	No	No	N/A	N/A
CYP2B7 *	3.87	5.67E-05	No	No	N/A	N/A
SULT1A1 *	3.81	6.08E-05	Yes	No	5.38	8.97E-06
SULT1A2 *	3.80	6.08E-05	Yes	Yes	5.01	1.79E-05
TIGD2	3.58	7.88E-05	No	No	2.48	1.10E-03
CHRNA5 *	3.37	1.05E-04	No	No	5.27	1.15E-05
BZRAP1	3.27	1.20E-04	No	Yes	−0.20	7.28E-01
GPX8 *	3.25	1.20E-04	No	No	N/A	N/A
TEKT3	3.19	1.31E-04	No	No	0.00	1.59E-01
SNRPB	3.06	1.63E-04	No	No	0.00	1.61E-01
ZNF652	3.03	1.69E-04	No	No	−0.02	2.69E-01
AHSA2 *	2.86	2.14E-04	No	No	2.22	1.63E-03
CDH23	2.82	2.21E-04	No	Yes	0.01	1.38E-01
NOP2	2.69	2.99E-04	No	No	N/A	N/A
AASDH	2.68	3.06E-04	No	No	2.45	1.14E-03
DAGLA	2.68	3.06E-04	No	No	N/A	N/A
IFI27L2 *	2.65	3.24E-04	No	No	2.90	5.98E-04
APIP	2.60	3.48E-04	No	No	2.52	1.03E-03
AXIN2	2.59	3.55E-04	No	No	−0.04	4.10E-01
WDR47	2.49	4.20E-04	Yes	No	N/A	N/A
C4orf33	2.41	4.74E-04	No	No	1.68	3.71E-03
HNRNPAB	2.34	5.23E-04	No	No	N/A	N/A
GFPT1	2.33	5.24E-04	Yes	No	−0.02	2.04E-01
LOC644172	2.32	5.30E-04	No	No	N/A	N/A
SNORD25	2.25	5.86E-04	No	No	N/A	N/A
PPAT	2.23	6.06E-04	Yes	No	−0.03	3.22E-01
FBRSL1	2.23	6.08E-04	No	No	−0.09	5.90E-01
FSTL5	2.22	6.14E-04	No	No	N/A	N/A
SMG6	2.18	6.44E-04	No	Yes	−0.01	1.85E-01
CHIAP2	2.09	7.58E-04	No	No	N/A	N/A
RPL23A	2.07	7.77E-04	Yes	No	N/A	N/A
C2orf74 *	2.06	7.85E-04	No	No	N/A	N/A
CTSH	2.04	8.17E-04	No	No	1.40	5.59E-03
UBE2J1	2.03	8.27E-04	Yes	No	N/A	N/A

Table 1 COPD genes identified in the Sherlock analysis *(Continued)*

Gene symbol	Total LBF score	Sherlock p value	Differentially expressed probe (p < 0.05)	Differentially methylated site (p < 0.05, effect > 5%)	GTEx V7 (cis-only, LBF score)	GTEx V7 (cis-only, p value)
AEN	2.01	8.50E-04	No	No	0.36	3.61E-02
CUL1	2.00	8.88E-04	No	No	−0.02	3.02E-01
DSP	2.00	8.91E-04	No	No	1.51	4.77E-03
MYCN	1.97	9.32E-04	No	No	−0.04	4.13E-01
TRIM4	1.96	9.43E-04	Yes	No	1.57	4.37E-03
ZNF57	1.94	9.64E-04	No	No	−0.02	2.16E-01
NARS2	1.94	9.74E-04	No	No	2.89	6.10E-04

LBF logarithm of Bayes factor
*Gene identified in the cis-eQTL-GWAS intersection in (Additional file 1: Table S4)

interaction with one of the three genes (*HHIP*, *FAM13A*, and *IREB2*) implicated by in-depth functional studies at COPD GWAS loci.

To validate the disease relevance of the communities, we calculated the differential expression and differential DNA methylation meta-analysis *p* values (see the "Methods" section) for these 16 communities. Seven communities were validated based on nominally significant (meta-*p* < 0.05) differential expression and differential methylation results (Table 2). These communities contain the Sherlock-derived genes *CDH23*, *CHRNA5*, *HNRNPAB*, *IREB2*, *PCBP2*, *ZNF652*, *ACVR1B*, and *RPL23A* (Figs. 3, 4, and 5 and Additional file 1: Figures S7–S8) or the interactors *HMGB1* and *CD79A*

(Additional file 1: Figures S9–S10). There was significant pathway enrichment (FDR *q* value < 0.05) using ConsensusPathDB [22] for two validated communities (ID = 222:*ACVR1B* and ID = 135:*CD79A*) in Table 2 (Additional file 1: Table S7), highlighting cGMP-PKG signaling, focal adhesion, and actin and immune system-related pathways. Six of the nine remaining communities, which were lacking joint evidence, had either nominally significant differential expression or differential methylation.

Discussion

Although many genome-wide significant loci from COPD GWAS were not eSNPs in lung tissue, we found

Table 2 CONDOR communities that contain Sherlock-derived genes or putative COPD GWAS gene interactors

Community ID	Sherlock or interactor gene(s)	Total SNPs	Sub-threshold SNPs	Total genes	Number of differentially expressed genes	Number of differentially methylated genes	Expression meta-p value	Methylation meta-p value
98**	HMGB1	143	0	4	3	1	2.26E-19	0.0028
113**	CDH23	489	0	12	2	1	0.0184	4.95E-05
135**	CD79A	1959	0	162	29	13	9.27E-11	4.27E-33
202**	CHRNA5, HNRNPAB, IREB2, PCBP2	293	57	17	4	1	0.0032	0.0026
218**	ZNF652	410	0	47	8	3	0.0017	4.85E-06
222**	ACVR1B	790	0	67	12	9	0.0003	8.23E-16
223**	RPL23A	509	4	32	10	6	3.26E-06	8.82E-18
20*	WDR47	476	0	6	3	0	0.0021	–
78*	CHIAP2	631	0	18	3	1	0.0907	0.0019
131	AHSA2 C2orf74	599	8	4	1	0	0.0634	–
161*	SMG6	633	0	18	1	2	0.3723	3.38E-09
179*	DSP	68	0	7	3	0	0.0060	–
181*	FSTL5	475	0	23	4	1	0.0503	0.0069
187*	SNRPB	178	0	14	1	2	0.5669	0.0001
210	CTSH	439	5	12	0	0	0.5741	–
249	TRIM4	555	0	11	3	0	0.0957	–

*Communities with either significant differential expression or differential methylation (p < 0.05)
**Communities with both significant differential expression and differential methylation (p < 0.05)

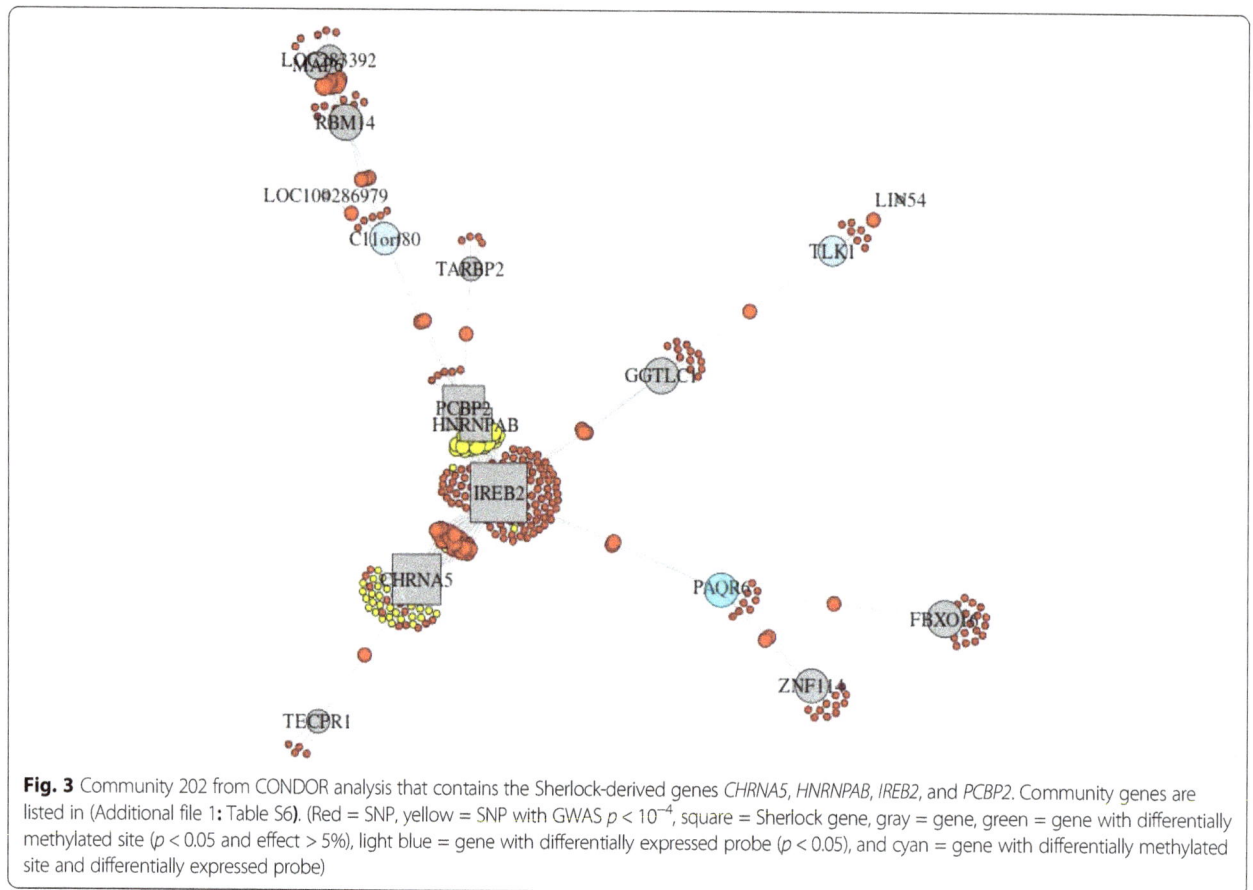

Fig. 3 Community 202 from CONDOR analysis that contains the Sherlock-derived genes *CHRNA5*, *HNRNPAB*, *IREB2*, and *PCBP2*. Community genes are listed in (Additional file 1: Table S6). (Red = SNP, yellow = SNP with GWAS $p < 10^{-4}$, square = Sherlock gene, gray = gene, green = gene with differentially methylated site ($p < 0.05$ and effect > 5%), light blue = gene with differentially expressed probe ($p < 0.05$), and cyan = gene with differentially methylated site and differentially expressed probe)

that the sub-threshold GWAS findings are enriched in eSNPs. We also observed that eQTLs with GWAS associations did not have eGenes significantly differentially expressed in severe COPD cases vs controls, demonstrating the complex nature of genetic control of gene expression. We employed an ensemble approach involving Bayesian and network methods to investigate these eQTL results, which yielded 16 relevant bipartite communities. Based on the differential gene expression and/or differential DNA methylation of all of the genes or CpG sites within each community, we validated the disease relevance for 13 of these communities, highlighting potential COPD genes within the significant and sub-threshold GWAS results.

One of the seven communities (community 202) which was validated by both differential expression and DNA methylation contains two previously identified COPD GWAS genes located in a genome-wide significant region: *IREB2* (iron responsive element binding protein 2) and *CHRNA5* (cholinergic receptor nicotinic alpha 5 subunit) [23–25]. The product of *IREB2* is known to interact with mRNA to influence translation or degradation. Two other Sherlock-derived genes in community 202 also have putative RNA binding activity, *PCBP2* (poly(rC) binding protein 2) and *HNRNPAB* (heterogeneous nuclear

ribonucleoprotein A/B). *PCBP2* plays a role in mRNA stability, and it has been suggested that deregulation of this stability may contribute to COPD pathogenesis [26]. A recent study of breast cancer highlighted the regulatory role of RNA binding by *PCBP3* (paralog of *PCBP1* along with *PCBP2*) on mRNA stability and induction of epithelial-mesenchymal transition (EMT) [27]. Additionally, *HNRNPAB* has been shown to induce EMT [28], a potential contributor to airway disease [29, 30]. Together, this suggests a role for this community in COPD pathogenesis. Community 222 contains the Sherlock-derived gene *ACVR1B* (activin A receptor type 1B), a gene identified in a previous eQTL study in blood and sputum in COPD [31]. *ACVR1B* was a sub-threshold finding in a GWAS of lung function in COPD [32] and was identified in our intersection of eQTLs with the sub-threshold GWAS of case-control status. The genes in community 222 were enriched for cGMP-PKG signaling, bacterial invasion of epithelial cells, and focal adhesion pathways [33], with possible relevance to COPD pathogenesis and exacerbations. Community 113 includes the Sherlock-derived gene *CDH23* (cadherin-related 23), involved in cell-cell adhesion and perhaps EMT as a calcium-dependent cell adhesion molecule [34]. This gene was contained within sub-threshold loci in GWAS of lung

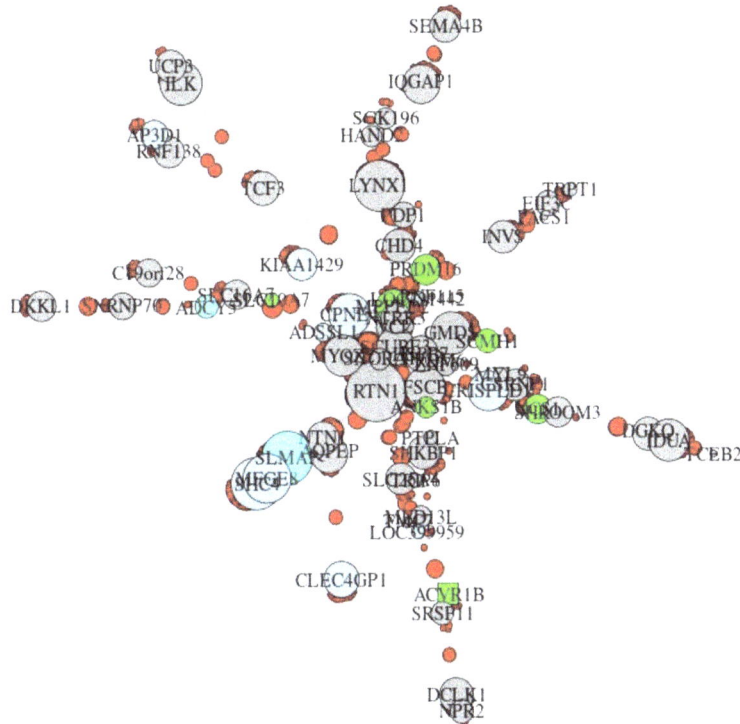

Fig. 4 Community 222 from CONDOR analysis that contains the Sherlock-derived gene *ACVR1B*. Community genes are listed in (Additional file 1: Table S6). (Red = SNP, yellow = SNP with GWAS $p < 10^{-4}$, square = Sherlock gene, gray = gene, green = gene with differentially methylated site ($p < 0.05$ and effect > 5%), light blue = gene with differentially expressed probe ($p < 0.05$), and cyan = gene with differentially methylated site and differentially expressed probe)

function decline [35], occupational asthma [36], and age at smoking initiation [37]. *DSP* (desmoplakin) was in a community (ID = 179) validated by differential expression but not differential methylation. *DSP* has been identified in a recent COPD GWAS meta-analysis [9] and in a study of interstitial lung disease [38]. Identifying this gene, which has only been highlighted in recent higher powered studies, supports our hypothesis that sub-threshold SNPs have the potential to confer disease susceptibility; genes in communities 222 and 113 may also be found significant in future GWAS.

The Sherlock analysis itself, prior to network integration, identified genes of interest that were not found through the simple intersection of eQTL and GWAS results. One of these genes, *MAPT* (microtubule associated protein tau), was previously found in a locus associated with extremes of lung function [39] and was suggestive in a recent COPD GWAS meta-analysis ($p = 4.5 \times 10^{-3}$) [9]. Genome-wide significant loci near *MAPT* were found to be associated with pulmonary fibrosis [38, 40]. In our previous gene expression profiling study, we observed a *MAPT* expression probe nominally differentially expressed ($p < 0.05$) in lung tissue of COPD cases vs. controls [21]. In the Sherlock analysis of the GTEx V7 results, we observed robust replication, with high scores from GTEx

(LBF > 2.1) for eight of our top ten findings. Overall, 17 of the 35 genes that overlap our top 50 Sherlock genes attained a LBF of 1.94 or higher in the GTEx data. Trans-eQTL results are not available in GTEx (see the "Methods" section), preventing a complete replication of our findings, as the trans-eQTLs contributed important information to the COPD lung tissue Sherlock analysis. In addition, seven of the COPD lung tissue Sherlock genes were not included in the GTEx Sherlock input and eight other genes were not available in GTEx V7 eQTL data.

Four genes in a complex region on chromosome 16 associated with COPD in an exome array study [41] were identified in the Sherlock analysis and in the eQTL-GWAS intersection: *TUFM* (Tu translation elongation factor, mitochondrial), *EIF3CL* (eukaryotic translation initiation factor 3 subunit C like), *SULT1A1* (sulfotransferase family 1A member 1), and *SULT1A2* (sulfotransferase family 1A member 2). Nominal associations ($p < 0.05$) for *SULT1A2* were found in both previous gene expression profiling [21] and DNA methylation profiling [42] studies; nominal results for only gene expression were observed for *SULT1A1* and *TUFM*. Two genes in the Sherlock results, *CYP2B7* (cytochrome P450 family 2 subfamily B member 7, pseudogene) and *C19orf54* (chromosome 19 open reading frame 54), are located in another complex COPD locus on chromosome 19

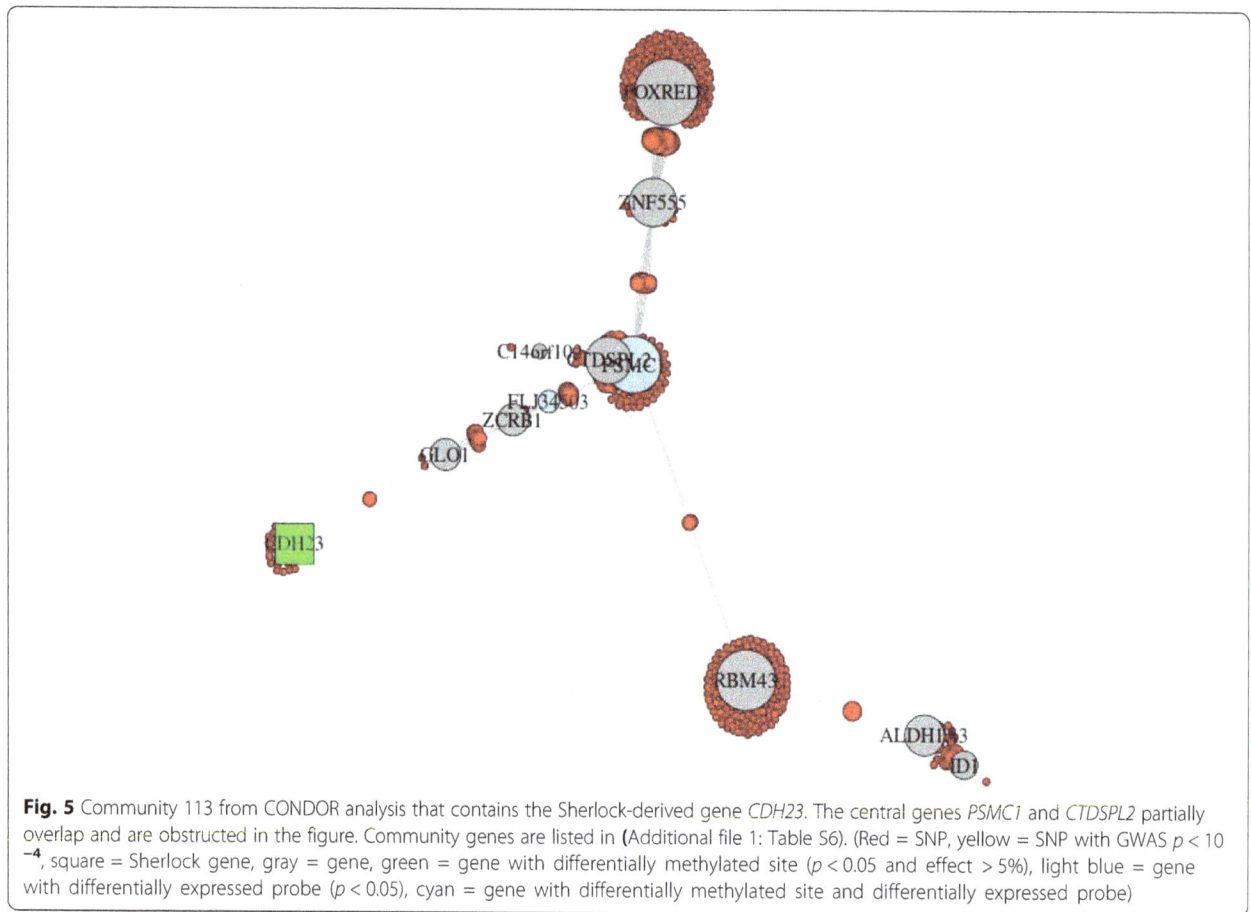

Fig. 5 Community 113 from CONDOR analysis that contains the Sherlock-derived gene *CDH23*. The central genes *PSMC1* and *CTDSPL2* partially overlap and are obstructed in the figure. Community genes are listed in (Additional file 1: Table S6). (Red = SNP, yellow = SNP with GWAS $p < 10^{-4}$, square = Sherlock gene, gray = gene, green = gene with differentially methylated site ($p < 0.05$ and effect > 5%), light blue = gene with differentially expressed probe ($p < 0.05$), cyan = gene with differentially methylated site and differentially expressed probe)

[7]. Further efforts will be required to determine which of these genes is relevant for COPD pathogenesis.

In a previous gene expression profiling study [21], we identified several putative interactors of three known COPD GWAS genes (*HHIP*, *FAM13A*, and *IREB2*). Communities harboring two of these interactors were identified in the current study. Both community 98 with *HMGB1* (high-mobility group box 1) and community 135 with *CD79A* (CD79a molecule) had evidence of differential expression and differential methylation. Additionally, there may also be a role for *HMGB1* in the development of EMT in airway epithelial cells [43].

Our study has several limitations. The omics datasets in this study were generated using homogenized lung tissue, so we could not determine the cellular specificity of the eQTLs, differential expression, and differential methylation. Studies in single lung cell types will address this cellular heterogeneity and provide validation of the findings. Our study focused on severe COPD and was enriched for subjects with emphysema and therefore may miss genes relevant for milder disease or other COPD phenotypes such as airway disease. Lastly, future integrative studies using these datasets will explore in more detail the gene regulatory impact of DNA methylation in lung tissue.

This study of the genetic control of gene expression in human lung has revealed potential genes of interest co-regulated with known COPD genes. The ensemble approach using statistical and network methods also pointed to specific genes in complex genomic regions found through prior GWAS, and genes within loci that would not meet strict thresholds for genome-wide significance, thereby extracting additional information from these results and supporting our hypothesis regarding the relevance of sub-threshold SNPs. We integrated three omics datasets, providing regulatory characterization of significant and sub-threshold GWAS variants, and highlighted genes for further functional investigation that may be involved in COPD pathogenesis. These genes would otherwise not have been identified through GWAS and could potentially meet the strict threshold for statistical significance in larger GWAS in COPD.

Methods

Study subjects

We collected lung tissue samples from former smokers undergoing thoracic surgery for lung transplantation, lung volume reduction surgery, or lung nodule resection

Ensemble genomic analysis in human lung tissue identifies novel genes for chronic obstructive...

117

at three medical centers; all subjects quit smoking at least 1 month prior to surgery [21, 42]. Distant normal tissue was sourced from lung nodule resection samples. The COPD subjects had severe airflow obstruction, with GOLD grade 3–4 spirometry (FEV1% predicted < 50% and FEV1/FVC < 0.7) and the controls had normal spirometry (FEV1% predicted ≥ 80% and FEV1/FVC ≥ 0.7). IRB approval was obtained at the three centers (Brigham and Women's Hospital, Boston, MA; St. Elizabeth's Hospital; Boston, MA; and Temple University Hospital, Philadelphia, PA), and subjects provided written informed consent.

eQTL analysis

Microarray expression profiling was available for 111 cases and 40 controls [21] (GEO Series GSE76925). Of the 32,831 expression probes, 24,495 had genomic location information and were retained for integration with genotyping data. Genome-wide SNP genotyping data was obtained from lung tissue DNA using the HumanOmni2.5Exome-8 V1.0 BeadChip (Illumina, Inc., San Diego, CA) as previously described [21]. After quality control, genotypes were phased using SHAPEIT2 [44] and imputed using IMPUTE2 [45, 46] with the 1000 Genomes Phase3 V5 reference. The analyses were performed using only data from the Caucasian subjects. Data for markers with an imputation info metric > 0.5 and minor allele frequency > 5% were retained for the 117 Caucasian subjects that had both high-quality genotyping and gene expression data (86 cases and 31 controls; Additional file 1: Table S8). To account for population stratification, two principal components (PC) based on the Tracy-Widom statistic for the Caucasian population were retained [47]. Both cis- and trans-eQTL analyses were performed using the R/Bioconductor package Matrix eQTL (version 2.1.1) [48]. A total window size of 1 million bases was used for the cis analysis (500 kb upstream and downstream from the gene); trans analysis was performed genome-wide. This analysis identifies associations between genotype dosage and gene expression levels, adjusting for age, sex, pack-years of smoking, and the two ancestry PCs. An iterative method was used to determine the number of PCs for the matrix of expression values to add as covariates to mitigate batch effects [21]; 13 PCs were included in the eQTL analyses. An eQTL association result consists of an eGene (microarray expression probe) and eSNP pair.

Integration using Sherlock

The Sherlock method performs genetic signature matching using a Bayesian statistical framework [19]. The hypothesis is that SNPs associated with expression of disease-relevant genes are also likely to influence disease risk and be identified through GWAS. Using Sherlock, we integrated the cis- and trans-eQTLs with all results from a published COPD GWAS [8]. Sherlock provides a total score for each gene, along with the score for each of the individual eQTL contributions. This total score is the sum of the LBFs (logarithm of Bayes factor) for each of these contributions. For interpretation of individual results, a value of 4.0 is typically required for significance. To output a p value, we created permuted GWAS results with similar linkage disequilibrium structure to the GWAS using the set of 379 EUR genotypes available in 1000 Genomes Phase1 V3 [49]. Specifically, we randomly permuted the case-control phenotypes 50 times as recommended in the Sherlock method (190 cases and 189 controls) and applied Plink2 [50] to calculate association p values for each iteration and used these results as inputs for Sherlock. Only overlapping SNPs (loci with rsIDs) present across the eQTL, GWAS, and permutation results were included in the analysis; minor allele frequencies for these markers were obtained from 1000 Genomes data. In the ensemble analysis, we applied a p value threshold of 10^{-3} to select a more significant set of Sherlock-derived genes for downstream analysis. We performed a replication of the Sherlock analysis using the GTEx V7 lung tissue eQTL results [51]. Only the GTEx markers found across the COPD GWAS [8] and our permutation results were included in the analysis. The GTEx project produced cis-eQTL results using a window of 1 million bases upstream and downstream. To align this Sherlock input with our study, we labeled eSNPs located 500 kb to 1 million bases from the gene transcription start site as trans-eQTLs.

Network construction

A bipartite network was constructed using the cis- and trans-eQTLs. Network nodes are eGenes represented by their gene symbol annotation and eSNPs represented by their rsIDs. Edges only connect eSNPs to eGenes; no edges are present between pairs of eSNPs or pairs of eGenes. Only eSNPs represented in the GWAS were included in the network. Cis- or trans-eQTLs with only a single edge between an eSNP and eGene were excluded, since they did not create additional connections in the network. We identified communities within this bipartite network using the R package CONDOR [20] and visualized them using the R package igraph [52], with the Fruchterman-Reingold algorithm. A differential expression meta-analysis p value was computed for each community of interest. Specifically, the differential expression p values from prior expression profiling [21] for each expression probe annotated to genes in the community were combined using Fisher's method via the R package metap. For differential DNA methylation, we used a similar approach based on prior methylation profiling results [42] for CpG sites annotated to genes in the community. In order to focus on CpG sites more likely to be biologically relevant, we required that the mean difference in methylation between cases and controls be greater than 5%.

Regulatory annotation

The R package Sushi [53] was used with gene annotation and regulatory information from Ensemble BioMart [54] (CTCF Binding Site, TF binding site, Open chromatin, Promoter and Enhancer information produced from EN-CODE, Roadmap Epigenomics, and Blueprint projects [55] for GRCh37) and DNaseI Hypersensitivity Clusters in 125 cell types from ENCODE (V3) from the UCSC database [56] (GRCh37). Linkage disequilibrium information in these regional plots was produced using correlation r^2 values for SNP pairs from PLINK, using genotyping data from 1000 Genomes Phase3 V5.

Acknowledgements
Funding: NIH grants K25 HL136846, P01 HL105339, R01 HL111759, R01 HL125583, R01 HL130512, P01 HL132825, R01 HL089856, R01 HL089897, and K25 HL133599 funded this study.
We thank Drs. Amund Gulsvik, Per Bakke, Augusto Litonjua, Pantel Vokonas, Ruth Tal-Singer, and the GenKOLS, NETT/NAS, ECLIPSE, and COPDGene studies for use of the GWAS meta-analysis data.
R01 HL089856 and R01 HL089897 are from the COPDGene study. NCT00608764 was funded by the National Institutes of Health is also supported by the COPD Foundation through contributions made to an Industry Advisory Board comprised of AstraZeneca, Boehringer Ingelheim, Novartis, Pfizer, Siemens, GSK, and Sunovion. The National Emphysema Treatment Trial was supported by the NHLBI N01HR76101, N01HR76102, N01HR76103, N01HR76104, N01HR76105, N01HR76106, N01HR76107, N01HR76108, N01HR76109, N01HR76110, N01HR76111, N01HR76112, N01HR76113, N01HR76114, N01HR76115, N01HR76116, N01HR76118, and N01HR76119; the Centers for Medicare and Medicaid Services; and the Agency for Healthcare Research and Quality. The Normative Aging Study is supported by the Cooperative Studies Program/ERIC of the US Department of Veterans Affairs and is a component of the Massachusetts Veterans Epidemiology Research and Information Center (MAVERIC). The Norway GenKOLS study (Genetics of Chronic Obstructive Lung Disease, GSK code RES11080), the ECLIPSE study (NCT00292552; GSK code SCO104960), and the ICGN study were funded by GlaxoSmithKline.

Authors' contributions
JM was responsible for the concept and design, analysis and interpretation of the data, manuscript preparation, and approval of final manuscript. MC contributed to the acquisition of the data, analysis and interpretation of the data, manuscript preparation, and approval of the final manuscript. JP contributed to the analysis and interpretation of data, statistical support, and approval of the final manuscript. XZ took part in the analysis and interpretation of the data, manuscript preparation, and approval of final manuscript. DD contributed to the acquisition of data, manuscript preparation, and approval of the final manuscript. WQ contributed to the analysis and interpretation of data, statistical support, and approval of the final manuscript. BC, NM, GC, and RB contributed to the acquisition of data, approval of final manuscript. GW took part in the acquisition of the data, analysis and interpretation of the data, and approval of final manuscript. KG contributed to the analysis and interpretation of the data, statistical support, manuscript preparation, and approval of the final manuscript. JQ provided statistical support and approval of the final manuscript. ES contributed to the concept and design, acquisition of the data, manuscript preparation, and approval of the final manuscript. CH was responsible for the concept and design, acquisition of the data, analysis and interpretation of data, manuscript preparation, and approval of the final manuscript.

Competing interests
Drs. Morrow, Platig, Zhou, Qiu, Marchetti, Criner, Celli, Glass, Quackenbush report no competing interests related to this manuscript.
Dr. Cho has received compensation from GSK.
Dr. DeMeo has received compensation from Novartis.
Dr. Bueno has received compensation from Myriad Genetics, Inc., Siemens, Verastem, Inc., Genentech, Inc., Gritstone Oncology, Inc., HTG Molecular Diagnostics, Inc., Neil Leifer, Esq, Morrison Mahoney, David Weiss, LLC, Balick & Balick, LLC, Hartford Hospital, Cleveland Clinic/Conference, Aspen Lung Conference, Case Western Reserve, North Shore University, Castle Bioscience, Novartis Institutes for Biomedical Research, AstraZebeca, imCORE/Roche, Arthur Tuverson, LLC, Ferraro Law Firm, Rice Dolan & Kershaw, Satterly & Kelly, LLC, Exosome, Inc.
Dr. Washko has received compensation from Boehringer Ingelheim, GlaxoSmithKline, Janssen Pharmaceuticals, BTG Interventional Medicine, Regeneron, Quantitative Imaging Solutions and ModoSpira, and his Spouse works for Biogen.
Dr. Silverman has received compensation from COPD Foundation, GlaxoSmithKline, Merck and Novartis,
Dr. Hersh has received consulting fees from AstraZeneca, Concert Pharmaceuticals, Mylan, and grant support from Boehrinher Ingelheim.

Author details
[1]Channing Division of Network Medicine, Brigham and Women's Hospital, 181 Longwood Avenue, Boston, MA 02115, USA. [2]Division of Pulmonary and Critical Care Medicine, Brigham and Women's Hospital, Boston, MA 02115, USA. [3]Department of Biostatistics and Computational Biology, Dana-Farber Cancer Institute, Boston, MA 02115, USA. [4]Division of Pulmonary and Critical Care Medicine, Temple University, Philadelphia, PA 19140, USA. [5]Division of Thoracic Surgery, Brigham and Women's Hospital, Boston, MA 02115, USA.

References
1. Vestbo J, Hurd SS, Agustí AG, Jones PW, Vogelmeier C, Anzueto A, et al. Global strategy for the diagnosis, management, and prevention of chronic obstructive pulmonary disease: GOLD executive summary. Am J Respir Crit Care Med. 2013;187:347–65.
2. Hersh CP, Hokanson JE, Lynch DA, Washko GR, Make BJ, Crapo JD, et al. Family history is a risk factor for copd. Chest. 2011;140:343–50.
3. McCloskey S, Patel B, Hinchliffe S, Reid E, Wareham N, Lomas D. Siblings of patients with severe chronic obstructive pulmonary disease have a significant risk of airflow obstruction. Am J Respir Crit Care Med. 2001;164: 1419–24.
4. Silverman EK. Genetics of chronic obstructive pulmonary disease. In: Organizer DC, Goode JA, editors. Chronic Obstr. Pulm. Dis. Pathog. Treat. John Wiley & Sons, Ltd; 2000. p. 45–64.
5. Silverman EK, Chapman HA, Drazen JM, Weiss ST, Rosner B, Campbell EJ, et al. Genetic epidemiology of severe, early-onset chronic obstructive pulmonary disease. Risk to relatives for airflow obstruction and chronic bronchitis. Am J Respir Crit Care Med. 1998;157:1770–8.
6. Cho MH, Boutaoui N, Klanderman BJ, Sylvia JS, Ziniti JP, Hersh CP, et al. Variants in FAM13A are associated with chronic obstructive pulmonary disease. Nat Genet. 2010;42:200–2.
7. Cho MH, Castaldi PJ, Wan ES, Siedlinski M, Hersh CP, Demeo DL, et al. A genome-wide association study of COPD identifies a susceptibility locus on chromosome 19q13. Hum Mol Genet. 2012;21:947–57.
8. Cho MH, McDonald M-LN, Zhou X, Mattheisen M, Castaldi PJ, Hersh CP, et al. Risk loci for chronic obstructive pulmonary disease: a genome-wide association study and meta-analysis. Lancet Respir Med. 2014;2:214–25.
9. Hobbs BD, de Jong K, Lamontagne M, Bossé Y, Shrine N, Artigas MS, et al. Genetic loci associated with chronic obstructive pulmonary disease overlap with loci for lung function and pulmonary fibrosis. Nat Genet. 2017;49:426–32.

10. Bjornsson H. An integrated epigenetic and genetic approach to common human disease. Trends Genet. 2004;20:350–8.

11. Feinberg AP. Epigenomics reveals a functional genome anatomy and a new approach to common disease. Nat Biotechnol. 2010;28:1049–52.

12. Wang X, Tucker NR, Rizki G, Mills R, Krijger PH, de Wit E, et al. Discovery and validation of sub-threshold genome-wide association study loci using epigenomic signatures. elife. 2016;5:e10557.

13. Bush WS, Moore JH. Chapter 11: genome-wide association studies. Lewitter F, Kann M, editors. PLoS Comput Biol. 2012;8:e1002822.

14. Civelek M, Lusis AJ. Systems genetics approaches to understand complex traits. Nat Rev Genet. 2013;15:34–48.

15. Li L, Kabesch M, Bouzigon E, Demenais F, Farrall M, Moffatt MF, et al. Using eQTL weights to improve power for genome-wide association studies: a genetic study of childhood asthma. Front Genet. 2013;4:103. doi:10.3389/fgene.2013.00103.

16. Nica AC, Montgomery SB, Dimas AS, Stranger BE, Beazley C, Barroso I, et al. Candidate causal regulatory effects by integration of expression QTLs with complex trait genetic associations. Gibson G, editor. PLoS Genet. 2010;6:e1000895.

17. Nicolae DL, Gamazon E, Zhang W, Duan S, Dolan ME, Cox NJ. Trait-associated SNPs are more likely to be eQTLs: annotation to enhance discovery from GWAS. PLoS Genet. 2010;6:e1000888.

18. Maurano MT, Humbert R, Rynes E, Thurman RE, Haugen E, Wang H, et al. Systematic localization of common disease-associated variation in regulatory DNA. Science. 2012;337:1190–5.

19. He X, Fuller CK, Song Y, Meng Q, Zhang B, Yang X, et al. Sherlock: detecting gene-disease associations by matching patterns of expression QTL and GWAS. Am J Hum Genet. 2013;92:667–80.

20. Platig J, Castaldi PJ, DeMeo D, Quackenbush J. Bipartite community structure of eQTLs. Markowetz F, editor. PLoS Comput Biol. 2016;12:e1005033.

21. Morrow JD, Zhou X, Lao T, Jiang Z, DeMeo DL, Cho MH, et al. Functional interactors of three genome-wide association study genes are differentially expressed in severe chronic obstructive pulmonary disease lung tissue. Sci Rep. 2017;7:44232.

22. Kamburov A, Stelzl U, Lehrach H, Herwig R. The ConsensusPathDB interaction database: 2013 update. Nucleic Acids Res. 2013;41:D793–800.

23. DeMeo DL, Mariani T, Bhattacharya S, Srisuma S, Lange C, Litonjua A, et al. Integration of genomic and genetic approaches implicates IREB2 as a COPD susceptibility gene. Am J Hum Genet. 2009;85:493–502.

24. Hardin M, Zielinski J, Wan ES, Hersh CP, Castaldi PJ, Schwinder E, et al. CHRNA3/5, IREB2, and ADCY2 are associated with severe chronic obstructive pulmonary disease in Poland. Am J Respir Cell Mol Biol. 2012;47:203–8.

25. Pillai SG, Ge D, Zhu G, Kong X, Shianna KV, Need AC, et al. A genome-wide association study in chronic obstructive pulmonary disease (COPD): identification of two major susceptibility loci. PLoS Genet. 2009;5:e1000421.

26. Navratilova Z, Krsjakova T, Novosadova E, Zatloukal J, Kolek V, Petrek M. Genes affecting mRNA stability and metalloproteinase inhibitor RECK are down-regulated in patients with COPD. Eur Respir J. 2013;42(Suppl 57):3512.

27. Hou P, Li L, Chen F, Chen Y, Liu H, Li J, et al. PTBP3-mediated regulation of ZEB1 mRNA stability promotes epithelial-mesenchymal transition in breast cancer. Cancer Res. 2017;canres.0883.2017.

28. Zhou Z-J, Dai Z, Zhou S-L, Hu Z-Q, Chen Q, Zhao Y-M, et al. HNRNPAB induces epithelial-mesenchymal transition and promotes metastasis of hepatocellular carcinoma by transcriptionally activating SNAIL. Cancer Res. 2014;74:2750–62.

29. Nowrin K, Sohal SS, Peterson G, Patel R, Walters EH. Epithelial-mesenchymal transition as a fundamental underlying pathogenic process in COPD airways: fibrosis, remodeling and cancer. Expert Rev Respir Med. 2014;8:547–59.

30. Sohal SS, Mahmood MQ, Walters EH. Clinical significance of epithelial mesenchymal transition (EMT) in chronic obstructive pulmonary disease (COPD): potential target for prevention of airway fibrosis and lung cancer. Clin Transl Med. 2014;3:33.

31. Castaldi PJ, Cho MH, Zhou X, Qiu W, Mcgeachie M, Celli B, et al. Genetic control of gene expression at novel and established chronic obstructive pulmonary disease loci. Hum Mol Genet. 2015;24:1200–10.

32. Lutz SM, Cho MH, Young K, Hersh CP, Castaldi PJ, McDonald M-L, et al. A genome-wide association study identifies risk loci for spirometric measures among smokers of European and African ancestry. BMC Genet. 2015;16(1):138.

33. Ezzie ME, Crawford M, Cho J-H, Orellana R, Zhang S, Gelinas R, et al. Gene expression networks in COPD: microRNA and mRNA regulation. Thorax. 2012;67:122–31.

34. Gheldof A, Berx G. Cadherins and epithelial-to-mesenchymal transition. Prog Mol Biol Transl Sci. 2013;116:317–36.

35. Imboden M, Bouzigon E, Curjuric I, Ramasamy A, Kumar A, Hancock DB, et al. Genome-wide association study of lung function decline in adults with and without asthma. J Allergy Clin Immunol. 2012;129:1218–28.

36. Yucesoy B, Kaufman KM, Lummus ZL, Weirauch MT, Zhang G, Cartier A, et al. Genome-wide association study identifies novel loci associated with diisocyanate-induced occupational asthma. Toxicol Sci. 2015;146:192–201.

37. Siedlinski M, Cho MH, Bakke P, Gulsvik A, Lomas DA, Anderson W, et al. Genome-wide association study of smoking behaviours in patients with COPD. Thorax. 2011;66:894–902.

38. Fingerlin TE, Murphy E, Zhang W, Peljto AL, Brown KK, Steele MP, et al. Genome-wide association study identifies multiple susceptibility loci for pulmonary fibrosis. Nat Genet. 2013;45:613–20.

39. Wain LV, Shrine N, Miller S, Jackson VE, Ntalla I, Artigas MS, et al. Novel insights into the genetics of smoking behaviour, lung function, and chronic obstructive pulmonary disease (UK BiLEVE): a genetic association study in UK Biobank. Lancet Respir Med. 2015;3:769–81.

40. Noth I, Zhang Y, Ma S-F, Flores C, Barber M, Huang Y, et al. Genetic variants associated with idiopathic pulmonary fibrosis susceptibility and mortality: a genome-wide association study. Lancet Respir Med. 2013;1:309–17.

41. Hobbs BD, Parker MM, Chen H, Lao T, Hardin M, Qiao D, et al. Exome array analysis identifies a common variant in *IL27* associated with chronic obstructive pulmonary disease. Am J Respir Crit Care Med. 2016;194:48–57.

42. Morrow JD, Cho MH, Hersh CP, Pinto-Plata V, Celli B, Marchetti N, et al. DNA methylation profiling in human lung tissue identifies genes associated with COPD. Epigenetics. 2016;11:730–9.

43. Chen Y-C, Statt S, Wu R, Chang H-T, Liao J-W, Wang C-N, et al. High mobility group box 1-induced epithelial mesenchymal transition in human airway epithelial cells. Sci Rep. 2016;6:18815. doi:10.1038/srep18815.

44. Delaneau O, Marchini J, Zagury J-F. A linear complexity phasing method for thousands of genomes. Nat Methods. 2011;9:179–81.

45. Howie B, Marchini J, Stephens M. Genotype imputation with thousands of genomes. Chakravarti a, editor. G3amp58 GenesGenomesGenetics. 2011;1:457–470.

46. Howie BN, Donnelly P, Marchini J. A flexible and accurate genotype imputation method for the next generation of genome-wide association studies. Schork NJ, editor. PLoS Genet. 2009;5:e1000529.

47. Price AL, Patterson NJ, Plenge RM, Weinblatt ME, Shadick NA, Reich D. Principal components analysis corrects for stratification in genome-wide association studies. Nat Genet. 2006;38:904–9.

48. Shabalin AA. Matrix eQTL: ultra fast eQTL analysis via large matrix operations. Bioinformatics. 2012;28:1353–8.

49. Auton A, Abecasis GR, Altshuler DM, Durbin RM, Abecasis GR, Bentley DR, et al. A global reference for human genetic variation. Nature. 2015;526:68–74.

50. Chang CC, Chow CC, Tellier LC, Vattikuti S, Purcell SM, Lee JJ. Second-generation PLINK: rising to the challenge of larger and richer datasets. GigaScience. 2015;4:7.

51. Aguet F, Ardlie KG, Cummings BB, Gelfand ET, Getz G, Hadley K, et al. Genetic effects on gene expression across human tissues. Nature. 2017;550:204–13.

52. Csardi G, Nepusz T. The igraph software package for complex network research. InterJournal 2006;Complex Systems:1695.

53. Phanstiel DH, Boyle AP, Araya CL, Snyder MP. Sushi.R: flexible, quantitative and integrative genomic visualizations for publication-quality multi-panel figures. Bioinformatics. 2014;30:2808–10.

54. Durinck S, Moreau Y, Kasprzyk A, Davis S, De Moor B, Brazma A, et al. BioMart and bioconductor: a powerful link between biological databases and microarray data analysis. Bioinformatics. 2005;21:3439–40.

55. Zerbino DR, Wilder SP, Johnson N, Juettemann T, Flicek PR. The Ensembl Regulatory Build. Genome Biol. 2015;16:56.

56. Rosenbloom KR, Sloan CA, Malladi VS, Dreszer TR, Learned K, Kirkup VM, et al. ENCODE Data in the UCSC Genome Browser: year 5 update. Nucleic Acids Res. 2013;41:D56–63.

12

The development of large-scale de-identified biomedical databases in the age of genomics— principles and challenges

Fida K. Dankar[1*] ⓘ, Andrey Ptitsyn[2] and Samar K. Dankar[3]

Abstract

Contemporary biomedical databases include a wide range of information types from various observational and instrumental sources. Among the most important features that unite biomedical databases across the field are high volume of information and high potential to cause damage through data corruption, loss of performance, and loss of patient privacy. Thus, issues of data governance and privacy protection are essential for the construction of data depositories for biomedical research and healthcare. In this paper, we discuss various challenges of data governance in the context of population genome projects. The various challenges along with best practices and current research efforts are discussed through the steps of data collection, storage, sharing, analysis, and knowledge dissemination.

Keywords: Biomedical database, Data privacy, Data governance, Whole genome sequencing

Background

Overview

Databases are both the result and the instrument of research. From the earliest times, assembling collections of samples and stories was essential for any research project. The results of research feeding back into the libraries and collections create a positive feedback in the accumulation of knowledge limited only by the technological platform for storage and retrieval of information. The modern times did not change the principle but further emphasized it with the advent of computers, mass information storage, and high-throughput research instrumentation. Modern biomedical databases may vary in size, specialization, and type of access but with a few exceptions are voluminous and include complex data from multiple sources. Arguably, the first integrated database of the population scale was initiated in Iceland when Decode Genetics started in 1996 [1]. This new generation of integrated biomedical databases incorporates both phenotype (medical records, clinical studies, etc.) and genotype (variation screening at

first, now increasingly shifting to whole exome and whole genome sequencing [2, 3]). The project started by Decode has generated one of the best resources for discovery in biomedical sciences and inspired development of multiple populational and national genomics projects, also feeding into integrated databases. Genomics England [4], Human Longevity [5], All of US (formerly known as Precision Medicine Initiative) [6], China's Precision Medicine Initiative [7], Korean Reference Genome Project [8], Saudi Human Genome Program [9], and Qatar Genome [10] programs are just a few recent examples of active large-scale projects generating enormous databases of complex biomedical information. Large-scale population genomics projects proliferating in the second decade of the twenty-first century show enormous diversity in goals and strategies. The Icelandic genome program has evolved from the largest population genetics study of the time and has primary objectives in advancing biomedical research. China's Precision Medicine Initiative is one of the most ambitious programs with an aim to sequence 100 million whole human genomes by 2030. The objective is to improve disease diagnosis, develop targeted treatments, and provide better wellness regimes. Genomics

* Correspondence: fida.dankar@uaeu.ac.ae
[1]College of IT, UAEU, Al Ain, UAE
Full list of author information is available at the end of the article

England is an augmented (100,000) research cohort study that implies sampling of the most common diseases and reflecting the genetic diversity of the population in Great Britain. The All of Us project has similar objectives and aims to collect a sufficiently large cohort (1,000,000). The numbers alone have a great ameliorating effect on statistical power of association studies. Deep phenotyping and follow-up sampling in All of Us are aiming to develop the new level of precision in diagnostic and treatment of multiple diseases. The declared aims of the Human Longevity project are even more focused on a specific range of age-associated diseases. To achieve its goals, Human Longevity plans to recruit about 1,000,000 donors. The Saudi Human Genome Program has a very different focus; it aims to develop effective methods and facilities for early diagnostics and treatment of heritable diseases. Such goal does not require the genome sequencing effort on the same scale as All of Us or Genomics England. The program implements only a small number of whole genome sequencing and up to 100,000 whole exome sequencing to collect the data reflecting local genetic variation and design a microarray chip for cost-effective mass neonatal screening. In contrast, the national genome program in Kuwait requires complete sampling of the entire population including nationals and non-citizen residents because the principal goal, according to the recently adopted DNA Law [11], is to counteract terrorist activity by precise unequivocal identification of every human being. The Qatar Genome Programme (QGP) aims to integrate genome sequencing information of all Qatari nationals with electronic medical records (EMRs) and results of clinical studies to provide quick and precise personalized diagnostic and treatment of diseases. The goal is to provide a solid basis for the biomedical research in the country.

These biomedical databases are often viewed as a platform for regional and worldwide collaborative research projects. Both the construction of these resources and serving them to a growing research community (national and international) present a significant challenge toward preserving the privacy of the participants.

Particularities of genomic data

In 2008, James Watson, a co-discoverer of the double-helix DNA model, opted to release his sequenced genome in a public database with the exception of his APOE gene (which has been associated with Alzheimer's disease). However, a statistical model was later developed that inferred the missing gene with a high degree of confidence [12]. This incident conveys one of many new privacy concerns that genomic data raises and that are difficult to deal with:

- First, genomic data is highly distinguishable. There is confirmation that a sequence of 30 to 80 SNPs could uniquely identify an individual [13]. Genomic data is also very stable [14]. It undergoes little changes over the lifetime of an individual and thus has a long-lived value (as opposed to other biomedical data such as blood tests which have expiry dates).

- Second, genetic data provides sensitive information about genetic conditions and predispositions to certain diseases such as cancer, Alzheimer, and schizophrenia. If breached, such information can be stigmatizing to participants and can be used against them in employment and insurance opportunities, even if these pre-dispositions never materialize.

- Third, genetic data does not only provide information about the sequenced individuals but also about their ancestors and off springs. Whole genome data increases our ability to predict information related to relatives' present and future health risks, which raises the question as to the obligation of a consented participant towards their family members (the authors in [15] describe privacy risks to family members of individuals who shared their genetic data for medical research).

- Finally, and most concerning, there is great fear from the potential information hidden within genomic data [16]. As our knowledge in genomics evolves, so will our view on the sensitivity of genomic data (in other words, it is not possible to quantify the amount and sensitivity of personal information that can be derived from it).

Paper outline

In this paper, we discuss various privacy and governance challenges encountered during the construction and deployment of population-scale sequencing projects. The various challenges are discussed through the stages of:

1. Initial data collection,
2. Data storage,
3. Data sharing (utilization), and
4. Dissemination of research findings to the community.

At each stage, we discuss current practices and challenges, as well as contemporary research efforts, with a particular interest in *data sharing for research purposes* [17]. We provide examples from a diversity of large-scale population sequencing projects and reflect on their scope and data governance models.

Note that the above division is simplistic as the different stages are not mutually exclusive; however, it makes for a simpler and more organized presentation of the different ideas.

Data collection

The data for the different genome projects is sought from the community and results from the efforts on part of the community. Thus, it is important to consult with the concerned population to establish the basic principles for data collection and research oversight. To achieve that, *a community engagement model* should be defined. The model should establish the basic principles for data collection and research oversight such as:

(i) *An advocating technique* for advertising the project to the community and raising the number of individuals who are aware of the project. Such technique should strive to reach different elements within the society, provide clear dissemination of risks and benefits, and establish methods for recurrent evaluation of the community attitudes and understanding of the project.

(ii) *Enrollment criteria* to define the basis for enrollment (should it be disease-based or volunteer-based) as well as the acceptable age for volunteers.

(iii) *An enrollment process* to define the scope of subjects' consent (a general opt in/out or an informed consent) and to set a clear boundary between research and clinical practice, and

(iv) *An institutional and community-based oversight process* to discuss and establish oversight for the program by the community and by independent ethics committees. The scope of these committees should include oversight on data repositories, oversight on research studies and oversight on any changes to the protocol (data use agreements, communications, etc.).

In many cases, regulations require the organization to establish an independent institutional review board, (IRB). The IRB's mandate (at the data collection and storage phases) is to review and approve all proposals related to the data collection protocol and to approve/ manage the participant's consent process for the data collection activity.

One of the most comprehensive community engagement models is that of the Electronic Medical Records and Genomics (eMERGE) network [18]. eMERGE, a National Institute of Health Initiative, is a consortium of nine US medical research institutes (including Vanderbilt Genome-Electronic Records (VGER) project and North Western University biorepository (NUgene)) that combine DNA repositories and EMR systems for advancing genetic research. In the case of VGER [19], the community engagement model was established in

consultation with the community through surveys, focus groups (from different ethnic, racial, and socio-economic backgrounds), posters, and in-person interviews. These activities helped in shaping the principles of data collection, data sharing, and community oversight. The established oversight bodies include The Vanderbilt IRB, the medical center's ethics committee, and several newly established ethics, scientific, and community advisory boards. The community advisory board's role is to evaluate the projects' adherence to the established security and privacy measures, to voice the concerns/issues of the community with regards to the use of their genetic information for research, and to monitor any social/ethical issues arising in the process and help in providing the necessary measures to resolve them [19].

In the case of the NUgene project (North Western University biorepository, another eMERGE network member), the NUMC (Northwestern Medical Center) scientific, medical, and ethics community; the North Western University IRB; community researchers; external advisors; and public health experts were all involved early in establishing issues of consent for genome-wide association studies (GWASs), means to inform participants about data sharing, means to keep participants informed about research activities, and means to engage participants and learn their concern regarding data sharing.

For the case of the Qatar Genome Programme, oversight is provided mainly by an IRB and an access committee (involving prominent members of the community). Although some effort was exercised to publicize the long-term goals and benefits of the project and to get the community involved, the major recruitment incentive is the comprehensive health check provided as part of the sample collection visits by the Qatar Biobank [10]. The appointment takes two 2 days and includes an extensive set of studies and measurement. The measurements include height, weight, blood pressure, grip strength, waist and hip measurements, and body fat composition. The study proceeds to lung function, ultrasound carotid artery scan, 12-lead electrocardiogram, full body iDXA scan, artery stiffness measurement, and treadmill walking test. Finally, samples of blood, saliva, and urine are collected and analyzed.

Most large-scale population genomics programs collect some phenotypic data; the type and volume adjusted to the goals of the study. For instance, the Estonian Genome Project data collection is performed by the Estonian Biobank. The emphasis is on collection of personal data by computer-assisted personal interview (CAPI) within hours of appointment at a doctor's office. The CAPI includes personal and genealogical data (place of birth, ethnicity, family history of medical conditions, etc.), educational and occupational history, and lifestyle data (physical activity, dietary habits, smoking, alcohol consumption, etc.). During the appointment, additional anthropometric, blood pressure, and heart rate data are collected along with the blood sample. The particular feature of the Estonian Genome Project is its strong association with electronic health records providing access to the past and current health status of each sample donor. However, the phenotype study is by far less intensive than that of the Qatar Genome Programme. Saudi Human Genome Program [20] collects virtually no individual phenotype data since this information is not essential to the goals of the program. In the most extreme example, the Kuwait DNA Law [11] showed no interest in phenotype data; mandatory DNA sampling from all residents and visitors also implied no need for consent on the part of the sample donor. Remarkably, after the international outcries pointing out potential abuse of such law, local protests, and challenge from the lawyers, the law has been amended in its most controversial parts.

Protecting participants' data from privacy breaches is a key issue to the success of any genome project. Prospective participants in research studies ranked privacy as one of their top worries and as a major determinant toward their participation in a study [21–23]. Privacy is a socially bound concept; it is deeply affected by language, religion, traditions, and cultural expectations. A simple question such as "how much rent do you pay?" is considered inappropriate in some societies while perfectly normal in others. In the Arab world, for example, personal reputation and family ties are among the highest moral values. As explained by Abokhodair and Vieweg [24], "membership in a family or tribe are of the utmost importance; there is no individual separate from a family ... asserting one's individuality is viewed in a negative light"; in fact, individuals often rely on their family members and communities for significant decisions, while in western societies, asserting one's individuality is celebrated. For these reasons, privacy breaches from genetic testing may differ in their impact on individuals from different backgrounds. Thus, it is important to investigate and understand the cultural values of concerned communities and to tailor the specifics of data collection and data sharing accordingly. Unfortunately, privacy is still treated as a universal notion, and little research has been done to understand the cultural impact.

In the next two sections, we discuss current practice and challenges in protecting participants' sensitive data while in storage (data storage) and while in use (data sharing).

Data storage

EMR and Biobank data are highly sensitive and require significant storage space (the total length of an individual genome is over 3 billion base pairs). As such, one of the biggest challenges for a data warehouse is to decide *where* and *how* to store this data.

Where to store the data?

Data storage presents a significant technological challenge for many large-scale genome projects. The total volume of deep whole genome sequencing (WGS) with raw read, aligned, and variant calling data can reach 0. 5 TB per genome. Phenotyping, imaging, and omics data add additional volume. The specific number may vary widely depending on the types of data collected. Questionnaires and physiological tests, even as comprehensive as those conducted by Qatar Biobank, when collecting samples for the Genome Sequencing Program, add only a small percent to the total volume. Digital images can potentially add large volumes on the same scale as genome sequencing (i.e., on TB scale). However, the real imaging data associated with a particular sample donor in current projects is relatively small and does not exceed gigabyte (GB) scale. Omics data (such as gene expression, methylation, or metabolomics) can also be as large as genome sequencing data. Some of such data is produced using similar next-generation sequencing techniques that result in the same volumes of raw data, which can be stored to reproduce the downstream analysis. Multiple tissue samples can be taken for omics analysis from different organs of the same donor, at different times or in different disease states. This potentially can multiply the volume of data by as many times as more samples are taken. However, at this time, this kind of data is rarely added in significant amounts due to the high costs of high-throughput methods. WGS data remains the most voluminous part of genomic databases. With reserve copy and redundancy, the overall data volume requires petabytes of storage space even for relatively small population studies with tens of thousands of samples. Data compression and selective saving of key data files (while other types of data can be reproduced from initial and intermediate data) can reduce the requirements. Nevertheless, the overall data storage demand in population sequencing is enormous. In the QGP example, it has been originally estimated as 300 PB. The challenge is further compounded by requirement of fast access to individual data files, high-throughput access to multiple genomes in research cohort studies, and long-term storage keeping the data safe and actively used for decades ahead. On the other hand, the price of storage has a hard ceiling dictated by the progress in sequencing technology: the price for data storage per gigabyte should not exceed (and better be significantly lower than) the price of sequencing of the same data from a stored sample. Such demands and limitations make engineering the data storage facility extremely challenging.

In general, the data can be outsourced to a cloud provider or stored on a private—locally managed—cloud. The former approach obscures the complexity of technology but demands highly developed broadband network infrastructure and limits the control over data security and access performance. The overall performance of a cloud-based data storage solution in a large-scale project is gated by the availability of broadband infrastructure. Nevertheless, when local conditions offer adequate answers to security and broadband infrastructure challenges, cloud solution can be very attractive. Genomics England with a goal of 100,000 WGS and full complement of phenotype data is the most brilliant example [25]. The latter approach can be more expensive in terms of engineering, capital expenses, and running costs. In the QGP example, the storage is engineered as a complex solution that involves multiple redundancy and multi-tier storage on different information carriers ranging from flash drives to tape libraries. However, the storage service is provided in a form of a single name space private cloud (see overview in Fig. 1).

In other examples of local storage solution for large-scale genomic and biomedical data, the technical details of storage architecture are rarely detailed and rely on the local policies of the data center for data integrity, security, and safety. Examples of such projects include the Estonian Genome Project and Saudi Human Genome Program [26, 27].

It is increasingly advocated that individuals should be the guardians of their own biomedical data. As such, they should have the ability to access, modify, and grant access (to family, health authorities, or research facilities) as they see fit. However, numerous challenges (in terms of data storage) have to be solved before such model can be adopted, such as:

1. Where should individual data be stored (individual's private PC or on a private access-controlled cloud?), and how to ensure the security of the data in either case?
2. How to grant access to different authorities and how to manage such access?
3. Should the data be backed up, where and how?
4. Does the individual have the right to withdraw authorized access or to delete their data, and how can either be done [28]?

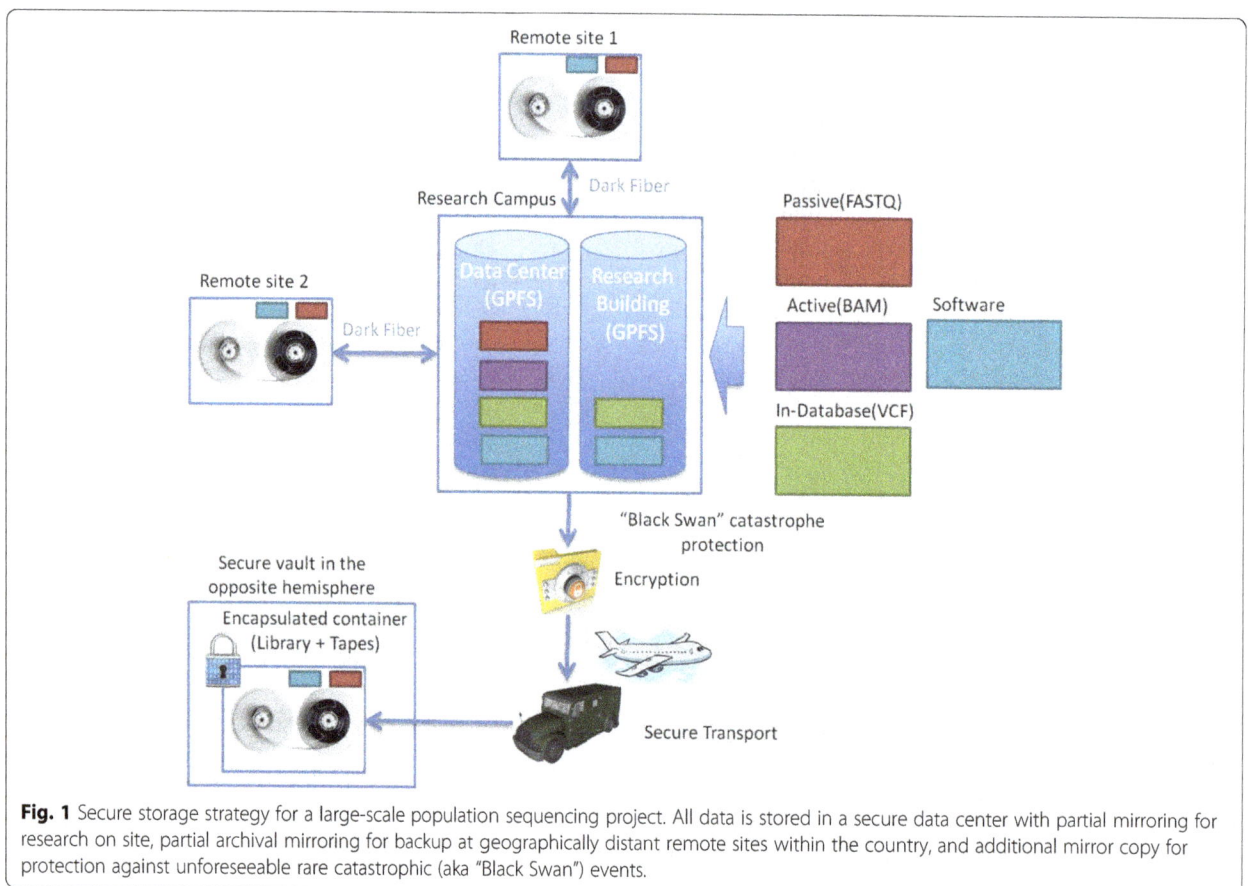

Fig. 1 Secure storage strategy for a large-scale population sequencing project. All data is stored in a secure data center with partial mirroring for research on site, partial archival mirroring for backup at geographically distant remote sites within the country, and additional mirror copy for protection against unforeseeable rare catastrophic (aka "Black Swan") events.

How to store the data?

To minimize the risk of harm, most research platforms store de-identified clinical and biobank data while retaining the link between both data sources (the de-identified EMR data and the biobank data). This can be achieved by applying the following two operations:

1. The first operation (known as pseudonymization) identifies a stable and unique identifier(s) (such as Social Security numbers and national IDs) that is included in both data sources and replaces it with a unique random ID or pseudonym (refer to Fig. 2). The pseudonym can be obtained by encrypting or hashing one or several identifiers. Decode genetics uses a symmetric encryption algorithm (TwoFish) to convert the Social Security number (SSN) to an alphabet-derived string. VGER hashes the medical record number using the public hashing algorithm SHA-512.

2. The second operation removes all uniquely identifying information (such as names, record number, and emails) from the structured data and masks all unique identifiers from the unstructured data (such as doctors' notes), (refer to Table 1 for examples of unique identifiers). Additional fields can be also removed from the data for added privacy; the VGER project, as an example, removes all geographic information smaller than a state and all elements of dates (except year) directly related to the individual (such as date of birth and date of death) and shifts all hospital visit dates by a random value between 1 and 364 days (the shift being the same across the record of the same patient to preserve temporal analysis).

Multiple aspects have to be considered when designing the pseudonymization operation; these include:

1. Ensuring that each subject is assigned the same random ID (pseudonym) across different data sources. This consistency will ensure that data belonging to a particular subject will always be mapped to one record.

2. Deciding whether the pseudonymization process should be reversible or not. Reversible systems allow reverting back to the identity of the subjects through a process called de-pseudonymization. For the case of Decode Genetics and QGP, reversibility was chosen because communication with patients was deemed to be a foreseen possibility (to communicate novel treatments and/or possible preventative measures). While for the VGER case, reversibility is not possible as the link between the pseudonym and the medical record number was not maintained.

3. When communication is forecasted, a secure de-pseudonymization mechanism should be specified; the mechanism should define (i) the cases for which de-identification can occur, (ii) the bodies that can initiate re-identification requests, (iii) those that rule and regulate these requests, and (iv) the actual re-identification mechanism.

Privacy breaches can occur if the data is leaked to an unauthorized party. Such leakage can happen if (i) the *stored data is hacked/handled recklessly* or if it is (ii) *shared with a pretentious/irresponsible third party*. After applying the pseudonymization process, the data remains vulnerable to de-identification attacks (in other words, although de-identification makes re-identification harder, it does not eliminate the risk). Thus, a strong security layer is needed to ensure that unauthorized individuals cannot access/modify the data. Encryption alone is not an adequate security solution, particularly for genomic data. As explained in [28], encryption schemes gradually weaken in the long run, while the information hidden inside a genome remains stable and is better interpreted with time. Thus, if encrypted genomes are available to an unauthorized third party, the party will be able to decrypt it with time (40–50 years).

Commercial cloud providers (such as IBM and Amazon) claim to employ foolproof security, but their models are not shared publicly and thus cannot be learned and evaluated. Security of the privately held infrastructure and private clouds depends on the proficiency of system administrators and security specialists

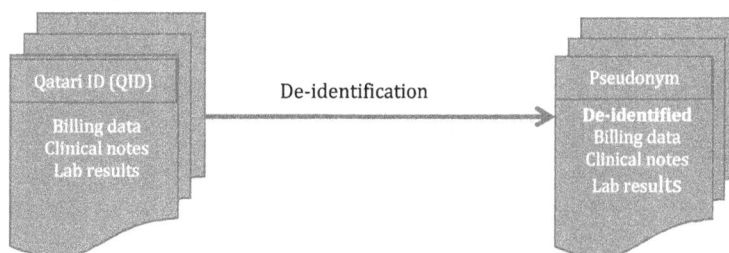

Fig. 2 De-identification of clinical data

Table 1 Examples of unique identifiers

Uniquely identifying fields	Remarks
National ID (or SSN)	
Name	Names of patients and caregivers
Email	
Source ID	Hospital/Biobank-assigned IDs
Passport number	
Exact address	

employed by the custodian organization. In some cases, like the Qatar Genome Programme, geographic location and state-regulated data access may provide additional protective layer against sporadic attacks and "social engineering" hacks. However, the ability of genomic data storage to withstand a determined and competent invasion is yet to be tested.

Data sharing

Electronic medical records (EMRs) hold diverse clinical information about large populations. When this information is coupled with genetic data, it has the potential to make unprecedented associations between genes and diseases. The incorporation of these discoveries into healthcare practice offers the hope to improve healthcare through personalized treatments. However, the availability of such data for widespread research activities is dependent *on the protection of a subject's privacy*. Current technological methods for privacy preservation are outdated and cannot provide protection for genomic and longitudinal data (EMR).

Access mechanisms and privacy

Data sharing mechanisms can be categorized into two broad categories: open-access and controlled-access. While both were widely used for regulating genomic data sharing, open-access datasets have been used in many more studies per year [29]. Open-access models either operate under a mandate from participants (who want to publish their genomic data in public platforms) or under the assumption that the shared data is de-identified and possibly aggregated [30]. However, as demonstrated by multiple recent studies, the risk of re-identification is strongly present. It was shown, in multiple independent studies, that it is possible to learn the identities of people who participate in research studies by matching their data with publicly available data [31]. In a recent study [32], the authors showed that they can infer the identity of 50 anonymous male subjects whose Y-chromosome has been sequenced as part of the 1000 Genomes Project. The researchers were not only able to discover the identities of these anonymized research participants but also their family members using available/public

pedigrees. In response to this study, the NIH removed the age information from the project's database. In another recent study, [33, 34], the authors reported that they can confirm whether a person participated in a genome-wide association study, by using information from the person's DNA sample, "even if the study reported only summary statistics on hundreds or thousands of participants" [31]. In response, the NIH shifted to a controlled access mechanism. In fact, currently, most human genome projects use controlled-access mechanisms.

The personal information derived from genomic data (and EMR data) can be very damaging to the participants. It can be used against them to limit insurance coverage, to guide employment decisions, or to apply social stigma. In [35], the authors report on a case of genetic discrimination by a railroad company. The case occurred in 2002 when the company forced its employees to undergo a genetic test; employees who refused to participate in the test were threatened with disciplinary actions. The company was later forced (in an out-of-court settlement) to compensate 36 of its employees. That is hardly a consolation because if such genetic data was obtained from online sources or breached through illegal means, the company may have been able to get away with its discrimination practices.

Regulations

In many countries, the use of sensitive human-subject data for research purposes has been studied extensively from the legal aspect. Resulting legislations aimed to ensure that private information is properly used and adequately protected when disclosed for research purposes [36, 37]. The legislations (such as the Common Rule [36], Health Information Portability and Accountability Act (HIPAA) [38], and EU data protection directive [39]) generally permit data sharing under one of the following guidelines:

G1. For the use of identifiable data, an approval from an Institutional Review Board (IRB) is required. To approve data requests, IRBs require:
   a. Informed consents from the participants for the specific data use, or
   b. When consents are deemed impractical, IRBs can grant data access if the study accrues more benefit than risk. Such decision requires a thorough and lengthy evaluation of each data access request from the IRB part.
G2. For adequately de-identified data, researchers can be exempt from IRB approval. The adequacy of the de-identification is generally established by the IRB or by pre-approved policies such as the United States HIPAA privacy rule [37].

Guideline G2 depends on the availability of robust de-identification techniques, but as current techniques are outdated, and unable to deal with genetic and EMR data (as evident from the privacy breaches cited earlier), G2 cannot be adopted. The Vanderbilt genome project is the only project we are aware of that was ruled by Vanderbilt IRB to be a "non-human subject data" as it was deemed to be properly de-identified. However, given the potential impact of the project on the community, guidelines adhering to G1.b were enforced.

Guideline G1.a requires informed consent from participants. The problem with such requirement is that data collectors have to forecast all possible uses of the data and create a comprehensive consent detailing the benefits and risks related to all different data uses. Something that is not easily achievable. In fact, most biobanks collect consents in the form of opt in/opt out [19]. The issues/challenges in implementing proper informed consent will be discussed in depth later in this section.

Almost all existing biomedical data warehouses that house (non-aggregate) genetic data coupled with EMR data follow guideline *G1.b*. These warehouses lightly de-identify their data and regulate investigators' access to the data through an IRB [18, 19, 40]. Only researchers with studies that involve less risk than benefit are allowed access to requested data and only after they pass a thorough identity check. However, IRB procedures are extensive and can obstruct timely research and discoveries [41–43]. Studies on platforms that rely on IRB for all data accesses reveal unsatisfied users. The application process is strenuous and approvals take a long time often delaying project initiation significantly [43, 44].

In Qatar, as an example, access to the biomedical data collected in Qatar is governed by the QSCH "guidelines, regulations and policies for research involving human subjects", which adheres to guideline *G1.b*. A recently formed IRB will regulate all accesses to the research data and services by all research institutes within Qatar and outside.

With such massive mandates, a principal feature for IRBs is to have the capacity to foster timely research and discoveries. Data application processes and approvals should be smooth and should not delay project initiation significantly. Thus, the traditional "IRB-based" data sharing will produce unsatisfied users.

Methods under investigation

The inadequacy of current de-identification methods and the delays in IRB processes prompted privacy experts to seek new solutions. Rapid progress is taking place in privacy research in the biomedical area, driven by the need to protect and benefit from the large biomedical data warehouses being built worldwide. The novel methods can be divided into two main categories, legislative and technical:

(i) *Legislative:* Legislative methods define privacy rights and responsibilities. Research in this area aims to understand and define individuals' privacy perspectives and expectations and to update policies and laws that govern data sharing. Genetic data introduces a difficult and unique regulatory situation (with respect to data collection laws and data sharing laws) that is not found with other types of health data [16]. So, until effective privacy protection solutions are made into law, scientists and civil right advocates are calling for the adoption of anti-genetic discrimination laws to mitigate the effect of genetic data breaches. An example is the Genetic Information Non-discrimination Act (GINA) adopted by the US government in 2008. GINA forbids discrimination by insurers or employers on the basis of genetic information. The problem with such regulations is that they are enforced only when discrimination on the basis of genetic information is proven, which necessitates the difficult task of proving malicious intentions.

(ii) *Technical:* Technical controls aim to create data sharing systems/methods that fulfill the requirements specified in privacy legislation. Current technical approaches to privacy, such as de-identification, are not effective in the genomic context (in fact, the genome is itself an identifier and as such cannot be de-identified (yet) while retaining its utility), thus the need for innovative methods to deal with our new data realities. We classify current research in privacy-preserving mechanisms into three categories: process-driven mechanisms, risk-aware systems, and consent-based systems. In process-driven mechanisms, such as differential privacy and cryptographic techniques, the dataset is held by a trusted server, users query the data through the server, and privacy is built into the algorithms that access the data. Risk-aware systems aim at speeding the IRB processes through partial/full automation, and consent-based systems aim to empower participants by allowing them to control how and by whom their data can be used. This is being done through the introduction of novel dynamic consent mechanisms.

In what follows, we briefly describe recent efforts within each of the three technical categories.

Dynamic consent

Consent-based mechanisms provide data subjects with control over who can access their stored data/specimens, for what purposes, and for how long. Thus, a researcher requesting access to data will receive the data records for which the consent is fulfilled.

The current (mostly paper-based) consent process is static and locks consent information to a single time point (typically during sample collection) [45], requiring all future data usages to be specified at the time of initial consent. This is not feasible with current (multi-purpose and evolving) biomedical data warehouses. The current process also requires limiting the amount of information conveyed to participants to ensure that their consent is informed (i.e., the educational program), since individuals can only absorb limited information at any one time. Re-contacting participants to obtain additional consents and/or to provide additional education materials is arduous, time-consuming, and expensive. Moreover, it can have a negative impact on the participants and on the enterprise.

Active research is underway to overcome this problem. It attempts to provide consent dynamicity to make it easier on the participants and data holders to continuously provide/update consent information. The authors of [46] are working on ways to represent and manage consent information. They focus on defining the different dimensions of a consent. Such dimensions include (i) the characteristics of the institutions that can access the patient's data, (ii) the level of details that each institution can access, and (ii) the type of research allowed on the data (all possible uses of the data). The authors' approach is to codify the different consent dimensions. The benefit of the codification "is to provide a common language to capture consented uses of data and specimens" and to "select those data for the investigator's study that are compliant with the subjects' consented uses and the investigator's permissions." Thus, given a particular study, the characteristics of the study could be matched against the subjects' codified consent to determine the data subset that conforms. In [47, 48], the authors discuss several challenges in designing dynamic consents, particularly, participant's consent withdrawal and its implications. It is worth noting that some commercial sequencing companies, such as 23andme [49], already provide a limited form of dynamic consent models through secure online portal systems. Such systems allow users to fill/change their consent information at their own will.

Additional aspects that need to be resolved are consent withdrawal, continuous participant education, and the cultural aspect of the consent:

- *Consent withdrawal:* Withdrawal is an essential motivator for research participation; thus, research participants must be allowed to withdraw their participation at any time without any penalties. However, withdrawal is complicated by the fact that participants' samples/data may already have been shared by other research organizations. Current best

practices recommend that any leftover specimens be discarded and that medical data no longer be updated or used but that shared samples and data do not necessarily need to be revoked [50]. It is important for the consent process to highlight these issues and to make sure that participants understand the limitations of consent withdrawal. Additionally, more investigation should be done around different forms of withdrawals to understand their impact on the willingness to participate and to update best practices accordingly.

- *Continuous participants' education:* Biomedical sciences are complex and are evolving very fast, which warrants the need for continuous participant education.

- *Cultural aspect:* The purpose of informed consent is to give the right of self-determination to individuals based on complete understanding of risks and benefits of research participation and without any interference or control by others. However, the right of self-determination is deeply affected by culture (some communities value the relationship with family members and turn to them for support when making critical decisions), and thus, consent should be adapted to the specifics of the underlying culture in terms of information sharing and disclosure [51].

Risk-aware access control

The risk of granting data access to a user depends on the characteristics of the request. For example, as stated in [52], "access to highly sensitive data at the data-holder's location by a trusted user is inherently less risky than providing the same user with a copy of the dataset. Similarly, access to de-identified clinical data from a secure remote system is inherently less risky than access to identifiable data from an unknown location." Risk-aware access control tries to quantify the risk posed by a data request and to apply mitigation measures on the data to counter the posed risk.

Risk aware access control received growing attention in the past few years. Several of the studies attempted to quantify/model privacy risk, both from the participants' perspective and the data holder's perspective. In [53], Adams attempts to model users' perceptions of privacy in multimedia environments. He identified three factors that determine users' perceptions of privacy: information sensitivity (user's perception of the sensitivity of the released information), information receiver (the level of trust the user has in the information recipient(s)), and information usage (costs and benefits of the perceived usages). Lederer [54] uses Adams' model as a framework for conceptualizing privacy in ubiquitous computing environments in addition to the Lessig model [55] for conceptualizing the influence of societal forces on the understanding of privacy. These efforts concentrate on privacy quantification from the participant perspective rather than the data holder.

Barker at al. [56] introduce a four-dimensional model for privacy: purpose (data uses), visibility (who will access the data), granularity (data specificity), and retention (time data is kept in storage). Barker et al.'s model was later used by Banerjee et al. [57] to quantify privacy violations. Along the same lines, and in multiple consecutive studies [58, 59], El Emam et al. defined three criteria that contribute to privacy risk; these are users' motives, the sensitivity of the requested data, and the security controls employed by the data requestor. The authors state that, according to their long experience in private data sharing [58, 60–62], these are the main criteria used (informally) by data holders.

Recently, in [52, 63], the authors defined a conceptual risk-based access model for a biomedical data warehouse; the model defines the risk posed by data requests using four dimensions:

1. Data sensitivity, or the extent of privacy invasion that would result from inappropriate disclosure of the requested data,
2. Access purpose, or the usages for which the data was requested,
3. Location of the investigator's institution, which is critical for checking the privacy legislation (if any) that applies at the data requester's end and whether the same laws are enforceable, and
4. User risk, which measures:
   a. The user's institution ability to secure the data (the research institution to which the user is affiliated). This is evaluated by looking at the privacy practices followed/enforced within their headquarters and
   b. The risk associated with the particular user/requestor; it is measured by tracking whether the user caused any past inconveniences.

Once calculated, the risk is fed into an access control decision module. The decision module imposes mitigation measures to counter the posed risk. The defined data-sharing mechanism would impose more mitigation measures on requests of higher sensitivity. The mitigations could manifest as reductions in the granularity of the data (de-identification) and/or as restrictions on when and how a user can access the data. The implementation of this model still requires significant efforts toward (i) assigning sensitivities to the different data attributes, (ii) assigning a score to institutions' privacy and security practices (such as certifications), and (iii) creating universal user records for storing data breach information.

The issue of assigning sensitivity to data attributes is gaining more consideration. In [64], the authors define a method to detect privacy-sensitive DNA segments in an input stream. In [65], the authors present a privacy test to distinguish degrees of sensitivity within different attributes recognized as sensitive.

Secure multiparty computation

Secure multiparty computations (SMCs) are an attractive approach that allows a researcher to run a function on data owned by multiple parties (each holding a fraction of the data to be analyzed). The calculation is carried out on the overall dataset without any party having to reveal any of their own raw data. Such scenario can be particularly useful for cross-institutional studies (or even cross-countries studies) particularly when no site has enough data to conduct the study in question (for example, studies on rare diseases).

Figure 3 illustrates the SMC concept. In the figure, a researcher wants to run a computation f over the private inputs of three remote databases (data1, data2, data3) while keeping these inputs private. The different parties are allowed to exchange messages with each other and with the researcher. However, such messages are encrypted so as to prevent the different parties from learning any private information through interaction.

SMC is gaining more popularity in the biomedical domain. SMCs are supported by robust mathematical proofs demonstrating their ability to securely protect privacy and thus proving their ability to support data sharing without fear of privacy abuse. In [66, 67], the authors designed a secure linear regression using homomorphic encryption for a multi-hospital quality improvement study. In [68], a secure genome-wide association study (GWAS) was designed using homomorphic

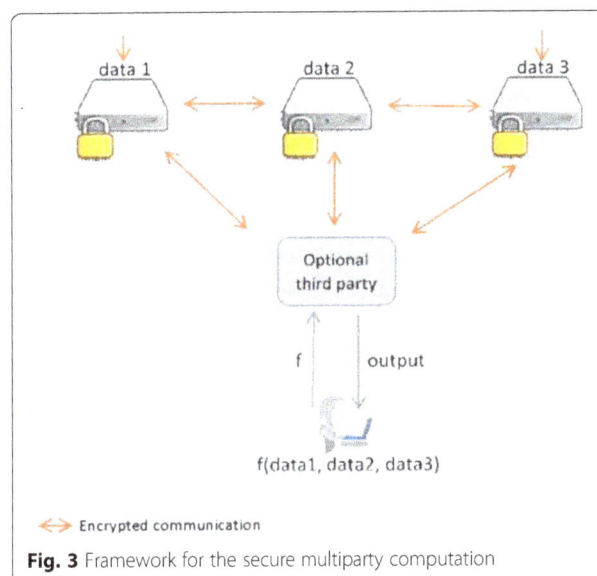

Fig. 3 Framework for the secure multiparty computation

encryption, and in [69], a GWAS protocol was designed using secret sharing. In [70], the authors use garbled circuits to perform metagenomics analysis.

In general, the protocols for secure computation have achieved outstanding results; it has been shown that any function (no matter how complex) can be computed securely. Efficiency however is the major drawback of these computations; they are much more complex than regular protocols (that do not provide any security) [71]. The complexity is driven by the extensive message passing between the involved parties as well as the cryptographic functions employed. Recently, the authors in [72] presented a fast and secure computation for linear regression over distributed data based on secure matrix multiplication. And, the authors in [73] designed another efficient secure multiparty linear regression protocol; their method was based on mathematical results in estimation theory. It remains to be seen whether these methods are generalizable to other estimators.

Dissemination of findings

Prior work demonstrated that in order to affirm the value of research participation and contribute to public education, it is important to have a mechanism for disseminating research findings to the public. This will keep the community aware of how their participation is facilitating research and improving knowledge in the biomedical field.

The mechanism should also tackle the issue of disseminating individual research findings to specific participants. The recommendations governing the return of individual results are usually driven by the psychological harm that could affect the subjects from knowing a result weighted by the benefits in learning it. As such, recommendations are usually aligned with returning "clinically actionable" results, that is, results that are considered *scientifically valid* and that constitute *valuable information* for the recipient, i.e., results associated with some kind of preventive/cautionary strategy.

For example, a finding of deleterious mutations in the BRCA1 or BRCA2 genes associates diagnosed women with high frequency of developing breast or ovarian cancer. Such valid findings help the participants choose to undergo more screening (yearly mammograms, yearly MRI), frequent clinical breast screenings, or bilateral risk-reducing mastectomy which is known to reduce the risk of cancer up to 95% [74–76].

Another example concerns the incidence of mutations in chromosome 12 in the gene coding for phenylalanine hydroxylase (PAH). The mutation may result in the absence of or a defect in PAH enzyme. Phenylketonuria (PKU) can be prevented if PKU is diagnosed soon after birth; children can be placed on diets low in phenylalanine and the detrimental effects of accumulated phenylalanine are avoided. Such highly valuable information for the recipient might prevent severe mental retardation as a result of PKU.

Other findings might not put the participants at risk of developing a disease but could give them the necessary information to guide some of their life choices; an example is whether the participant is a carrier for albinism.

The American College of Medical Genetics and Genomics (ACMG) published a policy statement in 2013 specifying the mutations that should be sought and reported back to the participants (in the context of clinical sequencing). ACMG updates these recommendations annually.

Although the ACMG recommendations were put forth by experts in the field, these underwent a thorough deliberation process and were reviewed (before publication) by external geneticists; they were criticized for excluding the community from the discussion [77]. In fact, there is a growing push to empower members of the public regarding genetic research in general and regarding the return of individual results to research participants in particular. Empirical studies have shown that the majority of participants would like to learn a broader array of genetic results than what is recommended and that they would like to be given the opportunity to decide on that matter [78]. This however necessitates the design of an educational and dynamic consent process to capture the informed (and fluctuating) choices of participants with regards to returning their interpreted data and to continuously educate participants (refer to the "Regulations" section). Such individual consent coupled with educational material could be provided to participants through a secure online portal system for them to complete at their own pace and as the need arises. This allows consent documents to be tied to real events as they occur in the data life cycle, rather than requiring all consent issues to be defined at the beginning of the study. Thus, for example, as new information is generated that changes a variant's status from ambiguous to actionable, additional educational programs and consent documents can be created to allow participants to decide if they want to receive information about the variant and/or to allow that information to be transmitted to their physicians.

Another difficult issue at the core of information dissemination is that of interpretation of the genome sequence information. Interpretation requires the storage of additional information in a form that is easily understood by medical doctors (and other caregivers). It also necessitates the continuous updating of this information with any relevant findings.

A table summarizing several characteristics of select genome projects is presented at the end of the manuscript (Table 2). For every project, it indicates the target number of genomes to be sequenced, the number of genomes sequenced to date, the project's context, the initiation date, the data access model (open versus controlled), the consent process, whether it supports notification (or dissemination) of relevant clinical data, and whether a de-identification mechanism is applied.

Conclusion

Biomedical sciences have been evolving faster than the societies' ability to cope with them. On one hand, current technical approaches to privacy are not adequate for modern biomedical data, and on the other hand, privacy laws have not been updated to deal with the special features of genomic data. As a result, common practice for biomedical data sharing is either rule-based or relies on an IRB for data-sharing decisions. These processes lack a clear and quantitative measurement of privacy risks.

Moreover, calls for participants' empowerment and data ownership are increasing. Data ownership gives the right to individuals to be the guardians of their own data, allowing them to access their data, modify it, set access rules, and modify the rules at will. Informed consent is believed to grant such right of self-determination to the individuals by specifying how they like their data to be accessed (data sharing) and what findings (from their data) they would like to receive back (data dissemination).

However, we cannot talk about participants' empowerment without talking about culture and education. As mentioned earlier in the paper, the right of self-determination is deeply affected by culture. More studies are needed to understand the role of religion, cultures, and traditions in constructing norms around privacy and self-determination.

On the education front, more effort should be made to (continuously and dynamically) educate the public and

Table 2 Characteristics of selected genome projects. In *opt-out* consent process, consent is presumed (for clinical data and left-over hospital samples) with an opportunity to opt out. *Opt-out* is usually coupled with *paper-based consent* for individuals who want to volunteer samples at the biobank. In *local access* model, researchers are not allowed to download the data; they can only access it on the data holder's site. – indicates missing information, *Intra-country* indicates that data is not allowed to leave the country (collaborations should be done through a local researcher)

Projects	Declared target #genomes/ exomes	#Genomes sequenced to date	Context	Start date	Data access model	Consent process	Notification of relevant data	De-identification process
Human Longevity	1000,000 WGS	–	Research	2013	Controlled	paper based	Yes	Yes
All of US	1000,000 WGS	0	Research	2017	Multi-tier (open to controlled), based on risk of request	Dynamic consent	Yes	Yes
Korean Genome Project	1000 WGS for 2016 10,000 WGS for 2018 50,000,000 WGS for 2030	1722	Research	2012	Open	–	–	Yes
QGP	300,000 WGS	4000	Research	2013	Controlled (multi-ethics/ review boards)	Paper-based (11 simple questions)	Yes	Yes
Estonian Genome Project	–	52,000[a] samples	Research	2000	Controlled (multi-ethics/ review boards	broad paper-based consent	Yes	Yes
Saudi Human Genome Program	100,000 WES	–	Research, diagnostic screening	2013	Controlled	Informed Paper based consent	Yes	Yes
Decode Genetics	300,000 WGS (with imputation)	160,000	Research	1996	Controlled (intra-country)	Opt-out/ paper-based consent	Yes	Yes
The Faroe Genome Project	50,000 WGS	–	Research	2011	Controlled (multi-ethics/ review boards)	Informed consent (one for each research project)	No[b]	Yes
Genomics England	100,000	52,065	Research	2015	Controlled (access committee)	Paper-based	Yes	Yes, coupled with local access

[a]The number of biological specimens collected up to date
[b]Upon participation in a research study, subjects may opt to receive notification about different genetic results that may be revealed

inform them about the great benefits arising from sharing their data and the potential risk and damage that could result on the individual and their close relatives should their information be breached.

On another related topic, that of genomic medicine, advancements are needed on many fronts to integrate genetic knowledge into medical practice. On one hand, consent issues regarding dissemination of findings should be resolved, and on the other hand, issues that require development are (i) genetic knowledge representation and the technical limitations of EMR systems, (ii) the lack of genetic training programs for practitioners, and (iii) the difficulty in interpreting genetic results (due to their probabilistic nature and their dependency on phenotypic data).

Abbreviations
ACMG: American College of Medical Genetics and Genomics; APOE: Apolipoprotein E; CAPI: Computer-Assisted Personal Anterview; DNA: DeoxyriboNucleic Acid; DXA: Dual X-ray Absorptiometry; eMERGE: Electronic Medical Records and Genomics; EMR: Electronic Medical Record; EU: European Union; GINA: Genetic Information Non-discrimination Act; GWAS: Genome-Wide Association Study; HIPAA: Health Information Portability and Accountability Act; IRB: Institutional Review Board; NIH: National Institute of Health; NUgene: North Western University biorepository; NUMC: North Western University Medical Center; PAH: PhenylAlanine Hydroxylase; PKU: PhenylKetonUria; PMI: Precision Medicine Initiative; QGP: Qatar Genome Programme; QSCH: Qatar Council for Healthcare Practitioners; SHA-512: Secure Hash Algorithm; SMC: Secure Multiparty Communication; SNP: Single Nucleotide Polymorphism; SSN: Social Security Number; VGER: Vanderbilt Genome-Electronic Records; WGS: Whole Genome Sequencing

Acknowledgements
We are deeply grateful to the late Professor Mahmud Micheal Barmada for the long informative discussions we had during his short time with us. He has shown, by his example, what a good scientist (and person) should be. Also, we would like to thank the two anonymous reviewers for their helpful comments/suggestions on earlier drafts of the manuscript.

Funding
This work is supported by the UAE University research grant #31T084 Research Start-up.

Authors' contributions
FKD designed the paper and contributed to writing and editing the manuscript. AP contributed to writing and editing the manuscript. SKD contributed to writing the manuscript. All authors read and approved the final manuscript.

Competing interests
The authors declare that they have no competing interests.

Author details
[1]College of IT, UAEU, Al Ain, UAE. [2]Gloucester Marine Genomics Institute, Gloucester, MA, USA. [3]Faculty of Sciences, University of Balamand, Souk El Ghareb, Lebanon.

References
1. Decode genetics. http://www.decode.com/.
2. Gulcher J, Stefansson K. An Icelandic saga on a centralized healthcare database and democratic decision making. Nat Biotechnol. 1999;17:620.
3. Gudbjartsson DF, Helgason H, Gudjonsson SA, Zink F, Oddson A, Gylfason A, et al. Large-scale whole-genome sequencing of the Icelandic population. Nat Genet. 2015;47:435–44.
4. Genome England. http://genomicsengland.co.uk.
5. Human Longevity. http://www.humanlongevity.com/.
6. Precision Medicine Initiative. http://www.nih.gov/precisionmedicine/.
7. Cyranoski D. China embraces precision medicine on a massive scale. Nat News. 2016;529:9.
8. Korean Reference Genome Project. http://152.99.75.168/KRGDB/menuPages/intro.jsp.
9. Abu-Elmagd M, Assidi M, Schulten H-J, Dallol A, Pushparaj PN, Ahmed F, et al. Individualized medicine enabled by genomics in Saudi Arabia. BMC Merd Genomics. 2015;8(Suppl 1):S3.
10. Qatar BioBank. http://www.qatarbiobank.org.qa/media-center/event-detail?item=33&backArt=29.
11. The DNA law. Kuwait Times. 2016. http://news.kuwaittimes.net/website/the-dna-law/. Accessed 26 Feb 2017.
12. Nyholt DR, Yu C-E, Visscher PM. On Jim Watson's APOE status: genetic information is hard to hide. Eur J Hum Genet. 2009;17:147.
13. El Emam K. Methods for the de-identification of electronic health records for genomic research. Genome Med. 2011;3:25.
14. Gelfand A. Privacy and biomedical research: building a trust infrastructure. 2012. http://biomedicalcomputationreview.org/content/privacy-and-biomedical-research-building-trust-infrastructure.
15. Cassa CA, Schmidt B, Kohane IS, Mandl KD. My sister's keeper?: genomic research and the identifiability of siblings. BMC Med Genomics. 2008;1. https://doi.org/10.1186/1755-8794-1-32.
16. Naveed M, Ayday E, Clayton EW, Fellay J, Gunter CA, Hubaux J-P, et al. Privacy in the genomic era. ACM Comput Surv CSUR. 2015;48:6.
17. Dankar FK, Al-Ali R. Building of a large scale de-identified biomedical database in Qatar—principles and challenges. Qatar Found Annu Res Conf Proc. 2016;2016:HBPP3324.
18. McCarty CA, Chisholm RL, Chute CG, Kullo IJ, Jarvik GP, Larson EB, et al. The eMERGE network: a consortium of biorepositories linked to electronic medical records data for conducting genomic studies. BMC Med Genomics. 2011;4:13.
19. Roden DM, Pulley JM, Basford MA, Bernard GR, Clayton EW, Balser JR, et al. Development of a large-scale de-identified DNA biobank to enable personalized medicine. Clin Pharmacol Ther. 2008;84:362–9.
20. All About The Human Genome Project (HGP). National Human Genome Research Institute (NHGRI). https://www.genome.gov/10001772/All-About-The%2D-Human-Genome-Project-HGP. Accessed 26 Feb 2017.
21. McGuire AL, Oliver JM, Slashinski MJ, Graves JL, Wang T, Kelly PA, et al. To share or not to share: a randomized trial of consent for data sharing in genome research. Genet Med. 2011;13:948–55.
22. McGuire AL, Hamilton JA, Lunstroth R, McCullough LB, Goldman A. DNA data sharing: research participants' perspectives. Genet Med. 2008; 10:46–53.
23. Oliver JM, Slashinski MJ, Wang T, Kelly PA, Hilsenbeck SG, McGuire AL. Balancing the risks and benefits of genomic data sharing: genome research participants' perspectives. Public Health Genomics. 2011;15:106–14.
24. Abokhodair N, Vieweg S. Privacy & social media in the context of the Arab Gulf. In: Proceedings of the 2016 ACM Conference on Designing Interactive Systems. New York: ACM; 2016. p. 672–83. https://doi.org/10.1145/2901790.2901873.
25. Hubbard T. HPC infrastructure at King's College London and Genomics England. In: Farr-ADRN-MB eInfrastructure Workshop. 2015.

26. Leitsalu L, Metspalu A. Chapter 8—from biobanking to precision medicine: the Estonian experience. In: Ginsburg GS, Willard HF, editors. Genomic and precision medicine. Third ed. Boston: Academic Press; 2017. p. 119–29. https://doi.org/10.1016/B978-0-12-800681-8.00008-6.

27. Abouelhoda M. The informatics side of the Saudi human genome project. In: GenoME. 2016.

28. Ayday E, Cristofaro ED, Hubaux JP, Tsudik G. The Chills and Thrills of Whole Genome Sequencing. IEEE Computer Magazine; 2013.

29. Wang S, Jiang X, Singh S, Marmor R, Bonomi L, Fox D, et al. Genome privacy: challenges, technical approaches to mitigate risk, and ethical considerations in the United States. Ann N Y Acad Sci. 2017; 1387:73–83.

30. ExAC Browser. http://exac.broadinstitute.org/about. Accessed 6 Mar 2018.

31. Check Hayden E. Privacy protections: the genome hacker. Nature. 2013;497: 172–4.

32. Gymrek M, McGuire AL, Golan D, Halperin E, Erlich Y. Identifying personal genomes by surname inference. Science. 2013;339;321–4.

33. Sweeney L, Abu A, Winn J. Identifying participants in the personal genome project by name. 2013.

34. Homer N, Szelinger S, Redman M, Duggan D, Tembe W, Muehling J, et al. Resolving individuals contributing trace amounts of DNA to highly complex mixtures using high-density SNP genotyping microarrays. PLoS Genet. 2008; 4:e1000167.

35. Malin B, Cassa C, Kantarcioglu M. A survey of challenges and solutions for privacy in clinical genomics data mining. In: Bonchi F, Ferrari E, editors. Privacy-Preserving Knowledge Discovery. New York: Chapman & Hall/CRC Press; 2011.

36. Federal policy for the protection of human subjects ('Common Rule'). http://www.hhs.gov/ohrp/humansubjects/commonrule/.

37. Sweeney L. Data sharing under HIPAA: 12 years later. In: Workshop on the HIPAA Privacy Rule's de-identification standard. 2010.

38. U.S. Department of Health & Human Services. http://www.hhs.gov/. Accessed 22 Sept 2015.

39. European Data Protection Directive. https://ico.org.uk/media/about-the-ico/documents/1042349/review-of-eu-dp-directive.pdf.

40. Murphy SN, Weber G, Mendis M, Gainer V, Chueh HC, Churchill S, et al. Serving the enterprise and beyond with informatics for integrating biology and the bedside (i2b2). J Am Med Inform Assoc JAMIA. 2010;17:124–30.

41. Wolf LE, Walden JF, Lo B. Human subjects issues and IRB review in practice-based research. Ann Fam Med. 2005;3(suppl 1):S30–7.

42. Graham DG, Spano MS, Manning B. The IRB challenge for practice-based research: strategies of the American Academy of Family Physicians National Research Network (AAFP NRN). J Am Board Fam Med. 2007;20:181–7.

43. He S, Narus SP, Facelli JC, Lau LM, Botkin JR, Hurdle JF. A domain analysis model for eIRB systems: addressing the weak link in clinical research informatics. J Biomed Inform. 2014;52:121–9.

44. Silberman G, Kahn KL. Burdens on research imposed by institutional review boards: the state of the evidence and its implications for regulatory reform. Milbank Q. 2011;89:599–627.

45. Appelbaum PS, Waldman CR, Fyer A, Klitzman R, Parens E, Martinez J, et al. Informed consent for return of incidental findings in genomic research. Genet Med. 2013;16:367–73.

46. Ohno-Machado L, Bafna V, Boxwala AA, Chapman BE, Chapman WW, Chaudhuri K, et al. iDASH: integrating data for analysis, anonymization, and sharing. J Am Med Inform Assoc. 2011;19(2):196-201.

47. Whitley EA, Kanellopoulou N, Kaye J. Consent and research governance in biobanks: evidence from focus groups with medical researchers. Public Health Genomics. 2012;15:232–42.

48. Steinsbekk KS, Myskja BK are, Solberg B. Broad consent versus dynamic consent in biobank research: is passive participation an ethical problem? Eur J Hum Genet 2013;21:897–902.

49. Goetz T. 23andMe will decode your DNA for $1,000: welcome to the age of genomics. Wired Mag. 2007. http://davehakes.com/weblog/wp-content/uploads/2007/11/11-17-07_wired_welcome_to_the_age_of_genomics.pdf. Accessed 26 Feb 2017.

50. McGuire AL, Beskow LM. Informed consent in genomics and genetic research. Annu Rev Genomics Hum Genet. 2010;11:361–81.

51. Grady, C. Enduring and emerging challenges of informed consent. New Engl J Med. 2015;372(9):855-62.

52. Dankar FK, Badji R. A risk-based framework for biomedical data sharing. J Biomed Inform. 2017;66:231–40.

53. Adams A. The implications of users' multimedia privacy perceptions on communication and information privacy policies. In: Proceedings of Telecommunications Policy Research Conference. 1999. http://www.researchgate.net/profile/Anne_Adams4/publication/228641284_The_Implications_of_Users'_Multimedia_Privacy_Perceptions_on_Communication_and_Information_Privacy_Policies/links/0046352a751ad9c417000000.pdf. Accessed 14 Jun 2015.

54. Lederer S, Dey AK, Mankoff J. A conceptual model and a metaphor of everyday privacy in ubiquitous. Berkeley: University of California at Berkeley; 2002.

55. Lessig L. Architecture of privacy. The Vand J Ent Pr. 1999;1:56.

56. Barker K, Askari M, Banerjee M, Ghazinour K, Mackas B, Majedi M, et al. A data privacy taxonomy. In: Dataspace: the final frontier. Springer; 2009. p. 42–54. http://link.springer.com/chapter/10.1007/978-3-642-02843-4_7. Accessed 7 Jul 2015.

57. Banerjee M, Adl RK, Wu L, Barker K. Quantifying privacy violations. In: Secure data management. Springer; 2011. p. 1–17. http://link.springer.com/chapter/10.1007/978-3-642-23556-6_1. Accessed 7 Jul 2015.

58. El Emam K, Dankar FK, Vaillancourt R, Roffey T, Lysyk M. Evaluating the risk of re-identification of patients from hospital prescription records. Can J Hosp Pharm. 2009;62:307.

59. El Emam K. Risk-based de-identification of health data. IEEE Secur Priv. 2010; 8:64–7.

60. El Emam K, Jonker E, Fineberg A. The case for de-identifying personal health information. Soc Sci Res Netw. 2011. http://papers.ssrn.com/sol3/papers.cfm?abstract_id=1744038. Accessed 18 Sep 2012.

61. Dankar FK, El Emam K, Neisa A, Roffey T. Estimating the re-identification risk of clinical data sets. BMC Med Inform Decis Mak. 2012;12:66.

62. El Emam K, Dankar FK, Neisa A, Jonker E. Evaluating the risk of patient re-identification from adverse drug event reports. BMC Med Inform Decis Mak. 2013;13:114.

63. Dankar FK, Al-Ali R. A theoretical multi-level privacy protection framework for biomedical data warehouses. Procedia Comput Sci. 2015;63:569–74.

64. Cogo VV, Bessani A, Couto FM, Verissimo P. A high-throughput method to detect privacy-sensitive human genomic data. In: Proceedings of the 14th ACM Workshop on Privacy in the Electronic Society. New York: ACM; 2015. p. 101–10. https://doi.org/10.1145/2808138.2808139.

65. Dyke SO, Dove ES, Knoppers BM. Sharing health-related data: a privacy test? Npj Genomic Med 2016;1:16024.

66. Dankar F, Brien R, Adams C, Matwin S. Secure multi-party linear regression. In: EDBT/ICDT workshops. 2014. p. 406–414. http://ceur-ws.org/Vol-1133/paper-68.pdf. Accessed 14 Jan 2015.

67. Dankar F. Privacy preserving linear regression on distributed databases. Trans Data Priv. 2015;8:3–28.

68. Ugwuoke C, Erkin Z, Lagendijk I. A Privacy-Preserving GWAS Computation with Homomorphic Encryption. 37th WIC Symposium on Information Theory in the Benelux/6th WIC/IEEE SP Symposium on Information Theory and Signal Processing in the Benelux, Louvain, Belgium. 2016. p. 166-73. https://pure.tudelft.nl/portal/files/11312239/11312198.pdf.

69. Kamm L, Bogdanov D, Laur S, Vilo J. A new way to protect privacy in large-scale genome-wide association studies. Bioinformatics. 2013;29:886–93.

70. Wagner J, Paulson JN, Wang X, Bhattacharjee B, Corrada Bravo H. Privacy-preserving microbiome analysis using secure computation. Bioinformatics. 2016;32(12):1873-9.

71. Lindell Y, Pinkas B. Secure multiparty computation for privacy-preserving data mining. J Priv Confidentiality. 2009;1:5.

72. de CM, Dowsley R, Nascimento ACA, Newman SC. Fast, privacy preserving linear regression over distributed datasets based on pre-distributed data. In: Proceedings of the 8th ACM Workshop on Artificial Intelligence and Security. New York: ACM; 2015. p. 3–14. https://doi.org/10.1145/2808769.2808774.

73. Dankar FK, Boughorbel S, Badji R. Using robust estimation theory to design efficient secure multiparty linear regression. In: Proceedings of the 2016 Joint EDBT/ICDT Workshops. 2016. http://ceur-ws.org/Vol-1558/paper33.pdf. Accessed 9 Sept 2016.

74. Rebbeck TR, Friebel T, Lynch HT, Neuhausen SL, van't Veer L, Garber JE, et al. Bilateral prophylactic mastectomy reduces breast cancer risk in BRCA1 and BRCA2 mutation carriers: the PROSE study group. J Clin Oncol. 2004;22: 1055–62.

75. Domchek SM, Friebel TM, Singer CF, Evans DG, Lynch HT, Isaacs C, et al. Association of risk-reducing surgery in BRCA1 or BRCA2 mutation carriers with cancer risk and mortality. JAMA. 2010;304:967–75.

13

A pipeline combining multiple strategies for prioritizing heterozygous variants for the identification of candidate genes in exome datasets

Teresa Requena[1*], Alvaro Gallego-Martinez[1] and Jose A. Lopez-Escamez[1,2]

Abstract

Background: The identification of disease-causing variants in autosomal dominant diseases using exome-sequencing data remains a difficult task in small pedigrees. We combined several strategies to improve filtering and prioritizing of heterozygous variants using exome-sequencing datasets in familial Meniere disease: an in-house Pathogenic Variant (PAVAR) score, the Variant Annotation Analysis and Search Tool (VAAST-Phevor), Exomiser-v2, CADD, and FATHMM. We also validated the method by a benchmarking procedure including causal mutations in synthetic exome datasets.

Results: PAVAR and VAAST were able to select the same sets of candidate variants independently of the studied disease. In contrast, Exomiser V2 and VAAST-Phevor had a variable correlation depending on the phenotypic information available for the disease on each family. Nevertheless, all the selected diseases ranked a limited number of concordant variants in the top 10 ranking, using the three systems or other combined algorithm such as CADD or FATHMM. Benchmarking analyses confirmed that the combination of systems with different approaches improves the prediction of candidate variants compared with the use of a single method. The overall efficiency of combined tools ranges between 68 and 71% in the top 10 ranked variants.

Conclusions: Our pipeline prioritizes a short list of heterozygous variants in exome datasets based on the top 10 concordant variants combining multiple systems.

Keywords: Exome sequencing, Variants filtering, Phenotype, Autosomal dominant diseases, Human phenotype ontology, Hearing loss, Meniere disease

Background

Whole-exome sequencing (WES) has become the preferred tool to discover new variants for the diagnosis of genetic diseases, since the protein-coding regions and their boundaries represent only 1.5–2% of the human genome and they accumulate most of the disease-causing mutations: missense and protein-truncating variants (frameshift, splice-acceptor, splice-donor, and nonsense variants) [1, 2]. On average, 45,000 single-nucleotide variants (SNVs) are obtained by WES, 39% are located in coding regions, while 4% are in untranslated regions (UTR), and 56% are in intronic regions near to UTR. In addition, ~90% of SNVs obtained by WES are described in dbSNP138 based in reference genome (GRCh37 hg19) [3]. However, novel and rare variants (minor allelic frequency (MAF) ≤0.01) identified by WES cannot be interpreted as pathogenic only with this information, and causality must be validated by replication in different individuals with the same phenotype and by functional studies in an appropriate cellular or animal model for each disease. Nevertheless, WES has already shown the efficiency to identify potential disease-causing variants in monogenic diseases [4, 5]. Particularly, WES has been successfully used in rare Mendelian disorders, since most of the disease-causing variants are located in protein-coding regions [5]. Recently, WES studies have been also extended for diagnosis

* Correspondence: mariateresa.requena@genyo.es
[1]Otology & Neurotology Group CTS495, Department of Genomic Medicine, GENYO - Centre for Genomics and Oncological Research – Pfizer/University of Granada/Junta de Andalucía, PTS, 18016 Granada, Spain
Full list of author information is available at the end of the article

in oligogenic and complex genetic disorders [6–10] and for predicting disease progression [11, 12]. However, when the disease is poorly characterized at the molecular level, the filtering and prioritizing of WES datasets requires a more elaborated search strategy based not only in single variant effects on protein structure or evolutionary conservation but also upon the phenotype description and mathematical interaction models.

The high efficiency of WES data in Mendelian disorders is explained because most of the causal variants in recessive disorders are rare homozygous variants or compound heterozygous variants observed in familiar cases, which are not found in healthy relatives or individuals in the same population [13]. However, the situation is more complex with autosomal dominant (AD) disorders, where a single heterozygous de novo variant can affect the gene function and hundreds of candidate variants need to be filtered. So, an improved workflow to identify potential candidate variants involved in the disease is needed. Software package as MendelScan try to solve this providing a composite score improved with tissue expression data [14]. However, systemic disease or disease involving tissues with multiple cells types and low-quality gene expression data as the cochlea are not easy to analyze with this approach.

Hearing and vestibular disorders are the most common sensory deficits in humans. Hearing loss affect around 5.3% of the world population according to the World Health Organization. Non-syndromic autosomal dominant sensorineural hearing loss (AD-SNHL) remains a challenge for genetic diagnosis, and 33 genes and 60 loci have been involved according to Hereditary Hearing loss Homepage [15], with a considerable overlap in the phenotype and pleiotropy [16].

Meniere's disease (MD) is clinically defined by episodes of vertigo, tinnitus, and SNHL (MD, [MIM 156000]) [17], and it has a prevalence about 0.5–1/1000 individuals. Most of the patients are considered sporadic, although around 8–10% are familial cases in European descendent population [18–20]. Previous linkage studies in familial MD (FMD) have found candidate loci at 12p12.3 in a large Swedish family [21] and 5q14-15 in another German family [22], but the involved genes were not identified. Recently, WES analyses have identified *DTNA*, *FAM136A*, and *PRKCB* as potential causal genes in FMD [9, 10]. MD is a clinical syndrome, and its phenotype may overlap with different conditions including vestibular migraine or autoimmune inner ear disease [16]. In contrast, other AD diseases with a more precise phenotype, such as Centro Nuclear Myopathy (CNM), an inherited neuromuscular disorder characterized by congenital myopathy with a histopathological diagnosis (centrally placed nuclei on muscle biopsy), have a reduced number of causal variants.

The aim of this study is to develop a workflow to improve the filtering and prioritizing of candidate variants and genes in AD disorders by using WES data. We focus mainly in AD familial MD, a complex clinical scenario with clinical and genetic heterogeneity, few cases per family, incomplete penetrance, and variable expressivity [23, 24]. The pipeline proposed is based on (1) the combination of several tools to score variants according to its effect on protein structure and phylogenetic conservation, (2) the ranking according to available information on phenotype databases, (3) the comparison with two integrated systems (CADD and FATHMM), and (4) the use of un-affected relatives as control to filter candidate variants. The pipeline is summarized in Fig. 1.

Results

Six prioritizing systems were selected and combined in the pipeline to filter and rank rare variants in exome sequencing data. Two of them were based upon protein structure and sequence conservation across species: (a) an in-house Pathogenic Variant (PAVAR) score and (b) the Variant Annotation Analysis and Search Tool (VAAST) [25], and the other two prioritize according to the Phenotype Ontology information: (c) Exomiser v2 [26] and (d) VAAST-Phevor [27]. And finally two integrated tools were compared and added to the system CADD [28] and FATHMM [29].

Comparison of prioritizing strategies with FMD exome datasets

Table 1 shows the number of variants obtained for each FMD dataset with the six systems after filtering by several control datasets. We included the number of ranked variants with enough score to be prioritized, according to each of the six systems (thresholds are described in the "Material and methods" section). Mean values obtained for each family dataset were highly variable for each system, and they were dependent on the number of cases and controls available for each family.

We selected the top 10, 20, and 50 ranked variants from each prioritizing system and filtered them using the different control datasets (F, T-F, and T) to analyze the concordance between methods. Figure 2 shows the concordance between all systems. Although PAVAR score and VAAST use a different methodology, both systems show the highest concordance rate to filter and prioritize the candidate variants. Between 20 and 55% of ranked variants were matched in top 10, top 20, and top 50. However, the observed variability in the ranked variants between the different systems is caused by the control datasets (F, T-F, or T) used to filter the variants. In contrast, Exomiser v2 and VAAST-Phevor prioritized according to the Phenotype Ontology information (HPO term) [30], but the maximum correlation between

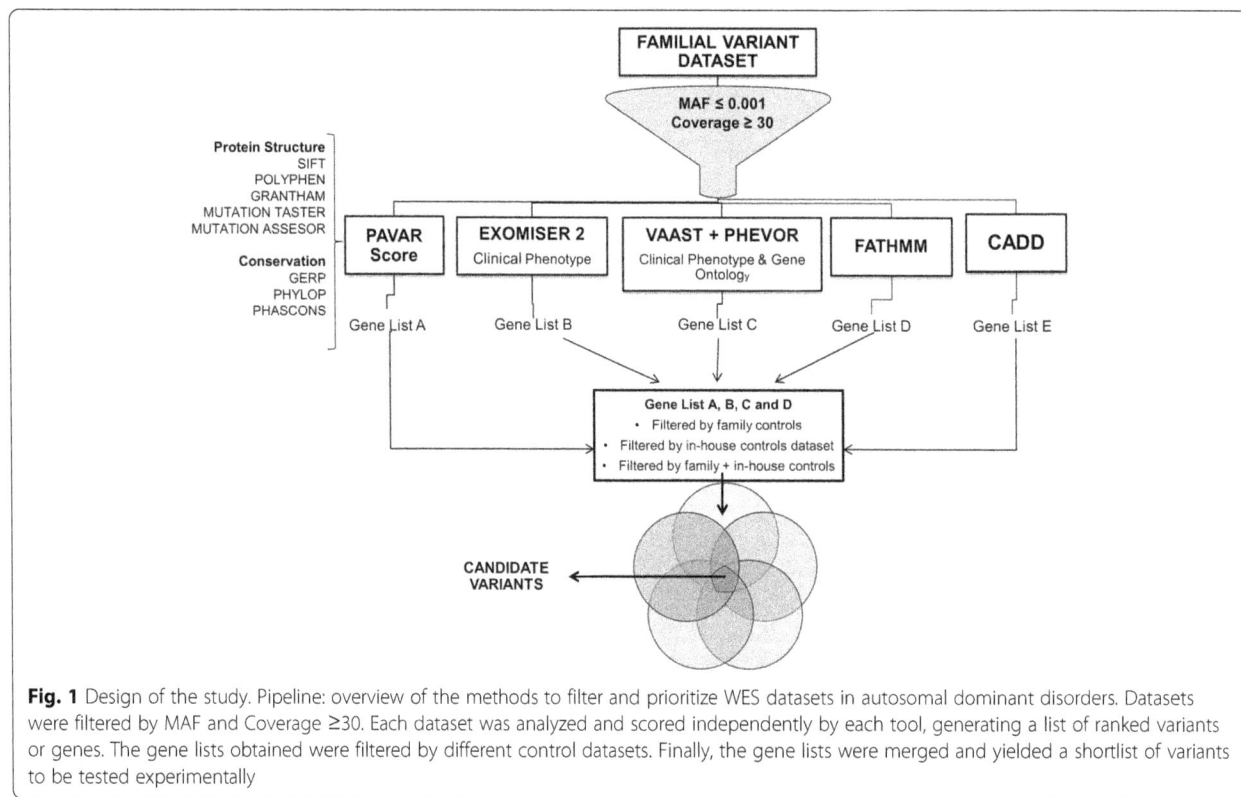

Fig. 1 Design of the study. Pipeline: overview of the methods to filter and prioritize WES datasets in autosomal dominant disorders. Datasets were filtered by MAF and Coverage ≥30. Each dataset was analyzed and scored independently by each tool, generating a list of ranked variants or genes. The gene lists obtained were filtered by different control datasets. Finally, the gene lists were merged and yielded a shortlist of variants to be tested experimentally

Table 1 Number of remaining variants per family dataset according to the filtering strategy

Family dataset	FMD exomes (N)	Control dataset (N)	PAVAR score ≥5 (N)	Exomiser score ≥1.46 × 10⁻⁵ (N)	VAAST (p value ≤1)	VAAST-Phevor (p value ≤1)	CADD score ≥15 (N)	FATHMM score ≤−1.5 (N)
1	3	F (1)	17 (134)	308 (1437)	40	39	15 (38)	7 (35)
		T-F (29)	15 (106)	78 (296)	48	44	18 (36)	7 (34)
		T (30)	10 (68)	42 (175)	27	27	12 (25)	5 (23)
2	2	F (3)	4 (58)	60 (270)	53	22	9 (18)	1 (14)
		T-F (27)	9 (73)	89 (369)	146	135	12 (28)	1 (25)
		T (30)	2 (34)	9 (39)	19	16	5 (13)	0 (11)
3	3	F (2)	9 (68)	151 (862)	23	23	9 (20)	1 (14)
		T-F (28)	13 (92)	67 (309)	38	38	17 (25)	5 (20)
		T (30)	6 (32)	24 (104)	16	16	7 (10)	1 (7)
4	3	F (0)	31 (283)	394 (2198)	54	46	34 (90)	4 (86)
		T (30)	4 (34)	20 (72)	19	17	5 (14)	1 (14)
5	3	F (3)	16 (83)	93 (391)	68	22	7 (20)	1 (15)
		T-F (27)	14 (113)	89 (430)	52	45	14 (35)	7 (28)
		T (30)	5 (36)	18 (67)	11	9	4 (9)	1 (6)
Mean (1–5)	21	F	15.4 ± 10.21 (125)	251.5 ± 143.83 (1032)	47 ± 16.95	30.4 ± 11.33	14.8 ± 9.96	2.8 ± 2.4
		T-F	12.75 ± 2.63 (96)	85 ± 28.66 (351)	71 ± 50.35	65.5 ± 46.44	13.5 ± 4.38	5.0 ± 2.44
		T	5.2 ± 2.97 (51)	31 ± 13.94 (155)	28.2 ± 5.81	5.81 ± 6.44	6.60 ± 2.87	1.6 ± 1.74

All variants with a MAF >0.001 were discarded. Setting for each software threshold is described in the "Material and methods" section

p values for VAAST and Phevor were not corrected since they were used as thresholds according to the user's guide

F family controls exome dataset, T-F in-house controls exome dataset without family control dataset, T in-house and family control datasets

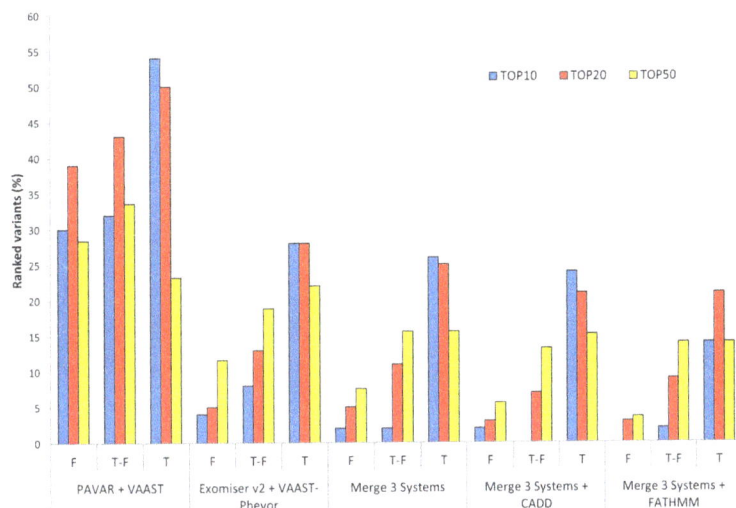

Fig. 2 Prioritized variants in FMD datasets. Percentage of the variants ranked and shared in top 10 (*blue*), 20 (*red*), and 50 (*yellow*) ranked variants by (a) PAVAR score and VAAST; (b) Exomiser v2 score and Phevor; (c) the combination of the three systems (PAVAR, Exomiser v2, VAAST, VAAST-Phevor); (d) the combination of the three systems (PAVAR, Exomiser v2, VAAST, VAAST-Phevor) and CADD; and (e) the combination of the three systems (PAVAR, Exomiser v2, VAAST, VAAST-Phevor) and FATHMM. F = family controls exome dataset, T-F = in-house controls exome dataset without family control datasets, and T = in-house and family control datasets

systems was 28% when the largest control dataset (T) was used to filter. Therefore, only the variants located in genes previously associated with the phenotype were matched by different systems. Consequently, the combinations of PAVAR, VAAST-Phevor, and Exomiser v2 only matched in few variants (2–26%), which were top ranked and highly related with MD HPO terms. A similar concordance was obtained between the combination of that three and other combined systems as CADD or FATHMM.

The maximum correlation between CADD and the merge of three systems was 24% in top 10, whereas for FATHMM was 21% in top 20. In both cases, this correlation was obtained after using the largest controls' dataset (T) to filter the variants.

Benchmark in exome datasets containing variants described in AD-SNHL and CNM genes

We compared the ability of these variant prioritizing tools to identify AD variants in small familial exome data files by a benchmarking procedure. Since the structure of the families as well as the number of cases and controls available for each pedigree could generate a bias in the benchmarking analyses, multiple families were tested.

Figure 3 shows the percentage of ranked variants in top 10, 20, and 50 by the six systems for both, hearing loss variants (Fig. 3a) and CNM variants (Fig. 3b). In top 10 and 20, the observed percentages were highly variable between each system, particularly depending on the control dataset used.

Next, we selected the top 10, 20, and 50 ranked variants from each prioritizing system and filtered them for

the different datasets (F, T-F, and T) to analyze the concordance between the different methods. Figure 4 illustrates a progressive increase of concordance between systems in the top 10, 20, and 50 ranked variants for both disorders. Exomiser v2 and VAAST-Phevor yielded higher correlations in the top 10 and 20, highlighting that both tools identify similar genes associated with the HPO term for a given phenotype. This pattern was more prominent in top 10 ranked variants for AD-SNHL datasets in the benchmarking, reaching a 50% of concordance (Fig. 4a), whereas in CNM datasets, only 34% of concordance was found (Fig. 4b). In contrast, low correlations were obtained between PAVAR score and VAAST (9–33%), mainly in the top 10 ranked, means that few variants are considered as candidates by both systems as real pathogenic variants. As a result, potentially pathogenic variants located in genes with HPO terms associated with the disease were shared by PAVAR, Exomiser v2, and VAAST-Phevor and tending to be ranked in the top 10.

A similar percentage was obtained when we add CADD to the combined system. However, the combination of multiple systems with CADD did not reduce the list of candidate variants in the top 10 ranking.

Next, 200 variants were randomly selected for each disease to build synthetic datasets. So, 42% for AD-SNHL and 25.5% CNM were previously described in HGDB as pathogenic (Additional file 1: Table S1 and S2). So, multiple logit regression models were performed to assess the accuracy to predict correctly candidate variants associated with each phenotype. The area under the curve

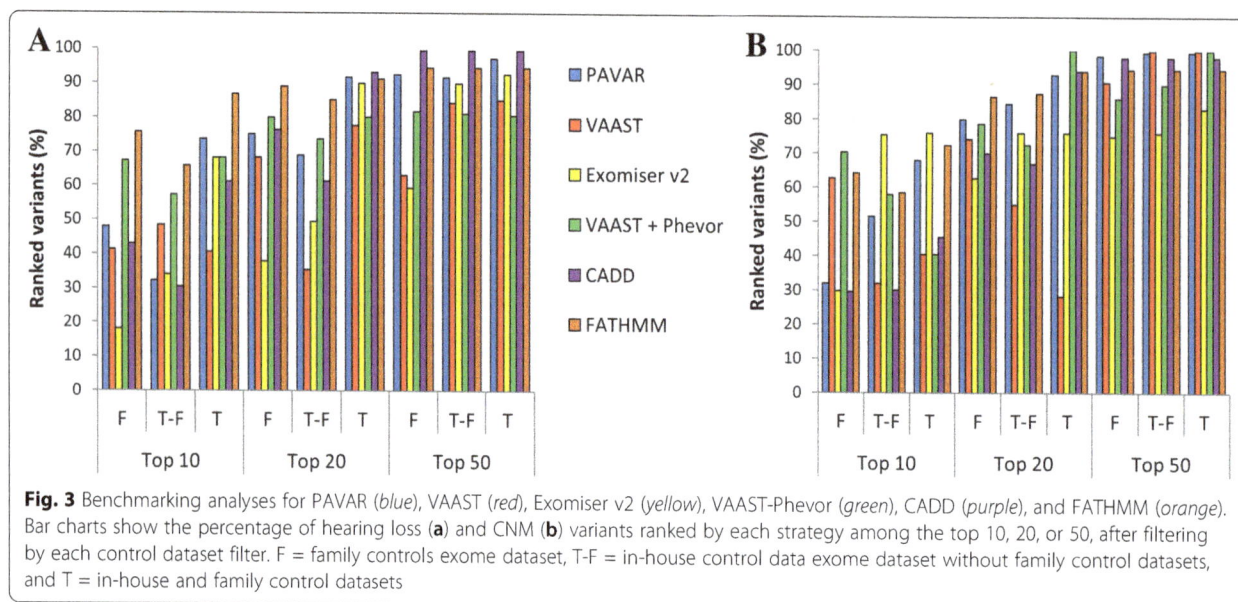

Fig. 3 Benchmarking analyses for PAVAR (*blue*), VAAST (*red*), Exomiser v2 (*yellow*), VAAST-Phevor (*green*), CADD (*purple*), and FATHMM (*orange*). Bar charts show the percentage of hearing loss (**a**) and CNM (**b**) variants ranked by each strategy among the top 10, 20, or 50, after filtering by each control dataset filter. F = family controls exome dataset, T-F = in-house control data exome dataset without family control datasets, and T = in-house and family control datasets

(AUC) for each system was calculated to assess the precision and accuracy to identify candidate variants for both diseases in several families (Additional file 1: Table S3). On average, the combination of PAVAR, Exomiser v2, VAAST-Phevor, CADD, and FATHMM predicts potentially pathogenic variants associated with the phenotype between 68 and 71% of times in top 10, for both diseases (Fig. 5a, b). These results were statistically significantly better than any single method (*p* values shown in Additional file 1: Table S3).

Discussion

The combination of linkage analysis and WES in large multicase pedigrees has shown a high effectiveness to

identify disease-causing variants in rare Mendelian disorders [4, 5]. However, small pedigrees with a few available cases are the most common clinical scenario and a challenge for the genetic diagnosis of dominant disorders, mainly those with overlapping phenotypes or incomplete penetrance such as AD-SNHL [31, 32], CNM [33], and MD [20]. Despite the increasing number of bioinformatics tools to analyze WES data [34, 35], the list of genes that must be experimentally validated for these diseases is too large.

The first issue to resolve for variant identification is the alignment of reads and variant calling algorithms. Current approaches have developed pipelines that combine tools to obtain consistent identification of variant

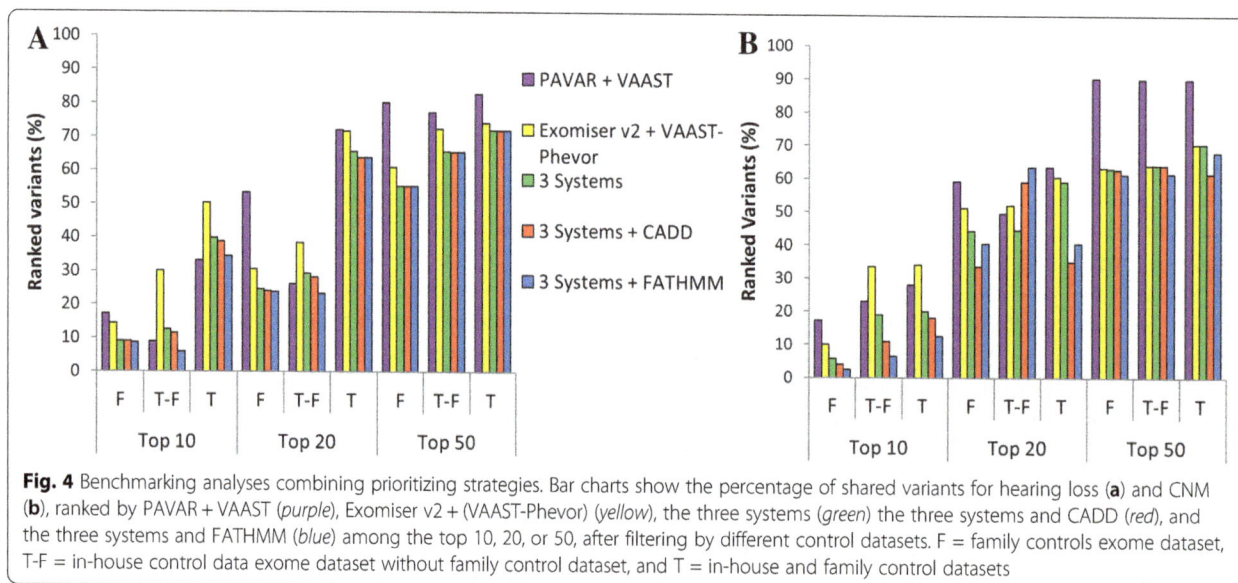

Fig. 4 Benchmarking analyses combining prioritizing strategies. Bar charts show the percentage of shared variants for hearing loss (**a**) and CNM (**b**), ranked by PAVAR + VAAST (*purple*), Exomiser v2 + (VAAST-Phevor) (*yellow*), the three systems (*green*) the three systems and CADD (*red*), and the three systems and FATHMM (*blue*) among the top 10, 20, or 50, after filtering by different control datasets. F = family controls exome dataset, T-F = in-house control data exome dataset without family control dataset, and T = in-house and family control datasets

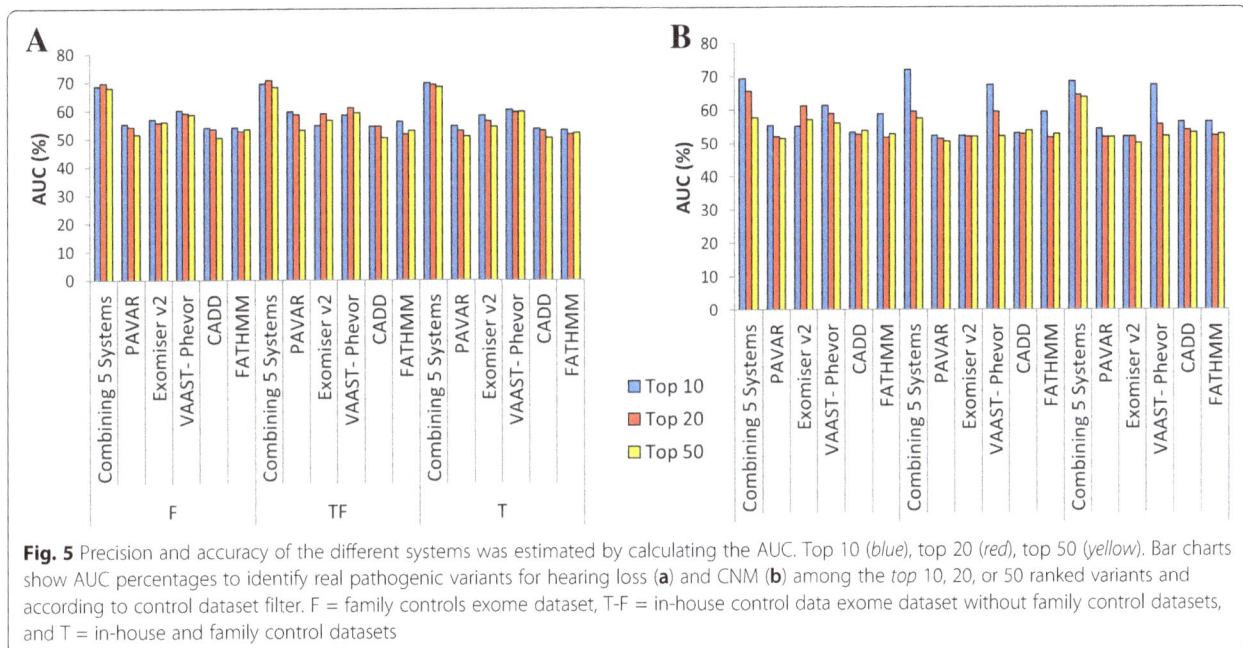

Fig. 5 Precision and accuracy of the different systems was estimated by calculating the AUC. Top 10 (*blue*), top 20 (*red*), top 50 (*yellow*). Bar charts show AUC percentages to identify real pathogenic variants for hearing loss (**a**) and CNM (**b**) among the *top* 10, 20, or 50 ranked variants and according to control dataset filter. F = family controls exome dataset, T-F = in-house control data exome dataset without family control datasets, and T = in-house and family control datasets

and facilitate the process [36, 37]. However, these pipelines do not provide functional annotation. Other pipelines go further, and they implement user-friendly graphic interface and include Annovar-based functional annotation [38]. However, our results show that the combination of multiple bioinformatics tools is a reliable strategy to reduce the list of candidate variants and to facilitate the identification of the disease-causing variants in small pedigrees. These results are consistent with previous studies designed to improve the yield of several prioritizing tools [39, 40].

The list of candidate variants generated by each system is usually too large to be validated experimentally (Table 1). So, the most common strategy is to filter by familiar controls to eliminate private familial variants and by controls' dataset from the same population to eliminate population-specific variants. However, the clinical evidence of incomplete penetrance or late age of onset of the disease should exclude the use of familial control datasets. Our results show that by combining five tools (PAVAR, Exomiser v2, VAAST-Phevor, CADD, FATHMM), the list of candidate variants is reduced and this facilitates the identification of potential disease-causing variants (Fig. 5).

Discrepancies between all the prioritization systems evaluated (PAVAR, VAAST, Exomiser v2, VAAST-Phevor, CADD, FATHMM) were found in the ranked results for all the diseases tested (Table 1 and Fig. 3). Consequently, systems based on the same criteria, protein structure, and sequence conservation or Phenotype Ontology information, were clustered to analyze the concordance between them in the top 10, 20, and 50

ranked variants. Although PAVAR and VAAST use a different methodology, both prioritize variants according to the intrinsic effect on the protein of the variants. Of note, MD, AD-SNHL, and CNM showed similar correlation scores between PAVAR and VAAST for top 10 and 20 ranked variants. Both systems were more concordant when in-house control datasets or the merge of in-house and family control datasets were used to filter. Although familial controls are important to filter private variants, a large control dataset of the same population is more effective to reduce the list of candidate variants list.

In contrast, the concordance between VAAST-Phevor and Exomiser v2 varies depending on the disease studied. Although both systems are based on phenotype, VAAST-Phevor has a balanced score between potential pathogenicity and the association with the phenotype whereas Exomiser v2 assigns more weight to the phenotype than the potential pathogenicity. Diseases with a well-characterized phenotype by several HPO terms or diseases with known involved genes show a high correlation between VAAST-Phevor and Exomiser v2, as our results confirm for AD-SNHL and CNM. However, since MD only has few HPO terms and no gene associated in public databases, our data show a reduced concordance. In particular, our results show that the correlation between both systems in well diseases with many HPO terms is twice than in disorders with limited phenotypic information such as diseases of the ear for all top 10, 20, and 50 ranked variants. Nevertheless, a high concordance between both systems does not indicate that those variants selected are really disease-causing variants. The degree of concordance between both systems only demonstrates that the candidate genes are associated with the phenotype, but not necessarily its pathogenicity.

Initially, our pipeline joins both approaches by the identification of variants ranked as potentially pathogenic by the PAVAR score and associated them with the phenotype by both Exomiser v2 and VAAST-Phevor. The combination of the three strategies gives few variants ranked in the top 10 or 20 and produces a short list of candidate variants to be validated experimentally [9, 10, 41]. In addition, other combined systems were added and the list was reduced. Logit regression models and benchmarking analyses show that the combination of PAVAR, Exomiser v2, VAAST-Phevor CADD, and FATHMM not only reduced the list of candidate variants to be validated; this combined approach is more efficient to predict potential diseases-causing variants than each system separately. This enhanced efficiency is observed independently of the type of control datasets used. Our results confirm previous studies showing that prioritizing tools have less ability to rank variants in disorders with no previously known candidate gene [42]. In addition, we demonstrate that the addition of more HPO terms improves the ranking of candidate genes. So, our pipeline allows to obtain a reduced list of variants when incomplete penetrance is found and familial control datasets cannot be used.

This combined strategy has a major limitation: a reduced phenotypic characterization of AD disorders (such as AD-SNHL or MD) will decrease the precision of the pipeline. So, a deep phenotyping and updating of HPO terms in major databases will improve the yield of the system. Although HPO project has been updated in 2017, ear diseases and, particularly, vestibular disorders still have a limited phenotype vocabulary and disease-phenotype annotations [43]. In addition, further improvements in the pipeline should be needed to include structural variants such as frameshift (insertions and deletions), synonymous variants, and copy number variants.

Conclusion

These results demonstrate that our pipeline combining multiple variant-prioritization algorithms is useful in small family-based analyses. We also showed that the model can reduce the number of variants in synthetic exome datasets with incomplete phenotypes without using familial controls. This approach will be useful when controls are not available or when incomplete penetrance is observed.

Material and methods

Patients

Four Spanish AD families with at least two patients with definite MD and a fifth family with monozygotic twins with MD, according to the diagnostic criteria of the Barany Society for familial MD [17], were selected for this study. The clinical phenotype and the pattern of inheritance in these families and their pedigrees were previously reported [10, 20, 41]. The number of asymptomatic relatives selected for WES in each family depended upon two criteria: (a) size and structure of the family, since some families showed patients with incomplete phenotype (i.e., SNHL without episodic vertigo), and (b) the availability to obtain samples from older asymptomatic relatives, which could be used as controls. All the procedures described were performed in accordance with the highest ethical standards on human experimentation, the Helsinki Declaration of 1975 and the EU regulations on biomedical research. In addition, this study was approved by the Review Board for Clinical Research of Instituto Biosanitario de Granada, and a written informed consent to donor biological samples was obtained from all subjects.

Whole exome sequencing (WES)

DNA was isolated from peripheral blood samples as previously described [9, 10] Exons and flanking intron regions were captured according to the methods previously described [9, 10]. Library products were sequenced with SOLiD 5500xl platform with Exact Call Chemistry and 200× of sequencing depth. A mean of 50–60 million of reads were obtained per sample. The quality of the reads was analyzed with SAMtools [44], MAQtools [45], and FastQC software (Babraham Bioinformatics), and shorter reads (<25) as well as all duplicate reads were deleted. The reads were aligned with the reference genome (GRCh37 hg19) with Bioscope™ (Applied Biosystems, Foster City, CA, USA) using the default settings. Results from Bioscope™ were filtered by depth >30 reads [46] and quality of the assigned genotype ≥100. This analysis identified SNVs, copy number variants, and frameshift variants (insertion and deletions). However, we only considered SNVs for this study.

Bioinformatics analysis

For each family, heterozygous SNVs found in all the affected cases with complete phenotype of the family were selected. The 1000 genome project [47], ExaAC database [48], and Exome Variant Server (EVS) were used to annotate the MAF and function for each variant (Additional file 1: Table S4). All SNVs were filtered by MAF. For MD and AD-SNHL, variants with MAF ≥0.001 were discarded, since MD has a prevalence of 10–225 cases/100,000 individuals [49, 50] and the low prevalence described for AD-SNHL [51]. For CNM, variants with MAF ≥0.0001 were also discarded, since CNM is considered as a rare disease with a very low prevalence (1/25,000 males).

The pipeline was designed using different strategies to filter and prioritize SNVs: (a) the calculation of a pathogenic variant (PAVAR) risk composite score; (b) Exomiser v2 software [26]; (c) VAAST annotation tool [25]; and (d) a combination of VAAST and Phevor tools [27]. However, Phevor returns the same results than VAAST, but ranked by phenotype. In addition, other composite algorithms were used CADD [28] and FATHMM [29]. So, the shared candidate variants were selected. All variants were considered as potentially pathogenic according to the ACMG Standards and Guidelines [52], and all digital resources used are listed in Additional file 1: Table S5.

In some AD diseases, incomplete penetrance was found; subsequently, familial controls could not be used to filter variants. Different control datasets collected for previous projects were used to evaluate the efficiency of our pipeline despite of the observed incomplete penetrance. F = family controls exome dataset, T-F = in-house control data exome dataset without familial control datasets, and T = in-house and family control datasets.

a) Pathogenic variant risk composite score (PAVAR score)

Functional annotation was used to prioritize SNVs, according to the effect on protein structure and phylogenetic conservation. Sequence conservation across species is a major criterium to assess the variant, and the number of compared species varies according to the tool. To estimate the risk of a SNV to become a pathogenic variant, we used a seven-point scoring system based upon open-access prediction bioinformatics tools. ANNOVAR and SeattleSeq Annotation tools were used to achieve the score of SIFT (Sort Intolerant from Tolerant) [53], PolyPhen2 (Polymorphism Phenotyping v2) [54], Grantham's Matrix [55], GERP++ (Genomic Evolutionary Rate Profiling) [56], Mutation taster [57], PhastCons, and PhyloP [58]. The threshold to consider each variant as pathogenic is described in Additional file 1: Table S6, according to the default settings suggested for each software developer. PAVAR score is calculated as the sum of the score obtained by seven systems. Each system adds one point if the variant is considered as potentially damaging and zero if it is benign. So, the higher the score is, the high the risk of pathogenicity for a given variant. PAVAR score cannot be calculated for nonsense variants, since protein structure tools cannot assign any value. Since nonsense variants can modify dramatically the sequence of the protein, they were considered directly as the maximum PAVAR score = 7. All the variants with a score ≥5 were not filtered, and they were considered as candidate variants.

b) Exomiser v2 software

Exomiser v2 prioritizes SNVs by comparing the phenotype across species, according to the inheritance pattern, using the mouse and fish as a model organism phenotype [26]. Variant Call Format (VCF) files were analyzed with the following parameters: (a) HPO terms, Vertigo (HP:0002321), Tinnitus (HP:0000360), and Hearing Impairment (HP:0000365), were selected for Clinical Phenotype and (b) AD inheritance model. Since there are only three HPO terms associated with MD according to the public Human Phenotype Ontology database, but no gene is still included on it, the "Exomiser Gene Combined Score" generated very low values. So, variants with a threshold ≥1.46×10^{-5} were considered as candidate variants. Exomiser v2 allows the use of several HPO terms, but Phevor only allows five HPO terms. To compare both systems, only five HPO terms were selected for the benchmarking analyses. The five HPO terms most commonly associated with each disease were selected (Additional file 1: Table S7 and S8).

c) VAAST annotation tool

The third approach was to annotate and filter SNVs, according to the dominant inheritance pattern by VAAST software [25]. All case and control VCF files were processed according to the manual provided in the official website. Case files from the same pedigree were combined by the VAAST selection tool (VST) into a single condenser file; SNVs found in all the affected cases were selected. The quality of the resulting files was measured using the background provided: 1KGv3_CG_Div_NHLBI_dbSNP_RefSeq. cdr. A p value >0.05 indicates that there is no significant difference between the files (Additional file 1: Table S9). The next step was to search for candidate genes and their potential disease-causing variants. Each family dataset was filtered with the following parameters: (a) dominant inheritance, (b) incomplete penetrance, (c) maximum combined population frequency for the disease-causing alleles >0.0005 [51], and (d) 1×10^6 permutations per analysis to achieve a significant p value after Bonferroni correction. Variants with an alpha error ≤1 were considered as possibly pathogenic.

d) Phevor tool

In the fourth approach, the list of the resulting genes generated by VAAST tool was uploaded to the Phevor Webtool (phenotype driven variant ontological re-ranking tool) to prioritize candidate genes, according to phenotype and HPO terms [30]. To run the analyses for MD, AD-SNHL, and CNM, the phenotypes were generated in Phevor using HPO term described in Additional file 1: Tables S7 and S8. Exomiser v2 only admits HPO term so to compare with Phevor; Disease Ontology Terms and Gene Ontology Terms were not used. No threshold value was applied in these analyses since the list of variants is generated from pre-filtered variants from VAAST.

e) Combined Annotation-Dependent Depletion (CADD)

CADD v1.3 [28, 59] is pre-computed score database that is based on classifier algorithms. The major goal of CADD is to predict the deleterious, functionally significant and pathogenic variants from diversified class of variants by integrative annotations. For each variant, CADD generates the combined annotation score (c-score) as an output and all scores were referenced against the pre-computed c-scores of 8.6 billion possible human SNPs. In CADD scoring criteria, functional variants should possess c-score greater than or equal to 10, whereas damaging variants show the c-score greater than or equal to 20 and the most lethal human variants show the c-score of greater than or equal to 30. To identify causal variants, a score ≥15 was considered as potentially pathogenic.

f) Functional Analysis through Hidden Markov Models (FATHMM)

FATHMM [29] predict the functional effects of protein missense mutations by combining sequence conservation within hidden Markov models (HMMs), representing the alignment of homologous sequences and conserved protein domains, with "pathogenicity weights", representing the overall tolerance of the protein/domain to mutations. The prediction outputs are scored, and the majority of disease-associated AASs fell below −3 and −1.5 threshold. To identify potential causal variants, a score ≤−1.5 was considered as potentially pathogenic.

Benchmarking procedures

The efficiency of the workflow was tested by benchmarking procedures in different synthetic family datasets with MD. In addition, a group of no familial healthy controls was tested to identify any bias caused for MD that could influence in the analysis. Moreover, two AD disorders were selected: (a) autosomal dominant sensorineural hearing loss (AD-SNHL) and (b) Central nuclear myopathy (CNM). AD-SNHL has 33 genes diseases, but the phenotype could overlap with MD. To avoid the bias of analyzing AD-SNHL and MD, we selected another disease (CNM) with no overlap in the phenotype with MD. CNM was selected because it has five different genes to perform the benchmarking analysis. The best characterized genes available for AD-SNHL included in the Hereditary Hearing Loss Homepage and CNM genes described in Orphanet were selected (Additional file 1: Table S5). For these genes, exome sequencing data of all

exonic variants, in VCF format, were obtained from the public ESP database. Next, 200 variants for each disease were randomly selected to perform benchmarking analyses, but we also checked that at least part of them were described as pathogenic or associated with the disease in human mutation database (HGMD) (Additional file 1: Table S1 and S2). To perform the analyses, the synthetic files were built inserting two random variants into real cases VCF files of each family. These synthetic family files for both diseases were analyzed with the six systems. The top 10, 20, and 50 ranked variants for AD-SNHL and CNM were analyzed by each separate system and by all combined strategies.

Statistical analysis

Logit regression model was built to assess the accuracy to predict correctly pathogenic variants associated with the phenotype. Firstly, variants selected for benchmarking analysis were classified as pathogenic or benign according to HGMD. The ranks conferred by each system were converted into ranks predictor-wise and normalized in [0, 1], according to top 10, 20, or 50. ROC curves were generated to determine the ability to predict real causal variants based on models consisting of the combination of the five systems (PAVAR, Exomiser v2, VAAST-Phevor, CADD, and FATHMM) and each individual system. In all the cases, the analyses were performed for the top 10, 20, and 50 ranked variants and using different control datasets to filter for private variants. AUCs were calculated for each ROC curves (Additional file 1: Table S3). The statistical differences between AUCs were calculated by analysis of variance. The logit regression models obtained, according to the different combinations and ROC curves, were analyzed with R version 3.0.3 and RStudio version 0.98.1102.

Abbreviations

AD: Autosomical dominant; AD-SNH: Non-syndromic autosomal dominant sensorineural hearing loss; CADD: Combined annotation-dependent depletion; CNM: Centro Nuclear Myopathy; FATHMM: Functional analysis through hidden markov models; FMD: Familial MD; HPO term: Human Phenotype Ontology term; MAF: Minor allelic frequency; MD: Meniere's disease; PAVAR: Pathogenic variant risk composite score; SNV: Single-nucleotide variants; UTR: Untranslated regions; VAAST: Variant annotation analysis and search tool; WES: Whole-exome sequencing

Acknowledgements

The authors would like to thank all patients and their relatives that participated in this study. We also thank the assistance of the Genomic and Bioinformatics staff at Genyo. Teresa Requena was a PhD student, and this work is part of her Doctoral Thesis.

Funding

This study was funded by EU-FEDER Funds for R+D+i by the Grants 2013-1242 from Instituto de Salud Carlos III and 2016-WES from The Meniere Society, UK.

Authors' contributions

This study was conceived and designed by TR and JALE. Selection of samples was performed by JALE. NGS libraries were prepared by TR. The bioinformatics pipeline and the NGS analysis were performed by TR and AGM. The manuscript was written by TR, AGM, and JALE. All aspects of the study were supervised by JALE. All authors read and approved the final manuscript.

Competing interests

The authors declare that they have no competing interests.

Author details

[1]Otology & Neurotology Group CTS495, Department of Genomic Medicine, GENYO - Centre for Genomics and Oncological Research – Pfizer/University of Granada/Junta de Andalucía, PTS, 18016 Granada, Spain. [2]Department of Otolaryngology, Complejo Hospitalario Universidad de Granada (CHUGRA), ibs.granada, 18014 Granada, Spain.

References

1. Ng SB, Turner EH, Robertson PD, Flygare SD, Bigham AW, Lee C, Shaffer T, Wong M, Bhattacharjee A, Eichler EE, et al. Targeted capture and massively parallel sequencing of 12 human exomes. Nature. 2009;461(7261):272–6.
2. Hodges E, Xuan Z, Balija V, Kramer M, Molla MN, Smith SW, Middle CM, Rodesch MJ, Albert TJ, Hannon GJ, et al. Genome-wide in situ exon capture for selective resequencing. Nat Genet. 2007;39(12):1522–7.
3. Robinson PN, Krawitz P, Mundlos S. Strategies for exome and genome sequence data analysis in disease-gene discovery projects. Clin Genet. 2011;80(2):127–32.
4. Ng SB, Buckingham KJ, Lee C, Bigham AW, Tabor HK, Dent KM, Huff CD, Shannon PT, Jabs EW, Nickerson DA, et al. Exome sequencing identifies the cause of a mendelian disorder. Nat Genet. 2010;42(1):30–5.
5. Rabbani B, Tekin M, Mahdieh N. The promise of whole-exome sequencing in medical genetics. J Hum Genet. 2014;59(1):5–15.
6. Do R, Kathiresan S, Abecasis GR. Exome sequencing and complex disease: practical aspects of rare variant association studies. Hum Mol Genet. 2012; 21(R1):R1–9.
7. Girard SL, Gauthier J, Noreau A, Xiong L, Zhou S, Jouan L, Dionne-Laporte A, Spiegelman D, Henrion E, Diallo O, et al. Increased exonic de novo mutation rate in individuals with schizophrenia. Nat Genet. 2011;43(9):860–3.
8. O'Roak BJ, Deriziotis P, Lee C, Vives L, Schwartz JJ, Girirajan S, Karakoc E, Mackenzie AP, Ng SB, Baker C, et al. Exome sequencing in sporadic autism spectrum disorders identifies severe de novo mutations. Nat Genet. 2011; 43(6):585–9.
9. Requena T, Cabrera S, Martin-Sierra C, Price SD, Lysakowski A, Lopez-Escamez JA. Identification of two novel mutations in FAM136A and DTNA genes in autosomal-dominant familial Meniere's disease. Hum Mol Genet. 2014. 15;24(4):1119–26.
10. Martin-Sierra C, Requena T, Frejo L, Price SD, Gallego-Martinez A, Batuecas-Caletrio A, Santos-Perez S, Soto-Varela A, Lysakowski A, Lopez-Escamez JA. A novel missense variant in PRKCB segregates low-frequency hearing loss in an autosomal dominant family with Meniere's disease. Hum Mol Genet. 2016;25(16):3407–15.
11. Haghighi A, Tiwari A, Piri N, Nurnberg G, Saleh-Gohari N, Haghighi A, Neidhardt J, Nurnberg P, Berger W. Homozygosity mapping and whole exome sequencing reveal a novel homozygous COL18A1 mutation causing Knobloch syndrome. PloS one. 2014;9(11):e112747.
12. Zhao S, Choi M, Heuck C, Mane S, Barlogie B, Lifton RP, Dhodapkar MV. Serial exome analysis of disease progression in premalignant gammopathies. Leukemia. 2014;28(7):1548–52.
13. Vermeer S, Hoischen A, Meijer RP, Gilissen C, Neveling K, Wieskamp N, de Brouwer A, Koenig M, Anheim M, Assoum M, et al. Targeted next-generation sequencing of a 12.5 Mb homozygous region reveals ANO10 mutations in patients with autosomal-recessive cerebellar ataxia. Am J Hum Genet. 2010; 87(6):813–9.
14. Koboldt DC, Larson DE, Sullivan LS, Bowne SJ, Steinberg KM, Churchill JD, Buhr AC, Nutter N, Pierce EA, Blanton SH, et al. Exome-based mapping and variant prioritization for inherited Mendelian disorders. Am J Hum Genet. 2014;94(3):373–84.
15. Smith RJH, Shearer AE, Hildebrand MS, et al. Deafness and Hereditary Hearing Loss Overview. 1999 Feb 14 [Updated 2014 Jan 9]. In: Pagon RA, Adam MP, Ardinger HH, et al., editors. GeneReviews® [Internet]. Seattle (WA):

University of Washington, Seattle; 1993-2017. Available from: https://www.ncbi.nlm.nih.gov/books/NBK1434/.
16. Vona B, Nanda I, Hofrichter MA, Shehata-Dieler W, Haaf T. Non-syndromic hearing loss gene identification: a brief history and glimpse into the future. Mol Cell Probes. 2015;29(5):260–70.
17. Lopez-Escamez JA, Carey J, Chung WH, Goebel JA, Magnusson M, Mandala M, Newman-Toker DE, Strupp M, Suzuki M, Trabalzini F, et al. Diagnostic criteria for Meniere's disease. J Vestib Res. 2015;25(1):1–7.
18. Vrabec JT. Genetic investigations of Meniere's disease. Otolaryngol Clin N Am. 2010;43(5):1121–32.
19. Morrison AW, Bailey ME, Morrison GA. Familial Meniere's disease: clinical and genetic aspects. J Laryngol Otol. 2009;123(1):29–37.
20. Requena T, Espinosa-Sanchez JM, Cabrera S, Trinidad G, Soto-Varela A, Santos-Perez S, Teggi R, Perez P, Batuecas-Caletrio A, Fraile J, et al. Familial clustering and genetic heterogeneity in Meniere's disease. Clin Genet. 2014;85(3):245–52.
21. Klar J, Frykholm C, Friberg U, Dahl N. A Meniere's disease gene linked to chromosome 12p12.3. Am J Med Genet B Neuropsychiatr Genet. 2006; 141B(5):463–7.
22. Arweiler-Harbeck D, Horsthemke B, Jahnke K, Hennies HC. Genetic aspects of familial Meniere's disease. Otol Neurotol. 2011;32(4):695–700.
23. Nadeau JH. Modifier genes and protective alleles in humans and mice. Curr Opin Genet Dev. 2003;13(3):290–5.
24. Nadeau JH. Modifier genes in mice and humans. Nat Rev Genet. 2001;2(3): 165–74.
25. Kennedy B, Kronenberg Z, Hu H, Moore B, Flygare S, Reese MG, Jorde LB, Yandell M, Huff C. Using VAAST to identify disease-associated variants in next-generation sequencing data. Current protocols in human genetics/editorial board, Jonathan L Haines [et al]. 2014;81:6 14 11-16 14 25.
26. Robinson PN, Kohler S, Oellrich A, Sanger Mouse Genetics P, Wang K, Mungall CJ, Lewis SE, Washington N, Bauer S, Seelow D et al. Improved exome prioritization of disease genes through cross-species phenotype comparison. Genome Res. 2014. doi:10.1101/gr.160325.113.
27. Singleton MV, Guthery SL, Voelkerding KV, Chen K, Kennedy B, Margraf RL, Durtschi J, Eilbeck K, Reese MG, Jorde LB, et al. Phevor combines multiple biomedical ontologies for accurate identification of disease-causing alleles in single individuals and small nuclear families. Am J Hum Genet. 2014;94(4): 599–610.
28. Kircher M, Witten DM, Jain P, O'Roak BJ, Cooper GM, Shendure J. A general framework for estimating the relative pathogenicity of human genetic variants. Nat Genet. 2014;46(3):310–5.
29. Shihab HA, Gough J, Cooper DN, Stenson PD, Barker GL, Edwards KJ, Day IN, Gaunt TR. Predicting the functional, molecular, and phenotypic consequences of amino acid substitutions using hidden Markov models. Hum Mutat. 2013; 34(1):57–65.
30. Kohler S, Doelken SC, Mungall CJ, Bauer S, Firth HV, Bailleul-Forestier I, Black GC, Brown DL, Brudno M, Campbell J, et al. The Human Phenotype Ontology project: linking molecular biology and disease through phenotype data. Nucleic Acids Res. 2014;42(Database issue):D966–74.
31. Schrijver I. Hereditary non-syndromic sensorineural hearing loss: transforming silence to sound. J Mol Diagn. 2004;6(4):275–84.
32. Chan DK, Schrijver I, Chang KW. Connexin-26-associated deafness: phenotypic variability and progression of hearing loss. Genet Med. 2010;12(3):174–81.
33. Bitoun M, Romero NB, Guicheney P. Mutations in dynamin 2 cause dominant centronuclear myopathy. Med Sci. 2006;22(2):101–2.
34. Bao R, Huang L, Andrade J, Tan W, Kibbe WA, Jiang H, Feng G. Review of current methods, applications, and data management for the bioinformatics analysis of whole exome sequencing. Cancer Informat. 2014;13 Suppl 2:67–82.
35. Precone V, Del Monaco V, Esposito MV, De Palma FD, Ruocco A, Salvatore F, D'Argenio V. Cracking the code of human diseases using next-generation sequencing: applications, challenges, and perspectives. Biomed Res Int. 2015;2015:161648.
36. Guo Y, Ding X, Shen Y, Lyon GJ, Wang K. SeqMule: automated pipeline for analysis of human exome/genome sequencing data. Sci Rep. 2015;5:14283.
37. Hwang S, Kim E, Lee I, Marcotte EM. Systematic comparison of variant calling pipelines using gold standard personal exome variants. Sci Rep. 2015;5:17875.
38. D'Antonio M, D'Onorio De Meo P, Paoletti D, Elmi B, Pallocca M, Sanna N, Picardi E, Pesole G, Castrignano T. WEP: a high-performance analysis pipeline for whole-exome data. BMC Bioinf. 2013;14 Suppl 7:S11.

39. Dong C, Wei P, Jian X, Gibbs R, Boerwinkle E, Wang K, Liu X. Comparison and integration of deleteriousness prediction methods for nonsynonymous SNVs in whole exome sequencing studies. Hum Mol Genet. 2015;24(8):2125–37.

40. Smedley D, Kohler S, Czeschik JC, Amberger J, Bocchini C, Hamosh A, Veldboer J, Zemojtel T, Robinson PN. Walking the interactome for candidate prioritization in exome sequencing studies of Mendelian diseases. Bioinformatics. 2014;30(22):3215–22.

41. Martin-Sierra C, Gallego-Martinez A, Requena T, Frejo L, Batuecas-Caletrio A, Lopez-Escamez JA. Variable expressivity and genetic heterogeneity involving DPT and SEMA3D genes in autosomal dominant familial Meniere's disease. Eur J hum genet. 2016;25(2):200–7.

42. Javed A, Agrawal S, Ng PC. Phen-Gen: combining phenotype and genotype to analyze rare disorders. Nat Methods. 2014;11(9):935–7.

43. Kohler S, Vasilevsky NA, Engelstad M, Foster E, McMurry J, Ayme S, Baynam G, Bello SM, Boerkoel CF, Boycott KM, et al. The Human Phenotype Ontology in 2017. Nucleic Acids Res. 2017;45(D1):D865–76.

44. Li H, Handsaker B, Wysoker A, Fennell T, Ruan J, Homer N, Marth G, Abecasis G, Durbin R. The sequence alignment/map format and SAMtools. Bioinformatics. 2009;25(16):2078–9.

45. Li H, Ruan J, Durbin R. Mapping short DNA sequencing reads and calling variants using mapping quality scores. Genome Res. 2008;18(11):1851–8.

46. Sims D, Sudbery I, Ilott NE, Heger A, Ponting CP. Sequencing depth and coverage: key considerations in genomic analyses. Nat Rev Genet. 2014; 15(2):121–32.

47. Genomes Project C, Auton A, Brooks LD, Durbin RM, Garrison EP, Kang HM, Korbel JO, Marchini JL, McCarthy S, McVean GA, et al. A global reference for human genetic variation. Nature. 2015;526(7571):68–74.

48. Lek M, Karczewski K, Minikel E, Samocha K, Banks E, Fennell T, O'Donnell-Luria A, Ware J, Hill A, Cummings B et al. Analysis of protein-coding genetic variation in 60,706 humans. bioRxiv. 2015. 18;536(7616):285–91.

49. Merchant SN, Adams JC, Nadol Jr JB. Pathophysiology of Meniere's syndrome: are symptoms caused by endolymphatic hydrops? Otol Neurotol. 2005;26(1):74–81.

50. Alexander TH, Harris JP. Current epidemiology of Meniere's syndrome. Otolaryngol Clin N Am. 2010;43(5):965–70.

51. Shearer AE, Eppsteiner RW, Booth KT, Ephraim SS, Gurrola 2nd J, Simpson A, Black-Ziegelbein EA, Joshi S, Ravi H, Giuffre AC, et al. Utilizing ethnic-specific differences in minor allele frequency to recategorize reported pathogenic deafness variants. Am J Hum Genet. 2014;95(4):445–53.

52. Richards S, Aziz N, Bale S, Bick D, Das S, Gastier-Foster J, Grody WW, Hegde M, Lyon E, Spector E, et al. Standards and guidelines for the interpretation of sequence variants: a joint consensus recommendation of the American College of Medical Genetics and Genomics and the Association for Molecular Pathology. Genet Med. 2015;17(5):405–23.

53. Choi Y, Sims GE, Murphy S, Miller JR, Chan AP. Predicting the functional effect of amino acid substitutions and indels. PloS one. 2012;7(10):e46688.

54. Adzhubei IA, Schmidt S, Peshkin L, Ramensky VE, Gerasimova A, Bork P, Kondrashov AS, Sunyaev SR. A method and server for predicting damaging missense mutations. Nat Methods. 2010;7(4):248–9.

55. Grantham R. Amino acid difference formula to help explain protein evolution. Science. 1974;185(4154):862–4.

56. Davydov EV, Goode DL, Sirota M, Cooper GM, Sidow A, Batzoglou S. Identifying a high fraction of the human genome to be under selective constraint using GERP++. PLoS Comput Biol. 2010;6(12):e1001025.

57. Schwarz JM, Rodelsperger C, Schuelke M, Seelow D. MutationTaster evaluates disease-causing potential of sequence alterations. Nat Methods. 2010;7(8):575–6.

58. Pollard KS, Hubisz MJ, Rosenbloom KR, Siepel A. Detection of nonneutral substitution rates on mammalian phylogenies. Genome Res. 2010;20(1):110–21.

59. Mather CA, Mooney SD, Salipante SJ, Scroggins S, Wu D, Pritchard CC, Shirts BH. CADD score has limited clinical validity for the identification of pathogenic variants in noncoding regions in a hereditary cancer panel. Genet Med. 2016; 18(12):1269–75.

14

Transcriptome sequencing of gingival biopsies from chronic periodontitis patients reveals novel gene expression and splicing patterns

Yong-Gun Kim[1,2†], Minjung Kim[3†], Ji Hyun Kang[4], Hyo Jeong Kim[4], Jin-Woo Park[1], Jae-Mok Lee[1], Jo-Young Suh[1], Jae-Young Kim[2,4], Jae-Hyung Lee[3,5*] and Youngkyun Lee[2,4*] (iD)

Abstract

Background: Periodontitis is the most common chronic inflammatory disease caused by complex interaction between the microbial biofilm and host immune responses. In the present study, high-throughput RNA sequencing was utilized to systemically and precisely identify gene expression profiles and alternative splicing.

Methods: The pooled RNAs of 10 gingival tissues from both healthy and periodontitis patients were analyzed by deep sequencing followed by computational annotation and quantification of mRNA structures.

Results: The differential expression analysis designated 400 up-regulated genes in periodontitis tissues especially in the pathways of defense/immunity protein, receptor, protease, and signaling molecules. The top 10 most up-regulated genes were *CSF3*, *MAFA*, *CR2*, *GLDC*, *SAA1*, *LBP*, *MME*, *MMP3*, *MME-AS1*, and *SAA4*. The 62 down-regulated genes in periodontitis were mainly cytoskeletal and structural proteins. The top 10 most down-regulated genes were *SERPINA12*, *MT4*, *H19*, *KRT2*, *DSC1*, *PSORS1C2*, *KRT27*, *LCE3C*, *AQ5*, and *LCE6A*. The differential alternative splicing analysis revealed unique transcription variants in periodontitis tissues. The EDB exon was predominantly included in *FN1*, while exon 2 was mostly skipped in *BCL2A1*.

Conclusions: These findings using RNA sequencing provide novel insights into the pathogenesis mechanism of periodontitis in terms of gene expression and alternative splicing.

Keywords: Periodontitis, Transcriptome sequencing, Alternative splicing, Gene expression profile

Introduction

Periodontitis is a chronic inflammatory disease of periodontium, characterized by massive destruction of both soft and hard tissues surrounding the teeth [1]. The current concept for the periodontal diseases involve complex interaction between the microbial biofilm and host immune responses that leads to the alteration of bone and connective tissue homeostasis [2, 3]. Understanding the

molecular mechanisms underlying the pathogenesis as well as development of efficient therapeutics is furthermore important since periodontitis is linked to other metabolic and/or systemic diseases including diabetes, cardiovascular diseases, and rheumatoid arthritis [4–6].

The analysis of transcriptome by microarrays has been a valuable tool to study the changes in gene expression profiles in gingival tissues of periodontitis patients [7–9]. However, recent advances in the high-throughput RNA sequencing technology revolutionarily enhanced our understanding on the complexity of eukaryotic transcriptome [10, 11]. RNA sequencing has several key advantages over the hybridization-based microarray techniques. First of all, direct sequencing enables an unbiased approach compared

---

* Correspondence: jaehlee@khu.ac.kr; ylee@knu.ac.kr
†Equal contributors
3Department of Life and Nanopharmaceutical Sciences, Kyung Hee University, Seoul 02447, Korea
2Institute for Hard Tissue and Bone Regeneration, Kyungpook National University, Daegu 41940, Korea
Full list of author information is available at the end of the article

with the microarrays that depends on the predetermined genome sequences. Secondly, RNA sequencing is highly accurate in detecting gene expression with very wide dynamic detection ranges with low background. Thus, RNA sequencing is not only useful to precisely determine gene expression profiles but also particularly powerful to detect novel transcription variants via alternative splicing [10].

In the present study, we analyzed the pooled transcriptome from gingival tissues of periodontitis patients and compared with that of healthy patients. The large sum of novel information on the gene expression profiles as well as novel transcripts through alternative splicing would provide not only insights into the pathogenesis of periodontitis but also basis for the development of biomarkers and therapeutic targets.

Materials and methods

Periodontitis patient characteristics and gingival tissue samples

Gingival tissue samples were collected from chronic periodontitis patients or healthy individuals. On the basis of clinical and radiographic criteria, the periodontitis-affected site had a probing depth of ≥4 mm, clinical attachment level of ≥4 mm, and bleeding on probing. A total of 10 gingival samples were collected from 9 periodontal healthy patients who visited Kyungpook National University Hospital. Similarly, a total of 10 periodontitis tissue samples were obtained from 4 periodontitis patients with pocket depth of 4~6 mm and 3 severe periodontitis patients with pocket depth of 7 mm or deeper. The patient characteristics are given in Additional file 1: Table S1. All patients were non-smoking and did not have untreated metabolic/systemic diseases nor associated with infection/autoimmune diseases at the time of tissue collection. The size of 3-mm^2 gingival biopsies were obtained from the marginal gingiva during periodontal flap surgery and immediately stored in RNAlater solution (Thermo Fisher Scientific, Waltham, MA) at −70 °C after removal of blood by brief washing in phosphate-buffered saline. The study was approved by the institutional review board of the Kyungpook National University Hospital with informed consent from all patients.

Isolation of RNA and RNA sequencing

Frozen tissues were disrupted in the lysis solution of mirVana RNA isolation kit (Thermo Fisher Scientific) using disposable pestle grinder system (Thermo Fisher Scientific). After RNA extraction, the same amount of total RNA isolated from each individual sample (1 μg) was pooled into 2 groups (healthy and periodontitis) and used for further analysis. The integrity of pooled total RNA was analyzed by Agilent 2100 Bioanalyzer (Agilent Technologies, Santa Clara, CA). After purification of mRNA molecules by poly-T oligo-attached magnetic

beads followed by fragmentation, the RNA of approximately 300-bp size was isolated using gel electrophoresis. The cDNA synthesis and library construction was performed using the Illumina Truseq RNA sample preparation kit (Illumina, San Diego, CA), following the manufacturer's protocol. The PCR-amplified cDNA templates on a flow cell was loaded and sequenced in the HiSeq 2000 sequencing system (Illumina) in the paired-end sequencing mode (2 × 101 bp reads).

Sequencing data analysis

All sequencing raw reads were aligned to the human genome reference hg19 using the GSNAP alignment tool (2013-11-27) [12]. Only uniquely and properly mapped read pairs were used for further analysis. The differentially expressed genes between gingival tissues from periodontal healthy patients and periodontitis patients were identified using the DESeq R package [13]. Differentially expressed genes were defined as those with changes of at least 2-fold between samples and at a false discovery rate (FDR) cutoff of 5 % based on DESeq adjusted p values. The analysis of alternative splicing events was performed using MATS software [14]. The differences in the alternative splicing in genes were considered significant when the inclusion difference between samples was equal or greater than 5 % at a 10 % FDR. Each alternative splicing change of the skipped exon vent was manually inspected in UCSC genome browser using the sequencing data. The functional classification analysis of differentially expressed genes was performed using the PANTHER tools (http://www.pantherdb.org). The GO term and KEGG pathway enrichment analysis was performed as described previously [15]. Briefly, the fraction of genes in a test set associated with each GO category was calculated and compared with that of control set comprised of randomly chosen genes of the same number and length of the test genes. The random sampling was repeated 100,000 times for the calculation of empirical p value. The significance of enriched GO terms or KEGG pathways were determined by the p value cutoff, which was 1/total number of GO terms considered.

Validation of differentially expressed genes and alternative splicing events

From the pooled RNA samples, 1 μg of RNA was reversed transcribed using the Superscript II Reverse Transcriptase (Thermo Fisher Scientific). Quantitative real-time PCR analysis was performed by the addition of 1 μg of cDNA and SYBR green master mix in MicroAMP optical tubes using the AB 7500 system (Thermo Fisher Scientific). The expression of genes relative to that of *HPRT1* was determined by the $2^{-\Delta\Delta C_T}$ method [16]. The differential alternative splicing events were confirmed via RT-PCR analysis with the addition of 1 μg of cDNA and Takara premix Taq polymerase (Takara Bio Inc, Shiga, Japan) for 33 cycles of

10 s at 98 °C, 30 s at 60 °C, and 1 min at 72 °C. The primers for the detection of alternative splicing were designed by the PrimerSeq software [17] in order that the PCR product to span the region of exon inclusion/skipping, enabling the differentiation of alternative splicing events by product size. The primer sequences for the real-time RT-PCR analysis of selected genes and those for the RT-PCR detection of alternative splicing events of *FN1* and *BCL2A1* gene were provided in the supplemental tables (Additional file 2: Table S2 and Additional file 3: Table S3).

Results

RNA sequencing results

Total RNA was extracted from 10 healthy gingival tissue samples and 10 chronic periodontitis-affected gingival tissues as described above. Then, cDNAs synthesized from the pooled RNA samples of both groups were sequenced using the Illumina HiSeq 2000 system, which generated approximately 80 million pairs of reads of 101 bp in size. When compared with the reference sequence of Genome Reference Consortium GRCh37 (hg19), more than 90 % of read pairs were uniquely mapped on the human genome (Table 1). Gene annotation using the Ensembl (release 75) identified that a total of 36,814 genes have at least 1 read mapped on the exonic regions. Among these, 4800 genes were unique to the periodontitis tissue sample, while 2811 transcripts were detected only in healthy gingival sample.

Identification and classification of differentially expressed genes between periodontitis and healthy gingiva

The differential expression of genes between periodontitis and healthy gingival samples was analyzed by DESeq package [13]. By applying the cutoff of at least twofold change in the number of reads with 5 % FDR, we found a total of 462 genes differentially expressed between the samples (Fig. 1a, volcano plot). While 400 genes were up-regulated in the periodontitis tissue sample, 62 genes were down-regulated compared with the healthy control (Additional file 4: Table S4). Previously, Davanian et al. reported the discovery of 381 genes up-regulated in the periodontitis-affected gingival tissues by RNA sequencing [18]. Notably, 182 genes among them were also found to be up-regulated in the present study (Additional file 5: Figure S1), demonstrating an overlap between the two sets of gene lists when analyzed by a hypergeometric test ($p < 2.2e^{-16}$) [19].

The top 20 up-regulated genes listed in Table 2 included cytokines and immune response-related genes (*CSF3*, *CR2*, *LBP*, *CXCL1*, and *IL19*), serum amyloid proteins (*SAA1*, *SAA4*, and *SAA2*), and proteases (*MME*, *MMP3*, *MME-AS1*, and *MMP7*). The 20 most down-regulated genes (Table 3) included peptidase inhibitors (*SERPINA12* and *SPINK9*) and structural proteins (*KRT2*, *KRT27*, *LCE3C*, *LCE6A*, *LCE1B*, *LCE2D*, and *KRT1*).

To classify the differentially expressed genes into functionally related subgroups, we utilized the PANTHER classification system (http://pantherdb.org). As a result, the 462 differentially expressed genes between periodontitis and healthy gingival tissues were segregated into 20 different classes of proteins. When we compared the composition of these protein classes, there was a significant difference in the number of genes between periodontitis and healthy gingival samples in 6 protein classes. In the periodontitis tissue, genes classified as defense/immunity protein, receptor, protease, and signaling molecules were significantly enriched (Fig. 1b). On the other hand, genes in the categories of cytoskeletal protein and structural protein were predominant in healthy tissue sample compared with periodontitis. Furthermore, functional annotation of GO and KEGG pathway enrichment analyses as previously described [15] revealed enhanced immune responses in the periodontal tissues, including NOD-like receptor signaling, cytokine and chemokine activities, response to lipopolysaccharide, Jak-STAT signaling pathway, and B cell receptor signaling pathway (Additional file 6: Table S5 and Additional file 7: Table S6).

Validation of differentially expressed genes between periodontitis and healthy gingiva by quantitative real-time PCR analysis

To validate the differential gene expression results by RNA sequencing analysis, we selected 10 up-regulated or down-regulated genes in periodontal tissue and assessed their expression by quantitative real-time RT-PCR analysis. Figure 1c shows that the examination of differential gene expression by both methods is significantly concordant, with the Pearson's correlation coefficient (R) value of 0.81 ($p = 0.005$). Since the current study design employed pooling of samples, we further validated the variations in gene expression in individual samples of healthy and periodontitis patients. The real-time RT-PCR analyses for selected genes (Additional file 8: Figure S2) mostly repeated the RNA sequencing results, showing significant reduction in *NOS1*, *CHP2*, *CDON*, and *MT4*. Similarly, significant

Table 1 Summary of RNA sequencing read mapping results

	Number of total sequencing pairs	Number of unique pairs	Number of unmapped pairs	Percentage of uniquely mapped pairs
Periodontitis tissue	87,118,086	80,778,080	6,340,006	92.72
Healthy tissue	72,014,202	67,035,158	4,979,044	93.09

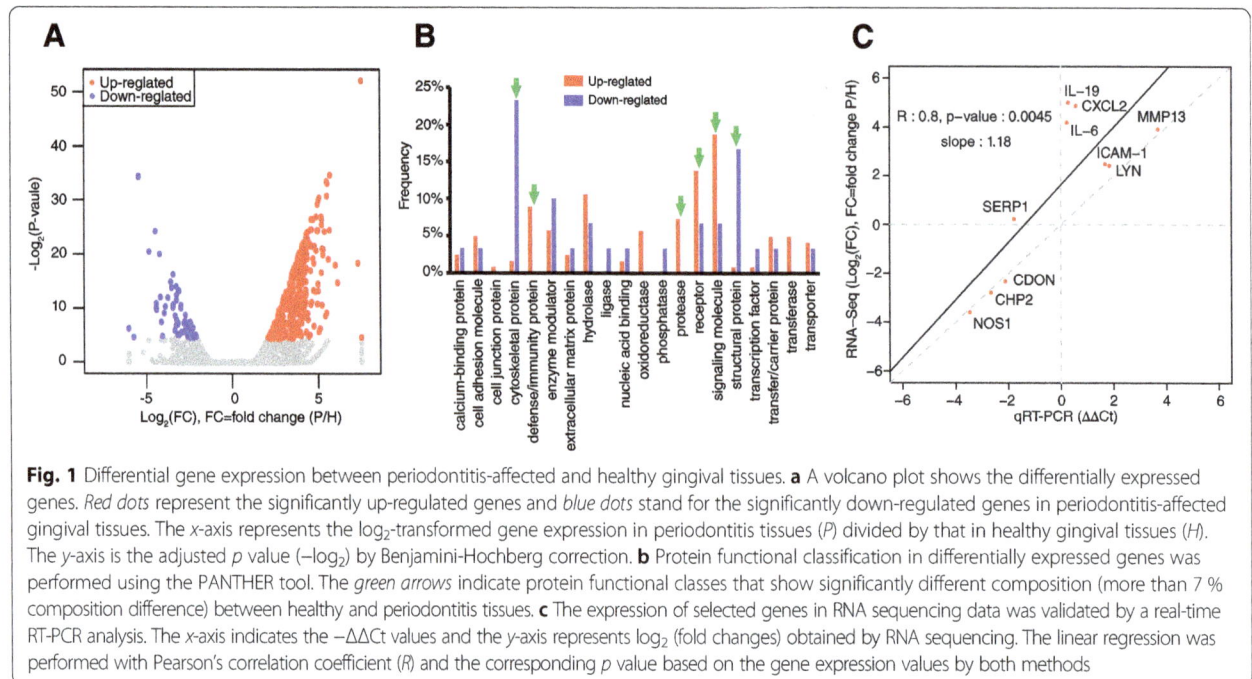

Fig. 1 Differential gene expression between periodontitis-affected and healthy gingival tissues. **a** A volcano plot shows the differentially expressed genes. *Red dots* represent the significantly up-regulated genes and *blue dots* stand for the significantly down-regulated genes in periodontitis-affected gingival tissues. The x-axis represents the log$_2$-transformed gene expression in periodontitis tissues (P) divided by that in healthy gingival tissues (H). The y-axis is the adjusted p value (−log$_2$) by Benjamini-Hochberg correction. **b** Protein functional classification in differentially expressed genes was performed using the PANTHER tool. The *green arrows* indicate protein functional classes that show significantly different composition (more than 7 % composition difference) between healthy and periodontitis tissues. **c** The expression of selected genes in RNA sequencing data was validated by a real-time RT-PCR analysis. The x-axis indicates the −ΔΔCt values and the y-axis represents log$_2$ (fold changes) obtained by RNA sequencing. The linear regression was performed with Pearson's correlation coefficient (R) and the corresponding p value based on the gene expression values by both methods

elevation was observed in *ICAM1*, *MMP13*, *LYN*, *CSF3*, *MMP3*, *LBP*, and CXCL2 while the expression of IL6 and IL19 only slightly increased. However, a large individual variation was observed in *SERP1* and *KRT2* expression.

Alternative splicing events in periodontitis and healthy gingival tissues

More than 90 % of human genes are alternatively spliced through different types of splicing [20, 21]. To identify the differential splicing events between the healthy and

Table 2 Top 20 up-regulated genes in periodontitis tissues

Ensemble ID	Gene symbol	Fold change	q value	Description
ENSG00000108342	CSF3	181.6	5.9E-21	Colony stimulating factor 3 (granulocyte)
ENSG00000182759	MAFA	157.5	8.2E-09	V-MAF avian musculoaponeurotic fibrosarcoma oncogene homolog A
ENSG00000117322	CR2	69.6	1.5E-07	Complement component (3D/Epstein Barr virus) receptor 2
ENSG00000178445	GLDC	50.8	2.6E-11	Glycine dehydrogenase (decarboxylating)
ENSG00000173432	SAA1	46.4	1.8E-14	Serum amyloid A1
ENSG00000129988	LBP	45.1	1.4E-05	Lipopolysaccharide binding protein
ENSG00000196549	MME	45.0	1.2E-14	Membrane metallo-endopeptidase
ENSG00000149968	MMP3	39.6	7.1E-10	Matrix metallopeptidase 3 (stromelysin 1, progelatinase)
ENSG00000240666	MME-AS1	38.8	2.1E-09	MME antisense RNA 1
ENSG00000148965	SAA4	37.3	4.7E-06	Serum amyloid A4, constitutive
ENSG00000137673	MMP7	37.1	4.5E-12	Matrix metallopeptidase 7 (matrilysin, uterine)
ENSG00000130513	GDF15	36.6	3.5E-08	Growth differentiation factor 15
ENSG00000134339	SAA2	36.4	2.6E-12	Serum amyloid A2
ENSG00000163739	CXCL1	33.3	1.6E-13	Chemokine (C-X-C motif) ligand 1 (melanoma growth stimulating activity, alpha)
ENSG00000117215	PLA2G2D	32.8	2.1E-04	Phospholipase A2, group IID
ENSG00000142224	IL19	32.4	5.3E-07	Interleukin 19
ENSG00000134873	CLDN10	31.8	1.8E-07	Claudin 10
ENSG00000255071	SAA2-SAA4	31.7	3.0E-11	SAA2-SAA4 readthrough
ENSG00000145113	MUC4	31.3	2.6E-11	Mucin 4, cell surface associated

Table 3 Top 20 down-regulated genes in periodontitis tissues

Ensemble ID	Gene symbol	Fold change	q value	Description
ENSG00000165953	SERPINA12	0.015	1.3E-04	Serpin peptidase inhibitor, clade A (alpha-1 antiproteinase, antitrypsin), member 12
ENSG00000102891	MT4	0.018	5.5E-04	Metallothionein 4
ENSG00000130600	H19	0.023	4.0E-15	H19, imprinted maternally expressed transcript (non-protein coding)
ENSG00000172867	KRT2	0.023	5.4E-15	Keratin 2
ENSG00000134765	DSC1	0.045	3.6E-11	Desmocollin 1
ENSG00000204538	PSORS1C2	0.046	7.2E-06	Psoriasis susceptibility 1 candidate 2
ENSG00000171446	KRT27	0.047	9.1E-06	Keratin 27
ENSG00000244057	LCE3C	0.053	1.8E-09	Late cornified envelope 3C
ENSG00000161798	AQP5	0.055	1.3E-06	Aquaporin 5
ENSG00000235942	LCE6A	0.057	5.3E-05	Late cornified envelope 6A
ENSG00000188959	C9orf152	0.059	4.2E-04	Chromosome 9 open reading frame 152
ENSG00000196734	LCE1B	0.067	5.4E-06	Late cornified envelope 1B
ENSG00000187223	LCE2D	0.073	1.5E-06	Late cornified envelope 2D
ENSG00000089250	NOS1	0.083	1.4E-07	Nitric oxide synthase 1 (neuronal)
ENSG00000204909	SPINK9	0.085	3.1E-07	Serine peptidase inhibitor, Kazal type 9
ENSG00000130595	TNNT3	0.091	6.7E-06	Troponin T type 3 (skeletal, fast)
ENSG00000110675	ELMOD1	0.091	4.1E-06	ELMO/CED-12 domain containing 1
ENSG00000167768	KRT1	0.091	4.5E-08	Keratin 1
ENSG00000237515	SHISA9	0.097	1.8E-04	Shisa family member 9

periodontitis gingival tissues, the inclusion level of alternative spliced exons was compared using the MATS tool [14] based on a statistical model that calculates the difference in the isoform ratio of a gene. The MATS analysis of RNA sequencing data revealed 183 significantly differential alternative splicing events in 155 genes with a cutoff of 5 % inclusion difference and 10 % FDR (Table 4 and Additional file 9: Table S7). The GO and KEGG pathway enrichment analyses for the determination of the biological relevance of those differentially spliced genes showed significant difference in the pathways including RNA splicing regulation, substrate adhesion-dependent cell spreading, response to wound healing, and positive regulation of cell migration (Additional file 10: Table S8 and Additional file 11: Table S9).

Among the genes that exhibited prominently novel included exons was *FN1* that encodes one of the major extracellular matrix protein fibronectin [22]. Fibronectin structure consists of 2 nearly identical ~250-kDa glycoprotein subunits with each monomer composed of repetitive units of type I, II, and III domains [23]. The type III domains contain 2 exons called extra domain A (EDA) and extra domain B (EDB), the latter showed significantly increased inclusion in periodontitis gingival tissues compared with healthy samples (Fig. 2a; left panel). The preferential formation of EDB-containing isoform in periodontitis was further corroborated by the RT-PCR analysis designed to amplify the included EDB exon regions (Fig. 2a; right panel). The analysis of alternative splicing events also indicated that *BCL2A1* (BCL2-related protein A1) exhibited prominently skipped exon 2 (Fig. 2b; left panel). RT-PCR analysis designed to amplify the skipped region revealed significantly increased shorter isoform (Fig. 2b; right panel). The individual variation between healthy and periodontitis tissues for these differences in the alternative slicing events was further confirmed by RT-PCR analyses (Additional file 12: Figure S3). For *FN1*, the inclusion of EDB exon was

Table 4 Summary of the differential alternative splicing event analysis

	Alternative 3' splicing sites	Alternative 5' splicing sites	Mutual exclusive exon	Retained intron	Skipped exon
Number of total alternative splicing events (genes)	3125 (2177)	2124 (1622)	4424 (2562)	2272 (1800)	32,824 (10,026)
% of total alternative splicing events (45,259)	6.9	4.7	9.8	6.1	72.5
Number of differential alternative splicing events (genes)	10 (10)	4 (4)	34 (32)	82 (77)	53 (42)
% of total differential alternative splicing events (183)	5.5	2.2	18.6	44.8	28.9

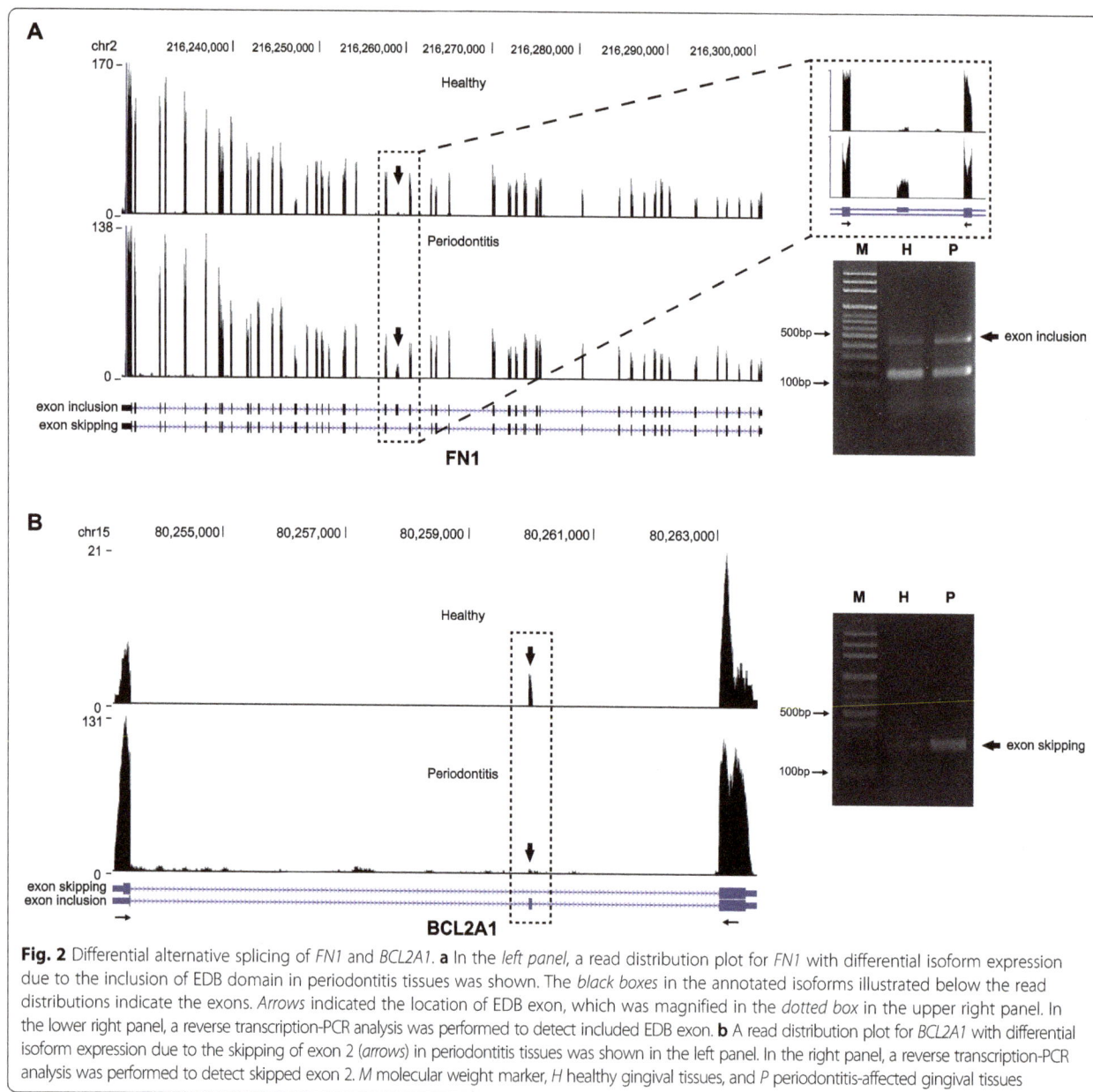

Fig. 2 Differential alternative splicing of *FN1* and *BCL2A1*. **a** In the *left panel*, a read distribution plot for *FN1* with differential isoform expression due to the inclusion of EDB domain in periodontitis tissues was shown. The *black boxes* in the annotated isoforms illustrated below the read distributions indicate the exons. *Arrows* indicated the location of EDB exon, which was magnified in the *dotted box* in the upper right panel. In the lower right panel, a reverse transcription-PCR analysis was performed to detect included EDB exon. **b** A read distribution plot for *BCL2A1* with differential isoform expression due to the skipping of exon 2 (*arrows*) in periodontitis tissues was shown in the left panel. In the right panel, a reverse transcription-PCR analysis was performed to detect skipped exon 2. *M* molecular weight marker, *H* healthy gingival tissues, and *P* periodontitis-affected gingival tissues

preferentially observed in periodontitis tissues (7/10) compared with healthy tissues (3/8) tested. Similarly, the skipping of exon 2 in *BCL2A1* was predominant in periodontitis tissues (9/10), compared with healthy tissues (2/8).

Discussion

Recent developments in the RNA sequencing technology and bioinformatics tools enabled elaborate analysis of gene expression in numerous human diseases. However, in periodontitis research, most RNA sequencing studies have focused on the identification of microbiome that constitutes periodontal biofilm, with little attention to the host responses against such microbial challenge. The

current study provides extensive information on gene expression as well as alternative splicing in periodontitis gingival tissues, which is crucial for the understanding the pathogenesis and development of biomarkers and therapeutic targets. The gene expression analysis revealed 62 down-regulated and 400 up-regulated genes in periodontitis tissues, suggesting the effectiveness of mRNA sequencing as a tool to scrutinize the differential gene expression during the development of periodontitis. Davanian et al. previously reported a series of up-regulated genes as well as enriched biological pathways in periodontitis [18]. When we compared these results with ours, the current results only partially overlap in terms of differential gene expression, possibly originated from the difference in the ethnic group of the subjects as well as in the methods to eliminate individual fluctuations in the gene expression. For example, Davanian et al. used healthy gingival tissue of the same periodontitis-affected individual as healthy control tissue. However, in the current study, the healthy and periodontitis tissues were pooled, allowing the dilution of individual differences in the gene expression. Indeed, the RNA sequencing analysis of pooled samples proved effective, since the expression levels of genes (except *IL6* and *IL19*) identified as differentially expressed by RNA sequencing were also significantly different between healthy and periodontitis samples, when we confirmed by real-time PCR analysis of individual samples (Additional file 8: Figure S2). Most of the top 20 up-regulated genes in periodontitis tissue (Table 2) were associated with inflammation and tissue degradation. Notably, serum amyloid A isoforms consisted 3 of 20 most up-regulated mRNAs, supporting the notion that these can serve as biomarkers for periodontitis-associated acute as well as chronic inflammation [24].

Until recently, gene expression analyses mostly focused on the genes whose expression was significantly increased in periodontitis. In line with this, 18 of top 20 up-regulated genes were associated with periodontal disease at least once by previous studies. The current study revealed 2 novel genes highly overexpressed in periodontitis tissues compared with healthy control. *MAFA* is a subgroup member of the basic leucine-zipper family transcription factor prominently known for its role in glucose-responsive insulin secretion [25]. *CLDN10* is an ion channel-forming member of claudin family, which is a constituent of tight junction [26]. The role of these genes in periodontitis is of great interest and requires further investigation.

In contrast to the highly expressed genes in periodontitis, fewer highlights have been drawn on the genes down-regulated in periodontal diseases. In accordance, most of the top 20 down-regulated genes (Table 3) have not been studied with regard to periodontitis, although investigating the role of those genes in periodontitis compared with that in normal tissues would greatly enhance our knowledge regarding the pathogenesis of periodontal diseases. Notably, keratin (*KRT2*, *KRT27*, and *KRT1*) and late cornified envelope (*LCE3C*, *LCE6A*, *LCE1B*, and *LCE2D*) genes constituted significant part of the down-regulated genes, suggesting the loss of epithelial barrier [27]. The causal relationship between the loss of these genes and the development of periodontal diseases requires further investigation.

It has long been suggested that different sites in the same individual exhibit different patterns of disease progression, morphology, and often response to therapy [28]. In addition, the oral microbiota responsible for the induction of periodontal diseases is distinct from site-to-site in the same individual [29, 30]. Accordingly, it is recommended to design clinical studies based on individual sites rather than individual person [31]. In agreement of this notion, the analysis of gene expression in individual sites by real-time RT-PCR (Additional file 8: Figure S2) revealed site-specific variation. In different sites from the same periodontitis patients (P2: P3, P7: P8, and P9: P10), it was clearly noticeable that *MMP3*, *MMP13*, and *LBP* expressions differ in a site-specific manner. An individual RNA sequencing study with larger number of patients is ongoing, which will further provide detailed information on the site specificity of periodontitis.

The gene ontology and KEGG pathway enrichment analyses revealed both innate and adaptive immune responses in the periodontal tissues, including NOD-like receptor signaling, response to lipopolysaccharide, cytokine and chemokine activities, and B cell receptor signaling pathways (Additional file 6: Table S5 and Additional file 7: Table S6). The NOD1 and NOD2 have been suggested to mediate the sensing of periodontal bacteria [32]. In addition, NOD2 has been linked to the *P. gingivalis*-induced bone resorption, since *NOD2* knockout mice were protected from bone loss in a periodontitis model [33]. Bellibasakis and Johansson showed that a periodontal pathogen *A. actinomyceptemcomitans* regulated NLRP3 and NLRP6 expression in human mononuclear cells [34]. Considering the existence of 22 human NOD-like receptor protein members and their crucial functions in immune diseases, it will be of great interest and importance to elucidate the involvement of these receptors in the pathogenesis of periodontitis.

In the periodontitis lesions, it has been estimated that more than 75 % of infiltrating immune cells are plasma cells and B cells, suggesting the importance of these cells in adaptive immunity during the development of periodontitis [35]. In accordance, molecules involved in B cell activation including *CD79*, *CD19*, *Lyn*, and *CR2* were significantly increased in periodontitis tissue. An increasing body of evidence indicates that B cells with autoreactive propensities might be linked to tissue destruction in periodontitis [36, 37]. Indeed, recent reports demonstrated that B cell-deficient mice were protected from alveolar bone loss in experimental periodontitis [38, 39].

Numerous studies attempted to delineate the role of T helper (Th) cell subsets in human periodontitis by examining the cytokine mRNA levels by RT-PCR, flow cytometry, and immunohistochemistry. However, those studies are incoherent in terms of Th1 and Th2 cytokine expression, although the Th17 cytokines are consistently increased [37]. The current study revealed that the levels of Th1 cytokines *IFNG* and *IL12* did not change between healthy and periodontitis-affected gingival samples while that of *TNF* slightly increased in periodontitis (Additional file 13: Table S10). The Th2 cytokines *IL10* and *IL33* remained unaltered in periodontitis patients. Interestingly, Th17 cytokines *IL6*, *IL23A*, and *IL17C* significantly increased in gingival tissues from periodontitis patients compared with those of healthy control, supporting the concept of Th17 cells as crucial mediators of inflammation, although it is still controversial whether these cells contribute to tissue destruction or protection in periodontitis [40, 41].

Alternative splicing of genes contribute to the diversity of proteome as well as genome evolution, control of developmental processes, and physiological regulation of various biological systems [42]. Not surprisingly, dysregulation of alternative splicing is often linked to various human diseases such as cancer, metabolic, neurological, and skeletal diseases [43–47]. However, alternative splicing events in the context of periodontitis has rarely been investigated. The current study uncovered significant differential alternative splicing events in *BCL2A1* and *FN1*. *BCL2A1* is a target gene of NF-kB, implicated in the survival of leukocytes thereby inflammation [48]. However, the role of alternative splicing on the activity of the protein has not been suggested until the present. Interestingly, recent discovery showed that *BCL2A1* was increased not only in periodontitis but also in systemic diseases such as cardiovascular diseases and ulcerative colitis [49]. Therefore, research regarding the multiple layers of regulatory mechanisms including mRNA expression and alternative splicing of *BCL2A1* are required to fully understand the role of this gene during the pathogenesis of periodontitis.

Parkar et al. previously suggested that *FN1* is differentially spliced in periodontitis [50]. Interestingly, the authors reported exon skipping of both EDA and EDB domain in periodontitis, while the current study showed conspicuously increased inclusion of EDB domain. Although whether these differences originated from the use of periodontal ligament [51] versus gingival tissues (the present study) yet to be cleared, it would be of great interest to fully identify the role of fibronectin isoforms in the pathogenesis of periodontitis considering the suggested role of EDA- and EDB-containing isoforms of fibronectin during embryonic development and tissue repair [23, 51].

In conclusion, the current study presented novel gene expression profiles as well as alternative splicing in gingival tissues from periodontitis patients by RNA sequencing experiments. Considering its effectiveness for whole transcriptome analysis, the use of RNA sequencing in periodontitis research would facilitate the elucidation of pathogenesis.

Additional files

Additional file 1: Table S1. The characteristics of patients involved in the current study. The information on age, gender, and disease severity is

Additional file 2: Table S2. Primer sequences used for the real-time RT-PCR validation of RNA sequencing differential gene expression results.

Additional file 3: Table S3. Primer sequences used for the RT-PCR validation of RNA sequencing alternative splicing results. The primer

Additional file 4: Table S4. The full list of differentially expressed genes in healthy and periodontitis tissues. This excel file contains the full list of

Additional file 5: Figure S1. Comparison of up-regulated genes in periodontitis with those of the previous study by Davanian et al. The Venn diagram shows the number of genes unique for each study and

Additional file 6: Table S5. The GO term analysis of genes of up- and down-regulated genes in periodontitis. This excel file contains the list of the differentially expressed genes, categorized according to the GO

Additional file 7: Table S6. The KEGG pathway analysis of genes of up- and down-regulated genes in periodontitis. This excel file contains the list of the differentially expressed genes, categorized according to the KEGG

Additional file 8: Figure S2. The expression levels of selected genes in individual samples. The individual variation in gene expression was examined by real-time RT-PCR analysis of individual healthy and periodontitis samples. The *p* values of the Wilcoxon rank-sum test between healthy and periodontitis

Additional file 9: Table S7. The full list of differential alternative splicing events in healthy and periodontitis tissues. This excel file contains the full list

Additional file 10: Table S8. The GO term analysis of genes with differential alternative splicing in periodontitis. This excel file contains the list of the genes with differential alternative splicing, categorized

Additional file 11: Table S9. The KEGG pathway analysis of genes with differential alternative splicing in periodontitis. This excel file contains the list of the genes with differential alternative splicing, categorized

Additional file 12: Figure S3. The alternative splicing events in individual samples. The individual variation in alternative splicing events in *FN1* and *BCL2A1* was examined by RT-PCR analysis of individual healthy

Additional file 13: Table S10. The expression of Th1, Th2, and Th17 cytokines in healthy and periodontitis tissues. This excel file contains the selected list of the Th1, Th2, and Th17 cytokine genes with their

Abbreviations
EDA, extra domain A; EDB, extra domain B; FDR, false discovery rate; GO, gene ontology; KEGG, kyoto encyclopedia of genes and genomes; PANTHER, protein analysis through evolutionary relationships

Acknowledgements
Not applicable.

Funding
This work was supported by grants from the National Research Foundation of Korea (NRF) funded by the Ministry of Science, ICT, and Future Planning (NRF-2012M3A9B6055415, NRF-2014R1A2A2A01004161, and NRF-2008-0062282 to YL). This work was also supported by grants from the Korea Health Technology R&D Project through the KHIDI, funded by the Ministry of Health & Welfare (HI14C0175 to J-HL).

Authors' contributions

Y-GK designed the experiments, collected the tissue samples, analyzed the data, and wrote the paper. MK analyzed the bioinformatics data and wrote the paper. JHK, HJK, J-YK, J-WP, J-ML, and J-YS performed the experiments and analyzed the data. J-HL designed and performed the experiments, analyzed the bioinformatics data, and wrote the paper. YL designed and performed the experiments, analyzed the data, and wrote the paper. All authors read and approved the final manuscript.

Competing interests

The authors declare that they have no competing interests.

Author details

[1]Department of Periodontology, School of Dentistry, Kyungpook National University, Daegu 41940, Korea. [2]Institute for Hard Tissue and Bone Regeneration, Kyungpook National University, Daegu 41940, Korea. [3]Department of Life and Nanopharmaceutical Sciences, Kyung Hee University, Seoul 02447, Korea. [4]Department of Biochemistry, School of Dentistry, Kyungpook National University, 2177 Dalgubeol-daero, Joong-gu, Daegu 41940, Korea. [5]Department of Maxillofacial Biomedical Engineering, School of Dentistry, Kyung Hee University, 26 Kyunghee-daero, Dongdaemun-gu, Seoul 02447, Korea.

References

1. Pihlstrom BL, Michalowicz BS, Johnson NW. Periodontal diseases. Lancet. 2005;366:1809–20.
2. Offenbacher S, Barros SP, Beck JD. Rethinking periodontal inflammation. J Periodontol. 2008;79:1577–84.
3. Garlet GP. Destructive and protective roles of cytokines in periodontitis: a re-appraisal from host defense and tissue destruction viewpoints. J Dent Res. 2010;89:1349–63.
4. Bullon P, Morillo JM, Ramirez-Tortosa MC, Quiles JL, Newman HN, Battino M. Metabolic syndrome and periodontitis: is oxidative stress a common link? J Dent Res. 2009;88:503–18.
5. Pischon N, Heng N, Bernimoulin JP, Kleber BM, Willich SN, Pischon T. Obesity, inflammation, and periodontal disease. J Dent Res. 2007;86:400–9.
6. Linden GJ, Lyons A, Scannapieco FA. Periodontal systemic associations: review of the evidence. J Periodontol. 2013;84:S8–19.
7. Abe D, Kubota T, Morozumi T, Shimizu T, Nakasone N, Itagaki M, Yoshie H. Altered gene expression in leukocyte transendothelial migration and cell communication pathways in periodontitis-affected gingival tissues. J Periodontal Res. 2011;46:345–53.
8. Beikler T, Peters U, Prior K, Eisenacher M, Flemmig TF. Gene expression in periodontal tissues following treatment. BMC Med Genomics. 2008;1:30.
9. Kim DM, Ramoni MF, Nevins M, Fiorellini JP. The gene expression profile in refractory periodontitis patients. J Periodontol. 2006;77:1043–50.
10. Wang Z, Gerstein M, Snyder M. RNA-Seq: a revolutionary tool for transcriptomics. Nat Rev Genet. 2009;10:57–63.
11. Garber M, Grabherr MG, Guttman M, Trapnell C. Computational methods for transcriptome annotation and quantification using RNA-seq. Nat Methods. 2011;8:469–77.
12. Wu TD, Nacu S. Fast and SNP-tolerant detection of complex variants and splicing in short reads. Bioinformatics. 2010;26:873–81.
13. Anders S, Huber W. Differential expression analysis for sequence count data. Genome Biol. 2010;11:R106.
14. Shen S, Park JW, Huang J, Dittmar KA, Lu ZX, Zhou Q, Carstens RP, Xing Y. MATS: a Bayesian framework for flexible detection of differential alternative splicing from RNA-Seq data. Nucleic Acids Res. 2012;40:e61.
15. Lee JH, Gao C, Peng G, Greer C, Ren S, Wang Y, Xiao X. Analysis of transcriptome complexity through RNA sequencing in normal and failing murine hearts. Circ Res. 2011;109:1332–41.
16. Livak KJ, Schmittgen TD. Analysis of relative gene expression data using real-time quantitative PCR and the $2^{(-\Delta\Delta C(T))}$ method. Methods. 2001;25:402–8.
17. Tokheim C, Park JW, Xing Y. PrimerSeq: design and visualization of RT-PCR primers for alternative splicing using RNA-seq data. Genomics Proteomics Bioinformatics. 2014;12:105 9.

18. Davanian H, Stranneheim H, Bage T, Lagervall M, Jansson L, Lundeberg J, Yucel-Lindberg T. Gene expression profiles in paired gingival biopsies from periodontitis-affected and healthy tissues revealed by massively parallel sequencing. PLoS One. 2012;7:e46440.
19. Fury W, Batliwalla F, Gregersen PK, Li W. Overlapping probabilities of top ranking gene lists, hypergeometric distribution, and stringency of gene selection criterion. Conf Proc IEEE Eng Med Biol Soc. 2006;1:5531–4.
20. Wang ET, Sandberg R, Luo S, Khrebtukova I, Zhang L, Mayr C, Kingsmore SF, Schroth GP, Burge CB. Alternative isoform regulation in human tissue transcriptomes. Nature. 2008;456:470–6.
21. Xiao X, Lee JH. Systems analysis of alternative splicing and its regulation. Wiley Interdiscip Rev Syst Biol Med. 2010;2:550–65.
22. Geiger B, Spatz JP, Bershadsky AD. Environmental sensing through focal adhesions. Nat Rev Mol Cell Biol. 2009;10:21–33.
23. White ES, Muro AF. Fibronectin splice variants: understanding their multiple roles in health and disease using engineered mouse models. IUBMB Life. 2011;63:538–46.
24. D'Aiuto F, Orlandi M, Gunsolley JC. Evidence that periodontal treatment improves biomarkers and CVD outcomes. J Periodontol. 2013;84:S85–105.
25. Hang Y, Stein R. MafA and MafB activity in pancreatic beta cells. Trends Endocrinol Metab. 2011;22:364–73.
26. Krug SM, Schulzke JD, Fromm M. Tight junction, selective permeability, and related diseases. Semin Cell Dev Biol. 2014;36:166–76.
27. Presland RB, Jurevic RJ. Making sense of the epithelial barrier: what molecular biology and genetics tell us about the functions of oral mucosal and epidermal tissues. J Dent Educ. 2002;66:564–74.
28. Socransky SS, Haffajee AD, Goodson JM, Lindhe J. New concepts of destructive periodontal disease. J Clin Periodontol. 1984;11:21–32.
29. Preza D, Olsen I, Willumsen T, Grinde B, Paster BJ. Diversity and site-specificity of the oral microflora in the elderly. Eur J Clin Microbiol Infect Dis. 2009;28:1033–40.
30. Aas JA, Paster BJ, Stokes LN, Olsen I, Dewhirst FE. Defining the normal bacterial flora of the oral cavity. J Clin Microbiol. 2005;43:5721–32.
31. Lindhe J, Socransky S, Wennstrom J. Design of clinical trials of traditional therapies of periodontitis. J Clin Periodontol. 1986;13:488–99.
32. Okugawa T, Kaneko T, Yoshimura A, Silverman N, Hara Y. NOD1 and NOD2 mediate sensing of periodontal pathogens. J Dent Res. 2010;89:186–91.
33. Prates TP, Taira TM, Holanda MC, Bignardi LA, Salvador SL, Zamboni DS, Cunha FQ, Fukada SY. NOD2 contributes to Porphyromonas gingivalis-induced bone resorption. J Dent Res. 2014;93:1155–62.
34. Belibasakis GN, Johansson A. Aggregatibacter actinomycetemcomitans targets NLRP3 and NLRP6 inflammasome expression in human mononuclear leukocytes. Cytokine. 2012;59:124–30.
35. Berglundh T, Donati M. Aspects of adaptive host response in periodontitis. J Clin Periodontol. 2005;32:87–107.
36. Berglundh T, Donati M, Zitzmann N. B cells in periodontitis: friends or enemies? Periodontol 2000. 2007;45:51–66.
37. Gonzales JR. T- and B-cell subsets in periodontitis. Periodontol 2000. 2015;69:181–200.
38. Abe T, AlSarhan M, Benakanakere MR, Maekawa T, Kinane DF, Cancro MP, Korostoff JM, Hajishengallis G. The B cell-stimulatory cytokines BLyS and APRIL are elevated in human periodontitis and are required for B cell-dependent bone loss in experimental murine periodontitis. J Immunol. 2015;195:1427–35.
39. Oliver-Bell J, Butcher JP, Malcolm J, MacLeod MK, Adrados Planell A, Campbell L, Nibbs RJ, Garside P, McInnes IB, Culshaw S. Periodontitis in the absence of B cells and specific anti-bacterial antibody. Mol Oral Microbiol. 2015;30:160–9.
40. Gaffen SL, Hajishengallis G. A new inflammatory cytokine on the block: re-thinking periodontal disease and the Th1/Th2 paradigm in the context of Th17 cells and IL-17. J Dent Res. 2008;87:817–28.
41. Cheng WC, Hughes FJ, Taams LS. The presence, function and regulation of IL-17 and Th17 cells in periodontitis. J Clin Periodontol. 2014;41:541–9.
42. Gamazon ER, Stranger BE. Genomics of alternative splicing: evolution, development and pathophysiology. Hum Genet. 2014;133:679–87.
43. Biamonti G, Catillo M, Pignataro D, Montecucco A, Ghigna C. The alternative splicing side of cancer. Semin Cell Dev Biol. 2014;32:30–6.

44. Tazi J, Bakkour N, Stamm S. Alternative splicing and disease. Biochim Biophys Acta. 2009;1792:14–26.

45. Juan-Mateu J, Villate O, Eizirik DL. Mechanisms in endocrinology: alternative splicing: the new frontier in diabetes research. Eur J Endocrinol. 2016;174:R225.

46. Raj B, Blencowe BJ. Alternative splicing in the mammalian nervous system: recent insights into mechanisms and functional roles. Neuron. 2015;87:14–27.

47. Fan X, Tang L. Aberrant and alternative splicing in skeletal system disease. Gene. 2013;528:21–6.

48. Vogler M. BCL2A1: the underdog in the BCL2 family. Cell Death Differ. 2012; 19:67–74.

49. Lundmark A, Davanian H, Bage T, Johannsen G, Koro C, Lundeberg J, Yucel-Lindberg T. Transcriptome analysis reveals mucin 4 to be highly associated with periodontitis and identifies pleckstrin as a link to systemic diseases. Sci Rep. 2015;5:18475.

50. Parkar MH, Bakalios P, Newman HN, Olsen I. Expression and splicing of the fibronectin gene in healthy and diseased periodontal tissue. Eur J Oral Sci. 1997;105:264–70.

51. White ES, Baralle FE, Muro AF. New insights into form and function of fibronectin splice variants. J Pathol. 2008;216:1–14.

15

Identification of a novel genetic locus underlying tremor and dystonia

Dorota Monies[1,2*†], Hussam Abou Al-Shaar[3], Ewa A. Goljan[1,2], Banan Al-Younes[1,2], Muna Monther Abdullah Al-Breacan[1], Maher Mohammed Al-Saif[4], Salma M. Wakil[1,2], Brian F. Meyer[1,2], Khalid S. A. Khabar[4] and Saeed Bohlega[2,3*†]

Abstract

Background: Five affected individuals with syndromic tremulous dystonia, spasticity, and white matter disease from a consanguineous extended family covering a period of over 24 years are presented. A positional cloning approach utilizing genome-wide linkage, homozygosity mapping and whole exome sequencing was used for genetic characterization. The impact of a calmodulin-binding transcription activator 2, (*CAMTA2*) isoform 2, hypomorphic mutation on mRNA and protein abundance was studied using fluorescent reporter expression cassettes. Human brain sub-region cDNA libraries were used to study the expression pattern of *CAMTA2* transcript variants.

Results: Linkage analysis and homozygozity mapping localized the disease allele to a 2.1 Mb interval on chromosome 17 with a LOD score of 4.58. Whole exome sequencing identified a G>A change in the transcript variant 2 5′UTR of *CAMTA2* that was only 6 bases upstream of the translation start site (c.-6G > A) (NM_001171166.1) and segregated with disease in an autosomal recessive manner. Transfection of wild type and mutant 5′UTR-linked fluorescent reporters showed no impact upon mRNA levels but a significant reduction in the protein fluorescent activity implying translation inhibition.

Conclusions: Mutation of *CAMTA2* resulting in post-transcriptional inhibition of its own gene activity likely underlies a novel syndromic tremulous dystonia.

Keywords: Dystonia, Tremor, Familial, Syndromic

Background

Currently, classification of dystonia relies upon phenomenology rather than etiology. A natural bifurcation is made based upon whether, with the exception of tremor, it is the sole motor feature (isolated dystonia) or is accompanied by other movement disorders including myoclonus (combined dystonia) [1]. Isolated dystonia may be subdivided into generalized or focal/segmental forms, with combined dystonia further categorized based upon the presence of myoclonus or Parkinsonism [2]. The advent of next generation sequencing has led to rapid expansion of phenotypic and genotypic subsets of

syndromes primarily characterized as isolated or combined dystonias with more than 20 loci (DYT1-DYT27; some are redundant) identified to date [2, 3].

Familial-isolated dystonias are predominantly inherited as incompletely penetrant autosomal dominant traits most frequently related to the DYT1 or DYT6 loci with mutations in *TOR1A* [4, 5] or *THAP1* [6, 7], respectively. Additional isolated dystonia loci include DYT23 (*CIZ1*) [8], DYT24 (*ANO3*) [9], and DYT25 (*GNAL*) [10, 11], all of which have recently been extensively reviewed [2]. DYT4 (*TUBB4A*) may present as an autosomal dominant disorder in adolescence or early adulthood with prominent laryngeal dysphonia and craniocervical, segmental, or generalized dystonia [12, 13]. A rare recessively inherited generalized isolated dystonia results from mutation of *PRKRA* (DYT16) and is characterized by early onset and frequent association with dystonia-Parkinsonism [2, 14, 15]. Two other recessively inherited

---

* Correspondence: moniesdm@gmail.com; boholega@kfshrc.edu.sa
†Equal contributors
[1]Department of Genetics, King Faisal Specialist Hospital, and Research Centre, PO Box 3354, Riyadh 11211, Saudi Arabia
[2]Saudi Human Genome Program, King Abdulaziz City for Science and Technology, Riyadh, Saudi Arabia
Full list of author information is available at the end of the article

isolated dystonias have also been described arising from mutation of DYT2 (*HPCA*) [16] or DYT27 (*COL6A3*) [15]. Like these, other dystonia loci such as DYT23 (*CIZ1*) and DYT24 (*ANO3*) are yet to be independently confirmed. Dystonic movements are also associated with mutations of *ADCY5*, identified as the likely cause of a novel movement disorder, familial dyskinesia with facial myokimia (FDFM) [17, 18].

We previously reported a consanguineous extended family having a novel autosomal recessive syndromic tremulous dystonia with spasticity and white matter disease [19]. In this study, we further delineate and genetically characterize the syndrome, identifying *CAMTA2* as a novel candidate gene for a syndromic tremulous dystonia, and describe its clinical course and prognosis over a long follow-up period.

Results

The families originated from the Eastern part of the Arabian Peninsula. Five patients were studied (Fig 1a); their current ages ranging from 33 to 46 years. The detailed clinical description was previously reported [19]. In summary, the disease onset was at 7–8 years of age with tremulous movement in fingers and arms that progressed to affect the face, neck, and trunk. Speech became dysarthric and tremulous. The volitional movement was exacerbated by posture and action. Initially, gait was not impaired. Intelligence, personality, and memory were not affected apart from paranoia and depression in two individuals. Patients exhibited a coarse generalized tremor of 4–5 Hz, present at rest, waxing, and waning in amplitude with side-to-side ("no no" type tremor). In addition, there was variable focal or segmental dystonia with retrocollis shoulder elevation and hyperextension of the fingers. There was generalized hyperreflexia with extensor planter response noted around the age of 15 or 16 years. Sensory examination was intact and there was no truncal ataxia. Patients were followed for up to 24 years with no noticeable increase in their movement disorder. The patients were cognitively intact, they were able to finish college, hold independent jobs, get married, and have children. However, all of them exhibited variable degrees of spasticity affecting their legs more than arms (Additional file 1) and two of them required walking aids in their 30's. Biochemical, organic acid, and lysosomal enzyme studies were normal. Visual and somatosensory evoke potentials showed evidence of prolonged central latencies. Accelerometric recording from the outstretched hand showed 4-Hz tremors. MRI of the brain showed similar abnormalities in all. There was mild symmetrical and confluent white-matter abnormalities sparing the U-fibers and involving the white matter of centrum semiovale, internal capsule, and ventral pons. These findings are not characteristic in

any of the classic leukodystrophies. No change was observed in subsequent MRI scans with more than 20 years of follow-up. MR spectroscopy showed no lactate peak or other abnormalities. Patients failed to respond to therapeutic trials of ethanol or anticholinergics. However, some symptomatic benefits were noted with high-dose propranolol, gabapentin, and clonazepam. Patient video. Patients exhibited a coarse generalized tremor of 4–5 Hz, present at rest, waxing and waning in amplitude with side-to-side ("no no" type tremor). In addition, there was variable focal or segmental dystonia with retrocollis shoulder elevation and hyperextension of the fingers. Patients exhibited generalized hyperreflexia with an extensor planter response being noted. (MOV 39038 kb).

Linkage analysis of the nuclear families with three and two affected individuals (Fig. 1a) resulted in independent LOD scores of 2.53 and 2.05, respectively, at rs11651665. Combined analysis (Fig. 1b) localized the disease to a region on chromosome 17 defined proximally by rs743646 and distally by rs34811366 (chr17:4,536,241-6,670,705) with a maximum LOD score of 4.58. Based upon runs of homozygosity shared by all the affected and absent in unaffected individuals (Fig. 1c; red rectangle), we refined the critical interval to a 2.1 Mb region (chr17:4,231,133-6,018,243) containing approximately 60 RefSeq genes (hg19).

Whole exome sequencing of individual IV:7 (Fig. 1a) identified 25,926 variants relative to the hg19 reference sequence, with 1498 variants on chr 17. These were further filtered to exclude all variants present outside our defined ROH (chr 17: 4,231,133-6,018,243) within which we identified 60 variants (Additional file 2). Within the critical interval (chr 17: 4,231,133-6,018,243), 99.42% of bases in the CDS and flanking regions of genes were covered at 30× or better with an average coverage of 425×. By excluding previously reported variants (present in dbSNP with incidence > 0.02; present in 1000 genomes with incidence > 0.02) and retaining those present at a frequency < 2% in more than 1000 Arab exomes held in an in-house database, the list was narrowed to 8. By only focusing on homozygous changes annotated as non-synonymous, splicing variants, frameshift insertions or deletions, and nonsense variants, we decreased the number of candidate variants to 1. It was a G>A change in the 5′UTR of transcript variant 2 of *CAMTA2* (c.-6G>A) (NM_001171166.1) (Fig. 2a). This homozygous variant was identified in 56 reads, was confirmed by Sanger sequencing (Fig. 2b), and segregated with disease in the extended family. *CAMTA2* has many transcript variants only six (1, 2, 3, 4, 7, and 10) of which are protein coding (https://www.proteinatlas.org/ENSG00000108509-CAMTA2/tissue). The aligned cDNA sequence of the translation start site and adjacent 5′ UTR of these six variants show considerable variation (Fig. 3a). The resulting amino terminus amino acid sequences of these transcript variants are aligned and show

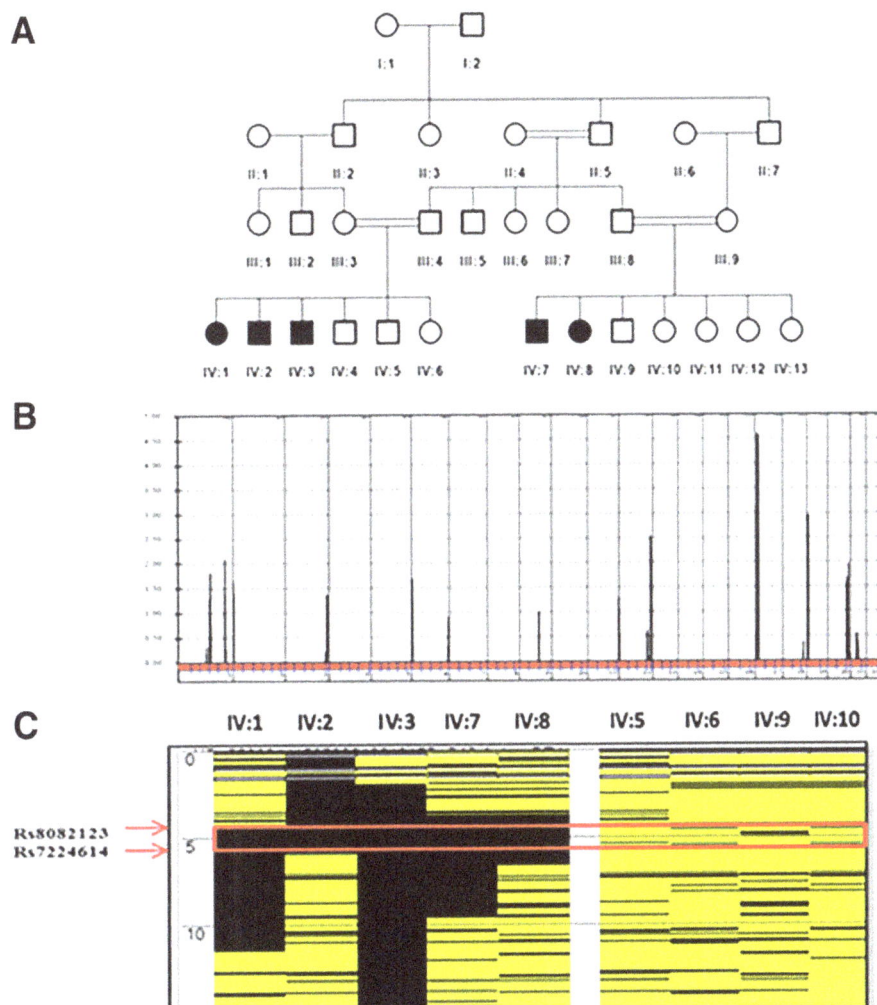

Fig. 1 Identification of a dystonia-associated locus on chromosome 17. **a** Pedigree of an extended family with novel syndromic familial tremulous dystonia. **b** Genome-wide linkage analysis revealed a maximal peak with a LOD score of 4.58 on chromosome 17. **c** AutoSNPa output for chromosome 17 reveals an ROH (boxed in red) shared among affected members (IV:1, IV:2, IV:3, IV:7, and IV:8) and not present in unaffected individuals (IV:4, IV:5, IV:6, and IV:9)

that the first 12 amino acids of transcript variant 2 are not shared by the other protein coding transcript variants (Fig. 3b). Despite the absence of linkage or homozygosity mapping data to suggest involvement of any known dystonia loci, WES of all affected individuals, parents, and unaffected siblings from both nuclear families was undertaken. There were no variants in any of the known dystonia genes (*TOR1A, TUBB4A, THAP1, CIZ1, ANO3, GNAL. SCGE, GCH1, TH, TITF1, TAF1, PRKRA, ATP1A3, SLC63, ADCY5*) that survived filtration that removed alleles present in public databases at a frequency > 2%, in any affected individual.

The wild-type *CAMTA2* 5′UTR 35 nt translation initiation region was subjected to analysis by a RNAdraw secondary structure program [20]. The structure obtained is a hairpin with three stems that is weakly stable (ΔG=11.1 kcal). The G>A variant 6 bases upstream of

the *CAMTA2* transcript variant 2 initiation AUG changed this structure to a more relaxed form (ΔG=9.5 kcal) compared to the wild type. More importantly, the mutant variant secondary structure has only two stems and a wider loop as opposed to the three stem-tight loop of the wild type (Fig. 4a).

In order to evaluate the effects of the *CAMTA2* transcript variant 2 mutation on 5′UTR-linked activities such as transcription and translation, we constructed a fluorescence reporter cassette that contained a 25 nt initiation region upstream of SGFP (Fig. 4b). We subsequently transfected HEK293 cells with the wild type or mutant *CAMTA2* transcript variant 2 5′UTR initiation region containing expression cassettes and measured both the mRNA (qRT-PCR) and protein levels (fluorescence). We observed significant reduction in protein

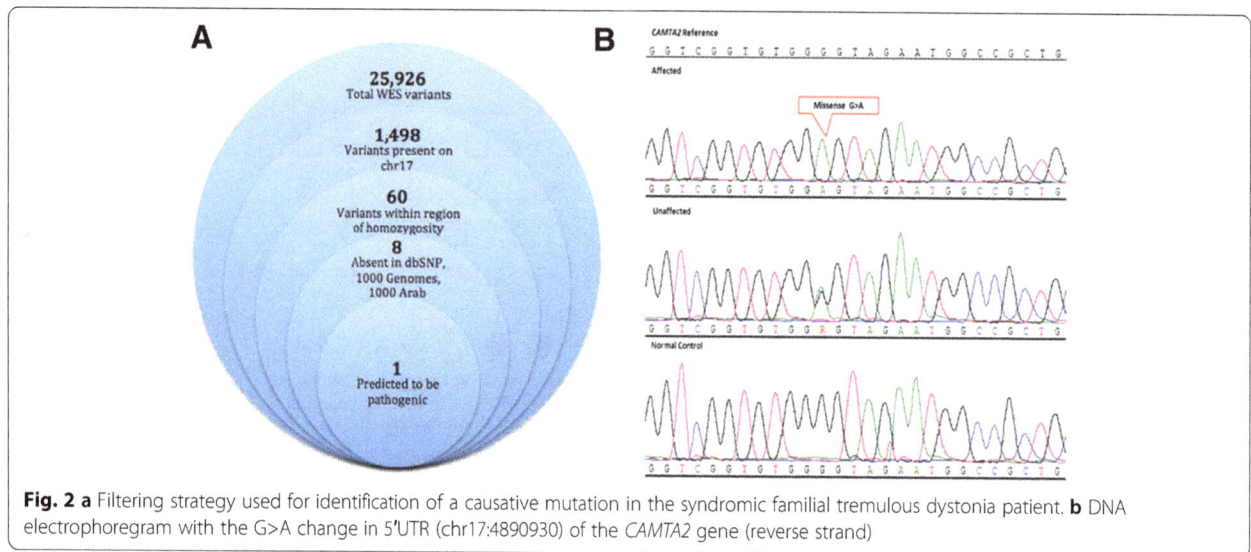

Fig. 2 a Filtering strategy used for identification of a causative mutation in the syndromic familial tremulous dystonia patient. **b** DNA electrophoregram with the G>A change in 5′UTR (chr17:4890930) of the *CAMTA2* gene (reverse strand)

(fluorescence levels; (Fig. 4c)) but not mRNA levels of the mutant *CAMTA2* transcript variant 2 expression cassette relative to its wild-type counterpart (Fig. 4d).

PCR amplification of each protein coding isoform of *CAMTA2* indicated differential expression of isoform 2 which was only detected in the vermis cerebellum, left and right cerebellum, cerebral cortex, olfactory lobe, and cerebellar peduncles. Expression of this variant was not detected in the corpus callosum, hippocampus, occipital, or frontal lobes (Fig. 5a). GAPDH expression was used as an internal control for PCR amplification and specificity for each isoform confirmed by Sanger sequencing of amplicons as shown for transcript variant 2 (Fig. 5b). Other protein coding transcript variants of CAMTA2 (1, 3, 4, 7, and 10) were ubiquitously expressed in most sub-regions of the brain tested (Additional file 3).

Discussion

We have described the clinical and genetic characteristics of a novel autosomal recessive familial tremulous dystonia syndrome, characterized by juvenile onset tremulous dystonia with spasticity and white matter disease. Phenotypically, the syndrome was heterogeneous within the families studied with all affected individuals displaying variable forms of both focal or segmental dystonia and coarse, asymmetrical, generalized tremor involving the head, neck and extremities [19]. Isolated dystonia is a classification reserved for exclusive occurrence of dystonia with the exception of tremor, whereas combined dystonia includes additional symptoms such as myoclonus or Parkinsonism by which it is further sub-classified [2].

Disease in the families we report is best characterized as a novel syndromic tremulous dystonia. The phenotype that combines dystonia, tremor, spasticity, and white matter disease clearly defines a novel clinical syndrome [19]. The novel nature of this syndrome is highlighted if not confirmed by identification of a previously undescribed single gene disorder segregating in an autosomal recessive manner within the families studied (LOD score 4.58; chr17:4,536,241-6,670,705). Whole exome and Sanger sequencing identified a homoallelic hypomorphic mutation (c.-6G>A) (NM_001171166.1) just upstream of the translation initiation site in the 5′UTR of *CAMTA2* transcript variant 2, with which disease segregated in the family studied. However, given the nature of WES where 100% coverage of the target region is almost never achieved and the coverage of only flanking regions (10–

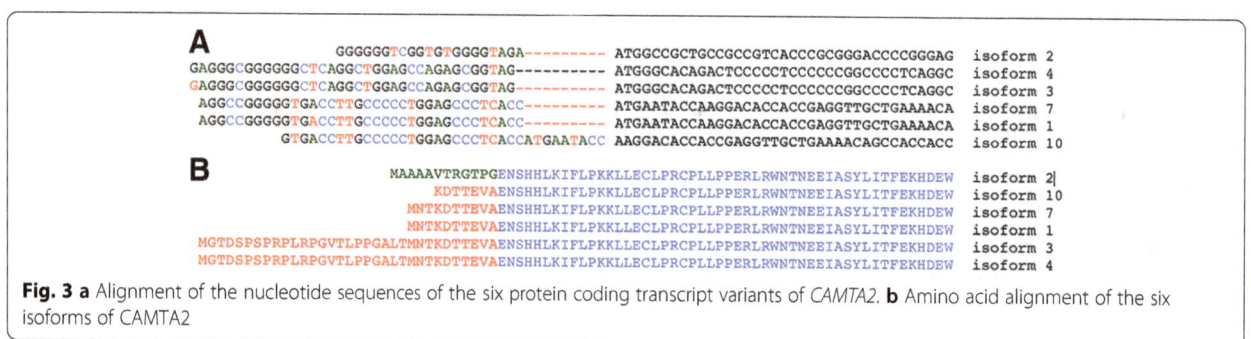

Fig. 3 a Alignment of the nucleotide sequences of the six protein coding transcript variants of *CAMTA2*. **b** Amino acid alignment of the six isoforms of CAMTA2

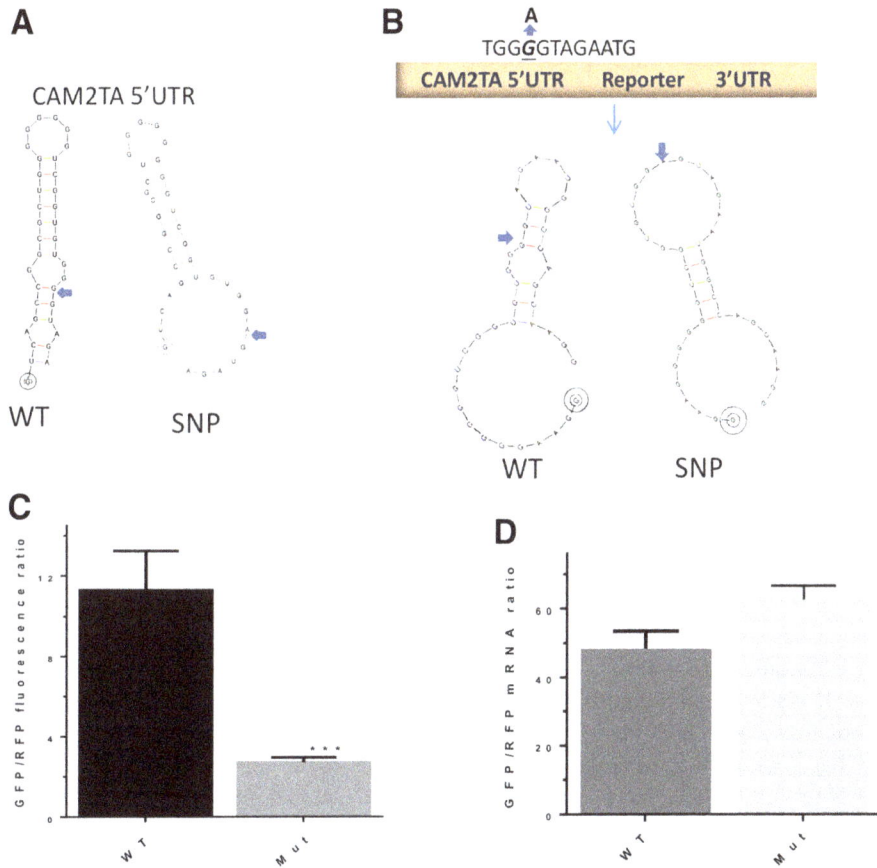

Fig. 4 SNPs nucleotide sequence variation-mediated translational inhibition of CAMTA2. **a** Predicted secondary structures for wild type and mutant initiation region of CAMTA2. **b** Schematic diagram showing the wild type and mutant containing 5'UTR reporter constructs. **c** HEK293 cells (3 × 10⁴ cells/ well) in 96-well plates were transfected with 75 ng of purified wild-type and mutant CAMTA2 5'UTR SGFP-expressing constructs along with control RFP expressing constructs (30 ng). After 20 h, fluorescence was quantified using automated image segmentation and quantification as described in the "Methods" section. The GFP/RFP expression ratio of WT and Mut of 5'UTR are shown as mean ± SD ($n = 6$). ***$p < 0.0001$ (Student's t test). **d** Real-time qRT-PCR for reporter mRNA levels. HEK293 cells were transfected with wild type and mutant *CAMTA2* 5'UTR reporters for 24 h. Total RNA was extracted, and qRT-PCR was performed using specific primers for SGFP and RFP as described in the "Methods" section. Data are presented as the mean ± SD of two independent experiments. **$p = 0.0014$ (Student's t test)

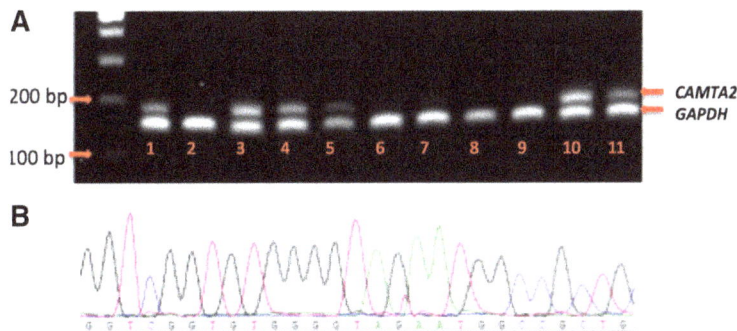

Fig. 5 Expression of *CAMTA2* transcript variant 2 in sub-regions of human brain. **a** PCR amplification of *CAMTA2* transcript variant 2 and *GAPDH* (housekeeping gene) in (1) vermis cerebella, (2) amygdala, (3) cerebellum left, (4) cerebellum right, (5) cerebral cortex, (6) corpus callosum, (7) hippocampus, (8) occipital lobe, (9) frontal lobe, (10) olfactory lobe, and (11) cerebellar peduncles. **b**. Sanger sequencing electrophrogram showing cDNA sequence uniquely identifying *CAMTA2* transcript variant 2

20 bp) of coding sequence in this study, and despite supporting functional evidence, we cannot exclude that a coding point mutation, CNV, deep intronic, or other mutation in the critical interval, in tight linkage disequilibrium with the reported variant, is the true causative mutation.

CAMTA proteins include multiple functional amino acid domains that are evolutionarily conserved including nuclear localization signals, nuclear export signals, a unique DNA binding domain CG-1, TIG-1 involved in protein dimerization, and ANK(ankyrin) repeats involved in protein-protein interactions [21–24]. CAMTA proteins also include a variable number of IQ motifs consisting of a repetitive sequence IQXXXRGXXX known to be associated with binding of Calmodulin (CaM) and CaM-like proteins. Transcription activation domains (TADS) have been reported in Arabadopsis AtCAMTA1, human HsCAMTA2, and functional support derived from reporter genes downstream of TAD's in plant protoplasts or mammalian cell cultures [25]. Cardiac hypertrophy as a consequence transcriptional reprogramming of cardiac gene expression by CAMTA2 interaction with class II histone deacetylase has been reported [26]. In drosophila, CAMTA is highly expressed in retinal cells and has been shown to induce dFbx14 that deactivates the G-protein coupled receptor (GPCR) rhodopsin. This is essential to maintaining Ca^{2+} homeostasis of the photo-transduction pathway, a central mechanism of which is light induced Ca2+ influx and efflux regulated through CaM and dmCAMTA [27]. It is not surprising that CAMTA2 is strongly expressed in both developing and adult murine retina; however, its function in this context remains unknown. Given the diverse expression and activity of GPCRs, it is reasonable to speculate that regulation of this class of molecule by CAMTA may modulate cellular growth and differentiation as evidenced in cardiac hypertrophy [26]. Both CAMTA1 and CAMTA2 are highly expressed in the heart and brain [27]. CAMTA2 has six protein coding isoforms (CAMTA2 ENSG00000108509) ranging from 178 to 1241 amino acids. The expression pattern and function of each isoform remains unknown.

In this study, we identified a G>A change in the 5' UTR of CAMTA2 transcript variant 2. The position of the variant, near a splice site (+ 30) and adjacent to the translation initiation site (– 6) suggested that it might impact CAMTA2 transcript variant 2 expression or translation. Our results clearly indicated that the CAMTA2 mutant affected processes downstream of mRNA transcription, most likely translation as protein levels were dramatically reduced while there was no effect on mRNA levels (Fig. 4c–d). As protein expression was severely impacted without any alteration in the coding region (i.e, no amino acid change), the hypomorphic

nature of the underlying mutation is clearly evident. It is known that secondary structures in the 5'UTR with stable high-energy forms ($\Delta G<-50$ kcal/mol) inhibit translation if near the mRNA methyl G cap [28]. Hairpin structures of weaker energy coupled with positions far away from the 5'end cap such as in our case, in contrast, enhance translation [28]. The wild-type CAMTA2 5' UTR-predicted structure is near the initiation codon and of weakly stable structure, thus may facilitate translation machinery entry and therefore enhances translation. These activities are lost in the case of the mutant variant. In general, mutations near initiation regions can dramatically affect translation. Context sequence upstream of the initiation codon can modulate the scanning activity of the 40S ribosomal subunit affecting translation; mutations in this region, such as those in the Kozak consensus sequence that direct ribosomes to initiate protein synthesis, negatively affect translation initiation [29].

Further support for the pathogenicity or association of the CAMTA2 variant with the phenotype described (for which we propose the name Bohlega Syndrome) in affected members of the family studied comes from the expression pattern of CAMTA2 transcript variant 2 in human brain sub-regions where it is expressed in the vermis cerebellum, left and right cerebellum, cerebral cortex, olfactory lobe, and cerebellar peduncles (Fig. 5a). Expression of this isoform was not detected in the corpus callosum, hippocampus, and occipital or frontal lobes (Fig. 5a). Other CAMTA2 protein coding transcripts were ubiquitously expressed in all brain sub-regions tested. In mouse brain, CAMTA2 is expressed in Purkinje cells and granule cells of the dentate gyrus, pyramidal layer, and cerebellum (Additional file 4), but the distribution of each isoform is not known. Dystonia and Parkinsonism, including tremor, have largely been attributed to dysfunction of the basal ganglia. However, more recently, the role of Purkinje cells, the cerebellum, and their links to the basal ganglia in dystonia and Parkinson's disease have been questioned [30–32]. Anatomical studies have identified connections from the basal ganglia and cerebellum via the thalamus to the cortex [33]. Of note, the ability of CAMTA2 knockout mice to mount a hypertrophic response to cardiac stress such as aortic banding is severely compromised [27]. There was no report of any tremor or dystonia in the CAMTA2 knockout mouse. In the affected individuals from our study, absence of any clinical cardiac symptoms extends the apparent discordance between the human and mouse phenotypes, albeit the mouse phenotype was induced by severe stress (aortic banding) [27]. However, the mouse ENCODE consortium mapped transcription factor binding and other regulatory domains across the mouse genome and compared them with the human genome. While they identified substantial conservation, they also identified a large degree of divergence between mouse and man in transcription and transcription regulation [34]. Therefore, differences in mouse and human phenotypes associated with genes such as *CAMTA2* involving transcription or transcription regulation should not be unexpected.

Conclusions

Our study identifies a novel dystonia locus *CAMTA2* that opens a new line of investigation associated with the role of CAMTA2 in the growth, differentiation, survival, and function of cells and their cellular mechanisms within the brain as related to movement disorders. It also highlights the value of rare inherited disorders in providing insight into more common disease states such as dystonia and tremor.

Methods

Subjects and nucleic acid extraction

Five patients from a consanguineous extended family (two nuclear families) (Fig. 1a) were examined in the Department of Neurosciences, King Faisal Specialist Hospital and Research Center (KFSHRC). They were diagnosed with familial tremulous dystonia. All subjects were enrolled under a KFSHRC IRB-approved (RAC# 2090011) protocol with full-written informed consent.

Genomic DNA extraction

Genomic DNA was extracted from peripheral blood samples of patients and family members using a Gentra Puregene Kit (QIAGEN GmbH, Hilden, Germany). Purity and quantity of DNA samples were assessed spectrophotometrically and stored at − 20 °C until required.

Clinical data and imaging

Patients were seen and examined in the neurology clinic of King Faisal Specialist Hospital and Research Centre (KFSHRC) by certified neurologists (H.A. and S.B.). Briefly, the clinical data was obtained from the charts of patients at the time of the study and during the 20 years of follow-up. Imaging was performed by magnetic resonance imaging (MRI) 3 T using the following sequences: T1, T2, FLAIR, DWI, ADC, and MR spectroscopy. The other clinical, neurophysiological, and laboratory methodology may be reviewed from the previously published clinical paper [19].

Linkage and Homozygosity mapping

All participating individuals (affected and unaffected) were genotyped using an Affymetrix Axiom Genome-Wide CEU array containing 587,353 markers (Affymetrix, Santa Clara, CA, USA) following the manufacturer's protocol (http://www.affymetrix.com/support/technical/manuals.affx).

Resulting genotypes were analyzed for shared runs of homozygosity (ROH) using autoSNPa (http://dna.leeds.ac.uk/autosnpa/). Linkage analysis was performed using the Allegro module of Easy Linkage assuming autosomal recessive inheritance and 100% penetrance (http://genetik.charite.de/hoffmann/easyLINKAGE/index.html). For linkage analysis, the extended family was broken down to reflect the two consanguineous nuclear families, with both independent LOD scores and a combined total LOD score being calculated, in a single multipoint analysis of both nuclear families.

Whole exome sequencing and analysis

DNA was amplified to obtain a whole exome Ion Proton AmpliSeq library which was further used for emulsion PCR on an Ion One Touch System followed by an enrichment process using an Ion OneTouch ES, both procedures following the manufacturer's instructions (Life Technologies, Carlsbad, CA, USA). The template-positive Ion PI Ion Sphere particles were processed for sequencing on the Ion Proton instrument (Life Technologies, Carlsbad, CA, USA). Approximately 15–17 Gb of sequence was generated per sequencing run. Reads were mapped to UCSC hg19 (http://genome.ucsc.edu/) and variants identified using the Ion Torrent pipeline (Life Technologies, Carlsbad, CA, USA). Based upon the consanguineous inbred pedigree and a clear autosomal recessive inheritance pattern in the family studied, the resultant variant caller file (vcf) was filtered to include only homozygous variants in the critical interval on chromosome identified by linkage and homozygosity mapping, within the pre-determined ROH shared by all affected individuals only. These were further filtered to only retain variants that were present in public databases including NHLBI Exome Sequencing Project, 1000 genomes project (phase 3), Exome Aggregation Consortium (ExAC) (version 0.3.1), dbSNP (build 141), and Kaviar (Known VARiants) (September 2015) databases at an incidence of < 2%. Included variants were further selected based upon pathogenicity predicted by Polyphen2 (http://genetics.bwh.harvard.edu/pph2/), SIFT (http://sift.jcvi.org/), and CADD (http://cadd.gs.washington.edu/info). Potential causative variant(s) were validated by Sanger sequencing and further vetted for familial segregation based upon autosomal recessive inheritance. For validation, an amplicon incorporating the variant of interest was amplified and sequenced using a BigDye Terminator kit (Applied Biosystems, Foster City, CA) and run on an ABI 3730xl automated sequencer (Applied Biosystems, Foster City, CA). SeqScape v.2.6 software (Applied Biosystems, Foster City, CA) was used to align sequence data and confirm variants. *CAMTA2* transcript variant 2 is a human isoform and aligns with the human reference sequence of this gene.

Expression constructs

The *CAM2TA* 5'UTR reporter expression constructs were generated by using a cloning-free PCR method [35]. The *CAM2TA* 5'UTR wild type and mutant sequences (underlined) were incorporated in the forward primer: CCTAT-CAGTGATAGGGCGGCTGGG*TATATAA*TGGAAG<u>GGGG GGTCGGTGTGGG</u>/<u>AGTAGA</u>ATGGCCAGCAAGG.

The sequence also contained a minimal promoter (TATA box in italics), 15 bases of complementary sequence to an expression vector containing strong modified EGFP, *UWr*-EGFP (SGFP), and a 3'UTR [36]. The reverse primer is complementary to a downstream region of the poly(A) site on the vector. Briefly, PCR was performed with the following conditions: 2.5 units of HotStart Taq(Qiagen) and 0.2 units of Pfx polymerase (Invitrogen, Carlsbad, CA) mix, 100 ng, template and cycle conditions: 95 °C for 12 min, 31 cycles of: 94 °C, 1 min., 55 °C, 1 min., 72 °C, 4 min., and final extension at 72 °C for 7 min. The PCR products were purified using Qiagen PCR purification columns and eluted in sterile water. The PCR products were run on a 1.2% agarose gel and visualized by ethidium bromide under UV light to verify size and quality. The resultant purified constructs contained a minimal promoter, *CAM2TA2* 5'UTR, SGFP reporter, and 3'UTR, and were used for transfection.

Cells and transfection

HEK293 was obtained from the ATCC (Rockville, MD) and cultured in DMEM medium (Invitrogen, Carlsbad, CA) supplemented with 10% FBS and antibiotics at 37 °C in 5% CO_2. Cells were seeded at 3×10^4 cells per well in 96-well clear-bottom black plates (Matrix technologies, Hudson, NH) and incubated overnight. Cells were transfected with purified reporter constructs. Transfections with *CAM2TA2 5'UTR*-SGFP reporter along with a normalization control RFP expression plasmid driven by constitutive yet non-inducible RPS30 promoter [37] were performed in serum-free medium for 4 h, using Lipofectinamine 2000 (Invitrogen) according to the manufacturer's instructions. Subsequently, the cell culture were replaced with completed DMEM medium and incubated further for 16 h. At these conditions, no effect on cell viability was observed. All transfections were performed in several replicates as indicated in the text. Fluorescence were acquired by the BD imaging pathway and quantified using the Proxcell imaging segmentation and quantification program [38]. The variance in GFP fluorescence among replicate microwells was < 10%. Data are presented as mean values ± standard deviation (SD) of total fluorescence intensity in each well, with at least six replicate readings.

Real-time RT-PCR

Quantitative real-time (qRT-PCR) was performed for SGFP and RFP reporter mRNA using SybrGreen Real-Time PCR. Briefly, total RNAs were treated with DNase I, and cDNAs were used with Lightcycler Faststart DNA master SYBR Green I, (Roche, USA). The following primers were used: SGFP forward: GCCAGGTCTTTTCTGCAGT-CACCG; reverse: GTAGTGCAGATGAACTTCAGG); human GAPDH forward: GGCAAATTCAACGGCACAGT; reverse: GATGGTGATGGGCTTCCC. In all cases, relative quantification of expression was determined using the standard curve method and the values obtained were within both detectable and linear range. Average concentrations were normalized to the endogenous GAPDH gene. The final results were converted to ratio ± SD of the specific mRNA levels to housekeeping mRNA levels. qRT-PCR was performed in multiplex using the Chroma 4DNA Engine thermocycler (Bio-Rad).

Amplification of *CAMTA2* protein coding isoforms from human cDNA libraries

We used cDNA libraries prepared from total RNA isolated from normal human adult brain tissues: vermis cerebelli, amygdala, cerebellum left, cerebellum right, cerebral cortex, corpus callosum, hippocampus, occipital lobe, frontal lobe, olfactory, and cerebellar peduncles (BioChain Institute, Newark, CA) to determine the expression pattern of CAMTA2 isoforms in human brain sub-regions, skeletal muscle, and cardiac muscle. The cDNA libraries were used as template for PCR amplification of protein coding *CAMTA2* isoforms (isoform 1, isoform 2, isoform 3, isoform 4, isoform 7, and isoform 10). Briefly, PCR mixtures containing 2.5 ng cDNA, 1× PCR buffer, 2.5 mM each dNTP, 0.5 µM each primer, and 0.25 U HotStar Taq polymerase (Qiagen) were cycled 30 times at 95 °C for 15 min, 95 °C for 45 s, 64 °C for 45 s, and 72 °C for 60 s. *GAPDH* was amplified in a multiplex reaction as an internal PCR control. Primer information is available on request. The resulting amplicons were evaluated by electrophoresis on a 2% agarose gel. Representative bands were sequenced to confirm amplicon specificity.

Acknowledgements

The authors would like to thank the family members for their participation in this study. We thank the Genotyping and Sequencing Core Facilities of King Faisal Specialist Hospital & Research Centre (KFSHRC) for their contributions.

Work described was supported by grants from KFSHRC (RAC#2090011) and King Abdulaziz City for Science and Technology (KACST) (KACST-12-BIO2943-20). We would also like to acknowledge the support of KACST through the Saudi Human Genome Project (SHGP).

Funding

This work was funded through grants from King Faisal Specialist Hospital & Research Centre (RAC#2090011) and King Abdulaziz City for Science and Technology (KACST-12-BIO2943-20).

Authors' contributions

DM contributed to the conception and design, acquisition and analysis of data, and drafting of the manuscript and figures. HA participated in the acquisition and analysis of data, and drafting of the manuscript and figures. EN participated in the acquisition and analysis of data and drafting of the manuscript and figures. BA contributed to the acquisition and analysis of data and drafting of the manuscript and figures. MAB contributed to the acquisition and analysis of data. MAS participated in the acquisition and analysis of data. SW contributed to the acquisition and analysis of data and drafting of the manuscript and figures. BM participated in the conception and design, acquisition and analysis of data and drafting of the manuscript and figures. KK participated in the conception and design, acquisition and analysis of data and drafting of the manuscript and figures. SB contributed to the conception and design, acquisition and analysis of data and drafting of the manuscript and figures. All authors read and approved the final manuscript.

Competing interests

The authors declare no competing interest regarding the production of this article. The authors have no personal financial or institutional interest in any of the drugs, materials, or devices described in this article.

Author details

¹Department of Genetics, King Faisal Specialist Hospital, and Research Centre, PO Box 3354, Riyadh 11211, Saudi Arabia. ²Saudi Human Genome Program, King Abdulaziz City for Science and Technology, Riyadh, Saudi Arabia. ³Department of Neurosciences, King Faisal Specialist Hospital and Research Centre, PO Box 3354, Riyadh 11211, Saudi Arabia. ⁴Biomolecular Medicine, Research Centre, King Faisal Specialist Hospital and Research Centre, Riyadh, Saudi Arabia.

References

1. Albanese A, Bhatia K, Bressman SB, et al. Phenomenology and classification of dystonia: a consensus update. Movement disorders : official journal of the Movement Disorder Society. 2013;28(7):863–73.
2. Balint B, Bhatia KP. Isolated and combined dystonia syndromes—an update on new genes and their phenotypes. European journal of neurology : the official journal of the European Federation of Neurological Societies. 2015;22(4):610–7.
3. Charlesworth G, Bhatia KP, Wood NW. The genetics of dystonia: new twists in an old tale. Brain : a journal of neurology. 2013;136(Pt 7):2017–37.
4. Ozelius LJ, Hewett J, Kramer P, et al. Fine localization of the torsion dystonia gene (DYT1) on human chromosome 9q34: YAC map and linkage disequilibrium. Genome Res. 1997;7(5):483–94.
5. Zirn B, Grundmann K, Huppke P, et al. Novel TOR1A mutation p.Arg288Gln in early-onset dystonia (DYT1). J Neurol Neurosurg Psychiatry. 2008;79(12):1327–30.
6. Clot F, Grabli D, Burbaud P, et al. Screening of the THAP1 gene in patients with early-onset dystonia: myoclonic jerks are part of the dystonia 6 phenotype. Neurogenetics. 2011;12(1):87–9.
7. Fuchs T, Gavarini S, Saunders-Pullman R, et al. Mutations in the THAP1 gene are responsible for DYT6 primary torsion dystonia. Nat Genet. 2009;41(3):286–8.
8. Xiao J, Uitti RJ, Zhao Y, et al. Mutations in CIZ1 cause adult onset primary cervical dystonia. Ann Neurol. 2012;71(4):458–69.
9. Charlesworth G, Plagnol V, Holmstrom KM, et al. Mutations in ANO3 cause dominant craniocervical dystonia: ion channel implicated in pathogenesis. Am J Hum Genet. 2012;91(6):1041–50.
10. Fuchs T, Saunders-Pullman R, Masuho I, et al. Mutations in GNAL cause primary torsion dystonia. Nat Genet. 2013;45(1):88–92.
11. Saunders-Pullman R, Fuchs T, San Luciano M, et al. Heterogeneity in primary dystonia: lessons from THAP1, GNAL, and TOR1A in Amish-Mennonites. Movement disorders : official journal of the Movement Disorder Society. 2014;29(6):812–8.
12. Hersheson J, Mencacci NE, Davis M, et al. Mutations in the autoregulatory domain of beta-tubulin 4a cause hereditary dystonia. Ann Neurol. 2013;73(4):546–53.
13. Wilcox RA, Winkler S, Lohmann K, Klein C. Whispering dysphonia in an Australian family (DYT4): a clinical and genetic reappraisal. Movement disorders : official journal of the Movement Disorder Society. 2011;26(13):2404–8.
14. Camargos S, Scholz S, Simon-Sanchez J, et al. DYT16, a novel young-onset dystonia-parkinsonism disorder: identification of a segregating mutation in the stress-response protein PRKRA. Lancet Neurol. 2008;7(3):207–15.
15. Zech M, Lam DD, Francescatto L, et al. Recessive mutations in the alpha3 (VI) collagen gene COL6A3 cause early-onset isolated dystonia. Am J Hum Genet. 2015;96(6):883–93.
16. Charlesworth G, Angelova PR, Bartolome-Robledo F, et al. Mutations in HPCA cause autosomal-recessive primary isolated dystonia. Am J Hum Genet. 2015;96(4):657–65.
17. Chen YZ, Friedman JR, Chen DH, et al. Gain-of-function ADCY5 mutations in familial dyskinesia with facial myokymia. Ann Neurol. 2014;75(4):542–9.
18. Chen YZ, Matsushita MM, Robertson P, et al. Autosomal dominant familial dyskinesia and facial myokymia: single exome sequencing identifies a mutation in adenylyl cyclase 5. Arch Neurol. 2012;69(5):630–5.
19. Bohlega S, Stigsby B, al-Kawi MZ, et al. Familial tremulous and myoclonic dystonia with white matter changes in brain magnetic resonance imaging. Movement disorders : official journal of the Movement Disorder Society. 1995;10(4):513–7.
20. Matzura O, Wennborg A. RNAdraw: an integrated program for RNA secondary structure calculation and analysis under 32-bit Microsoft Windows. Computer applications in the biosciences : CABIOS. 1996;12(3):247–9.
21. Aravind L, Koonin EV. Gleaning non-trivial structural, functional and evolutionary information about proteins by iterative database searches. J Mol Biol. 1999;287(5):1023–40.
22. Bouche N, Scharlat A, Snedden W, Bouchez D, Fromm H. A novel family of calmodulin-binding transcription activators in multicellular organisms. J Biol Chem. 2002;277(24):21851–61.
23. Muller CW, Rey FA, Sodeoka M, Verdine GL, Harrison SC. Structure of the NF-kappa B p50 homodimer bound to DNA. Nature. 1995;373(6512):311–7.
24. Sedgwick SG, Smerdon SJ. The ankyrin repeat: a diversity of interactions on a common structural framework. Trends Biochem Sci. 1999;24(8):311–6.
25. Finkler A, Ashery-Padan R, Fromm H. CAMTAs: calmodulin-binding transcription activators from plants to human. FEBS Lett. 2007;581(21):3893–8.
26. Schwartz RJ, Schneider MD. CAMTA in cardiac hypertrophy. Cell. 2006;125(3):427–9.
27. Song K, Backs J, McAnally J, et al. The transcriptional coactivator CAMTA2 stimulates cardiac growth by opposing class II histone deacetylases. Cell. 2006;125(3):453–66.
28. Babendure JR, Babendure JL, Ding JH, Tsien RY. Control of mammalian translation by mRNA structure near caps. RNA. 2006;12(5):851–61.
29. Kozak M. Regulation of translation via mRNA structure in prokaryotes and eukaryotes. Gene. 2005;361:13–37.
30. Babij R, Lee M, Cortes E, Vonsattel JP, Faust PL, Louis ED. Purkinje cell axonal anatomy: quantifying morphometric changes in essential tremor versus control brains. Brain : a journal of neurology. 2013;136(Pt 10):3051–61.
31. Lewis MM, Galley S, Johnson S, Stevenson J, Huang X, McKeown MJ. The role of the cerebellum in the pathophysiology of Parkinson's disease. The Canadian journal of neurological sciences. J Can Sci Neurol. 2013;40(3):299–306.
32. Prudente CN, Hess EJ, Jinnah HA. Dystonia as a network disorder: what is the role of the cerebellum? Neuroscience. 2014;260:23–35.
33. Middleton FA, Strick PL. Basal ganglia and cerebellar loops: motor and cognitive circuits. Brain Res Brain Res Rev. 2000;31(2–3):236–50.
34. Yue F, Cheng Y, Breschi A, et al. A comparative encyclopedia of DNA elements in the mouse genome. Nature. 2014;515(7527):355–64.
35. al-Haj L, Al-Ahmadi W, Al-Saif M, Demirkaya O, Khabar KS. Cloning-free regulated monitoring of reporter and gene expression. BMC Mol Biol. 2009;10:20.
36. Al-Saif M, Khabar KS. UU/UA dinucleotide frequency reduction in coding regions results in increased mRNA stability and protein expression. Molecular therapy : the journal of the American Society of Gene Therapy. 2012;20(5):954–9.
37. Hitti E, Al-Yahya S, Al-Saif M, et al. A versatile ribosomal protein promoter-based reporter system for selective assessment of RNA stability and post-transcriptional control. RNA. 2010;16(6):1245–55.
38. Mahmoud L, Al-Saif M, Amer HM, Sheikh M, Almajhdi FN, Khabar KS. Green fluorescent protein reporter system with transcriptional sequence heterogeneity for monitoring the interferon response. J Virol. 2011;85(18):9268–75.

16

An efficient method for protein function annotation based on multilayer protein networks

Bihai Zhao, Sai Hu*, Xueyong Li, Fan Zhang, Qinglong Tian and Wenyin Ni*

Abstract

Background: Accurate annotation of protein functions is still a big challenge for understanding life in the post-genomic era. Many computational methods based on protein-protein interaction (PPI) networks have been proposed to predict the function of proteins. However, the precision of these predictions still needs to be improved, due to the incompletion and noise in PPI networks. Integrating network topology and biological information could improve the accuracy of protein function prediction and may also lead to the discovery of multiple interaction types between proteins. Current algorithms generate a single network, which is archived using a weighted sum of all types of protein interactions.

Method: The influences of different types of interactions on the prediction of protein functions are not the same. To address this, we construct multilayer protein networks (MPN) by integrating PPI networks, the domain of proteins, and information on protein complexes. In the MPN, there is more than one type of connections between pairwise proteins. Different types of connections reflect different roles and importance in protein function prediction. Based on the MPN, we propose a new protein function prediction method, named function prediction based on multilayer protein networks (FP-MPN). Given an un-annotated protein, the FP-MPN method visits each layer of the MPN in turn and generates a set of candidate neighbors with known functions. A set of predicted functions for the testing protein is then formed and all of these functions are scored and sorted. Each layer plays different importance on the prediction of protein functions. A number of top-ranking functions are selected to annotate the unknown protein.

Conclusions: The method proposed in this paper was a better predictor when used on *Saccharomyces cerevisiae* protein data than other function prediction methods previously used. The proposed FP-MPN method takes different roles of connections in protein function prediction into account to reduce the artificial noise by introducing biological information.

Background

The accurate annotation of protein functions is the key to understanding life at the molecular level and has great biomedical and pharmaceutical implications. Due to high-throughput biological technologies, a large number of protein sequences [1] are available, while majority of their functions are still unknown. With its inherent difficulty and expense, experimental characterization of protein functions cannot accommodate the ever-increasing number of sequences and structures produced by Genomics Centers. Recent developments in experiments such as

yeast two-hybrid [2], tandem affinity purification [3] and mass spectrometry [4] have resulted in the publications of many high-quality, large-scale protein-protein interaction (PPI) data, which make it possible and feasible to use computational methods to predict functions for un-annotated proteins [5].

The past decade has witnessed a rapid development of computational methods for predicting protein functions from PPI datasets. A neighbor counting (NC) method proposed by Schwikowski et al. [6] predicted an un-annotated protein with the functions that occurred most frequently among its neighbor proteins. However, this method ignored the background frequency of different function annotations. Hishigaki et al. [7] improved the

* Correspondence: husaiccsu@163.com; wenyinccsu@163.com
Department of Mathematics and Computing Science, Changsha University, Changsha, Hunan 410022, China

neighbor counting method by using the Chi-Square statistics instead of frequency as a scoring function. Besides direct neighbors, Chua et al. [8] inferred the functional information within both direct (level 1) and indirect (level 2) neighbors by giving them different weights. Prior methods typically measured proximity as the shortest-path distance in the network, while most proteins are close to each other. Cao et al. [9] introduced diffusion state distance (DSD), a new metric based on a graph diffusion property, designed to capture finer-grained distinctions in proximity for transferring functional annotation in PPI networks. Other methods have been introduced to make functional prediction by getting the most consistent agreement throughout the whole PPI networks [10]. Chi et al. [11] proposed an approach that predicted protein functions iteratively. This iterative approach incorporated the local and global semantic influence of protein functions into the prediction. Some kind of network-based methods partitioned proteins in PPI networks into several function modules [12], and the proteins in the same modules are assigned with the same functions. Lee et al. [13] applied a novel method that generated improved modularity solutions, and developed a better method to use this community information to predict protein's functions.

Taking both high noise in PPI data and insufficient number of available annotated proteins into account, some researchers have tried to improve the prediction performance by incorporating other heterogeneous data sources. Cozzetto et al. [14] proposed an integrative approach for addressing annotation challenge, which combines into a wide variety of biological information sources encompassing sequence, gene expression, and PPI data. Zhang et al. [15] presented a novel protein function prediction method that combined protein domain composition information and PPI networks. Domain combination similarity (DCS) [16] was applied to predict protein function by integrating PPI networks and proteins' domain information. Different from Zhang's, DCS changed the method to calculate domain context similarity and combined the domain compositions of both proteins and their neighbors. Liang et al. [17] built a network model called protein overlap network (PON) using domain co-occurrence information. In a PON, each node represented a protein and two nodes were connected with an edge if they share a common domain. The function of a protein can be predicted by counting the occurrence frequency of gene ontology (GO) terms associated with domains of direct neighbors in the PON. Recently, some new algorithms are proposed to predict protein function from PPI networks. Gong et al. [18] developed a method named GoFDR for predicting GO-based protein functions. The input for GoFDR is simply a query sequence-based multiple sequence alignment (MSA) produced by PSI-BLAST (Position-Specific Iterated BLAST). Kumar et al.

[19] proposed an improved approach for protein function prediction by exploiting the connectivity properties of prominent proteins. Yu et al. [20] proposed a method called Predicting Protein Function using Multiple Kernels (ProMK). ProMK iteratively optimizes the phases of learning optimal weights and reduces the empirical loss of multi-label classifier for each of the labels simultaneously.

In conclusion, many computational methods that integrate heterogeneous data for predicting protein (or gene) functions have been suggested. Most of these techniques follow the same basic paradigm: firstly, they generate various functional association networks by analyzing implicit information of shared functions of proteins from different data sources. Then these individual networks are combined into a composite and highly reliable network through a weighted sum. The weight of each individual network represents the contribution of the corresponding data source to the function prediction. A correct setting of these weights is thought to be the key to designing an effective function prediction method. In general, the weights adjustment of individual networks is mainly influenced by human experience and statistical analysis. The major drawback of how each network is weighted is that it varies between different datasets. Furthermore, functions of proteins are diverse and some of them only occur under specific conditions. Different functional association networks play different roles and have varying importance in function prediction. Combining a heterogeneous data source into a single weighted network could obscure the inherent nature of the protein function.

To address these difficulties, we construct a multilayer protein network which integrates PPI network topology, domain information, and protein complexes. Additionally, we propose an efficient protein function annotation method, named FP-MPN (function prediction based on multilayer protein networks). FP-MPN takes into account the varying influences by multiple connections in the prediction of protein function. Given an un-annotated protein, FP-MPN generates candidate functions by examining multilayer networks systematically in turn. The performance of FP-MPN was tested on the well-studied species of *Saccharomyces cerevisiae*. Compared to several previously reported protein function prediction algorithms, FP-MPN achieved a greater degree of accuracy in predicting protein function. The experimental results demonstrate that this method, which distinguishes different types of connections in function prediction, is more robust and effective than those methods combining multiple interactions, and that FP-MPN is a good example of this.

Materials and methods
Assessment criteria
Cross-validation is a widely used method to evaluate the performance of protein function prediction algorithms.

The proteins in the PPI network are partitioned into two subsets, the training set and the testing set. Functions are removed from the part of proteins in the PPI network artificially. These proteins consist of the testing set and the rest proteins form the training set. Functions of proteins in the testing set are predicted, using functional information of proteins in the training set. Finally, the comparing results of predicted functions with actual functions are used to evaluate the performance of protein function prediction algorithms. The cross-validation methods can be classified into two categories: leave-one-out cross-validation and leave-percent-out cross-validation. The leave-one-out cross-validation method puts one protein into the testing set and the remaining proteins into the training set, while the leave-percent-out cross-validation method randomly selects a percentage of proteins as the testing set and then puts other proteins into the training set. Each function of proteins in the testing set is assigned with a probability, according to the functions of proteins in the training set. Then a number of top-ranking functions are selected to annotate the protein with unknown functions. The quality of prediction depends on the matching results of predicted functions with actual ones. There are two widely used criteria to measure the predicted results. The one is Precision which measures the percentage of predicted functions that match the known functions. The other is Recall which measures the fraction of known functions that are matched by the predicted ones. They can be calculated as follows:

$$\text{Precision} = \frac{TP}{TP + FP} \quad (1)$$

$$\text{Recall} = \frac{TP}{TP + FN} \quad (2)$$

where TP (true positive) is the number of predicted functions matched by known functions. FP (false positive) is the number of predicted functions that are not matched by known functions. FN (false negative) is the number of known functions that are not matched by predicted functions. Selecting more functions can improve the recall, but it may lead to the reduction of precision. F-measure, as the harmonic mean of precision and recall, is another measure to evaluate the performance of a method synthetically, which is calculated as follows:

$$F\text{-measure} = \frac{2 \times \text{Precision} \times \text{Recall}}{\text{Precision} + \text{Recall}} \quad (3)$$

At the same time, the coverage rate (CR) [21] is also used to evaluate a function prediction algorithm, which shows how many functions of proteins in the testing set can be covered by predicted functions. Given a testing protein set TP = {tp$_1$, tp$_2$, ..., tp$_n$}, KF = {kf$_{11}$, kf$_{12}$,..., kf$_{ij}$,

..., kf$_{nm}$} is a list of known function sets of TP, KF$_i$ = {kf$_{i1}$, kf$_{i2}$,..., kf$_{il}$} is a known function set of the protein tp$_i$. PF = {pf$_{11}$, pf$_{12}$,..., pf$_{ij}$, ..., pf$_{nm}$} is a list of predicted function sets of TP, PF$_i$ = {pf$_{i1}$, pf$_{i2}$,..., pf$_{il}$} is a predicted function set of the protein tp$_i$. The coverage rate is then defined as

$$CR = \sum_{i=1}^{n} |KF_i \cap PF_i| / \sum_{i=1}^{n} |KF_i| \quad (4)$$

Motivation

Some methods try to reconstruct more reliable networks by integrating PPI networks and biological information, in order to reduce the impact of random noise on predicting performance. There exist complex and diverse relationships between proteins as demonstrated after integrating biological information. For example, proteins can interact with each other through physical interactions which can be identified by biological experiments, co-expression based on time course gene expression data [22, 23], or co-annotation based on gene ontology [24, 25], etc. Most of these methods generate various functional association networks, such as co-expression networks and co-annotation networks. Then a single network can be constructed through a weighted sum of these individual networks. The weight assigned to each individual network reflects its contribution towards protein function annotation, which is computed by a specific similar metric for the related biological data.

Figure 1 describes an example of constructed networks by integrating the PPI network and heterogeneous data. Figure 1a shows an original physical PPI network, which was derived from experimental methods. In the co-annotation network, as shown in Fig. 1b, there exists a connection between a pair of proteins if they perform the same functions. As for the co-expressed network, it is based on time course gene expression data. For a protein v, its gene expression at n different times is denoted as a variate:Gen(v) = {T(v, 1), T(v, 2), ..., T(v, n)}, T(v, i) denotes the expression level of gene v at the time point i. Generally, the Pearson correlation coefficient [26] is used to assess the probability of whether two particular proteins are co-expressed. If the Pearson correlation coefficient of two proteins over all time points is greater than 0.8, then they are considered to be co-expressed and are connected in the co-expressed network. The network shown in Fig. 1d is a reconstructed network based on three networks currently used. This network shows that proteins could have a diversity of functions when exposed to different conditions or at different time points. Therefore, the importance and roles of different types of interactions between proteins are not the same for the protein function prediction. When functions are predicted for the unknown protein YJL115W using the

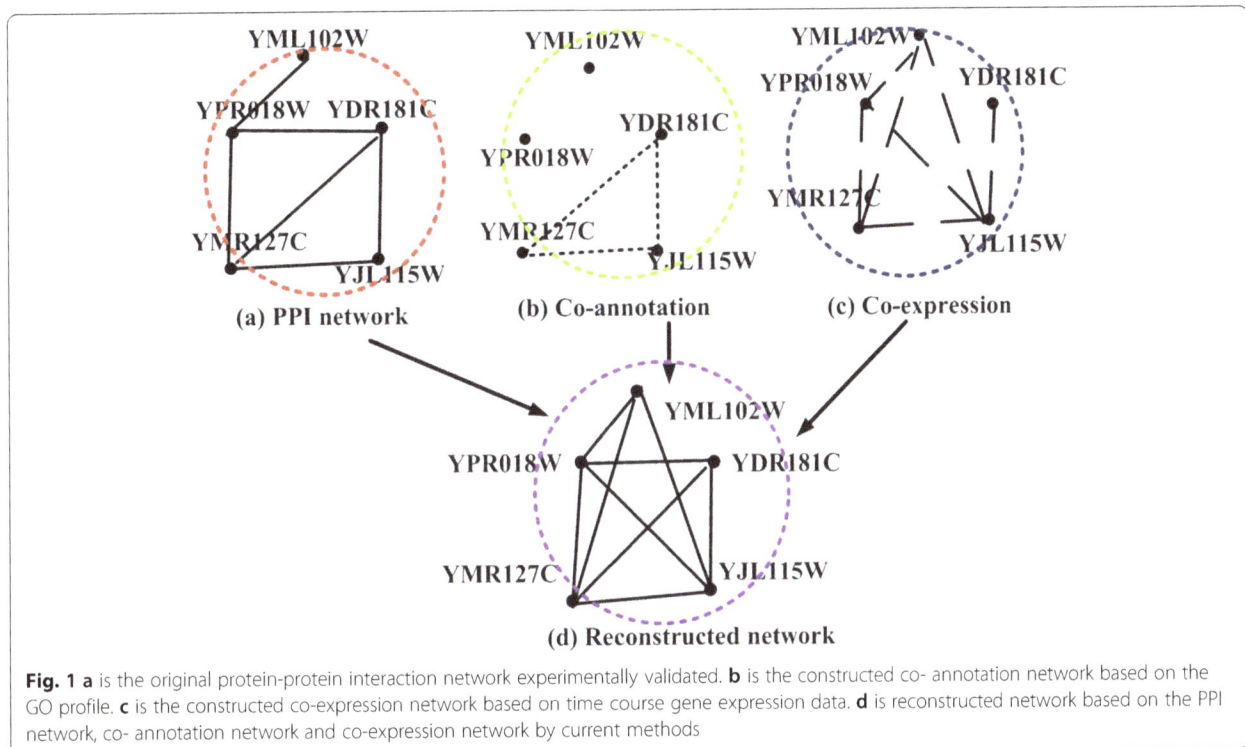

Fig. 1 a is the original protein-protein interaction network experimentally validated. **b** is the constructed co-annotation network based on the GO profile. **c** is the constructed co-expression network based on time course gene expression data. **d** is reconstructed network based on the PPI network, co-annotation network and co-expression network by current methods

constructed network in Fig. 1d, YPR018W and YDR181C are treated in the same way. The connection (YPR018W, YJL115W) and (YDR181C, YJL115W) has the same status and reliability (they both have an edge clustering coefficient [27] of one). After analyzing the original PPI network, co-annotation network, and co-expression network as shown in Fig. 1, it is demonstrated that the connection (YDR181C, YJL115W) is more reliable than (YPR018W, YJL115W), due to its occurrence in all three networks. YPR018W and YJL115W are only co-expressed at the gene expression level, based on gene expression data. Therefore, YDR181C should contribute more to the function prediction of YJL115W, than the protein YPR018W. Connections between YDR181C and YJL115W overlap in the reconstructed network; therefore, it is difficult to determine their relationship. The information mentioned above was obtained from the reconstructed network.

The analysis of this experiment suggests that existing methods have two deficiencies. Different biological data sources (i.e., PPI networks, protein domains, and subcellular information) often describe protein properties in different ways and have different correlations with different GO terms. Combining multiple biological data into a single network can not only enhance the matching accuracy (i.e., recall, which measures the fraction of known functions that are matched to the predicted ones) to a certain extent but also introduce a lot of noise functions and reduce predicting accuracy (i.e., precision, which measures the percentage of predicted functions which match the known

functions). As a result, the comprehensive performance improvement is not apparent. Current methods set different weights for heterogeneous data based on the quality of data sources in order to integrate them into a single network. Setting the weighting system for multiple biological data is the key to ensuring the accuracy of protein function prediction. These optimal weighting methods rely on empirical analysis and have differences between datasets. Furthermore, these weighting methods may also lead to the inconsistency of these prediction algorithms.

In conclusion, it is inappropriate to combine multiple interactions or connections between two proteins, as they often occur under different conditions and play different roles in protein function prediction. In this paper, we describe a multilayer protein network developed by integrating PPI network topology and heterogeneous data. In the constructed network, a pair of proteins has more than one connection which is connected through multiple links. Based on the multilayer protein network, we propose a new method for predicting protein functions, named FP-MPN.

Multilayer protein networks construction

The complex network is a hot, new research area as a result of the increased use of networks in various fields, such as mathematics, social science, and life science. The features of many real-life complex networks are that they are small-world (i.e., high clustering coefficient and small average path length) and scale-free (i.e., follow the power-law distributions in node degree and display the growth and preferential attachment). In reality, connections among nodes in complex networks are diversified. For instance, in social networks, people can contact each other via emails, telephones or MSN, etc., and hence make up a complex network with multi-links. Similarly, in biological networks there are diverse links among proteins via co-expression or co-annotation of the proteins. Multilayer networks are more complex than those with single link.

We consider a multilayer network $G = (V, E)$, where $V = \{v_1, v_2, ..., v_n\}$ represents a set of proteins, the edge set $E = \{Me_1, Me_2, ..., Me_m\}$ consists of edges of L different types representing different relations. That is, $Me_i = \{e_{i1}, e_{i2}, ..., e_{iL}\}$ $(0 < i <= m)$, e_{ij} $(0 < j <= L)$ represents the ith connection in the jth layer of G. We can view the multilayer network as a graph with vector valued edge information, i.e., the adjacency matrix A consists of elements A_{ij}, who are themselves L dimensional vectors: $A_{ij} = \{A_{ij}^{(1)}, A_{ij}^{(2)}, ..., A_{ij}^{(L)}\}$. An alternative way to approach the problem is to view the multi-graph as a collection of L, $N \times N$ adjacency matrices $\{A^{(1)}, A^{(2)}, ..., A^{(L)}\}$, each corresponding to one type of relation. Figure 2 describes an example of a multilayer network according to Fig. 1. The multilayer network consists of five nodes and three

layers. Each layer represents a different level of connection or relationship between nodes.

Functions are often performed by proteins physically interacting with each other, located within the same complex, or by having similar structures. A protein consists of one or more domains which have independent functions. There may be discrepancies within domain combinations among different proteins and it is of great significance to recognize these. In this paper, we develop a multilayer network by integrating the PPI network, protein domain information, and protein complexes. The multilayer network consists of three layers, which include the physical interaction layer (PIL), sharing domain layer (SDL), and sharing complex layer (SCL). The physical interaction layer is derived from original PPI networks. On the SDL, two proteins are physically connected if there is at least one domain common to both of them. On the SCL, each node represents a protein and two nodes are physically connected if they are contained in a common complex. Our previous research on protein complex prediction [28] and essential protein identification [26] suggests that the performance of the prediction algorithm based on weighted networks is superior to that based on un-weighted networks. An

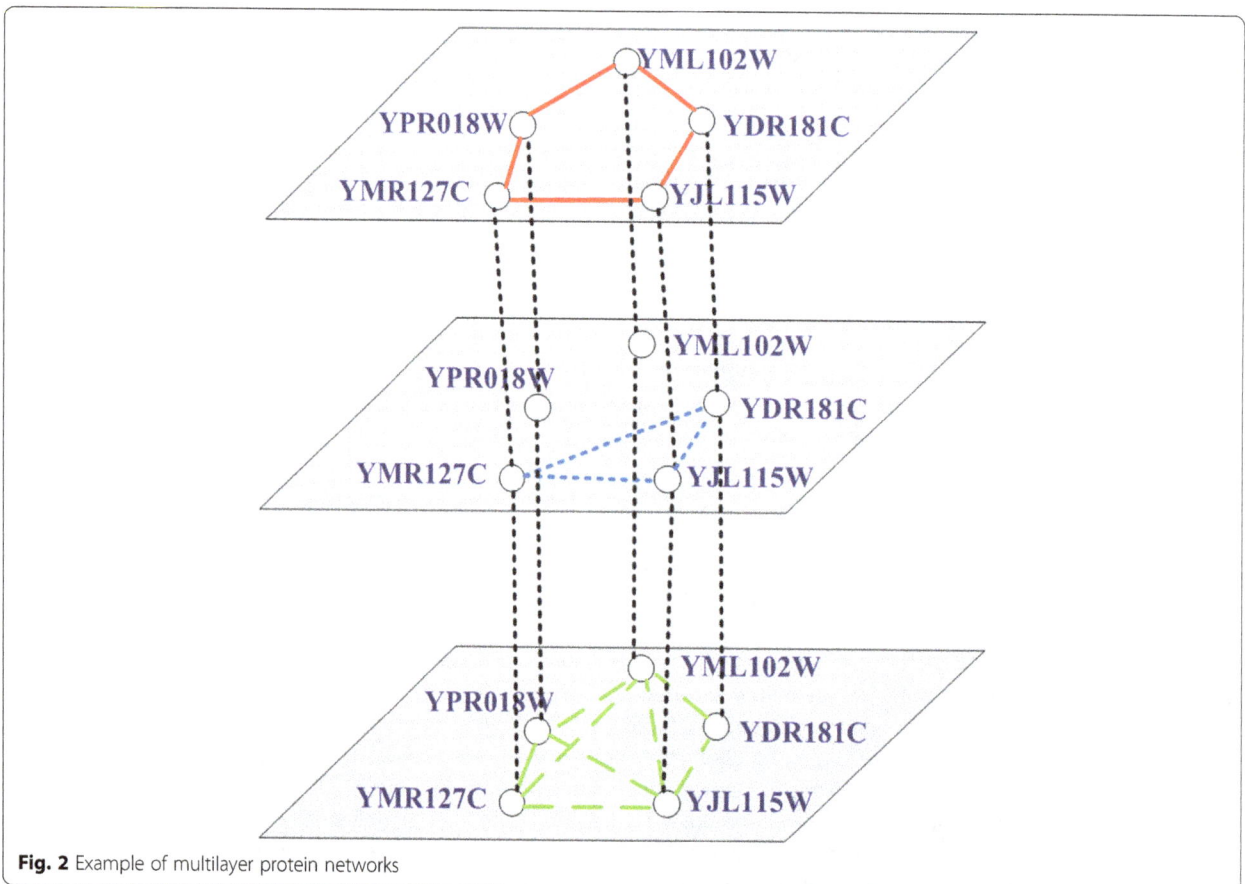

Fig. 2 Example of multilayer protein networks

explanation for this could be that the weight stands for the reliability of interactions and therefore, weighted networks can be more useful than un-weighted networks in the representative of PPI networks. In this work, appropriate weighting methods for the three types of connections are developed for the multilayer network.

Methods of Zhang and DCS successfully integrated domain information and PPI networks, improving the performance of protein function prediction. The two methods rely on the same principle, which is to implement function prediction by way of computing similarities between the two proteins. The two methods differ in that the method described by Zhang only computes similarity through the domain information of the protein itself, while the DCS method expands on the extra domain information of the neighbors surrounding it. The two methods are all based on the computing similarity of the combination formula. However, they have the problem of being highly complex to program. To balance the pros and cons of the two methods, this study has set up the weighting computational formula aiming at the interaction of shared domain as follows:

$$W(v_i, v_j) = \begin{cases} \dfrac{|D_i \cap D_j|^2}{|D_i| \times |D_j|} &, \quad D_i \neq \emptyset \text{ and } D_j \neq \emptyset \\ 0 &, \quad \text{otherwise} \end{cases} \quad (5)$$

where D_i and D_j are sets of distinct domain types of v_i and v_j, respectively.

In a similar way, the weight of sharing complexes between v_i and v_j on the SCL can be calculated as follow:

$$W(v_i, v_j) = \begin{cases} \dfrac{|C_i \cap C_j|^2}{|C_i| \times |C_j|} &, \quad C_i \neq \emptyset \text{ and } C_j \neq \emptyset \\ 0 &, \quad \text{otherwise} \end{cases} \quad (6)$$

where C_i and C_j are the sets of protein complexes that contained v_i and v_j, respectively, and $C_i \cap C_j$ denotes the set of common protein complexes.

As for the weight of connections on the PIL, we suggest that the weight of an interaction can be reflected by the number of common neighbors between the proteins. Here we use a variant of edge clustering coefficient (ECC) [27] to calculate the weight of protein pairs. Given a pair of proteins v_i and v_j, the weight of edge (v_i, v_j) on the PIL is defined as follows:

$$W(v_i, v_j) = \begin{cases} \dfrac{|N_i \cap N_j|^2}{(|N_i|-1) * (|N_j|-1)} &, \quad |N_i| > 1 \text{ and } |N_j| > 10, \text{otherwise} \end{cases}$$

$$\quad (7)$$

where N_i and N_j are sets consisting of all neighbors of v_i and v_j, respectively.

Figure 3 is the visualization of our constructed multilayer protein network. The network consists of three layers, i.e., PIL, SDL, and SCL. There are the same set of proteins and different connections sets on these three layers. The multilayer protein network can be modeled as $G = (V, E)$, where $V = \{v_1, v_2,..., v_n\}$, $E = \{Me_1, Me_2,..., Me_m\}$. $Me_i = \{e_{i1}, e_{i2}, e_{i3}\}$ $(0 < i <= m)$, e_{ij} $(0 < j <= 3)$ represents the ith connection in the jth layer of G.

FP-MPN algorithm

Based on the weighted multilayer protein network, we propose a new method for protein functional prediction, named FP-MPN. How to deal with the multilayer networks is the first problem to be addressed. Current algorithms combine different connections into a single connection when dealing with these complex biological networks. In reality, it is inappropriate to combine multiple connections between two proteins, as they often occur under different conditions and play different roles in protein function prediction. The influences of different types of interactions in protein function prediction are not the same. Combining different interactions into a single event can lead to false positive results. So, it is necessary to deal with multilayer networks in another way.

The different connections among proteins may have different impacts on function prediction. To address this, FP-MPN visits each layer of the multilayer network in turn to generate candidate functions. Each layer has different contribution to predict ion of functions for an un-annotated protein. The FP-MPN algorithm operates in two stages, pre-processing data and predicting functions.

To assign functions of proteins in the testing of a set of probabilities, pre-processing of the multilayer protein network is required. The constructed multilayer protein network can be represented as a tensor $A = (a_{i,j,k})_{n \times n \times m}$, where n is the number of proteins and m is the number of types of interconnections. If node i is connected to node j by the kth type link, $a_{i,j,k}$ is equal to 1; otherwise, it equals 0. Figure 4 depicts the tensor representation of the multilayer network as shown in Fig. 2. Given a tensor A, we can get a new tensor $A^{(1)}$, which is calculated as follows:

$$a_{i,j,k}^{(1)} = \begin{cases} a_{i,j,k} / \sum_{j=1}^{n} a_{i,j,k}, & \sum_{j=1}^{n} a_{i,j,k} > 0, \text{otherwise} \end{cases} \quad (8)$$

Therefore, for each row i of the tensor $A^{(1)}$, $\sum_{j=1}^{n} a_{i,j,k}^{(1)} = 1$ or

$\sum_{j=1}^{n} a_{i,j,k}^{(1)} = 0$.

The second stage of FP-MPN is predicting functions for un-annotated proteins. The FP-MPN method visits each layer of the corresponding multilayer network of the tensor $A^{(1)}$, Given that the proteins interact with each other under different conditions or stimuli in order to perform different functions, FP-MPN generates predicted functions across all layers. While the importance of each layer to the prediction is not the same. We assign different importance

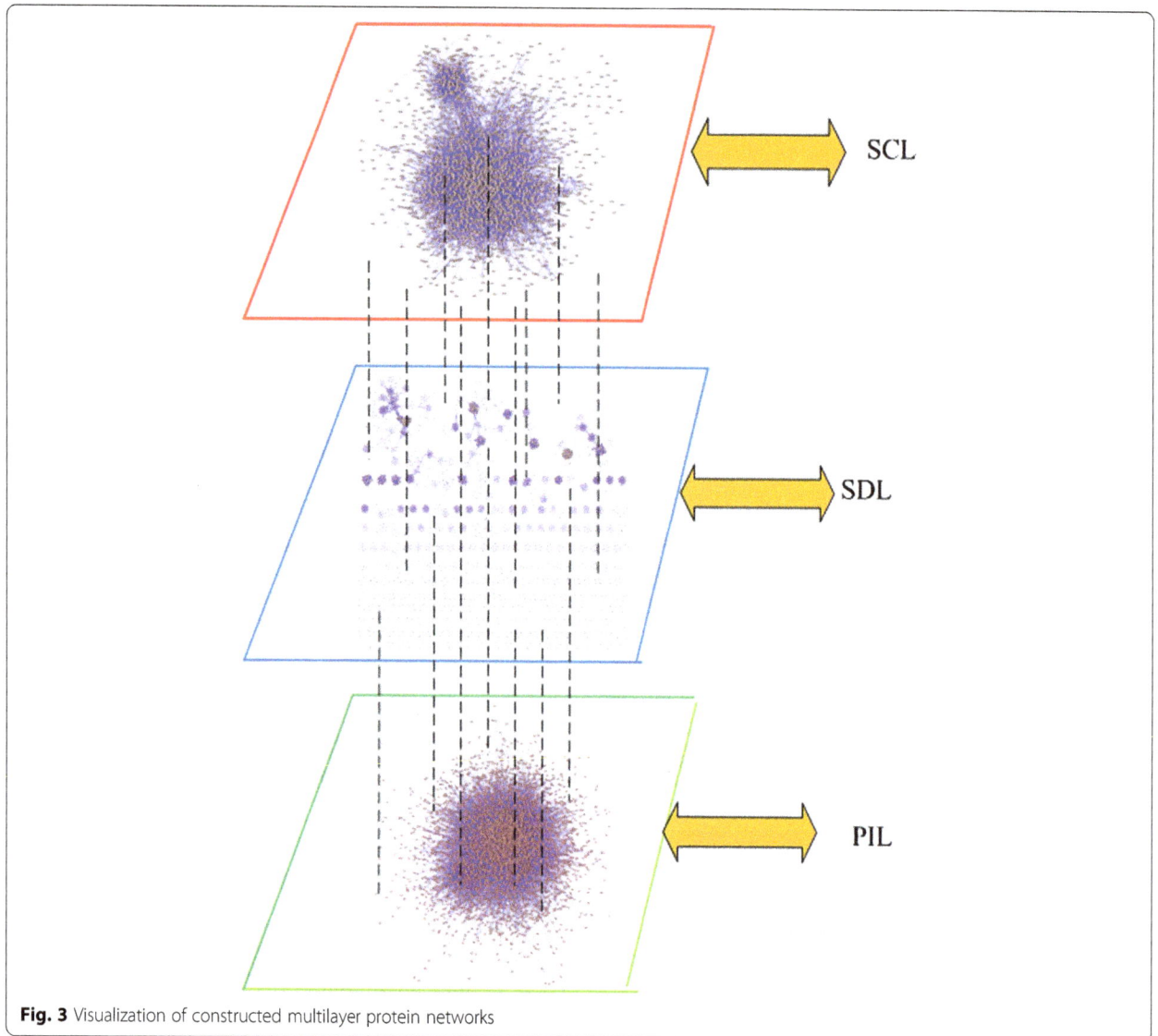

Fig. 3 Visualization of constructed multilayer protein networks

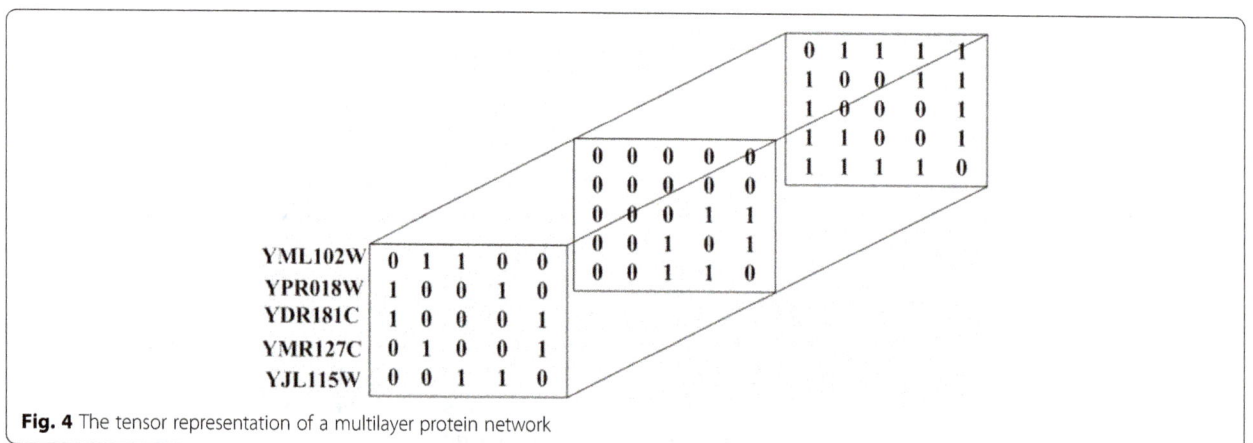

Fig. 4 The tensor representation of a multilayer protein network

coefficient (IC) for each layer of the MPN. For the ith layer, its IC value can be calculated as follow:

$$\mathrm{IC}(i) = \frac{1}{2^i} \quad (9)$$

The final score of a predicted function is the weighed sum of scores achieved from all layers. The IC value of a layer is used to present the weight. The layer accessed firstly has higher IC value than that rest of the layers. For this reason, the set up access sequence of each layer in the MPN is critical for the FP-MPN method. This paper addresses the problem of the impact of each layer on the accuracy of function predictions using statistical analysis. More detailed statistical results can be found in Table 1.

In this experiment, we used the NC [6] method on the SDL, SCL, and PIL to annotate all unknown proteins, using leave-one-out cross-validation. Then, we calculate the average Precision, Recall, and F-measure to evaluate the significance of each layer for function prediction. The original PPI network consisted of 5093 proteins with 24,743 interactions. For the PIL, SDL, and SCL, there are 13,871, 23,749, and 7337 connections, respectively. Using PIL, there are 2388 proteins, which had at least one neighbor. The number of nodes with neighbors on the SDL and SCL is 2972 and 1494, respectively. From Table 1, it can be seen that SCL archives the highest F-measure among the three layers. In addition, 73.83 % (1103/1494 = 73.83 %) of proteins with neighbors on the SCL have been annotated as at least one function. While the proportion of PIL and SDL is 53.35 % (1274/2388 = 53.35 %) and 40.88 % (1215/2972 = 40.88 %), respectively. The SDL gets the second highest F-measure and Recall after SCL among all the layers. Thus, we assigned the highest access sequence to SCL, the second highest priority to SCL, and the lowest order to PIL.

The second stage of FP-MPN consists of two major steps. The first step is to search its neighbors in the MPN for a particular protein u with unknown function, to generate candidate functions. Starting from the layer in MPN which has the highest access sequence, the FP-MPN method creates a functions list PF. These lists of functions are derived from neighbors of the testing protein u. Assume that $P = \{p_1, p_2,..., p_n\}$ is a set of neighbors of the protein u on the first layer, $F = \{f_1, f_2,..., f_m\}$ is a set of functions of all these proteins in P. The score of

a certain function f_j in F can be calculated by the following formula:

$$S(f_j) = \sum_{i=1}^{n} W(u, p_i) \times t_{ij}, \quad (j \in [1, m]) \quad (10)$$

where $W(u, p_i)$ represents the weight of the connection between u and p_i. If p_i contains function f_j, then $t_{ij} = 1$, otherwise $t_{ij} = 0$. Then, the FP-MPN enters the next layer of MPN and continues to predict functions. If a function has been predicted on previous layers, its score is accumulated. This process is repeated for the next layer etc., until all the layers are traversed. For a predicted function f, its final score is the weighed sum of scores on all layers and can be calculated as follow:

$$\mathrm{Score}(f) = \sum_{i=1}^{L} IC(i) * S(f_i) \quad (11)$$

where L is the number of layers, IC(i) is the IC value of the ith layer, and $S(f_i)$ is the score of function f on the ith layer calculated using Equation (10). From Equation (9), it is not difficult to deduce the formula $\sum_{i=1}^{m} IC(i) < 1$, thus ensuring that Score(f) is less than 1 and can be used as a probability of the function f. Figure 5 illustrates how the FP-MPN method gets the predicted functions list. Figure 5a depicts the constructed multilayer protein network. Numbers on the edges of each layer in the MPN represent their corresponding weights. Figure 5b is the tensor representation of MPN after pre-processing, using Equation (8). Figure 5c shows the predicted functions list for the unknown protein A generated by the FP-MPN method. In this example, FP-MPN predicts functions $f3$ and $f4$ according to its neighbors on the SCL. FP-MPN computes the scores of $f3$ and $f4$ on the SCL by Equation (10), which is 1 and 1, respectively. Then, FP-MPN enters the SDL and continues to generate functions. The candidate function set of A's neighbors on SDL consists of $\{f1, f2, f3, f4\}$. The score of $f1, f2, f3, f4$ on the SDL is 0.28, 0.28, 0.72, and 0.72, respectively. In a similar way, FP-MPN records the functions $\{f1, f2, f3, f4, f5\}$ on the PIL. Scores of the five functions are the same that is 0.5. According to Equation (11), the final score of $f3$ can be calculated as follow:

$$\mathrm{Score}(f_3) = 1 * \frac{1}{2} + 0.72 * \frac{1}{2^2} + 0.5 * \frac{1}{2^3} = 0.7425$$

The final score of $f1, f2, f4, f5$ is 0.1325, 0.1325, 0.7425, and 0.0625, respectively.

The last step of the second stage is to rank functions according to their scores and select a top N of the ranked functions for the protein with unknown function. This is a key factor which influences the performance of the function prediction algorithm. Existing methods for function selection

Table 1 Statistical analysis of the influence of three layers

Layers	Annotated proteins	Precision	Recall	F-measure
PIL	1274	0.3791	0.1094	0.1697
SDL	1215	0.3595	0.1538	0.2154
SCL	1103	0.3404	0.1829	0.238

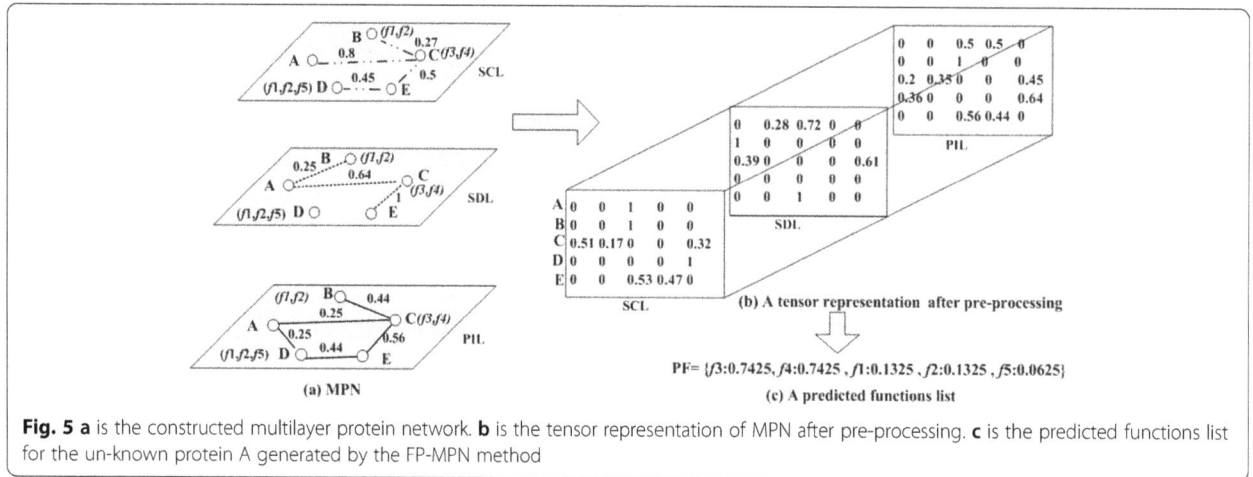

Fig. 5 a is the constructed multilayer protein network. **b** is the tensor representation of MPN after pre-processing. **c** is the predicted functions list for the un-known protein A generated by the FP-MPN method

are mainly implemented in two ways: one is represented by the methods of Zhang [15] and DCS [16], which computes the similarity between proteins and endow all functions of the protein with the highest similarity to the protein with unknown function. Another is represented by the method of NC, which forms candidate functions set by all the functions of the neighbors, then grades and ranks these functions according to a strategy. We have performed statistical analysis for the overlap of functions between the annotated proteins, in order to determine a solution to function selection, as shown in Table 2.

The first column in Table 2 refers to the function overlap between each pair of proteins. The function overlap score of two proteins u and v is defined as follows [28]:

$$OS(u, v) = \frac{|F_u \cap F_v|^2}{|F_u| \times |F_v|} \qquad (12)$$

where F_u and F_v is the function set of proteins u and v, respectively. The second column in Table 2 has shown statistical results of overlaps of all pairs of proteins with shared functions, among which the overlap score of 54.22 % protein pairs has exceeded 0.8. As many proteins have only one function, we made statistics again after excluding those with only one function (the result is shown in the third column). It turned out that the overlap score of more than half of the protein pairs falls in (0.4, 0.6], and

the protein pairs with overlap score over 0.6 accounts for only 11.99 %. Based on these statistical results, the FP-MPN method adopts the second strategy of function selection mentioned above.

All functions are sorted in descending order according to their scores. The top N of these functions can be selected to annotate the testing protein u, where N is the number of functions of the protein most closely associated with u. In this paper, we used the highest weight of a pair of proteins to evaluate the close degree of all their layers. We limited the number of predicted functions to be less than or equal to that of the annotated GO terms in the protein with highest weight to u. Algorithm FP-MPN illustrates the overall framework to predict protein functions based on multilayer protein networks.

Table 2 Statistical analysis of overlaps of functions

OS	Proportion (all proteins)	Proportion (proteins with more than one function)
(0, 0.2]	2.81 %	5.64 %
(0.2, 0.4]	13.90 %	27.95 %
(0.4, 0.6]	27.05 %	54.41 %
(0.6, 0.8]	2.02 %	4.06 %
(0.8, 1]	54.22 %	7.93 %

FP-MPN Algorithm

Input: A PPI network $G = (V, E)$

Output: The set of predicted functions PF

1. Generate a weighted multilayer protein network WG by Equation (5-7);
2. FOR each un- annotated protein u DO
3. $\quad$ $PF = \Phi$; // initialization;
4. $\quad$ FOR $J = 1$ TO 3 DO
5. $\quad\quad$ $CP = \{v_i \mid dis(v_i, u) = 1\} \cup \{u\}$
6. $\quad\quad$ $CF = \{f_i \mid \exists v_i, v_i \in CP, f_i$ is a function of $v_i\}$
7. $\quad\quad$ FOR each function f_i in CF DO
8. $\quad\quad\quad$ IF $f_i \notin PF$ THEN
9. $\quad\quad\quad\quad$ $Score(f_i) = \frac{1}{2^j} \times \sum_{i=1}^{n} W(u, p_i) \times t_{ij}, \ (p_i \in CP)$;
10. $\quad\quad\quad\quad$ insert f_i into PF;
11. $\quad\quad\quad$ ELSE
$\quad\quad\quad\quad$ $Score(f_i) = Score(f_i) + \frac{1}{2^j} \times \sum_{i=1}^{n} W(u, p_i) \times t_{ij}, \ (p_i \in CP)$
12. $\quad\quad\quad$ END IF
13. $\quad\quad$ END FOR
14. $\quad$ END FOR
15. $\quad$ Sort functions in PF descendant by their score
16. $\quad$ Select Top N functions from PF; //N is the number of functions of the protein, which has close degree with u on all layers.
17. $\quad$ Output PF
18. END FOR

Results and discussion

Experimental data

The *S. cerevisiae* (yeast) PPI networks are widely used in the research of network-based function prediction methods, because the species of yeast has been well characterized by knockout experiments and is the most complete and convincible. Here, we also adopt the yeast PPI network to test our method. We have applied our method and four other competing algorithms by integrating network topological features, domain information, and protein complexes data: Zhang [15], DCS [16], domain combination similarity in context of protein complexes (DSCP) [16], and PON [17] on DIP data [29]. DSCP is a variant of DSC, which combines protein complex information. The DIP dataset, updated to Oct. 1, 2014, consists of 5017 proteins and 23,115 interactions among the proteins. The self-interactions and the repeated interactions are filtered out in DIP data. The annotation data of proteins used for method validation is the latest version (2012.3.3) downloaded from GO official website [30]. The GO system consists of three separate categories of annotations, namely molecular function (MF), biological process (BP), and cellular component (CC). The predictions are validated separately for each of the three GO categories. To avoid too special or too general, only those GO terms that annotate at least 10 and at most 200 proteins will be kept in the experiments. After processing by this step, the number of GO terms is 267. The domain data is derived from Pfam database [31], including 1107 different types of domains among 3056 proteins. As for the protein complex information, we used the dataset CYC2008 [32], which consists of 408 protein complexes involving 1492 proteins in the yeast PPI network. The GO data and Pfam domain data are transformed to use the ensemble genome protein entries because the original PPI network uses such a labeling system.

Effect of access sequence of each layer

The access sequence of each layer in the MPN plays an important role in the performance of the proposed FP-MPN method. In this paper, the priority of each layer was determined using statistical analysis. Different schemes were used to sequence layers of the MPN and then compare these results to verify the effectiveness of the FP-MPN method. Table 3 depicts the results of FP-MPN when different schemes were adopted. Table 3 demonstrates that the first scheme (SCL → SDL → PIL), in which SCL was visited first and the SDL was visited second, performed the highest in terms of BP (biological process), MF (molecular function), and CC (cellular component). The comparison of these results with the statistical results show they are in agreement. Experimental results also verify the method used to access the sequence of each layer in the FP-MPN.

Table 3 The influence of access sequence

Categories	Schemes	Precision	Recall	F-measure	CR
BP	SCL → SDL → PIL	0.444	0.427	0.435	0.426
	SCL → PIL → SDL	0.462	0.401	0.429	0.374
	SDL → PIL → SCL	0.452	0.404	0.426	0.396
	SDL → SCL → PIL	0.442	0.424	0.433	0.422
	PIL → SDL → SCL	0.453	0.404	0.427	0.397
	PIL → SCL → SDL	0.459	0.398	0.426	0.372
MF	SCL → SDL → PIL	0.569	0.544	0.556	0.508
	SCL → PIL → SDL	0.566	0.535	0.55	0.495
	SDL → PIL → SCL	0.585	0.54	0.561	0.505
	SDL → SCL → PIL	0.568	0.543	0.555	0.507
	PIL → SDL → SCL	0.584	0.539	0.561	0.504
	PIL → SCL → SDL	0.573	0.541	0.557	0.5
CC	SCL → SDL → PIL	0.463	0.439	0.451	0.415
	SCL → PIL → SDL	0.468	0.43	0.448	0.4
	SDL → PIL → SCL	0.473	0.424	0.447	0.402
	SDL → SCL → PIL	0.461	0.439	0.45	0.413
	PIL → SDL → SCL	0.473	0.424	0.448	0.403
	PIL → SCL → SDL	0.467	0.429	0.447	0.4

Leave-one-out cross-validation

A representative set of function prediction algorithms was run: FP-MPN, Zhang, DCS, DSCP, and PON, and their performance was examined using the leave-one-out cross-validation method. In the DIP PPI network, 2870, 1592, and 2427 proteins from a total of 5017 proteins were annotated by BP, MF, and CC, respectively. We analyzed the overall prediction performance of FP-MPN on these annotated proteins, as well as four other

Table 4 Overall comparisons of various methods

Categories	Methods	MP	Precision	Recall	F-measure	CR
BP	FP-MPN	1595	0.444	0.427	0.435	0.426
	Zhang	810	0.225	0.220	0.222	0.216
	DCS	1148	0.312	0.314	0.313	0.327
	DSCP	1298	0.357	0.359	0.358	0.363
	PON	572	0.150	0.140	0.145	0.161
MF	FP-MPN	995	0.569	0.544	0.556	0.508
	Zhang	608	0.332	0.332	0.332	0.316
	DCS	839	0.461	0.462	0.461	0.441
	DSCP	927	0.518	0.515	0.516	0.489
	PON	413	0.223	0.216	0.22	0.228
CC	FP-MPN	1265	0.463	0.439	0.451	0.415
	Zhang	561	0.197	0.196	0.197	0.198
	DCS	876	0.306	0.309	0.307	0.315
	DSCP	1014	0.364	0.363	0.364	0.356
	PON	440	0.148	0.138	0.143	0.158

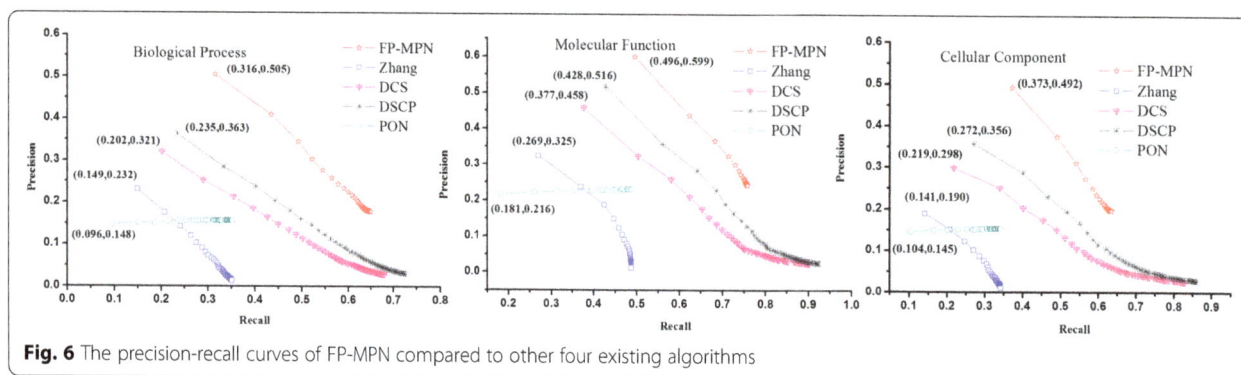

Fig. 6 The precision-recall curves of FP-MPN compared to other four existing algorithms

methods. The results are shown in Table 4, which include the average Precision, Recall, and *F*-measure and coverage rate (CR) of the various algorithms.

In Table 4, MP is the number of proteins which have been matched to at least one function with known function. Among the five methods, FP-MPN and PON are two methods of selecting top-ranking functions from the set of candidate functions, whereas the methods of Zhang, DCS, and DSCP are three methods of endowing un-annotated proteins with all functions of proteins with the highest similarity values. From Table 4, we can see that FP-MPN can predict functions for more proteins and archive higher performance than the other four methods, with respect to BP, MF, and CC. For BP, the *F*-measure of FP-MPN is 95.95, 38.98, 21.51, and 200 % higher than Zhang, DCS, DSCP, and PON, respectively. After integrating protein complexes and domains, DSCP improves the performance compared to DCS. FP-MPN outperforms DSCP, including the *F*-measure and coverage rate. When looking at MF, the performances of these five methods are better. The *F*-measure of FP-MPN is 67.47, 20.61, 7.75, and 152.73 % higher than the results using the methods of Zhang, DCS, DSCP, and PON, respectively. As for CC, the *F*-measure of FP-MPN is 128.93, 46.91, 23.9, and 215.38 % higher than the results using the methods of Zhang, DCS, DSCP, and PON, respectively. Compared to BP and MF, FP-MPN had a higher *F*-measure growth rate compared to other methods.

A comprehensive comparison of the performances of these five methods was undertaken using a Precision-Recall (PR) curve to evaluate the global performance of every method in terms of the different strategies of function selection adopted by the five prediction methods. The same number of functions was chosen for each method, i.e., the top K functions of each prediction method. When examining the methods of Zhang, DCS, and DSCP, the top M ($M < =K$) proteins which had the highest similarity value were selected and the top K functions from the function list as a predictor of functions was listed in descending order according to the maximum value of protein similarity (e.g., given a certain function F_i found in more than one protein, the score of F_i is the similarity value of this protein when compared to the tested proteins). As for the FP-MPN and PON methods, the top K GO terms are chosen to assign functional properties to the unknown proteins (K ranges from 1 to 50). The areas under the curve (AUC) for FP-MPN and other methods are used to compare their performance. AUC is considered to be a standard method to assess the accuracy of predictive distribution models. From Fig. 6, we can see that FP-MPN outperforms other methods in terms of BP, MF, and CC. For example, on the BP, the AUC of FP-MPN is 347.67, 53.76, 31.76, and 195.46 % higher than Zhang, DCS, DSCP, and PON, respectively.

The number of incorrect predicted functions when matching a function correctly using these methods was

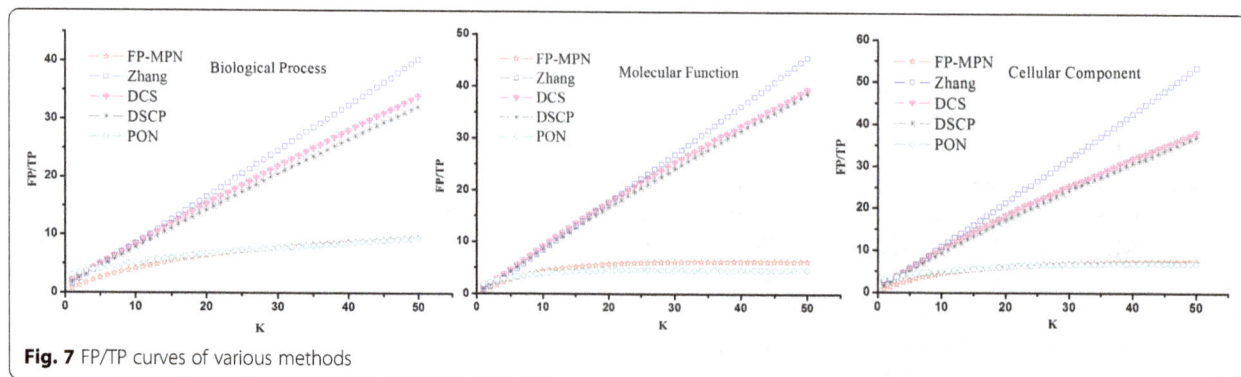

Fig. 7 FP/TP curves of various methods

Table 5 Statistical analysis of FP/TP of various methods

Categories	Methods	Maximum	Minimum	Average	Middle
BP	FP-MPN	9.44	0.72	6.48	7.18
	Zhang	40.29	1.59	20.96	21.04
	DCS	33.94	2.12	18.64	18.94
	DSCP	32.14	1.75	17.49	17.75
	PON	9.39	3.07	6.98	7.41
MF	FP-MPN	6.19	0.53	5.23	5.99
	Zhang	45.5	0.9	22.81	22.71
	DCS	39.41	1.18	21.28	21.88
	DSCP	38.54	0.94	20.4	20.73
	PON	4.57	1.85	4.2	4.57
CC	FP-MPN	7.39	0.72	5.88	6.59
	Zhang	53.51	2.12	27.29	27.09
	DCS	38.15	2.36	21.49	22.25
	DSCP	37.02	1.81	20.45	21.04
	PON	6.88	3.07	6.02	6.57

determined. For each testing protein, the top K functions are selected as its predicted ones, and TP and FP values are calculated according to its known functions. The TP and FP values of all testing proteins are added to calculated TP and FP pairs. Selecting different values of K (ranging from 1 to 50), a FP/TP curve can be generated with different TP and FP pairs, as shown in Fig. 7. Figure 7 clearly shows that the curvature of FP-MPN curve is the lowest as compared to others, which means that, if matched functions are the same, the number of functions incorrectly matched by FP-MPN is the least. Table 5 lists the statistical results of the various FP/TP curves, including maximum value, the minimum value, the average value, and the middle value. These results indicates that to match a protein function correctly, the number of average noise functions (i.e., predicted function incorrectly matched) produced by FP-MPN is smaller compared to the Zhang, DCS, and DSCP methods. FP-MPN has comparable results with PON's. For example, on the BP, the number of average noise functions of the

methods of FP-MPN, Zhang, DCS, DSCP, and PON is 7, 21, 19, 18, and 7, respectively. The results illustrate that FP-MPN has the high prediction efficiency and accuracy.

Tenfold cross-validation

The performance of FP-MPN was tested using leave-one-out validation. Experimental results demonstrate improvements when predicting protein functions by the FP-MPN method compared to competing methods. However, in practical applications, there are much more proteins without annotations, instead of one unknown protein. In this section, we will use the leave-percent-out cross-validation method to verify the effectiveness of FP-MPN on PPI networks that have less functional information. Tenfold cross-validation is a widely used leave-percent-out cross-validation, which is used in this paper. The tenfold cross-validation requires the entire set of examples to be divided into ten equal sets randomly. Nine of the ten parts are used for training, and one part is used for testing. This is repeated ten times, each time using another testing set. We evaluate the performance of each method using area under precision-recall (PR) curve. Figure 8 illustrates the PR curve using tenfold cross-validation, in terms of biological processes, molecular functions, and cellular components. When compared to the results of leave-one-out cross-validation, the performance of all methods using tenfold cross-validation decrease slightly, due to the decrease of the number of training proteins. It appears that Fig. 8 is very similar to Fig. 6, except for the coordinate values of the various methods. Figure 8 demonstrates that FP-MPN still outperforms other methods when tenfold cross-validation is used to test all methods.

Analysis of the overlaps and differences between FP-MPN and other methods

To further analyze the differences between the FP-MPN and other methods, we selected 12 testing proteins and predicted their functions using the five methods. Table 6 lists the functions of these selected proteins predicted by

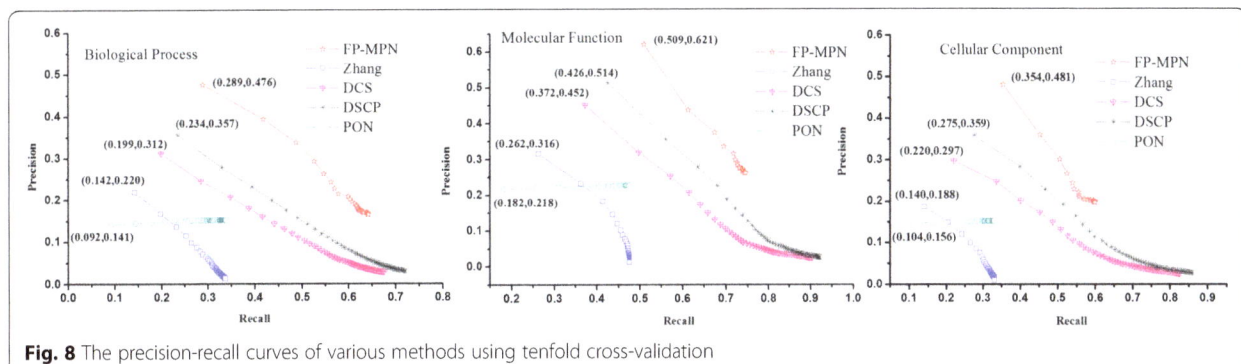

Fig. 8 The precision-recall curves of various methods using tenfold cross-validation

Table 6 Selected functions predicted by various methods

Categories	Proteins	FP-MPN	Zhang	DCS	DSCP	PON
BP	YGL100W (8 GO terms)	*GO:0006409* *GO:0006607* *GO:0006913* *GO:0006999* *GO:0006406* *GO:0006609* *GO:0006611* *GO:0006407* *GO:0000973* *GO:0000055*	GO:0000723 GO:0006348 GO:0006355 GO:0051568	GO:0043161	GO:0043161	GO:0000001 GO:0000002 GO:0000027 GO:0000055 GO:0000082 GO:0000086 GO:0000122 GO:0000209
	YNL262W (7 GO terms)	*GO:0006272* *GO:0006273* *GO:0006289* *GO:0006298* *GO:0000084*	*GO:0006273* *GO:0000084* *GO:0006270*	*GO:0006273* *GO:0000084* *GO:0006270*	*GO:0006273* *GO:0000084* *GO:0006270*	*GO:0006272* *GO:0006273* *GO:0006289* GO:0000084 GO:0006260 GO:0006270 GO:0006284
	YLR321C (6 GO terms)	*GO:0006337* *GO:0006368* *GO:0043044* *GO:0000086*	*GO:0006302* *GO:0043044* GO:0006338 GO:0042766 GO:0045944	*GO:0006302* *GO:0043044* GO:0006338 GO:0042766 GO:0045944	*GO:0006302* *GO:0043044* GO:0006338 GO:0042766 GO:0045944	*GO:0006302* *GO:0043044* GO:0006338 GO:0042766 GO:0045944
	YBR278W (5 GO terms)	GO:0006272 GO:0006273 GO:0006289 GO:0006298 GO:0006348 GO:0006303 GO:0007064		*GO:0006348* *GO:0000723* *GO:0006281* *GO:0007064* *GO:0030466*	*GO:0006348* *GO:0000723* *GO:0006281* *GO:0007064* *GO:0030466*	
MF	YBR114W (3 GO terms)	*GO:0004842* *GO:0003684* *GO:0008094*	*GO:0008094*	*GO:0008094*	*GO:0008094*	GO:0000386 GO:0000990 GO:0001102
	YJR052W (3 GO terms)	*GO:0004842* *GO:0003684* *GO:0008094*		GO:0008134	GO:0043130	
	YJR140C (3 GO terms)	*GO:0003677* *GO:0031491* *GO:0003714*		GO:0046933 GO:0046961	*GO:0003677* *GO:0031491*	
	YBL021C (2 GO terms)	*GO:0001077* *GO:0000978*	GO:0003713 GO:0003714	GO:0003713 GO:0003714	GO:0003713 GO:0003714	GO:0003713 GO:0003714
CC	YNL161W (6 GO terms)	*GO:0005933* *GO:0005934* *GO:0005935* *GO:0043332*	*GO:0005935* GO:0005816	*GO:0005935* GO:0005816	*GO:0005935* GO:0005816	*GO:0000131* GO:0000139 GO:0000142 GO:0000307 GO:0000324 GO:0000329
	YBR198C (3 GO terms)	GO:0000124 GO:0046695 GO:0005669	GO:0070210	GO:0070210	GO:0070210	*GO:0000124* GO:0000139 GO:0000228
	YDR167W (3 GO terms)	GO:0000124 GO:0046695 GO:0005669		GO:0005666	*GO:0000124* *GO:0046695*	
	YNL273W (3 GO terms)	*GO:0031298* *GO:0000228* *GO:0043596*		GO:0005751	GO:0005751	

various methods. The third to the seventh column of Table 6 lists functions predicted by the FP-MPN, Zhang, DCS, DSCP, and PON methods, respectively. In this table, functions in italics represent the matched functions of the testing proteins, the rest are mismatched functions. In Table 6, we can see that FP-MPN can record more correct functions and fewer error functions compared to the other competing methods.

In addition, we continued to look for sources of functions predicted by various methods. For the protein YGL100W, the functions set predicted by the method of Zhang consists of GO:0000723, GO:0006348, GO:0006355, and GO:0051568, which were derived from the protein YAR003W. In this study, YAR003W is regarded as having the most similar domain to YGL100W among all the proteins. Unfortunately, these predicted functions are mismatched by the real functions of YGL100W. As for DCS and DSCP, the protein YCL039W is considered to be the most similar in domain to YGL100W than the other known proteins. Similarly, the predicted functions of GO:0043161, which were derived from YCL039W, created errors in predicted functions for YAR003W. Predicted functions by PON were GO:0000001, GO:0000002, GO:0000027, GO:0000055, GO:0000082, GO:0000086, GO:0000122, and GO:0000209, which were derived from YBR234C, YJL112W, YKL021C, YDR267C, YDR364C, YFL009W, YLR055C, and YIL046W, respectively. All of these proteins have at least one domain with YGL100W. So, we can draw a conclusion that we cannot predict functions for the protein YGL100W based on domain information only. Our FP-MPN predicts ten functions, in which eight are matched and two are mismatched. These matched functions were derived from protein YDL116W, which is located in the transcription factor TFIID complex with the YGL100W protein. FP-MPN successfully matched eight functions for the protein YGL100W, with the help of protein complexes information. The results suggest that complexes information improves the accuracy of protein function prediction. However, protein complexes data is also used in the DSCP methods, which has a different predictor results compared to that of FP-MPN. This could be due to the difference in how the data is used between the two methods. For the protein YNL262W, the methods of Zhang, DCS, and DSCP created the same function lists, consisting of GO:0006273, GO:0000084, and GO:0006270. These three functions are derived from the protein YNL102W, which has common domains with the protein YNL262W. In the predicted functions list, only GO:0006273 is correct as a function for the protein YNL102W. Compared to the methods of Zhang, DCS, and DSCP, PON can identify two other correct functions GO:0006273 and GO:0006289 from another protein YDL102W, which shares domains with the protein YNL102W. The result suggests that annotating proteins according to multiple known proteins is more reliable than predicting functions from a single protein. Besides the three matched functions identified by other methods, FP-MPN identifies a new correct function GO:0006298. In this example, FP-MPN predicts more matched functions compared to other methods, due to the domain and complexes information being used. This phenomenon suggests that proper use of multiple heterogeneous biological data can effectively improve the performance of function prediction algorithms. The analysis for the rest of the ten proteins described above is consistent with that of YGL100W and YNL262W.

Efficiency analysis

To compare the efficiency of these methods, we ran FP-MPN and competing methods under the same conditions and looked at their running time. All methods in this paper were run on a notebook computer with Inter(R) Core(TM) i5-4300M 2.6 GHz CPU and 4 GB RAM. Figure 9 illustrates a comparison of the running time of FP-MPN and the other four methods used for predicting protein functions. The methods of Zhang, DCS, and DSCP are all based on combined number computation. So, they have the disadvantage of being time consuming. From Fig. 9, it can be seen that FP-MPN is extremely fast, 25, 52, 55, and 0.8 times faster than the methods of Zhang, DCS, DSCP, and PON, respectively. As protein-protein interactions are accumulating, FP-MPN can be used in larger scale PPI networks.

Conclusions

Different types of interactions or connections play different roles in protein function prediction. Combining multiple interactions or connections between two proteins could reduce the impact of false negatives and increase the number of correct predicted functions. However, there appears to be more false functions identified compared to positive functions, thus the overall performance of function prediction would not be improved greatly. In this paper, multilayer protein networks (MPN) are constructed based on topological characteristics, protein domain information, and protein complex information, with each layer given various priorities. Based on the constructed networks, we proposed a new method, named FP-MPN, to predict the functions of a particular protein. The proposed

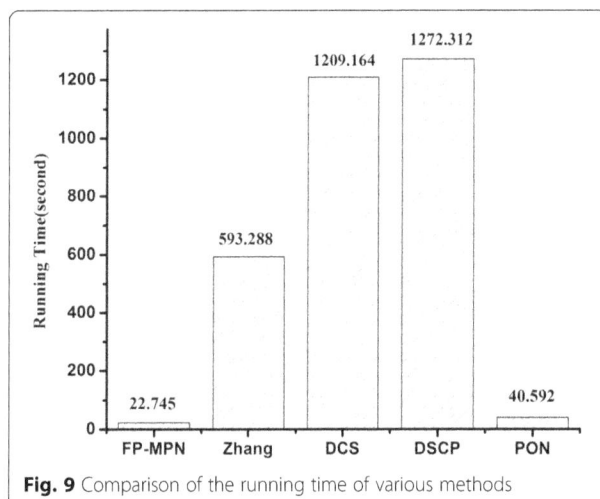

Fig. 9 Comparison of the running time of various methods

method is based around visiting each layer of the MPN in turn and forming a set of candidate neighbors with known functions. The set of predicted functions is then formed and all of these functions are scored and sorted. Each layer contributes differently to the predicted functions in the un-annotated protein. The experimental results indicate that it is an effective method to predict protein functions.

Acknowledgements
Not applicable

Funding
This work is supported in part by the National Natural Science Foundation of China under Grant No. 11501054; the Science and Technology Plan Project of Hunan Province, China No. 2015GK3072; the Natural Science Foundation of Hunan Province, China No. 2016JJ3016; the National Scientific Research Foundation of Hunan Province Education Department, China No. 16A020, 16B028, No. 16C0133, No. 16C0137; and the Education Scientific Planning Project of Hunan Province, China No. XJK016BGD078.

Authors' contributions
BHZ and SH obtained the protein-protein interaction data, gene ontology annotation data, protein complex data, and domain data. BHZ and SH designed the new method, FP-MPN, and analyzed the results. BHZ, XYL, and SH drafted the manuscript together. FZ, QLT, and WYN participated in revising the draft. All authors have read and approved the manuscript.

Competing interests
The authors declare that they have no competing interests.

References
1. Liu B, Fang L, Liu F, Wang X, Chen J, Chou K-C. Identification of real MicroRNA precursors with a pseudo structure status composition approach. PLoS One. 2015;10(3):e0121501.
2. Ito T, Chiba T, Ozawa R, et al. A comprehensive two-hybrid analysis to explore the yeast protein interactome. Proc Natl Acad Sci. 2001;98(8):4569–74.
3. Uetz P, Giot L, Cagney G, et al. A comprehensive analysis of protein–protein interactions in Saccharomyces cerevisiae. Nature. 2000;403(6770):623–7.
4. Gavin AC, et al. Functional organization of the yeast proteome by systematic analysis of protein complexes. Nature. 2002;415(6868):141–7.
5. Enright AJ, Van Dongen S, Ouzounis CA. An efficient algorithm for large-scale detection of protein families. Nucleic Acids Res. 2002;30(7):1575–84.
6. Schwikowski B, Uetz P, Fields S. A network of protein–protein interactions in yeast. Nat Biotechnol. 2000;18(12):1257–61.
7. Hishigaki H, Nakai K, Ono T, et al. Assessment of prediction accuracy of protein function from protein–protein interaction data. Yeast. 2001;18(6):523–31.
8. Chua HN, Sung WK, Wong L. Exploiting indirect neighbours and topological weight to predict protein function from protein–protein interactions. Bioinformatics. 2006;22(13):1623–30.
9. Cao M, Zhang H, Park J, et al. Going the distance for protein function prediction: a new distance metric for protein interaction networks. PLoS One. 2013;8(10):e76339.
10. Nabieva E, Jim K, Agarwal A, et al. Whole-proteome prediction of protein function via graph-theoretic analysis of interaction maps. Bioinformatics. 2005;21 suppl 1:i302–10.
11. Chi X, Hou J. An iterative approach of protein function prediction. BMC Bioinformatics. 2011;12(1):437.
12. Wu Z, Zhao X, Chen L. Identifying responsive functional modules from protein-protein interaction network. Mol Cells. 2009;27(3):271–7.
13. Lee J, Gross SP, Lee J. Improved network community structure improves function prediction. Sci Rep. 2013;3:2197.
14. Cozzetto D, Buchan DWA, Bryson K, et al. Protein function prediction by massive integration of evolutionary analyses and multiple data sources. BMC Bioinformatics. 2013;14 Suppl 3:S1.
15. Zhang S, Chen H, Liu K, et al. Inferring protein function by domain context similarities in protein-protein interaction networks. BMC Bioinformatics. 2009;10(1):395.
16. Peng W, Wang J, Cai J, et al. Improving protein function prediction using domain and protein complexes in PPI networks. BMC Syst Biol. 2014;8(1):35.
17. Liang S, Zheng D, Standley DM, et al. A novel function prediction approach using protein overlap networks. BMC Syst Biol. 2013;7(1):61.
18. Gong Q, Ning W, Tian W. GoFDR: a sequence alignment based method for predicting protein functions. Methods. 2016;93:3-14.
19. Kumar DS, Reddy PK. Improved approach for protein function prediction by exploiting prominent proteins: IEEE International Conference on Data Science and Advanced Analytics (DSAA). 2015. p. 1–7.
20. Yu G, Rangwala H, Domeniconi C, et al. Predicting Protein Function Using Multiple Kernels. IEEE/ACM Trans Comput Biol Bioinform. 2015;12(1):219–33.
21. Wu M, Li X, Kwoh CK, et al. A core-attachment based method to detect protein complexes in PPI networks. BMC Bioinformatics. 2009;10(1):169.
22. Wang J, Peng X, Li M, et al. Construction and application of dynamic protein interaction network based on time course gene expression data. Proteomics. 2013;13(2):301–12.
23. Zhao BH, Wang JX, Li XY, et al. Essential Protein Discovery based on a Combination of modularity and conservatism. Methods. 2016. doi:10.1016/j.ymeth.2016.07.005.
24. Liu W, Li D, Zhu Y, et al. Reconstruction of signalling network from protein interactions based on function annotations. IEEE/ACM Trans Comput Biol Bioinform. 2013;10(2):514–21.
25. Zhao BH, Wang JX, Li M, et al. A new method for predicting protein functions from dynamic weighted interactome networks. IEEE Trans NanoBioscience. 2016;15(2):415–24.
26. Zhao BH, Wang JX, Li M, et al. Prediction of essential proteins based on overlapping essential modules. IEEE Trans NanoBioscience. 2014;13(4):415–24.
27. Peng W, Wang J, Zhao B, et al. Identification of protein complexes using weighted PageRank-Nibble algorithm and core-attachment structure. IEEE/ACM Trans Comput Biol Bioinform. 2015;12(1):179–92.
28. Zhao B, Wang J, Li M, et al. Detecting protein complexes based on uncertain graph model. IEEE/ACM Trans Comput Biol Bioinform. 2014;11:486–97.
29. Xenarios X, et al. DIP: the database of interacting proteins. Nucleic Acids Res. 2000;28:289–91.
30. Ashburner M, Ball CA, Blake JA, et al. Gene ontology: tool for the unification of biology. Nat Genet. 2000;25(1):25–9.
31. Bateman A, Coin L, Durbin R, et al. The Pfam protein families database. Nucleic Acids Res. 2004;32 suppl 1:D138–41.
32. Pu S, Wong J, Turner B, et al. Up-to-date catalogues of yeast protein complexes. Nucleic Acids Res. 2009;37:825–31.

17

Computational analysis of mRNA expression profiling in the inner ear reveals candidate transcription factors associated with proliferation, differentiation, and deafness

Kobi Perl[1,2], Ron Shamir[1*] and Karen B. Avraham[2*] (iD)

Abstract

Background: Hearing loss is a major cause of disability worldwide, impairing communication, health, and quality of life. Emerging methods of gene therapy aim to address this morbidity, which can be employed to fix a genetic problem causing hair cell dysfunction and to promote the proliferation of supporting cells in the cochlea and their transdifferentiation into hair cells. In order to extend the applicability of gene therapy, the scientific community is focusing on discovery of additional deafness genes, identifying new genetic variants associated with hearing loss, and revealing new factors that can be manipulated in a coordinated manner to improve hair cell regeneration. Here, we addressed these challenges via genome-wide measurement and computational analysis of transcriptional profiles of mouse cochlea and vestibule sensory epithelium at embryonic day (E)16.5 and postnatal day (P)0. These time points correspond to developmental stages before and during the acquisition of mechanosensitivity, a major turning point in the ability to hear.

Results: We hypothesized that tissue-specific transcription factors are primarily involved in differentiation, while those associated with development are more concerned with proliferation. Therefore, we searched for enrichment of transcription factor binding motifs in genes differentially expressed between the tissues and between developmental ages of mouse sensory epithelium. By comparison with transcription factors known to alter their expression during avian hair cell regeneration, we identified 37 candidates likely to be important for regeneration. Furthermore, according to our estimates, only half of the deafness genes in human have been discovered. To help remedy the situation, we developed a machine learning classifier that utilizes the expression patterns of genes to predict how likely they are to be undiscovered deafness genes.

Conclusions: We used a novel approach to highlight novel additional factors that can serve as points of intervention for enhancing hair cell regeneration. Given the similarities between mouse and human deafness, our predictions may be of value in prioritizing future research on novel human deafness genes.

Keywords: Inner ear, Cochlea, Hearing, Balance, Deafness, Transcriptome, Regeneration

* Correspondence: rshamir@tau.ac.il; karena@tauex.tau.ac.il
[1]Blavatnik School of Computer Science, Tel Aviv University, 6997801 Tel Aviv, Israel
[2]Department of Human Molecular Genetics and Biochemistry, Sackler Faculty of Medicine and Sagol School of Neuroscience, Tel Aviv University, 6997801 Tel Aviv, Israel

Background

Hearing and balance are fundamental processes that are essential for communication and for orientation within space. The inner ear is composed of the auditory system, which is responsible for hearing, and the vestibular system, which is responsible, in part, for balance. While these systems display extensive similarities, there are also structural and functional differences. The organ of Corti in the cochlea is unique to the auditory system and contains the sensory epithelium responsible for hearing. In contrast, the vestibular system contains five organs: the three semicircular canals lined with cristae sensory epithelium that detect angular acceleration by fluid motion, and the saccule and utricle, which contain the macula sensory epithelium that can sense linear acceleration due to gravity. The development of the inner ear requires a complex dynamic process to produce the final sensory organ with both hearing and balance capabilities [1].

The mouse has long served as a model for studying human inner ear structure and function, in part because of the ability to breed and select offspring with desired traits, including those affecting hearing and balance [2]. More recently, the similarities between the genomes, and the ability to manipulate the mouse phenotype by gene-targeted mutagenesis and genome editing, have reaffirmed the mouse as an ideal vehicle for studying human auditory and vestibular dysfunction [3, 4]. As a result, mouse inner ear development has been studied in detail on a molecular level [5, 6]. This includes the elucidation of transcriptional pathways that govern the differentiation of the otocyst towards sensory or nonsensory regions during early development (reviewed in [7]). A number of temporal and spatial triggers of development and maturation have been characterized, including the molecular controls on patterning, hair bundle height, and numbers of stereocilia. Information about the active transcriptional pathways has laid the groundwork for establishing the nature of the early and late developmental pathways of the inner ear. Mutations in some of these critical developmental genes are now known to lead to defects in the mouse [8] and human inner ear and to cause deafness [9].

Regeneration after cellular damage shares some similarities with normal organ development. In birds, regeneration of hair cells involves proliferation of nearby epithelial supporting cells, which then differentiate to form replacement hair cells and supporting cells [10, 11]. However, while mature mammalian vestibular organs are also able to regenerate at least a subpopulation of hair cells after damage [12–14], the adult cochlea is incapable of any regeneration. It should be noted that there is some evidence that the cochlea may contain supporting cells with the ability to form new hair cells in very young animals [15] or upon misexpression of *Atoh1* [16]. Given the

limitations in the mammalian systems, the resemblance of the auditory sensory epithelia and cochlea between birds and mammals [5], and the ability of birds to regenerate hair cells in the cochlea and vestibule, it is relevant to compare the gene expression profiles of the mammalian and avian inner ears. To this end, we applied systemic transcriptomic approaches to decipher the regulatory pathways of the auditory system and make relevant comparisons to the avian transcriptome.

Sensorineural hearing loss most commonly results from degeneration of cochlear hair cells. As mentioned, if these are lost through damage or the natural aging process, they are not replaced. Gene therapy could potentially be used to induce hair cell regeneration [17]. For many tissues, reprogramming and regeneration is achieved by coordinated manipulation of multiple factors. Initial evidence shows this approach might be successful in the cochlea. In embryonic and neonatal mouse cochlear tissue, ectopic expression of *ETV4*, *TCF3*, *GATA3*, *MYCN*, or *ETS2* in combination with *ATOH1* yielded more hair cell-like cells than did overexpression of *ATOH1* alone [18, 19]. The efficacy of these interventions is partial, rendering the search for other transcription factors (TFs) that can be manipulated to enhance this process extremely relevant. As the number of TFs in human is estimated to be in the range of a few thousands [20], one cannot perform an exhaustive experimental search on all possible manipulations of TFs and their combinations. Instead one should focus its efforts on TFs that are more likely to participate in tissue differentiation. In the aforementioned studies [18, 19], the manipulation was performed on TFs that have conserved binding sites near ATOH1 on the POU4F3 gene. Here, we suggest yet another method to identify these candidate TFs, which focus on the concordance between TFs involved in tissue identity in early stages of development, and those participating in avian hair cell regeneration.

The main purpose of this research was to elucidate transcriptional pathways that govern auditory versus vestibular functions or control cell cycle exit. We report the characterization of transcriptional profiles for mouse cochlea and vestibule sensory epithelium at embryonic day (E)16.5 and postnatal day (P)0, time points chosen because they correspond to developmental stages before and during the acquisition of mechanosensitivity [21]. Genes differentially expressed between the tissues, and between the developmental ages, could be associated with the activity of specific TFs. Our analysis identified a number of regulators that are already known, while others are novel. The identified regulators were compared with TFs already known to alter their expression during avian hair cell regeneration [22, 23], allowing us to detect TFs involved either in proliferation or in differentiation of the inner ear. To our knowledge, this is the first study in the inner ear to integrate expression data from a developmental study in the mouse with data from a regeneration experiment in the chick in the search for TFs governing regeneration.

In addition, our analysis identified a number of candidate genes as involved in inner ear defects. For this purpose, we developed a machine learning classifier, which utilized the expression patterns of genes to predict their probabilities of being yet undiscovered deafness genes. Our predictions allow for prioritizing of candidate genes by their probability to be involved in deafness. The development of a classifier for deafness genes is another unique contribution of this study. Our predictions of novel deafness genes and of TFs with a role in regeneration can be helpful in advancing gene therapy research.

Results

Tissue source and age are associated with differences in transcription

Sensory epithelia were dissected from the cochlea and vestibule of mice at two stages of development, embryonic day 16.5 (E16.5) and postnatal day 0 (P0). This was followed by RNA-seq, as previously described [24, 25]. Our analysis identified 39,178 Ensembl genes (including non-coding genes and pseudogenes), 15,206 of which have at least one read per million in three or more of the samples. A principal component analysis (PCA) plot demonstrated four well separated groups (Fig. 1). The first principal component (PC1) explained almost half the variance and is associated with the age of the sample, whereas PC2 explained about a quarter of the variance and is associated with the originating tissue (F test on associations, p values = 1.99×10^{-5}, 1.31×10^{-5}, respectively). Additional PCs were not associated with either tissue or age (p value ≥ 0.05). The E16.5 genes displayed a lower intra-group variability than at P0. This might reflect differences in the rate of development of the

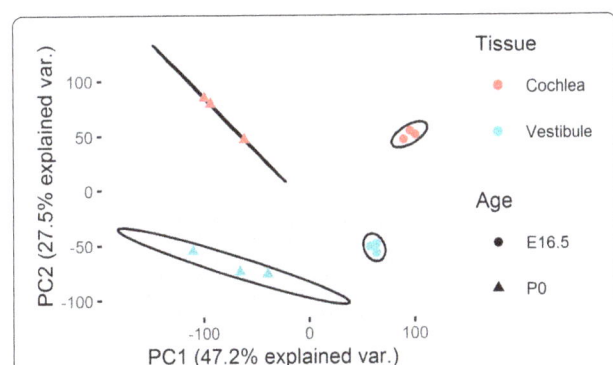

Fig. 1 PCA plot comparing samples in the different ages and tissues according to their mRNA expression. The x- and y-axes are the first and second coordinates, respectively. The samples are colored according to their originating tissue, while the marker shape relates to age. A normal contour line is drawn at 68% probability for each group

different organs between mice from the same population in the period between E16.5 and P0.

We used linear mixed models to estimate the percentage of variance that can be attributed to age, tissue, or the interaction of age and tissue (Additional file 1: Supplementary Methods). According to our estimates, the majority of variance can be attributed to either age (44.0 ± 6.5) or tissue (39.6 ± 5.4) (mean percentage ± standard deviation). The remaining non-negligible percentage can be attributed to the interaction term (8.0 ± 1.5), and a model with this interaction term describes the data better according to a restricted likelihood ratio test (p value $\leq 2.2 \times 10^{-16}$). Less than 10% of the variance was left unexplained (8.4 ± 1.08).

We selected genes that were differentially expressed between tissues or between ages, and genes for which the interaction of tissue and age was significant in determining expression. Our results identified 3306 upregulated genes and 6890 downregulated genes at P0 compared to E16.5. Four thousand one hundred fifty-nine genes were found to be upregulated and 2382 were downregulated in the vestibule compared to the cochlea. For 745 genes, the cochlea to vestibule expression ratio increased over development, and it decreased for 1211 genes. We performed gene ontology (GO) and Kyoto Encyclopedia of Genes and Genomes (KEGG) enrichment analyses on genes from the six identified sets (Additional file 2: Table S1). The enrichment results are summarized below.

Expression changes with age

Genes that were upregulated at E16.5 are enriched for terms related to cell cycle, DNA replication, cytoskeleton organization, and other terms that are in accordance with a highly proliferative state. In contrast, genes that were upregulated at P0 are enriched for ribosomes, indicating high protein synthesis, mainly of plasma membrane and extracellular matrix proteins. The lipid and oxphos-related metabolic activities are also high in this group. The cells at this stage of development are more adhesive, communicate more with one another, and are more responsive to external cues. They are also responsive to a variety of signaling receptors, including calcium signaling, and have high ion transport activity. The upregulated terms are typical of a less proliferative environment, where the highly expressed genes promote homeostatic processes and inhibit peptidase activity. Some terms show signs of cell specialization, in terms of sensory perception, cartilage-related metabolism, and the regulation of ossification; the last might indicate a cross-talk between sensory epithelium cells and endochondral cells. Another marker for the more differentiated state is an up-regulation of the MHC protein complex. In summary, the enrichment suggests that the inner ear is in a more proliferative state at E16.5 than at P0, whereas at P0 the tissues are more differentiated and exhibit specialization for sensory perception.

KEGG enrichment generally confirmed the aforementioned differences and provided more details regarding specific metabolic processes activated at P0. For example, we could attribute the enriched lipid metabolism to sphingolipids, arachidonic acid, and retinol, the enriched aminoglycan metabolism to glycan degradation, and the biosynthesis of chondroitin and keratan sulfate. Pathways enriched at P0 suggest that the activity of the immune system increases during development, with leukocytes migrating into the tissue and intercellular communication using cytokines. As the complement and coagulation cascades and the renin-angiotensin system are also enriched at P0, we can hypothesize that the inner ear is more exposed to blood circulation at this age.

Expression change between tissues

According to the enrichment analysis (Additional file 2: Table S1), a number of the differentially expressed (DE) genes in both the cochlea and vestibule are involved in signal transduction. In the cochlea, the majority of the signaling is mediated by voltage- and ligand-gated ion channels and can be attributed to neuron-neuron synaptic transmission. In agreement with this finding, other upregulated activities are neurogenesis and neuron projection. In contrast, the signaling in the vestibule is probably required for the coordination of both innate and acquired immune responses, an observation that relates to the main function enriched in this tissue. The signaling, some of which involves purinergic receptors, plays a role in the response to external stimulus and stress, and also in taxis. Another function enriched in the vestibule is locomotion, with the cilium and the axoneme being two enriched cellular components related to the movement of the hair cells' stereocilia. The vestibule is richer in blood vessel formation and hematopoiesis, and the extracellular matrix is more evolved than in the cochlea. Together with the high immune-related activity, these factors may explain why the vestibular cells are more adhesive. We also detected enrichment for replacement ossification, suggesting the development of bone. As a generalization, upregulated genes were associated with neurological terms in the cochlear, but to vascular, structural, and immunological terms in the vestibule. This partitioning was not perfect as we could detect enrichment for mesenchymal cell differentiation in the cochlea, and 3.1% of the upregulated genes in the vestibule were annotated for a role in sensory perception.

The KEGG enrichment data also agreed with the characterization of the cochlea as more neurological versus a more vascular vestibule. In addition, the data provided more information about the typical signaling in each apparatus. Neuroactive ligand signaling was identified in both, although the cochlea was associated with the TGF-beta, MAPK, and ErbB signaling pathways, while cytokine-mediated, calcium, and Toll-like receptor signaling were more important in the vestibule. Three pathways shown to be unique to the cochlea affect cell proliferation, survival, differentiation, and migration [26–28], suggesting that these developmental processes are more activated in the cochlea. Other unique metabolic pathways enriched in the cochlea were O-glycan and chondroitin sulfate biosynthesis. The vestibule, on the other hand, was enriched for glycan degradation and metabolic pathways concerning arachidonic acid, retinol, and glutathione.

Tissue expression ratio change with age

Genes for which the cochlea to vestibule expression ratio increased with age $\left(\frac{Cochlea}{Vestibule}\uparrow\right)$ were enriched for processes related to sensory perception and central nervous system development, as well as signaling through G-coupled receptors, ligand-gated ion channels, or calcium. Accordingly, a significant number of genes were annotated to be in the apical part of the cell. Other genes annotated to the extracellular region might mediate the biological adhesion, which increases during development. Another enriched component was identified as the sarcomere, which most closely resembles the stereocilia in the inner ear.

We can envision two possible scenarios for each of these enrichments. The first option is that genes annotated for enrichment are upregulated in the cochlea at E16.5 and the gap between the cochlea and the vestibule increases during development. The second option is that these genes are upregulated in the vestibule at E16.5 and the gap between the cochlea and the vestibule decreases during development. To distinguish between the two, we compared the expression of all genes that are annotated for each GO term. The median expression log-ratio between the cochlea and the vestibule at P0 was plotted against the value of the same parameter at E16.5 (Fig. 2, circles). The plot only contains the terms for which the gap between the cochlea and the vestibule significantly increases with age. More precisely, only terms for which the log-ratios at P0 were larger than their paired values at E16.5 were included (Wilcoxon signed rank test, q values ≤ 0.05).

Interestingly, the vestibule is appeared to be more specialized for sensory perception at E16.5 than the cochlea, as manifested by a negative median log-ratio for terms sensory perception, mechanoreceptor differentiation, and detection of stimulus involved in sensory perception. However, by P0, the cochlea surpassed the vestibule in all of these fields. In contrast, ligand-gated ion channel activity was already higher in the cochlea at E16.5, and the gap only increased with development.

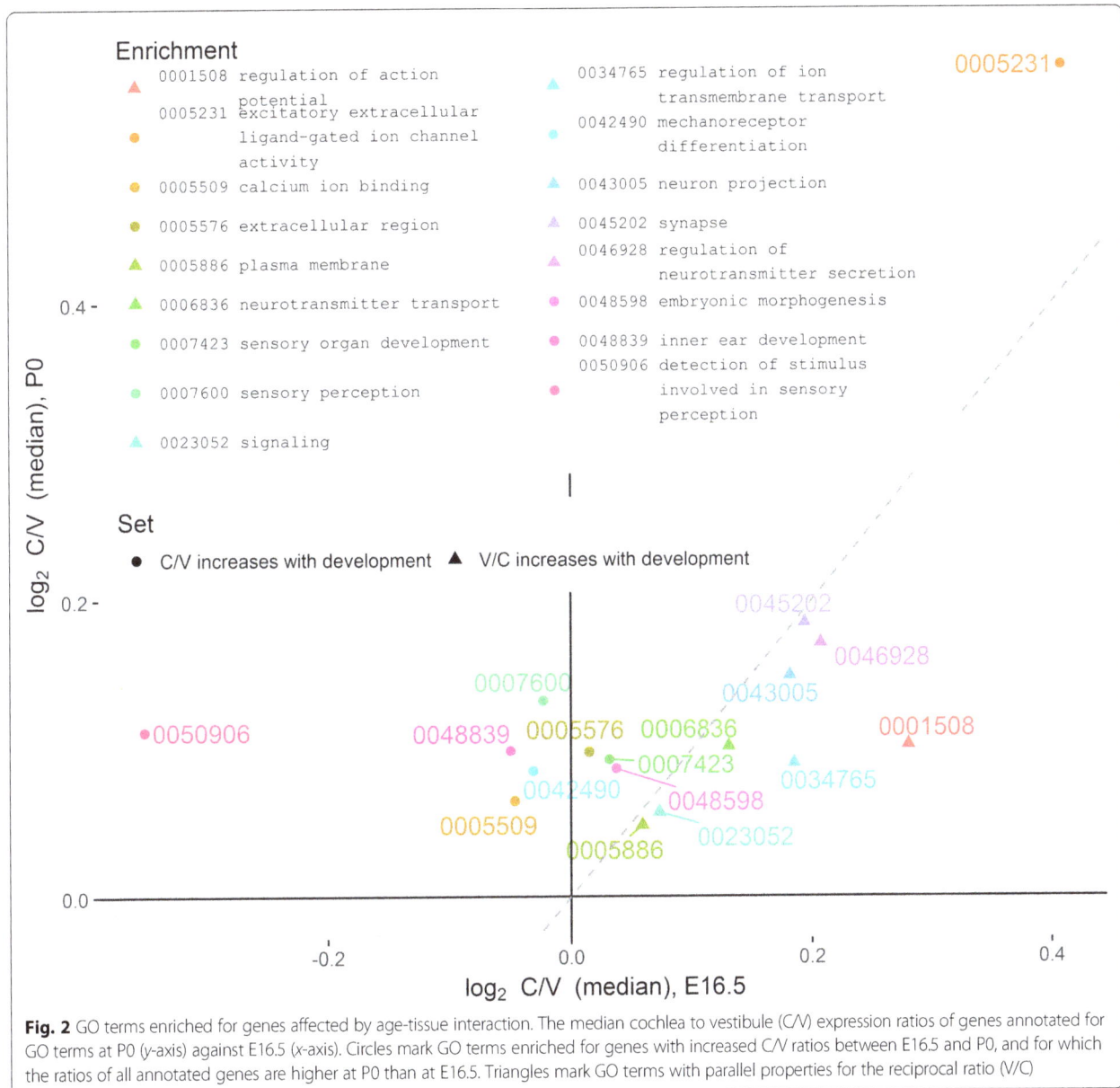

Fig. 2 GO terms enriched for genes affected by age-tissue interaction. The median cochlea to vestibule (C/V) expression ratios of genes annotated for GO terms at P0 (y-axis) against E16.5 (x-axis). Circles mark GO terms enriched for genes with increased C/V ratios between E16.5 and P0, and for which the ratios of all annotated genes are higher at P0 than at E16.5. Triangles mark GO terms with parallel properties for the reciprocal ratio (V/C)

Genes for which the vestibule to cochlea ratio increased with age $\left(\frac{Vestibule}{Cochlea}\uparrow\right)$ were enriched for signaling, neuron projection, neurotransmitter transport, and secretion. These are all functions that are higher in the cochlea at E16.5, and for which the difference between the vestibule and the cochlea decreases with time (Fig. 2, triangles).

Deafness genes can be predicted using expression patterns

A list of 140 genes associated with human deafness was compiled from a public dataset (http://hereditaryhearingloss.org/; Additional file 3: Table S2). Expression data for 130 orthologous mouse genes are available in our dataset. Of these genes, mutations in 25 orthologs are associated with syndromic deafness in human, 96 with non-syndromic deafness, and nine with both types of deafness and are treated as syndromic deafness genes (DGs) in subsequent analyses. It should be noted that we found no ortholog for any of the five mitochondrial DGs.

We observed general patterns of expression for these syndromic and non-syndromic DGs. First, when comparing vestibular and cochlear expression, the absolute values of the fold change (FC) of the DGs were higher than for the background FCs (p value = 1.98×10^{-5}, one-sided Wilcoxon rank sum test; Fig. 3, upper subfigure). In addition, the absolute FCs of non-syndromic DGs were slightly higher than the FCs of syndromic DGs (p value = 7.00×10^{-2}, same test). That is, DGs tend

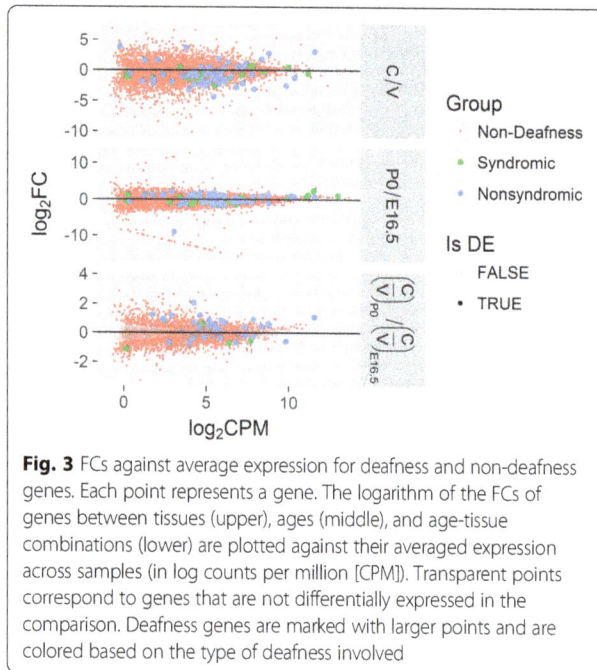

Fig. 3 FCs against average expression for deafness and non-deafness genes. Each point represents a gene. The logarithm of the FCs of genes between tissues (upper), ages (middle), and age-tissue combinations (lower) are plotted against their averaged expression across samples (in log counts per million [CPM]). Transparent points correspond to genes that are not differentially expressed in the comparison. Deafness genes are marked with larger points and are colored based on the type of deafness involved

to be tissue-specific, with the non-syndromic genes possibly being even more specific. Interestingly, the majority of the DE DGs were higher in the vestibule than in the cochlea, despite the acknowledged role of the cochlea in hearing (57 out of 76, p value $= 2.19 \times 10^{-5}$, two-sided proportion test).

Second, when comparing P0 and E16.5 expression, DGs tended to have higher FCs compared to background FCs (p values $= 6.32 \times 10^{-6}$, one-sided Wilcoxon rank sum test; Fig. 3, middle subfigure). This indicates that their expression tends to increase with development. Third, their cochlea to vestibule expression ratio tended to increase with development compared to background (p values $= 5.15 \times 10^{-6}$, same test; Fig. 3, lower subfigure). Moreover, the increase in the ratio of non-syndromic DGs was higher than that for syndromic genes (p value $= 3.48 \times 10^{-3}$, same test).

Deafness gene prediction

We used the three types of FC and the averaged expression (see the "Methods" section), to build a classifier that can predict whether a gene is a DG. The classifier achieved a ROC score of 0.66 ± 0.04 across repeated training/test splits. A ROC score of greater than 0.5 indicates that the expression data have some predictive value for the relation of a gene to deafness. This classifier performs better than a similar version that used the averaged RPKM values in each condition (ROC score 0.60 ± 0.05). Removing one or more of the four feature types from the original classifier resulted in a lower score.

It must be appreciated that genes not marked as DGs might still represent undiscovered DGs. For this reason, it was important to train our classifier to distinguish between known DGs and genes with an unknown role in deafness. The first group of genes is termed positive, and those in the second group are classified as unlabeled. We wished to adapt our positive unlabeled (PU) classifier to output the probability that an unlabeled gene is a positive gene. This type of classification is referred to as transductive PU learning [29]. Supposing that the known DGs are a random subset of all DGs, i.e., the features we explore impose no bias over which of the positive genes are labeled, then, the probability that the PU classifier assigns to the positivity of new genes both (i) correctly ranks the genes and (ii) the probabilities are only off by a constant factor (see [30] for details). We used a bagging-like algorithm similar to the one presented in [29] in order to calculate the probabilities for the set of unlabeled genes. Some modifications in our system are described in the "Methods" section. One main difference between our approach and the previously reported version in [29] was that we kept the same proportion of positive (labeled) samples in the training set as in the test set, whereas in [29], all positive samples were included in training. This property allowed us to address the issue of biases in the probabilities, albeit at the price of losing some predictive power. One source of bias was due to undersampling in the learning process [31]. A second source of bias was the one described above for a PU classifier. We addressed the latter using methods presented in [30].

To gain some insight about the accuracy of our estimator, in spite of the lack of a definitive classification of the unlabeled set, we downloaded lists of genes associated with hearing loss according to the text mining tools DigSeE [32], DisGeNET [33], and DISEASES [34]. We refer to these genes as deafness-associated genes (DAGs). By these means, we obtained 1313 genes that were associated with deafness according to at least one tool. These included 115 known DGs, accounting for 82% of all reported DGs. The respective numbers of mouse orthologs were 1021, 106, and 82%. See Additional file 1: Supplementary Results, Figure S1 for a comparison of the lists of genes provided by the tools.

Applying our bagging-like algorithm resulted in a PU classifier with a ROC score of 0.694 where the probabilities from this native classifier were probably biased upward due to undersampling. Correcting for this bias resulted in a better calibration of the probabilities, as demonstrated by a calibration plot (Additional file 1: Figure S2, left), and the lowering of the Brier score (BS) from 2.07×10^{-1} to 8.47×10^{-3}. We employed three different methods (e1, e2, e3; see [30]) to correct the bias in the probabilities caused by the PU scenario. In order to perform the calibration, all three methods first estimate the probability that a known DG is labeled $p(s = 1|$ $y = 1)$. The estimates for this probability, according to e1, e2, and e3, were 0.032 ± 0.014, 0.022 ± 0.007, and 0.518 ± 0.248, respectively. The estimates made by e1 and e2 support the existence of a few thousand DGs, compared to the few hundred predicted according to e3 (4.1×10^3, 5.9×10^3, and 2.5×10^2, respectively). We believe that given the status of deafness research, the last estimate is the most reasonable. To investigate the issue further, we re-evaluated the calibration of the probabilities produced by each method. For this purpose, we assumed that all the DAGs are in fact deafness genes. With this assumption, the e3 method resulted in the best calibration, as demonstrated by a calibration plot (Additional file 1: Figure S2, right), and the lowest BS (scores 6.64×10^{-2}, 1.20×10^{-1}, 2.84×10^{-1}, 6.45×10^{-2} for no fix, e1, e2, and e3, respectively). Hence, we decided to use e3 probabilities in all subsequent analyses and let p_g be the probability that gene g is positive according to e3.

We then reran our bagging-like algorithm, but this time, we chose to treat a gene g as positive with probability p_g, and as negative with probability $1 - p_g$. This reassignment was performed before each iteration. Finally, we recalculated the ROC score of our classifier. In this case, we ignored known DGs in order to make a proper separation between training and test stages. The rerun achieved a slightly better ROC score (0.602 vs 0.600, $p < 0.05$, DeLong's test for two correlated ROC curves [35]). We chose to continue with the rerun classifier and added a correction for undersampling to the resultant probabilities. The predictions for both human genes and mouse orthologs are available in Additional file 4: Table S3. The 20 mouse genes with the highest predicted probabilities include the known non-syndromic DGs *Smpx*, and *Ptprq*, seven DAGs (*Gfi1*, *Lhx3*, *Erbb4*, *Ephx1*, *Il33*, *Slc52a3*, and *Ttr*), and nine genes not associated with deafness (*Mlf1*, *Nell1*, *Espnl*, *Rbm24*, *Lrrc10b*, *Agr3*, *Tgm2*, *Id4Cd164l2*, and *Faim2*).

For the purpose of selecting a discrimination threshold for our binary classifier, we can consider two plots, which demonstrate how well our classifier predicts DAGs (again while ignoring known DGs). The first is a ROC curve, which visualizes the balance between specificity and sensitivity (Fig. 4, top). The threshold maximizing the sum of these two parameters is suggested as a candidate threshold. A disadvantage of a ROC curve, in our context, is that it ignores the association scores provided by the text mining tools. In order to account for these scores, we can consider a range of values of the threshold and use a non-parametric test (one-tailed Wilcoxon rank sum test) to compare the association scores of the genes with probabilities higher than the threshold, with all the others. We hypothesized that

genes above the "right" threshold would tend to have higher association scores. We analyzed the association scores from each tool separately and together (see the "Methods" section) and plotted $-\log_2 P$ – value against the threshold (Fig. 4, bottom). The value giving the lowest p value for the combined scoring was proposed as a candidate threshold. Four thousand six hundred seventy-four and 1934 genes passed the thresholds suggested by the ROC curve (0.027) and the Wilcoxon test (0.043), respectively. Other thresholds may also be considered, depending on the required number of candidates, specificity, and sensitivity. We recommend choosing thresholds that give local maxima on either curve (available in Additional file 4: Table S3).

Transcription factors affecting expression

When we screened for enrichment of transcription factor (TF) binding sites in three sets of DE genes (Additional file 5: Table S4) we could identify six motifs that were associated with changes in expression during development, 43, between tissues, and 10, across an age-tissue interaction (i.e., the change in the cochlea to vestibule expression ratio throughout development). This 7-fold increase in tissue-specific motifs over those associated with a developmental stage was very surprising, in view of the fact that the absolute number of tissue-specific DE genes identified was about 35% less than the number that changed during development. In total, we identified 50 unique motifs across all comparisons and manually connected them to 64 mouse TFs (i.e., a few motifs were associated with multiple TFs).

For each TF, we tested whether the TF gene itself was DE under the same conditions as the gene it regulates (Additional file 5: Table S4). This property interests us for three reasons: (i) It indicates whether the regulation of the TF activity is (at least partially) transcriptional. Knowing how a TF is regulated makes it a better candidate for experimental interventions. (ii) The direction (upregulation or downregulation) in which a TF is DE implies whether it functions as a repressor or an activator. (iii) It strengthens our faith that the associated motif is important for regulation, and not a false-positive. In our analysis, 30 of the 64 TFs identified were DE (in at least one comparison).

In order to investigate how the levels of the TFs affect their targets, we plotted the median FC of *all* targets of a specific motif, against the median FC of the TFs associated with that motif (Additional file 1: Figure S3). In all cases, we observed a positive, although insignificant, correlation between the two values (Pearson's $r = 0.51$, 0.05, or 0.52 for the comparisons between tissues, across age, and for age-tissue interaction, respectively; combined p value (22) = 0.15) [36]. Among the factors that contribute to the incomplete correlation is the

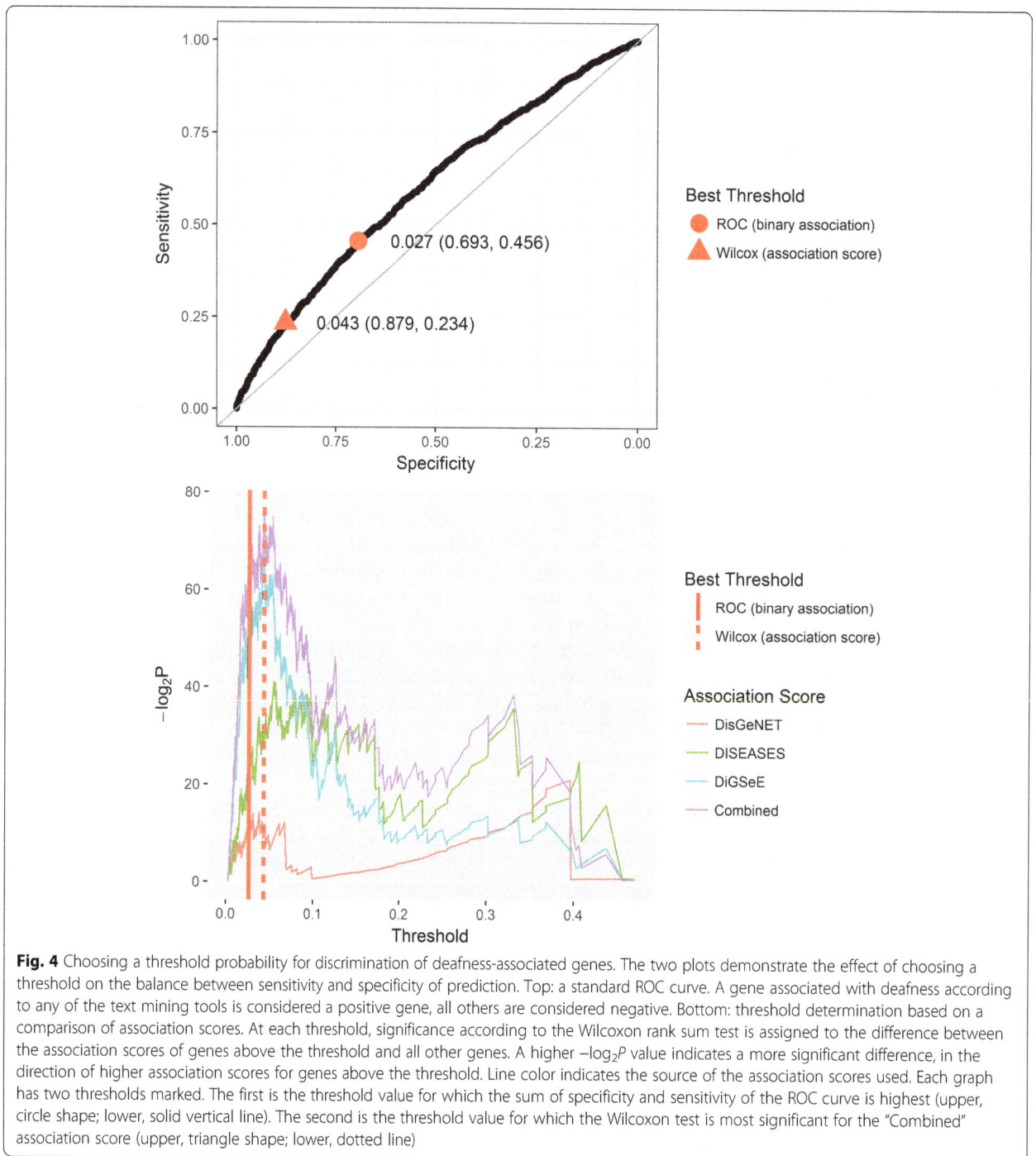

Fig. 4 Choosing a threshold probability for discrimination of deafness-associated genes. The two plots demonstrate the effect of choosing a threshold on the balance between sensitivity and specificity of prediction. Top: a standard ROC curve. A gene associated with deafness according to any of the text mining tools is considered a positive gene, all others are considered negative. Bottom: threshold determination based on a comparison of association scores. At each threshold, significance according to the Wilcoxon rank sum test is assigned to the difference between the association scores of genes above the threshold and all other genes. A higher $-\log_2 P$ value indicates a more significant difference, in the direction of higher association scores for genes above the threshold. Line color indicates the source of the association scores used. Each graph has two thresholds marked. The first is the threshold value for which the sum of specificity and sensitivity of the ROC curve is highest (upper, circle shape; lower, solid vertical line). The second is the threshold value for which the Wilcoxon test is most significant for the "Combined" association score (upper, triangle shape; lower, dotted line)

post-transcriptional regulation of TFs, which reduces the correlation between the transcript levels and TF activity. In addition, while most TFs activate the transcription of the targets, certain factors can repress the transcription of some or all of their targets. Moreover, taking the median FC of the TFs associated with a motif ignores the possibility of complex interrelationships, such as the ability of a subset of the TFs to activate transcription alone (an example for the motif AHRHIF is discussed later).

The TFs identified as being associated with development were compared with TF genes shown to change their expression during avian regeneration of inner ear sensory epithelia in one of two experiments conducted in chick. The first experiment measured expression of TFs after either laser "wounding" cultured sensory epithelia or treating inner ear organs with the ototoxic antibiotic neomycin [22]. The sampling time points after the laser lesion (30 min, 1 h, 2 h and 3 h) were chosen in order to provide insights into the very early signaling events that occur after epithelial injury, while the sampling time points after a 24-h incubation of inner ear organ cultures with neomycin (immediately after incubation, and after 24 and 48 h in neomycin-free medium) were chosen to cover the period of the S-phase entry by supporting cells, which peaks at about 48 h after ototoxic injury in vitro. Unlike the first experiment, which measured responses to lesions in both cochlear and vestibular cultures, the second regeneration experiment [23] from the same group only measured expression in chick utricles. Also, the second experiment only explored the effect of an ototoxic antibiotic on gene expression. Still, this study had several advantages over [22]. First, it followed the expression changes across a 7-day time course, with more frequent measures in the 48–72 h window of regeneration, a period characterized by highly dynamic patterns of expression for many genes. Second, it employed RNA-seq instead of microarrays for the expression measuring, allowing the authors to obtain a comprehensive transcriptome, instead of specifically focusing on transcription factors expression as was done in the first experiment.

The comparison of the TFs was designed to detect pathways that are common to inner ear development and regeneration and specifically to reveal genes essential for either proliferation of supporting cells, or for transdifferentiation to hair cells. Out of 712 DE TFs in the first regeneration experiment [22], we mapped 596 to orthologous mouse genes. Intersection with our list of 64 TFs yielded 33 TFs that are involved in both development and regeneration (Additional file 1: Figure S4). Significantly, eight of these are also DE. The overlap with the later avian transcriptome experiment [23] was far more limited. Out of 212 DE TFs found in the experiment, we mapped 208 to orthologous mouse genes, of which only six appear also in our list of TFs (Additional file 1: Figure S5), and five of them are also DE. The TFs SMAD9 and SPI1 were DE in both avian experiments and were associated with enriched motifs in our developmental study.

Finally, we performed a comprehensive literature search for the motifs found in the context of inner ear development. For a small subset, the results are detailed in the following sections, with a more complete list available in Additional file 1: Supplementary Results.

Transcription factors affecting expression changes with age
The set of genes that were upregulated at E16.5 was enriched for binding sites for the motifs: Elk-1, Nrf-1, E2F-1, E2F, NF-Y, and AHRHIF of which, the subset Elk-1, Nrf-1, NF-Y, E2F-1 and some TFs associated with the motifs AHRHIF (Arnt and AhR) were upregulated together with their regulated genes. Upregulation of

Hif1a, another motif associated with AHRHIF, could be detected at P0, suggesting that the upregulation of Arnt controlled genes is achieved by an increase in the formation of the heterodimer Arnt:AhR and not Arnt:Hif1a [37]. There was no enrichment of binding sites detected in the genes upregulated at P0.

ELK1 and TFs associated with AHRHIF are known to change their expression during regeneration. The expression of ELK1 was reported to increase 30 min after wounding cochlear hair cells with a laser, marking an early signaling event that occurs after epithelial damage [22]. Another TF that was increased after cellular insult was the AHRHIF TF, ARNT whose expression increased 24 h after exposing cochlear hair cells to neomycin, only to decrease again by 48 h, together with HIF1A and AHR. These time points reflect a change of expression in the supporting cells [22]. The transient increase of ARNT during regeneration resembles its transient expression pattern during normal inner ear development, between E13 and E17 in mouse cochlear epithelial cells [38]. Interestingly, the three TFs (ARNT, HIF1A, and AHR) were also reported to respond to tissue damage caused by a different toxic compound (TCDD [39]). E2F1 is an important pro-apoptotic TF [40], and under some mitochondrial stress, it engages apoptotic signals to cause deafness [41]. Regulation of transcription during the cell cycle is under the control of E2 factors (E2Fs), often in cooperation with nuclear factor Y (NF-Y) [42], another TF highlighted in this comparison. In utricle hair cell regeneration [23], E2F1 is changing its expression in a pattern that is associated with cell cycle genes. As mentioned, this TF and its targets are upregulated in E16.5, an age when we see enrichment for cell cycle activity.

Transcription factors affecting expression change between tissues
In contrast to the genes differentially expressed during the development, the set of genes upregulated in the cochlea was enriched for binding sites for the motifs: HIC1, E2F, ZNF219, ZF5, UF1H3BETA, MOVO-B, MAZ, VDR, MAZR, MTF-1, c-Myc:Max, AP-2, CAC-binding protein, ETF, E47, Lmo2 complex, RREB-1, LBP-1, CP2/LBP-1c/LSF, and Spz1. TFs associated with E2F, ZF5, and MAZ were significantly upregulated in the cochlea, while TFs associated with MOVO-B, VDR, and Lmo2 complex were upregulated in the vestibule. TFs associated with 11 of these 20 motifs (LBP-1, Lmo2 complex, E47, E2F, ZNF219, ZF5, VDR, MTF-1, c-Myc:Max, AP-2, CP2/LBP-1c/LSF) have been previously reported to change their expression during the regeneration of inner ear sensory epithelia [22, 23].

Focusing on genes that are altered both during development and regeneration, the enrichment of E2F noted indicates the presence of proliferation in the cochlea at the relevant period of development. Given the role of this TF family in inducing proliferation, their involvement in hair cell regeneration is not surprising and is currently the focus of active research [43]. In contrast, *ZF5* is known primarily as a repressor of transcription and specifically as a regulator of cell cycle progression (through *c-myc* [44]), and cognitive development (through *FMR1* [45]). Thus, the upregulation of expression in the cochlea, where its targets are also upregulated, was unexpected. This might indicate the existence of an additional activating role for *ZF5*, or that another TF is activating the transcription of these targets, and *ZF5* is upregulated as part of a negative feedback loop. In avian hair cell regeneration, the expression of *ZF5* in the cochlea increases late in the recovery from neomycin damage, suggesting a role in cochlear hair cell differentiation. Another TF with the same pattern of expression during hair cell regeneration is *LMO2*. Enrichments for *LMO2* binding sites were found in the list of upregulated genes from both the cochlea and the vestibule. While the results of the regeneration experiment support a function for *LMO2* in the cochlea, the expression of the TF in our experiment was higher in the vestibule. A possible explanation for this duality could be that LMO2 interacts with different partners in the two tissues, and thus, a different subset of genes is increased in each case. The Lmo2 complex typically contains a single GATA factor and a single TAL1/E47 heterodimer, but the GATA factor can be replaced by an additional TAL1/E47 heterodimer, resulting in a change in the genes regulated [46]. As *Gata2* and *Gata3* are upregulated in the vestibule and *Tal1* is upregulated in the cochlea (DE q-values = 7.32×10^{-18}, 1.67×10^{-175}, and 5.29×10^{-7}, respectively), the complexes formed in each tissue might differ in composition. *VDR* is a transcription factor regulated by vitamin D levels [47]. Hypo- and hypervitaminosis D can cause sensorineural hearing loss [48]. The downregulation of the gene in the cochlea, where its targets are upregulated, suggests a repressor role for this TF, which is supported by existing literature [49]. In utricle hair cell generation [23], *VDR*'s expression peaks in the 54–72 h window after the aminoglycoside damage. This pattern makes it a candidate for playing a role in the phenotypic conversion process from supporting cells to hair cells in the vestibule. According to our experiment, it might fulfill a similar role in the vestibular development.

In the set of genes upregulated in the vestibule, we could detect enrichment for binding sites for the 21 motifs: HNF4, SREBP-1, NF-1, PEA3, TEF-1, AP-2rep, NF-kappaB (p65), LBP-1, LUN-1, E2A, PU.1, MyoD, Nrf2, Lmo2 complex, COUPTF, ISRE, HEB, E47, SMAD, AML-1a, and c-Ets-1. TFs associated with five motifs

(TEF-1, PU.1, Nrf2, Lmo2 complex, and ISRE) were significantly upregulated in the vestibule, while TFs associated with four other motifs (PEA3, COUPTF, most SMADs, and AML-1a) were upregulated in the cochlea. TFs associated with 15 of the 21 enriched motifs (HNF4, SREBP-1, PEA3, NF-kappaB p65, LBP-1, E2A, PU.1, MyoD, Nrf2, Lmo2 complex, COUPTF, ISRE, HEB, E47, SMAD, c-Ets-1) displayed a change in expression during the regeneration experiments [22, 23].

The upregulation of TFs associated with the motifs *Spi1* [PU.1] and *Nfe2l2* [Nrf2] in the vestibule supports their role as inducers of transcription. However, the decrease seen in the cochlear expression in late (48 h) recovery from neomycin [22] suggests that their repression is required for proper differentiation of supporting cells to cochlear cells. *SPI1* is known to be involved in hematopoietic development and induces proliferation of immune cells [50] and therefore might upregulate the immune functions that are enriched in the vestibule. Similarly, *NFE2L2* can upregulate functions related to stress response and specifically to antioxidant defense [51]. The expression pattern of *Nr2f1* and *Nr2f2* associated with the COUPTF motif is in agreement with their suggested role as repressors of transcription, as they are downregulated in the vestibule, although the motif as a whole is enriched in the genes upregulated in the vestibule. Following laser damage, the expression of *NR2F2* increases in the cochlea for 3 h and an increase in cochlear expression is also evident in late (48 h) recovery from neomycin [22]. *Nr2f2* is known to work as a repressor of myogenesis, inhibiting *MyoD* [52], another TF whose targets are upregulated in the vestibule. Our data suggest that their repressive effect might have a role in cochlea development.

SMADs are intracellular proteins that transduce extracellular signals from transforming growth factor beta (TGF-β) ligands to the nucleus, where they activate downstream gene transcription [53]. Although TGF-β signaling is thought to be active in the cochlea, our results show rather that the downstream targets of this pathway are enriched in the vestibule. In order to address this issue, we examined the expression levels of individual SMADs. Most receptor-regulated SMADs (R-SMADs) were upregulated in the cochlea (*Smad1*, *Smad2*, *Smad5*, *Smad9*), in agreement with the hypothesis of higher TGF-β activity in the cochlea. However, inhibitors of this signaling pathway (*Smad6* and *Smad7*) were also upregulated in the cochlea, and with relatively high FCs (1.9 and 1.6, respectively), and may be responsible for decreasing the transcription of the downstream genes in the cochlea compared to the vestibule. The story becomes more complex with the two intracellular pathways involving SMADs. The R-SMADS *Smad2* and *Smad3* mediate the response to TGF-β ligands, which participate in the regulation of inner ear development by retinoic acid [54]. *Smad2* was upregulated in the cochlea, while *Smad3* was upregulated in the vestibule. In the regeneration experiment [22], *SMAD2* expression in the vestibule increased in a late response to neomycin damage in the utricle, emphasizing the importance of TGF-β signaling for vestibular differentiation. In a different pathway, the R-SMADS *Smad1*, *Smad5*, and *Smad9* mediate the response to bone morphogenetic proteins (BPMs), which are involved in generation of inner ear sensory epithelia [55], as well as chondrogenesis [56]. All three were upregulated in the cochlea, with *Smad9* showing a very impressive FC of 3.4. *SMAD9* was also increased in response to late neomycin damage in the cochlea [22]. This, together with its high cochlear levels, implies that it plays a role in cochlear differentiation.

SPI1 and *SMAD9* also change in expression during utricle hair cell regeneration [23]. The patterns of the expression are complex. Notably, their maximal deviations from the control are at time point 66 h, where *SPI1* is upregulated and *SMAD9* is downregulated. These changes are of opposite directions to those observed in cochlear regeneration in [22], agreeing with the tissue-specific roles of the two TFs.

Transcription factors affecting expression ratio change with age

In the set of genes for which the cochlea to vestibule expression ratio increases with age ($\frac{Cochlea}{Vestibule}\uparrow$), we could detect enrichment for the binding sites for the motifs HNF4, E47, and a group of nuclear receptors (LXR, PXR, CAR, COUP, RAR), AP-4, and SMAD. The expression ratio of *Nr2f1*, a COUP TF, increased significantly in the same direction as its targets, which might have a positive downstream effect on retinoic acid receptor (RAR) signaling [57]. Interestingly, TFs associated with all the motifs changed their expression during the regeneration of inner ear sensory epithelia [22].

Retinoid signaling is critical during inner ear embryonic development, as well as in the postnatal maintenance of its function [58]. Both vitamin A deficiency and intake of excess retinoic acid (RA) during pregnancy have been shown to cause malformations in ear development. In rodents, in utero exposure of fetuses to RA negatively affected the semicircular canals and the cochlea. Key components in retinoid signaling show spatiotemporal expression patterns, and the interactions that excess RA interferes with are dependent on the developmental stage. KEGG enrichment of our DE genes showed that metabolism of RA was higher in the vestibule and at P0. Taken together with the motif enrichment, we deduce that retinoid signaling is important to both cochlear and vestibular development, with its role

in the cochlea becoming more prominent in the period between E16.5 and P0. In the hair cell regeneration experiment, the cochlear expression of the retinoid receptor *RARA* decreased 24 h after neomycin damage, but by 48 h, *NR2F1* expression increased [22]. This later increase might mimic the increase in retinoid signaling seen in normal development.

Interestingly, we could detect enrichment of binding sites for AML-1a, LEF1, LBP-1, HEB, and POU6F1 in the set of genes for which the vestibule to cochlea expression ratio increases with age ($\frac{Vestibule}{Cochlea}\uparrow$). The expression ratio of *Runx1* [AML-1a] increased significantly in the same direction as its targets. TFs associated with LBP-1 and HEB also changed their expression during the regeneration of inner ear sensory epithelia.

Comparison with transcription factors known to enhance mammalian hair cell regeneration

Previous studies that induced hair cell regeneration by coordinated manipulation of multiple factors, showed a better efficacy for the ectopic expression of *ETV4*, *TCF3*, *GATA3*, *MYCN*, or *ETS2* in combination with *ATOH1* over the overexpression of *ATOH1* alone [18, 19]. In retrospect, our method identifies some of the TFs that were mentioned earlier for their ability to induce differentiation. Specifically, it singles out *Etv4* [PEA3] and *Tcf3* [E47]; *Gata3* is a partner of the highlighted *Lmo2*; and *Mycn* and *Ets2* have similar targets as *c-myc* [59] and *Ets1* [60], respectively. Moreover, four out of five of the TF genes are DE between the cochlea and the vestibule (*Etv4*, *Gata3*, *Mycn*, and *Ets4*; *q* value ≤ 0.05), which makes them good candidates for experimental interventions, as explained above.

Change in the proportion of hair cells in sensory epithelia

Because of the difficulty of dissecting out the sensory epithelia and separating the hair cells from the adjacent supporting cells, all tissue samples of this type contain varying amounts of both hair cells and supporting cells. This complicates conclusions as to whether differential expression can be attributed to differences in the expression profiles or to variability in the cell mixture composition. In order to address this issue, we produced expression signatures of hair cells and supporting cells from a previous experiment [21] and used them to compute the proportion of each type in each preparation. We also evaluated the heterogeneity of cell types assuming that the cochlear sample is contaminated by cells from the vestibule (or utricle) and vice versa.

A different subset of genes was used to create the signatures for E16.5 and P0. For each age, we ranked the genes in decreasing order of expression variance across the four reference samples (cochlear and vestibular GFP

+ and GFP− samples). We then took the expression of the first k genes in the list, where k equals 453 for E16.5, and 193 for P0. The value of k was chosen so that it minimized the estimated percentage of contamination in our mixed data, i.e., the estimated percentage of cochlear cells in vestibular samples plus the estimated percentage of vestibular cells in cochlear samples. We predicted that this heuristic approach would improve the overall prediction accuracy, although it did not directly optimize the precision of estimation of the percentage hair cells, which was our main goal. We used DeconRNASeq to estimate the mixing proportions [61].

The estimated proportions of hair cells were similar in both scenarios (Fig. 5), which allows us to ignore the issue of possible tissue contamination. The estimated percentages (±SD) are 32.6 (± 1.6) and 23.8 (± 1.0) in the cochlea and the vestibule at E16.5 and 44.0 (± 1.1) and 40.1 (± 0.2) in the cochlea and the vestibule at P0, respectively. These results indicate that the percentage of hair cells is higher in the cochlea at both ages and increases with development in both tissues, with the increase in the vestibule being more prominent (1.9-fold increase compared to 1.4-fold in the cochlea). Strikingly, in all estimations, the percentage of supporting cells was higher than 50%, suggesting that these cells have a dominant influence on the expression profiles.

Even with the value of k selected to minimize the contamination, our calculation gives 51.8% contamination in the cochlea at P0. We are unsure how to interpret this high number. Possible causes for an overestimate of contamination could be (1) experimental noise, either in our data or the data used to generate the expression signatures at P0, or (2) inaccuracy of the deconvolution method when the signatures are similar. The similarity of the signatures of the same cell type in the cochlea and the vestibule can be seen by the high correlation values ($r = 0.65$, or 0.83 for signatures of hair cells and supporting cells, respectively).

Discussion

In this study, we analyzed sensory epithelia RNA-seq data from mouse at E16.5 and P0, which correspond to developmental stages before and during the acquisition of mechanosensitivity. By exploring these data with considerations of developmental age and tissue type, we provided extensive information about the development of the inner ear. Moreover, we identified multiple transcription factors that are involved in transcriptional regulation, and a comparison with previous reports [22, 23] enabled us to focus on those that are also involved in regeneration of the avian inner ear after damage.

The sensory epithelium constitutes a heterogeneous tissue composed of hair cells and supporting cells, which cannot be easily separated by mechanical means. Although some previous experiments (e.g., [21]) employed FACS sorting to obtain pure populations, the analysis of data from the native tissue has the advantage of summarizing the expression of the hair cells and the milieu with which they interact. Although we did not physically separate the cells by type, we did estimate the contributions of each cell type by using expression deconvolution. Our results indicated a higher hair cell content in the cochlea compared to the vestibule, a content, which increased further during development in both tissues, albeit with a relatively larger increase in the vestibule.

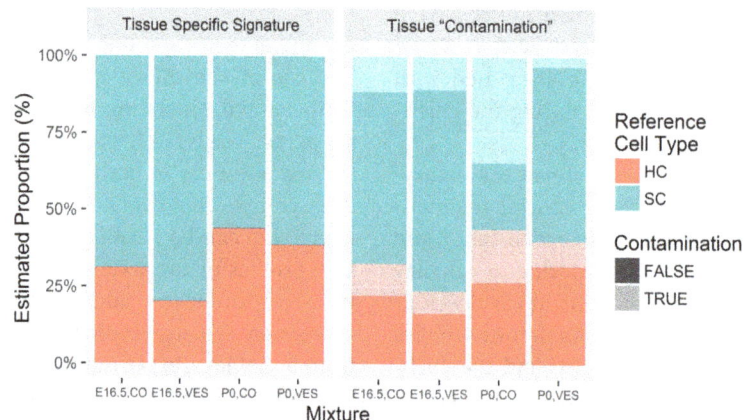

Fig. 5 Estimated proportions of hair cells and supporting cells in various samples. This estimated proportion of each cell type in each of the groups is displayed in a stack bar chart, where the color of a stack identifies the cell type. On the left side, the cells composing a tissue were confined to originating from that tissue, without allowing cross-tissue contamination, whereas on the right side, cross-tissue contamination is assumed to occur. A light color indicates the amount of contamination. For example, focusing on the cochlear tissue at age P0 (P0.CO), the estimated proportion of hair cells, when contamination is not allowed, is 44.1% (in red). When contamination is allowed, the estimated proportion of hair cells decreases slightly to 44.0% and is composed of 26.6% cochlear hair cells (in dark red) and 17.4% contaminating vestibular hair cells (in light red). The three other samples show a majority of non-contaminated tissue (darker colors). HC hair cells, SC supporting cells

Nearly 75% of the variation in the gene expression of our samples was explained by principal components associated with age ($\sim 47.5\%$) or tissue ($\sim 27.5\%$). Our analysis therefore focused on expression comparisons during development and across tissues. We also analyzed the more complex interaction of age and tissue. Our results showed that both cochlear and vestibular tissues become less proliferative with development and more differentiated in order to acquire the specialization required for their roles in sensory perception. According to our estimations, this specialization is accompanied by an increase in the relative proportion of hair cells in the sensory epithelia.

More surprising results were obtained from a comparison between tissues. While the cochlea was characterized mainly by neurological GO terms, the vestibule was shown to be enriched for vascular, structural, and immunological functions. Some of these differences could be attributed to alterations in the relative proportion of hair cells, which are presumed to be the dominant cell type in the cochlea. This finding has medical implications, as the higher vascularization of the vestibule, and its accessibility to immune cells, might impact the susceptibility of the tissues to ototoxic medications and inner ear infections.

With respect to the interaction of tissue and age, one notable finding was the delay in the development of sensory perception in the cochlea compared to the vestibule. This finding is supported by a delayed acquisition of mechanosensitivity in the cochlea (between P0 and P2 [62]) compared to the vestibule (between E16 and E17 [63]). In contrast, neuron projection and signaling at E16.5 is less developed in the vestibule than the cochlea, although the gap decreases by P0. This decrease can be attributed to the relatively larger increase in the proportion of hair cells in the vestibule compared to the cochlea.

Known DGs tended to be differentially expressed between the tissues. From E16.5 to P0, there was an increase both in expression and in the cochlear to vestibular expression ratio. In order to predict the probabilities of unidentified genes being yet undiscovered DGs, we built a classifier based on expression patterns. This classifier achieved a ROC score of 0.602 in predicting which genes are associated with deafness when validated by text mining tools. While the list of deafness-associated genes produced might not accurately reflect the genes that are essential for hearing, we believe it to be a good proxy for the true list. Ranking genes according to their algorithm estimated probability of being DGs can be useful in prioritizing candidate DGs in a real-world scenario, e.g., when multiple candidates arise from a familial segregation study.

We used enrichment analysis to identify TFs that are responsible for differences in expression between across tissues or developmental stages. Some of the TFs we

identified as controlling expression were already known, e.g., the E2F family of TFs, which is responsible for promoting proliferation in the sensory epithelia and is controlled by retinoblastoma 1 during this stage of development [7], or the retinoic acid nuclear receptors, which are essential for the proper morphogenesis of the ear [58]. Our analysis not only strengthens the evidence connecting these known TFs to inner ear development, but also emphasizes their additional roles in hair cell regeneration in birds (see below). We also identified a number of TFs that do not have a known function in the inner ear. These include *Arnt*, which activates the transcription of its target genes in E16.5; COUP TFs, which we speculate to have a dual role, with *Nr2f2* in inhibiting myogenesis in the cochlea and *Nr2f1* in promoting retinoid signaling; and the hemopoiesis agent *Lmo2* [46], which we believe may interact with different coactivators in the vestibule and the cochlea.

To learn about the possibilities of regeneration of hearing in humans, it might be beneficial to mimic the regulation of transcription during a response to inner ear damage in birds and follow the ability of avian cochlear hair cells to regenerate [22]. Two experiments measured changes in TFs expression during such a response. The two complement each other, as the first [22] follows the response in both cochlear and vestibular tissues to either immediate laser damage or after a long exposure to ototoxic antibiotic, while the second [23] focuses only on vestibular response to an ototoxic antibiotic, but includes more frequent sampling, across a longer time period, using newer, more sensitive technologies, including RNA-seq. In these experiments, significant changes in hundreds of TFs were identified during the regenerative response. These factors were intersected with our list of developmental TFs, in order to highlight genes likely to be involved in either proliferation or differentiation. Although we could detect dozens of overlapping TFs, we focused only on those with differential expression, because this facilitates the interpretation of how the genes are regulated and suggests the possibility to influence this regulation through interventions.

To date, only a few TFs known to enhance mammalian cochlear hair cell regeneration were detected [18, 19]. For each of them, our method succeeded in detecting either the TF, a TF with a very similar motif or an interaction partner. Most of them showed differential expression, supporting our choice to further focus on TFs with this property. Moreover, our method highlighted the complex Arnt:AhR, which we believe is important in early development and undergoes a transient increase during regeneration of avian hair cells. We also concluded that an increase in the genes *Zbtb14* [ZF5], *Lmo2*, *Nr2f1*, *Nr2f2*, and *Smad9* and a decrease in *Spi1* [PU.1], *Nfe2l2* [Nrf2], and *Mafk* [Nrf2] are required for proper differentiation of the cochlea or hair cell regeneration. An increase in *Smad2* and *VDR* is involved in the parallel processes in the vestibule. Noteworthy, *Smad9* and *Spil* were DE in both avian regeneration experiments in directions that fit their suggested tissue specific roles.

The discussion has been concerned above with reprogramming of embryonic and neonatal tissue. Overcoming the limits of aging on reprogramming cochlear cells might be essential for clinical purposes because human cochleae become functionally mature neonatally and because sensorineural hearing loss is most prevalent in older adults [64]. Lately, it was shown that co-manipulation of *ATOH1* and $p27^{kip1}$ creates new cochlear hair cells in adult mice [64]. In contrast to known functions of *p27*, the authors did not observe proliferation of supporting cells or converted hair cells following its deletion and concluded that *p27* plays a cell cycle-independent role in preventing *ATOH1*-mediated conversion of adult supporting cells to hair cells by repressing *GATA3* expression. Only a limited number of converted hair cells could be produced in the models suggested in the article, and some of the converted hair cells exhibited clear signs of apoptotic cell death. We believe that by inducing a more proliferative environment, the numbers of new hair cells generated would increase and their survival would improve. For this purpose, it might be beneficial to ectopically express TFs that are active in the highly proliferative age E16.5 and are also upregulated in hair cell regeneration, especially in the immediate response phase. According to these criteria, *Elk1* and *Arntl* are the most prominent candidates. Suppression of the pro-apoptotic *E2f1* might contribute as well.

Conclusions

We found the cochlea to be more enriched in neurological functions, and to contain a higher percentage of hair cells than the vestibule, but also to display delayed development of sensory perception compared with the vestibule. The vestibule, on the other hand, was shown to be more vascular and more accessible to the immunological system. The majority of TFs we predict to be key regulators of the differentiation process have known functions that agree with this dichotomistic characterization. Selected TFs identified here may have potential as future candidates for inducing hair cell regeneration. Given the parallels between the mouse and human inner ear, in structure, function, genes, and mechanisms of pathogenesis leading to deafness, several of these candidates may be relevant for human hearing loss.

Methods

Generation of mRNA data

Data generation for E16.5 and P0 samples is described in our previous articles [24, 25, 65]. The datasets are available in the Gene Expression Omnibus (GEO) repository under accession numbers GSE97270 (E16.5) GSE76149 (P0) and are available on the gene Expression Analysis Resource web portal, gEAR, http://umgear.org/p?s=ace02363 (SVG); http://umgear.org/p?s=1e3f9408 (bar graph). Sequence data was analyzed as previously described [24].

Principal component analysis

Principal components were calculated with R, after scaling and centering the log2-transformed RPKM values and plotted using ggbiplot (http://github.com/vqv/ggbiplot). Swamp (http://CRAN.R-project.org/package=swamp) was used to test the association between the principal components and annotations of sample age and tissue.

Differential expression

Differential expression analysis was done using edgeR [66]. The design formula included the combination of age and tissue of each sample. The tested contrasts were the average difference between the two ages across tissues, the average difference between the two tissues across ages, and the difference of the differences at both ages. This last contrast is sometimes referred to as the interaction term of tissue and age. edgeR detection threshold was q value ≤ 0.05. An FDR correction was applied for each contrast separately.

GO and KEGG enrichment analysis

We performed the enrichment analysis using the Expander software [67], exploring all GO ontologies, "biological process" (BP), "molecular function" (MF), and "cellular component" (CC) (corrected p value ≤ 0.05), and KEGG pathways (q value ≤ 0.01). For each contrast, we looked separately for enrichments in the set of genes upregulated and downregulated, using as a background set all the genes that were tested for differential expression.

Illustrating age-tissue interacting GO terms

We calculated the expression ratios between the cochlea and the vestibule for E16.5 and P0 separately, using edgeR [66]. We then z-scored the ratios at each age, to allow a fair comparison of the ages. These ratios were used both to select which GO terms to display and to calculate a median ratio for each of these terms.

To select GO terms, we began with the lists of terms enriched in genes with increased cochlear to vestibular (C/V) or vestibular to cochlear (V/C) ratios between E16.5 and P0 (see GO and KEGG enrichment analysis). From each of these lists separately, we filtered only the GO terms for which the expression ratios of annotated genes are higher at P0 than at E16.5 (one-sided Wilcoxon signed rank test at the respected direction, q value ≤ 0.05). An FDR correction was applied for each list separately.

TF enrichment analysis

We performed the enrichment analysis using PRIMA [68] with detection threshold q value ≤ 0.1. An FDR correction was applied for each list separately.

Deafness genes expression patterns

One hundred forty DGs were manually curated from http://hereditaryhearingloss.org/ (updated 3/13/17). Using BioMart [69], we mapped 133 of the genes to mouse orthologs. Three genes were filtered out due to missing expression data of their homologs. To resolve multiple mapping, we preferably mapped to orthologs for which we have expression data. The DGs were annotated according to the type of deafness, as syndromic, non-syndromic, or mitochondrial. Genes that were associated with both syndromic and non-syndromic deafness were treated as if they were syndromic in subsequent analyses.

Classifying deafness genes by expression

We built a classifier in order to categorize each gene as DG or non-DG. We are aware that some of the genes currently categorized as non-DGs are in fact DGs that have not yet been discovered. Our classifier thus learned to distinguish between positive and unlabeled genes. For every gene, the features for the classifier were (1) the averaged expression over all samples, in log counts per million (CPM), (2) the logarithm of the fold change (FC) of expression between the ages, (3) the logarithm of FC of expression between the tissues, and (4) the logarithm of the FC of the tissue expression ratio between the ages [i.e., log (cochlea to vestibule expression ratio at P0)/ (cochlea to vestibule expression ratio at E16.5)]. This last feature represents the interaction of age and tissue. All four features were computed using edgeR [66]; specifically, the FCs were obtained from the model presented in the 'Differential expression' section. We trained the classifier with 75% of the genes, reserving the remaining 25% for testing purposes. Our classifier bagged over 1000 decision trees. Downsampling was used to account for the imbalance in the frequencies of the deafness and non-DGs (130 and 15,076 genes respectively). That is, to build each decision tree, we chose 130 non-DGs at random and used them together with all DGs in the building process. The R package caret was used for machine learning [70].

We used only 25 repeated training/test splits to compare the classifier with a classifier using the averaged RPKM values in each condition as features. Two thousand repeated splits were used to assign gene probabilities, although internal testing revealed that the ROC score reached a plateau after about 150 iterations. In each iteration, we used the classifier to predict the probabilities in the test set, corrected these probabilities for the undersampling bias, and corrected them again for the bias caused by the PU scenario. The correction methods are detailed below.

The correction of the biases did not affect the ranking of the genes in that iteration and was performed in order to produce well-calibrated probabilities. We averaged the probabilities over all iterations. The averaging caused minor differences in ranking between different methods of calibration, but the ROC score did not change significantly ($p > 0.05$, DeLong's test for two correlated ROC curves [35]). We then assessed the calibration of the probabilities produced by each method. Under the assumption that most DGs are yet to be discovered, calibration curves that treat only known DGs as positive cases will falsely inflate the probabilities. For this reason, we downloaded lists of genes that were associated with hearing loss according to the text mining tools and assumed that these deafness-associated genes together with the known DGs comprise the full list of DGs. The annotation of DAGs and the comparison of the calibration are detailed below. An illustration of the classification process is provided in Additional file 1: Figure S6.

We then used these probabilities to build an improved classifier where p_g represents our estimation of the probability of gene g. We reran our bagging-like algorithm, but this time, we chose to treat a gene g as a positive example with probability p_g and as a negative example with probability $1 - p_g$. This reassignment was performed before each iteration, independently for each gene, and only for the unlabeled genes. Labeled genes were always treated as positive examples. This idea is inspired by [30] where the authors achieved slightly better results by rerunning their classifier with weights based on the initial probabilities learnt, after adjusting for the PU bias. Instead of reweighing the samples, we decided to reassign their classes, as reassignment (of only a few hundred genes) still allows us to perform undersampling. We again used 2000 repeated splits and averaged the probabilities over all iterations. We did not perform any bias correction until the end of the run, when we performed a correction only due to undersampling, as detailed below. We compared the ability of the initial classifier and the "rerun" classifier to predict DAGs among all unlabeled genes using DeLong's test for two correlated ROC curves [35]. Assuming a considerable portion of DAGs are undiscovered DGs, we wished our algorithm to rank those higher than genes that are neither known DGs nor deafness-associated. It should be noted that the probabilities assigned by the classifiers to known DGs are ignored in this comparison, because the annotation of these genes as positive in the training of the initial classifier can lead to an artificial inflation of the probabilities assigned by the "rerun" classifier. An illustration of the classification process improvement is provided in Additional file 1: Figure S7.

Finally, we converted the mouse genes back to human genes and resolved multiple mapping by averaging the assigned probabilities.

Calibration of the estimator

The calibration of the probabilities was tested using calibration plots produced with the R package caret. The prediction space was discretized into 11 bins. Cases with a predicted value between 0 and 0.09 fell in the first bin, between 0.09 and 0.18 in the second bin, etc. For each bin, the mean predicted value was plotted against the true fraction of positive cases, together with the 95% binomial confidence interval. If the model is well calibrated, the points should fall near the diagonal line. We also used the BS to measure probabilities calibration [71]. The lower the BS, the more accurate are the probabilistic predictions of a model. Let $\widehat{p}(y_i|x_i)$ be the probability estimate of sample x_i to have class $y_i \in \{0, 1\}$. Then BS is defined as:

$$BS = \frac{1}{N} \sum_{i=1}^{N} \{y_i - \widehat{p}(y_i|x_i)\}^2$$

Correcting undersampling bias

Undersampling creates an upward bias of the probabilities. To correct for this bias, we used the transformation suggested in [31] where p_s is the probability assigned by the model learnt on the balanced training set. p' is the bias-corrected probability obtained from p_s:

$$p' = \frac{\beta p_s}{\beta p_s - p_s + 1}$$

where β is the probability of selecting a negative instance with undersampling.

We used this method in two iterations. First, we adapted our PU classifier. Since we know whether each gene is positive or unlabeled ("negative"), then the estimation of β is trivial. We set $\beta = \frac{N^+}{N^-}$, with $N^+ = 130$ and $N^- = 15{,}076$. Second, we adapted the "rerun" classifier, which used initial, well-calibrated probabilities as input. The expected number of DGs according to these input probabilities was $E(N^+) = 435$. We thus set $\beta \cong \frac{E(N^+)}{15{,}206 - E(N^+)}$.

Correcting positive-unlabeled bias

PU classifiers create a downward bias of the probabilities. If x is an example, then let $y \in \{0, 1\}$ be a binary label. Let $s = 1$ if the example x is labeled and let $s = 0$ if x is unlabeled. According to [30], $p(y = 1|x) = p(s = 1|x)/c$ where $c = p(s = 1|y = 1)$. Our PU classifier estimates $p(s = 1|x)$, the probability of the example to be labeled. In order to

obtain an estimate for $p(y = 1|x)$, the positivity probability, we need to divide the first probability by an estimate of c. Three estimators were suggested for c:

$$e_1 = \frac{1}{n} \sum_{x \in P} g(x)$$

$$e_2 = \sum_{x \in P} g(x) / \sum_{x \in V} g(x)$$

$$e_3 = \max_{x \in V} g(x)$$

where $g(x) = p(s = 1|x)$ is the posterior probability according to the PU classifier, V is the validation set, and P is the subset of examples in V that are labeled. We used the same set V for validation (estimating c) and for testing (estimating probabilities).

Methods e_1 and e_2 can give estimated probabilities higher than 1. For the calibration plots and calculation of BSs, we truncated them at 1 which gave us 1128 and 1897 probabilities that exceeded 1 for e_1 and e_2, respectively.

We note that e_1 should theoretically have a lower variance than e_3, since it involves averaging multiple samples instead of using just one [30]. However, we cannot assume that e_1 is necessarily more accurate than e_3, especially as the number of positive samples in a validation set used for e_1 calculations is only 32 whereas the e_3 set has a maximum of 3801 probabilities, and as such, might be more accurate. In practice, we used all three estimates and chose the one that produced the most calibrated probabilities to be e_3.

Deafness-associated gene annotation

We downloaded lists of genes that were associated with hearing loss according to the text mining tools DigSeE [32], DisGeNET [33], and DISEASES [34]. We searched the disease terms "Hearing Loss" in DigSeE and DisGeNET and the "Sensorineural Hearing Loss" in DISEASES. We then converted the human genes returned by the searches to mouse orthologs using BioMart [69]. In DisGeNET and DISEASES, an association has a score, but in DiGSeE, the association of gene g is characterized by the number of articles $n_{g, a}$ and the number of sentences within articles $n_{g, s}$ supporting it. We assigned this association the score $n_{g,a} + \frac{n_{g,s}}{\max_{x \in G} n_{x,s} + 1}$, i.e., the number of sentences served as a tie breaker if two genes had the same number of articles. In order to calculate the ROC scores and BSs, we treated association as a binary trait and in order to demonstrate the effect of choosing different thresholds, we used Wilcoxon signed-rank test to compare the scores of genes with a probability above the threshold with the rest. The score of a gene not associated with deafness was set to 0. In this analysis, we also used a combined association score, which is the mean rank across the three lists of scores. We set the minimum "Combined" score to zero.

Deconvolution of heterogeneous tissue samples

Using RNA-seq expression data from [21], we created an expression signature for each combination of tissue (cochlea/utricle), age (E16/P0), and type (GFP+/GFP−; GFP was specifically expressed in hair cells in the transgenic mouse used). For the process of deconvolution of heterogeneous tissue data, limiting signatures to a few hundred genes, which best separate the reference cell types, can provide accurate predictions [72, 73]. We therefore selected a separate subset of genes for each age using the following heuristics. First, we ranked the genes in decreasing order of expression variance across the four reference samples. Then, we took the first k genes in the list, with k selected to minimize a specific error in the deconvolution of our mixed data. The error measure used provides signatures that differentiate well between cochlear and vestibular origins of tissue (described below). Once k was determined, we built the expression signatures, and used them to assess the proportion of cells, under two different scenarios. In the first, we limited the cells composing a tissue to cells that originated from that tissue, while in the other, we allowed the inclusion of foreign cells mimicking a contaminated sample. The property we minimized in the selection of k was the estimated percentage of contamination in our mixed data under this second scenario, i.e., the estimated percentage of cochlear cells in vestibular samples plus the estimated percentage of vestibular cells in cochlear samples. We tested all possible ks in the range 1...1000. For E16.5, we chose the minimizing $k = 453$, but for P0, we ignored the first local minimum, which was narrow (~ 5 genes), and instead chose $k = 193$ (Additional file 1: Figure S8).

The expression data of the mixture was given in units of RPKM, and of the reference in counts per million (CPM). We did not normalize the reference data to the gene length, because the technique used in [61] of sequencing the 3′ end is not biased by gene length. Before building a signature, we filtered out genes for which the CPM was less than 1 in any of the conditions (within an age). The calculation of the variance in the expression of a gene was done on log-transformed expression.

We used DeconRNASeq to estimate the mixing proportions [61] with the default setting of the R package, except that we chose not to scale the data. We performed the deconvolution on the log-transformed expression. This is not generally recommended, specifically for microarray data, as it introduces a bias [74]. However, when we tried to work with the expression in the linear scale without log transformation, our results deviated extremely from what is known about the ratio of

hair cell to supporting cells in both ages. To be specific, the estimated percentage of hair cells at E16.5 and P0 were ~ 12.5 and $\sim 70\%$ in both tissues. The gap is higher than expected, and, also, the second estimate is much higher than parallel quantities in other species. In adult humans between the ages of 27 and 67, 46.5% of the cells of the crista ampullaris are hair cells [75], and in hatched chicks, 28.2% of the cells in the utricular macula are hair cells [76]. Reference samples from E16 were used to estimate the proportions in our E16.5 samples. In addition, reference samples originating from the utricle were used to estimate the composition of our whole-vestibule samples. The estimation was done for each sample separately, and the predictions were subsequently averaged across each group.

Additional files

Additional file 1: Supplementary Data. Supplementary table legends,

Additional file 2: Enrichment Analysis. Enrichments in genes differentially expressed between ages, tissues, and the interaction of age

Additional file 3: Deafness genes. Genes associated with deafness compiled from www.hereditaryhearingloss.org (updated 3/13/17), and the differential expression results for the mouse orthologs of the

Additional file 4: Deafness genes prediction. Probabilities assigned to

Additional file 5: Transcription factors affecting transcription. Motifs enriched in genes differentially expressed between ages, tissues, and the interaction of age and tissue, and the expression of the TFs associated

Abbreviations
BS: Brier score; DAG: Deafness-associated gene; DE: Differentially expressed; DG: Deafness gene; E: Embryonic day; FC: Fold change; GO: Gene ontology; KEGG: Kyoto Encyclopedia of Genes and Genomes; P: Postnatal day; PCA: Principal component analysis; RA: Retinoic acid; TF: Transcription factor

Acknowledgements
We would like to thank Kathy Ushakov, Tal Koffler, and Ofer Yizhar-Barnea for their help with the experimental aspects of this work previously published. This work was performed in partial fulfillment of the requirements for a Ph.D. degree by Kobi Perl at the Sackler Faculty of Medicine, Tel Aviv University, Israel.

Funding
This work was supported by the National Institutes of Health (NIDCD) [grant number R01DC011835 to K.B.A.]; Israel Science Foundation [ISF-NSFC joint program to R.S., 2033/16 to K.B.A]; United States-Israel Binational Science Foundation [grant number 2013027 to K.B.A.], the Raymond and Beverly Sackler Chair in Bioinformatics (R.S.); the Drs Sarah and Felix Dumont Chair for Research of Hearing Disorders (K.B.A.); and the Edmond J. Safra Center for Bioinformatics at Tel Aviv University (K.P.).

Authors' contributions
KP, KBA, and RS conceived the study. KP, KBA, and RS wrote the manuscript. KP performed the computational analysis. All authors read and approved the final manuscript.

Ethics approval
All animal procedures from [24, 25, 62] were approved by the Animal Care and Use Committee at Tel Aviv University (M-10-087, M-13-114, 01-13-115).

Competing interests
The authors declare that they have no competing interests.

References

1. Petit C, Richardson GP. Linking genes underlying deafness to hair-bundle development and function. Nat Neurosci. 2009;12:703–10.
2. Friedman LM, Dror AA, Avraham KB. Mouse models to study inner ear development and hereditary hearing loss. Int J Dev Biol. 2007;51:609–31.
3. Platt RJ, Chen S, Zhou Y, Yim MJ, Swiech L, Kempton HR, Dahlman JE, Parnas O, Eisenhaure TM, Jovanovic M, et al. CRISPR-Cas9 knockin mice for genome editing and cancer modeling. Cell. 2014;159:440–55.
4. Zou B, Mittal R, Grati M, Lu Z, Shu Y, Tao Y, Feng Y, Xie D, Kong W, Yang S, et al. The application of genome editing in studying hearing loss. Hear Res. 2015;327:102–8.
5. Groves AK, Fekete DM. Shaping sound in space: the regulation of inner ear patterning. Development. 2012;139:245–57.
6. Wu DK, Kelley MW. Molecular mechanisms of inner ear development. Cold Spring Harb Perspect Biol. 2012;4:a008409.
7. Kelley MW. Regulation of cell fate in the sensory epithelia of the inner ear. Nat Rev Neurosci. 2006;7:837–49.
8. Kiernan AE, Ahituv N, Fuchs H, Balling R, Avraham KB, Steel KP, Hrabe de Angelis M. The notch ligand Jagged1 is required for inner ear sensory development. Proc Natl Acad Sci U S A. 2001;98:3873–8.
9. Vahava O, Morell R, Lynch ED, Weiss S, Kagan ME, Ahituv N, Morrow JE, Lee MK, Skvorak AB, Morton CC, et al. Mutation in transcription factor POU4F3 associated with inherited progressive hearing loss in humans. Science. 1998; 279:1950–4.
10. Corwin JT, Cotanche DA. Regeneration of sensory hair cells after acoustic trauma. Science. 1988;240:1772–4.
11. Ryals BM, Rubel EW. Hair cell regeneration after acoustic trauma in adult Coturnix quail. Science. 1988;240:1774–6.
12. Forge A, Davies S, Zajic G. Characteristics of the membrane of the stereocilia and cell apex in cochlear hair cells. J Neurocytol. 1988;17:325–34.
13. Kawamoto K, Izumikawa M, Beyer LA, Atkin GM, Raphael Y. Spontaneous hair cell regeneration in the mouse utricle following gentamicin ototoxicity. Hear Res. 2009;247:17–26.
14. Golub JS, Tong L, Ngyuen TB, Hume CR, Palmiter RD, Rubel EW, Stone JS. Hair cell replacement in adult mouse utricles after targeted ablation of hair cells with diphtheria toxin. J Neurosci. 2012;32:15093–105.
15. Cox BC, Chai R, Lenoir A, Liu Z, Zhang L, Nguyen DH, Chalasani K, Steigelman KA, Fang J, Rubel EW, et al. Spontaneous hair cell regeneration in the neonatal mouse cochlea in vivo. Development. 2014;141:816–29.
16. Kawamoto K, Ishimoto S, Minoda R, Brough DE, Raphael Y. Math1 gene transfer generates new cochlear hair cells in mature Guinea pigs in vivo. J Neurosci. 2003;23:4395–400.
17. Chien WW, Monzack EL, McDougald DS, Cunningham LL. Gene therapy for sensorineural hearing loss. Ear Hear. 2015;36:1–7.
18. Masuda M, Pak K, Chavez E, Ryan AF. TFE2 and GATA3 enhance induction of POU4F3 and myosin VIIa positive cells in nonsensory cochlear epithelium by ATOH1. Dev Biol. 2012;372:68–80.
19. Ikeda R, Pak K, Chavez E, Ryan AF. Transcription factors with conserved binding sites near ATOH1 on the POU4F3 gene enhance the induction of cochlear hair cells. Mol Neurobiol. 2015;51:672–84.
20. Vaquerizas JM, Kummerfeld SK, Teichmann SA, Luscombe NM. A census of human transcription factors: function, expression and evolution. Nat Rev Genet. 2009;10:252–63.
21. Scheffer DI, Shen J, Corey DP, Chen ZY. Gene expression by mouse inner ear hair cells during development. J Neurosci. 2015;35:6366–80.
22. Hawkins RD, Bashiardes S, Powder KE, Sajan SA, Bhonagiri V, Alvarado DM, Speck J, Warchol ME, Lovett M. Large scale gene expression profiles of regenerating inner ear sensory epithelia. PLoS One. 2007;2:e525.
23. Ku YC, Renaud NA, Veile RA, Helms C, Voelker CC, Warchol ME, Lovett M. The transcriptome of utricle hair cell regeneration in the avian inner ear. J Neurosci. 2014;34:3523–35.
24. Perl K, Ushakov K, Pozniak Y, Yizhar-Barnea O, Bhonker Y, Shivatzki S, Geiger T, Avraham KB, Shamir R. Reduced changes in protein compared to mRNA levels across non-proliferating tissues. BMC Genomics. 2017;18:305.

25. Rudnicki A, Isakov O, Ushakov K, Shivatzki S, Weiss I, Friedman LM, Shomron N, Avraham KB. Next-generation sequencing of small RNAs from inner ear sensory epithelium identifies microRNAs and defines regulatory pathways. BMC Genomics. 2014;15:484.
26. Cargnello M, Roux PP. Activation and function of the MAPKs and their substrates, the MAPK-activated protein kinases. Microbiol Mol Biol Rev. 2011; 75:50–83.
27. Wieduwilt MJ, Moasser MM. The epidermal growth factor receptor family: biology driving targeted therapeutics. Cell Mol Life Sci. 2008;65:1566–84.
28. Derynck R, Zhang YE. Smad-dependent and Smad-independent pathways in TGF-beta family signalling. Nature. 2003;425:577–84.
29. Mordelet F, Vert J-P. A bagging SVM to learn from positive and unlabeled examples. Pattern Recogn Lett. 2014;37:201–9.
30. Elkan C, Noto K. Learning classifiers from only positive and unlabeled data. Proceedings of the 14th ACM SIGKDD international conference on Knowledge discovery and data mining; 2008. p. 213–20.
31. Dal Pozzolo A, Caelen O, Johnson RA, Bontempi G. Calibrating probability with undersampling for unbalanced classification. IEEE Symp Ser. 2015: 159–66.
32. Kim J, Kim JJ, Lee H. An analysis of disease-gene relationship from Medline abstracts by DigSee. Sci Rep. 2017;7:40154.
33. Pinero J, Queralt-Rosinach N, Bravo A, Deu-Pons J, Bauer-Mehren A, Baron M, Sanz F, Furlong LI. DisGeNET: a discovery platform for the dynamical exploration of human diseases and their genes. Database (Oxford). 2015; 2015:bav028.
34. Pletscher-Frankild S, Palleja A, Tsafou K, Binder JX, Jensen LJ. DISEASES: text mining and data integration of disease-gene associations. Methods. 2015;74: 83–9.
35. DeLong ER, DeLong DM, Clarke-Pearson DL. Comparing the areas under two or more correlated receiver operating characteristic curves: a nonparametric approach. Biometrics. 1988;44:837–45.
36. Han C-P. Combining tests for correlation coefficients. Am Stat. 1989;43:211.
37. Jain S, Maltepe E, Lu MM, Simon C, Bradfield CA. Expression of ARNT, ARNT2, HIF1 alpha, HIF2 alpha and Ah receptor mRNAs in the developing mouse. Mech Dev. 1998;73:117–23.
38. Aitola MH, Pelto-Huikko MT. Expression of Arnt and Arnt2 mRNA in developing murine tissues. J Histochem Cytochem. 2003;51:41–54.
39. Mimura J, Fujii-Kuriyama Y. Functional role of AhR in the expression of toxic effects by TCDD. Biochim Biophys Acta. 2003;1619:263–8.
40. Matsumura I, Tanaka H, Kanakura Y. E2F1 and c-Myc in cell growth and death. Cell Cycle. 2003;2:333–38.
41. Raimundo N, Song L, Shutt TE, McKay SE, Cotney J, Guan MX, Gilliland TC, Hohuan D, Santos-Sacchi J, Shadel GS. Mitochondrial stress engages E2F1 apoptotic signaling to cause deafness. Cell. 2012;148:716–26.
42. Caretti G, Salsi V, Vecchi C, Imbriano C, Mantovani R. Dynamic recruitment of NF-Y and histone acetyltransferases on cell-cycle promoters. J Biol Chem. 2003;278:30435–40.
43. Tarang S, Doi SM, Gurumurthy CB, Harms D, Quadros R, Rocha-Sanchez SM. Generation of a retinoblastoma (Rb)1-inducible dominant-negative (DN) mouse model. Front Cell Neurosci. 2015;9:52.
44. Sobek-Klocke I, Disque-Kochem C, Ronsiek M, Klocke R, Jockusch H, Breuning A, Ponstingl H, Rojas S, Overhauser J, Eichenlaub-Ritter U. The human gene ZFP161 on 18p11.21-pter encodes a putative c-myc repressor and is homologous to murine Zfp161 (Chr 17) and Zfp161-rs1 (X Chr). Genomics. 1997;43:156–64.
45. Orlov SV, Kuteykin-Teplyakov KB, Ignatovich IA, Dizhe EB, Mirgorodskaya OA, Grishin AV, Guzhova OB, Prokhortchouk EB, Guliy PV, Perevozchikov AP. Novel repressor of the human FMR1 gene—identification of p56 human (GCC)(n)-binding protein as a Kruppel-like transcription factor ZF5. FEBS J. 2007;274:4848–62.
46. Chambers J, Rabbitts TH. LMO2 at 25 years: a paradigm of chromosomal translocation proteins. Open Biol. 2015;5:150062.
47. Carlberg C, Campbell MJ. Vitamin D receptor signaling mechanisms: integrated actions of a well-defined transcription factor. Steroids. 2013;78:127–36.
48. Zou J, Minasyan A, Keisala T, Zhang Y, Wang JH, Lou YR, Kalueff A, Pyykko I, Tuohimaa P. Progressive hearing loss in mice with a mutated vitamin D receptor gene. Audiol Neurootol. 2008;13:219–30.
49. Sanchez-Martinez R, Zambrano A, Castillo AI, Aranda A. Vitamin D-dependent recruitment of corepressors to vitamin D/retinoid X receptor heterodimers. Mol Cell Biol. 2008;28:3817–29.

Computational analysis of mRNA expression profiling in the inner ear reveals candidate transcription...

197

50. Celada A, Borras FE, Soler C, Lloberas J, Klemsz M, van Beveren C, McKercher S, Maki RA. The transcription factor PU.1 is involved in macrophage proliferation. J Exp Med. 1996;184:61–9.

51. Ma Q. Role of nrf2 in oxidative stress and toxicity. Annu Rev Pharmacol Toxicol. 2013;53:401–26.

52. Bailey P, Sartorelli V, Hamamori Y, Muscat GE. The orphan nuclear receptor, COUP-TF II, inhibits myogenesis by post-transcriptional regulation of MyoD function: COUP-TF II directly interacts with p300 and myoD. Nucleic Acids Res. 1998;26:5501–10.

53. Massague J, Wotton D. Transcriptional control by the TGF-beta/Smad signaling system. EMBO J. 2000;19:1745–54.

54. Butts SC, Liu W, Li G, Frenz DA. Transforming growth factor-beta1 signaling participates in the physiological and pathological regulation of mouse inner ear development by all-trans retinoic acid. Birth Defects Res A Clin Mol Teratol. 2005;73:218–28.

55. Li H, Corrales CE, Wang Z, Zhao Y, Wang Y, Liu H, Heller S. BMP4 signaling is involved in the generation of inner ear sensory epithelia. BMC Dev Biol. 2005;5:16.

56. Yoon BS, Ovchinnikov DA, Yoshii I, Mishina Y, Behringer RR, Lyons KM. Bmpr1a and Bmpr1b have overlapping functions and are essential for chondrogenesis in vivo. Proc Natl Acad Sci U S A. 2005;102:5062–7.

57. Lin B, Chen GQ, Xiao D, Kolluri SK, Cao X, Su H, Zhang XK. Orphan receptor COUP-TF is required for induction of retinoic acid receptor beta, growth inhibition, and apoptosis by retinoic acid in cancer cells. Mol Cell Biol. 2000; 20:957–70.

58. Romand R, Dolle P, Hashino E. Retinoid signaling in inner ear development. J Neurobiol. 2006;66:687–704.

59. Adhikary S, Eilers M. Transcriptional regulation and transformation by Myc proteins. Nat Rev Mol Cell Biol. 2005;6:635–45.

60. John S, Russell L, Chin SS, Luo W, Oshima R, Garrett-Sinha LA. Transcription factor Ets1, but not the closely related factor Ets2, inhibits antibody-secreting cell differentiation. Mol Cell Biol. 2014;34:522–32.

61. Gong T, Szustakowski JD. DeconRNASeq: a statistical framework for deconvolution of heterogeneous tissue samples based on mRNA-Seq data. Bioinformatics. 2013;29:1083–5.

62. Lelli A, Asai Y, Forge A, Holt JR, Geleoc GS. Tonotopic gradient in the developmental acquisition of sensory transduction in outer hair cells of the mouse cochlea. J Neurophysiol. 2009;101:2961–73.

63. Geleoc GS, Holt JR. Developmental acquisition of sensory transduction in hair cells of the mouse inner ear. Nat Neurosci. 2003;6:1019–20.

64. Walters BJ, Coak E, Dearman J, Bailey G, Yamashita T, Kuo B, Zuo J. In vivo interplay between p27(Kip1), GATA3, ATOH1, and POU4F3 converts non-sensory cells to hair cells in adult mice. Cell Rep. 2017;19:307–20.

65. Ushakov K, Koffler-Brill T, Aviv R, Perl K, Ulitsky I, Avraham KB. Genome-wide identification and expression profiling of long non-coding RNAs in auditory and vestibular systems. Sci Rep. 2017;7:8637.

66. Robinson MD, McCarthy DJ, Smyth GK. edgeR: a Bioconductor package for differential expression analysis of digital gene expression data. Bioinformatics. 2010;26:139–40.

67. Ulitsky I, Maron-Katz A, Shavit S, Sagir D, Linhart C, Elkon R, Tanay A, Sharan R, Shiloh Y, Shamir R. Expander: from expression microarrays to networks and functions. Nat Protoc. 2010;5:303–22.

68. Elkon R, Linhart C, Sharan R, Shamir R, Shiloh Y. Genome-wide in silico identification of transcriptional regulators controlling the cell cycle in human cells. Genome Res. 2003;13:773–80.

69. Durinck S, Spellman PT, Birney E, Huber W. Mapping identifiers for the integration of genomic datasets with the R/Bioconductor package biomaRt. Nat Protoc. 2009;4:1184–91.

70. Kuhn M. Building predictive models in R using the caret package. J Stat Soft. 2008;28:119804.

71. Brier GW. Verification of forecasts expressed in terms of probability. Mon Weather Rev. 1950;78:1–3.

72. Newman AM, Liu CL, Green MR, Gentles AJ, Feng W, Xu Y, Hoang CD, Diehn M, Alizadeh AA. Robust enumeration of cell subsets from tissue expression profiles. Nat Methods. 2015;12:453–7.

73. Gong T, Hartmann N, Kohane IS, Brinkmann V, Staedtler F, Letzkus M, Bongiovanni S, Szustakowski JD. Optimal deconvolution of transcriptional profiling data using quadratic programming with application to complex clinical blood samples. PLoS One. 2011;6:e27156.

74. Zhong Y, Liu Z. Gene expression deconvolution in linear space. Nat Methods. 2011;9:8–9. author reply 9

75. Lopez I, Ishiyama G, Tang Y, Tokita J, Baloh RW, Ishiyama A. Regional estimates of hair cells and supporting cells in the human crista ampullaris. J Neurosci Res. 2005;82:421–31.

76. Goodyear RJ, Gates R, Lukashkin AN, Richardson GP. Hair-cell numbers continue to increase in the utricular macula of the early posthatch chick. J Neurocytol. 1999;28:851–61.

18

Associations of high-altitude polycythemia with polymorphisms in *PIK3CD* and *COL4A3* in Tibetan populations

Xiaowei Fan[1,2†], Lifeng Ma[1,2†], Zhiying Zhang[1,2†], Yi Li[3,5], Meng Hao[3], Zhipeng Zhao[1,2], Yiduo Zhao[1,2], Fang Liu[1,2], Lijun Liu[1,2], Xingguang Luo[4], Peng Cai[1,2], Yansong Li[1,2] and Longli Kang[1,2*]

Abstract

Background: High-altitude polycythemia (HAPC) is a chronic high-altitude disease that can lead to an increase in the production of red blood cells in the people who live in the plateau, a hypoxia environment, for a long time. The most frequent symptoms of HAPC include headache, dizziness, breathlessness, sleep disorders, and dilation of veins. Although chronic hypoxia is the main cause of HAPC, the fundamental pathophysiologic process and related molecular mechanisms responsible for its development remain largely unclear yet.

Aim/methods: This study aimed to explore the related hereditary factors of HAPC in the Chinese Han and Tibetan populations. A total of 140 patients (70 Han and 70 Tibetan) with HAPC and 60 healthy control subjects (30 Han and 30 Tibetan) were recruited for a case-control association study. To explore the genetic basis of HAPC, we investigated the association between HAPC and both phosphatidylinositol-4,5-bisphosphonate 3-kinase, catalytic subunit delta gene (*PIK3CD*) and collagen type IV α3 chain gene (*COL4A3*) in Chinese Han and Tibetan populations.

Results/conclusion: Using the unconditional logistic regression analysis and the false discovery rate (FDR) calculation, we found that eight SNPs in *PIK3CD* and one SNP in *COL4A3* were associated with HAPC in the Tibetan population. However, in the Han population, we did not find any significant association. Our study suggested that polymorphisms in the *PIK3CD* and *COL4A3* were correlated with susceptibility to HAPC in the Tibetan population.

Keywords: High-altitude polycythemia, PIK3CD, COL4A3

Introduction

High-altitude polycythemia (HAPC) is a chronic high-altitude disease, characterized by excessive erythrocytosis. The clinical HAPC is diagnosed by a hemoglobin concentration ≥ 19 g/dL for females and ≥ 21 g/dL for males, according to the criteria established in the VI World Congress on Mountain Medicine and High-altitude Physiology in 2004 [1]. More than 140 million people are living at high altitudes above 2500 m worldwide, majorly in the Andes, Ethiopian Highlands, and Qinghai-Tibet Plateau

[2]. The Qinghai-Tibet Plateau is the highest plateau in the world, which covers a large area with low oxygen in natural environment, and millions of people are living and working in this region. It is well known that the body's hemoglobin concentration increases due to the hypoxic environment of high altitude, and therefore, this response is crucial for people who adapt to live at high altitudes. Some studies show that a number of populations suffer from chronic mountain sickness because they stay long at high altitudes [3]. HAPC mainly leads to a significant increase in blood viscosity, causing damage to microcirculatory and immune response disturbances such as vascular thrombosis, extensive organ damage, and sleep disorders [4, 5]. It is reported that the prevalence of HAPC in the Qinghai-Tibet Plateau is around 5 to 18% [1], and the prevalence of HAPC increases with the altitude. As the construction of the Qinghai-Tibet Railway has been

* Correspondence: longli_kang@163.com
†Xiaowei Fan, Lifeng Ma and Zhiying Zhang contributed equally to this work.
[1]Key Laboratory for Molecular Genetic Mechanisms and Intervention Research on High Altitude Disease of Tibet Autonomous Region, School of Medicine, Xizang Minzu University, Xianyang 712082, Shaanxi, China
[2]Key Laboratory of High Altitude Environment and Genes Related to Diseases of Tibet Autonomous Region, School of Medicine, Xizang Minzu University, Xianyang 712082, Shaanxi, China
Full list of author information is available at the end of the article

completed, a number of Han populations migrate to Tibet. The incidence of HAPC among immigrants is significantly higher than the high-altitude natives [6]. As the Tibetan population keeps genetic adaptations, they can easily adapt to the high-altitude hypoxia environment, for example, showing lower hemoglobin levels and lower hematocrit. Many studies have noted that there are some significant differences in the genomes between immigrants and high-altitude natives, which indicates that genetic factors may contribute to the development of HAPC, although the molecular mechanisms and pathogenesis are still under study. In our study, we aimed to investigate the associations between susceptibility to HAPC and two new candidate genes that are related to the oxygen metabolism in red blood cells but have not been reported before.

The first candidate, *PIK3CD*, encodes the p110δ catalytic subunit of phosphoinositide 3-kinaseδ (PI3Kδ), a member of a big family of metalloenzymes. PI3Kδ is a heterodimer comprising the p110δ and p85 family regulatory subunit and expressed predominantly in leukocytes. Therefore, it plays an important role in the proliferation, survival, and activation of leukocytes [7–9]. The expression pattern and functions of *PIK3CD* are very important in PI3K/Akt pathway. Recently, research studies revealed that PI3K/Akt mediated the stabilization of HIF-1α (hypoxia-inducible factors-1α) [10], and it was also involved in the increase of HIF-1α protein level [11]. Meanwhile, HIF-1α plays an important role in transcriptionally upregulating erythropoietin (EPO) in hypoxia and affecting the amount of red blood cells [12].

The second candidate, *COL4A3*, encodes a subunit of type IV collagen that is a structural protein of the alveolar extracellular matrix (ECM) and mostly found in the kidney, lung, and basement membranes. It is located at 2q35-q3 and mainly contains 51 exons [13]. Type IV collagen is involved in various physiological conditions, including aging, diabetes, kidney disease, scarring, and pulmonary fibrosis [14]. The ECM is important to the structure and function of cell types. It contributes to many processes, such as cellular proliferation, differentiation, migration, and apoptosis [15].

Results

The demographics of HAPC patients and controls are shown in Table 1. The basic characteristics of candidate SNPs in the Han and Tibetan subjects are summarized in Table 2 (Fig. 1) and Table 3 (Fig. 2). We analyzed the associations between SNPs and HAPC using unconditional logistic regression analysis. In the Han population, rs72633866 ($P1 = 0.033$ before adjustment and $P2 = 0.014$ after adjustment for age), rs9430220 ($P1 = 0.081$

Table 1 Demographics of the control individuals and patients with high-altitude polycythemia

Variables	Han		Tibetan	
	Case ($n = 70$)	Control ($n = 30$)	Case ($n = 70$)	Control ($n = 30$)
Male	35	15	35	15
Female	35	15	35	15

and $P2 = 0.029$), rs199962152 ($P1 = 0.024$ and $P2 = 0.034$), and rs10864435 ($P1 = 0.013$ and $P2 = 0.002$) in *PIK3CD* were significantly associated with HAPC. In the Tibetan subjects, rs2230735 ($P1 = 0.008$ and $P2 = 0.008$), rs28730671 ($P1 = 0.007$ and $P2 = 0.007$), rs111888887 ($P1 = 0.034$ and $P2 = 0.034$), rs28730674 ($P1 = 0.007$ and $P2 = 0.007$), rs371870925 ($P1 = 0.007$ and $P2 = 0.007$), rs199962152 ($P1 = 0.045$ and $P2 = 0.040$), rs77571929 ($P1 = 0.005$ and $P2 = 0.005$), rs117226273 ($P1 = 0.007$ and $P2 = 0.007$), rs28730676 ($P1 = 0.007$ and $P2 = 0.007$), and rs28730677 ($P1 = 0.007$ and $P2 = 0.007$) in *PIK3CD* were significantly associated with HAPC. Furthermore, rs34505188 ($P1 = 0.028$ and $P2 = 0.028$), rs11677877 ($P1 = 0.013$ and $P2 = 0.013$), rs34019152 ($P1 = 0.018$ and $P2 = 0.018$), and rs28381984 ($P1 = 0.001$ and $P2 = 0.001$) in *COL4A3* were associated with HAPC.

After using FDR to correct for multiple comparisons, in the Tibetan subjects, we found that rs2230735 (OR = 0.844, 95% CI = 0.337–2.079, $P = 0.046$), rs28730671 (OR = 0.821, 95% CI = 0.324–2.035, $P = 0.046$), rs28730 674 (OR = 0.821, 95% CI = 0.324–2.035, $P = 0.046$), rs371870925 (OR = 0.812, 95% CI = 0.320–2.017, $P = 0.046$), rs77571929 (OR = 0.814, 95% CI = 0.320–2.024, $P = 0.046$), rs117226273 (OR = 0.821, 95% CI = 0.324–2.035, $P = 0.046$), rs28730676 (OR = 0.821, 95% CI = 0.324–2.035, $P = 0.046$), rs28730676 (OR = 0.821, 95% CI = 0.324–2.035, $P = 0.046$), and rs28730677 (OR = 0.821, 95% CI = 0.324–2.035, $P = 0.046$) in *PIK3CD* were significantly associated with HAPC. Furthermore, rs28381984 (OR = 0.761, 95% CI = 0.294–1.928, $P = 0.035$) in *COL4A3* was associated with HAPC in the Tibetan population. But in the Han population, we did not find any significant association. In addition, using haplotype analysis, two blocks were detected among the *PIK3CD* SNPs (Fig. 3): block 1 contains rs7518602, rs7516138, rs7516214, and rs11805716 and block 2 contains rs79190623, rs72633866, rs2230735, rs182137610, rs188191807, rs28730671, rs111888887, rs9430220, rs28 730674, rs371870925, rs199962152, rs77571929, rs117 226273, rs28730676, rs10864435, and rs28730677. Two blocks were detected among the *COL4A3* SNPs too (Fig. 4): block 1 contains rs10178458 and rs6436669 and block 2 contains rs55703767, rs10205042, rs34505188, rs11677877, and rs34019152. These SNPs within the same genes showed strong linkage in-between.

Table 2 Basic information of candidate SNPs in Han subjects

SNP_ID	Gene	Alleles A/B	Case (N)			Control (N)			OR (95% CI)	P	P1	P2
			AA	AB	BB	AA	AB	BB				
rs7518602	PIK3CD	C/T	4	16	50	0	6	23	3.899 (1.515–10.290)	0.961	0.261	0.425
rs7516138	PIK3CD	G/A	4	19	47	0	11	18	4.150 (1.615–10.989)	0.993	0.959	0.800
rs7516214	PIK3CD	G/A	4	19	46	0	11	18	4.070 (1.582–10.786)	0.993	0.924	0.829
rs11805716	PIK3CD	T/C	13	17	32	3	9	14	3.610 (1.335–10.014)	0.961	0.516	0.488
rs11806839	PIK3CD	G/C	7	11	12	2	6	6	2.800 (0.640–12.570)	0.993	0.627	0.616
rs79190623	PIK3CD	C/T	63	7	0	23	6	0	3.952 (1.533–10.448)	0.766	0.160	0.245
rs72633866	PIK3CD	G/A	64	4	0	22	6	0	5.107 (1.892–14.498)	0.236	0.033	0.014
rs2230735	PIK3CD	A/G	63	7	0	23	6	0	3.952 (1.533–10.448)	0.766	0.160	0.245
rs182137610	PIK3CD	A/C	63	7	0	24	5	0	3.961 (1.540–10.444)	0.961	0.321	0.510
rs188191807	PIK3CD	G/A	57	3	0	23	3	0	4.280 (1.564–12.125)	0.961	0.287	0.486
rs28730671	PIK3CD	C/T	65	5	0	23	6	0	3.808 (1.463–10.129)	0.509	0.061	0.129
rs111888887	PIK3CD	T/C	65	5	0	24	5	0	3.816 (1.471–10.117)	0.821	0.141	0.312
rs9430220	PIK3CD	T/C	37	28	4	9	18	2	5.044 (1.871–14.464)	0.245	0.081	0.029
rs28730674	PIK3CD	A/G	65	5	0	23	6	0	3.808 (1.463–10.129)	0.509	0.061	0.129
rs371870925	PIK3CD	T/C	65	3	0	24	5	0	4.016 (1.520–10.884)	0.509	0.050	0.112
rs199962152	PIK3CD	A/G	63	2	0	22	5	0	3.065 (1.118–8.502)	0.245	0.024	0.034
rs77571929	PIK3CD	T/C	64	5	0	23	6	0	3.737 (1.439–9.970)	0.509	0.065	0.132
rs117226273	PIK3CD	G/T	65	5	0	23	6	0	3.808 (1.439–10.129)	0.509	0.061	0.129
rs28730676	PIK3CD	T/C	65	5	0	23	6	0	3.808 (1.436–10.129)	0.509	0.061	0.129
rs10864435	PIK3CD	C/T	63	7	0	20	9	0	6.247 (2.235–18.787)	0.051	0.013	0.002
rs28730677	PIK3CD	G/A	65	5	0	24	5	0	3.816 (1.471–10.117)	0.821	0.141	0.312
rs10178458	COL4A3	T/C	0	9	61	0	4	25	4.116 (1.069–10.826)	0.993	0.900	0.803
rs6436669	COL4A3	A/G	0	9	61	0	4	25	4.116 (1.069–10.826)	0.993	0.900	0.803
rs80109666	COL4A3	G/A	49	19	2	22	7	0	3.984 (1.545–10.552)	0.993	0.433	0.707
rs55703767	COL4A3	G/T	53	15	2	21	7	1	4.088 (1.600–10.732)	0.993	0.732	0.762
rs10205042	COL4A3	C/T	2	15	53	1	7	21	4.073 (1.592–10.704)	0.993	0.732	0.869
rs34505188	COL4A3	G/A	46	19	5	18	11	0	4.214 (1.637–11.199)	0.993	0.787	0.587
rs11677877	COL4A3	A/G	46	19	5	17	12	0	4.187 (1.625–11.138)	0.993	0.997	0.725
rs34019152	COL4A3	G/A	46	19	5	18	11	0	4.214 (1.637–11.199)	0.993	0.787	0.587
rs28381984	COL4A3	C/T	27	32	11	9	16	4	4.160 (1.623–10.984)	0.993	0.711	0.599

SNP single-nucleotide polymorphism, *OR* odds ratio, *95% CI* 95% confidence interval, *P value* FDR-calculated *P* value, *P1* *P* value calculated by unconditional logistic regression analysis, *P2* *P* value adjusted for age

Discussion

Tibet covers a vast area with a harsh hypoxic natural environment. According to a report in 2006, approximately 12 million people permanently settled down in this region. This number constantly increases every year; the increase mainly comes from the Han population that are emigrating from plain areas [16]. HAPC is a serious disease that threatens the health of people in the plateau area, especially those who have emigrated from a low-altitude area. In the past, a large number of patients with HAPC have been investigated with a focus on the pathophysiologic mechanisms of this disease. Nevertheless, a lot of questions remain to be elucidated. With the completion of the human genome project, much research has been shifted to human genetic variation, which was one of NIH's Roadmap Initiatives for 2008 [17]. As we all know, in Tibet, in order to adapt to altitude hypoxia, the body increases the hemoglobin concentration to increase the efficiency of carrying oxygen, and this response is crucial for the Han population who adapt to live at high altitudes. Compared with the Han people, the Tibetan population keeps genetic adaptations; they can easily adapt to the high-altitude hypoxia environment. Several studies have indicated that natural selection associated with high-altitude adaptation appears to act on genes in the hypoxic response pathway

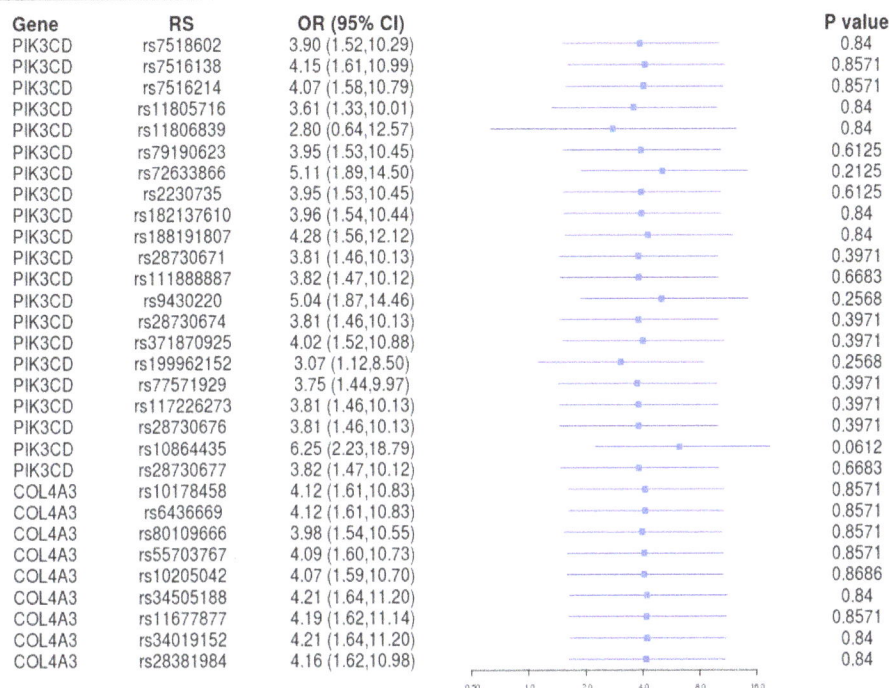

Gene	RS	OR (95% CI)	P value
PIK3CD	rs7518602	3.90 (1.52,10.29)	0.84
PIK3CD	rs7516138	4.15 (1.61,10.99)	0.8571
PIK3CD	rs7516214	4.07 (1.58,10.79)	0.8571
PIK3CD	rs11805716	3.61 (1.33,10.01)	0.84
PIK3CD	rs11806839	2.80 (0.64,12.57)	0.84
PIK3CD	rs79190623	3.95 (1.53,10.45)	0.6125
PIK3CD	rs72633866	5.11 (1.89,14.50)	0.2125
PIK3CD	rs2230735	3.95 (1.53,10.45)	0.6125
PIK3CD	rs182137610	3.96 (1.54,10.44)	0.84
PIK3CD	rs188191807	4.28 (1.56,12.12)	0.84
PIK3CD	rs28730671	3.81 (1.46,10.13)	0.3971
PIK3CD	rs111888887	3.82 (1.47,10.12)	0.6683
PIK3CD	rs9430220	5.04 (1.87,14.46)	0.2568
PIK3CD	rs28730674	3.81 (1.46,10.13)	0.3971
PIK3CD	rs371870925	4.02 (1.52,10.88)	0.3971
PIK3CD	rs199962152	3.07 (1.12,8.50)	0.2568
PIK3CD	rs77571929	3.75 (1.44,9.97)	0.3971
PIK3CD	rs117226273	3.81 (1.46,10.13)	0.3971
PIK3CD	rs28730676	3.81 (1.46,10.13)	0.3971
PIK3CD	rs10864435	6.25 (2.23,18.79)	0.0612
PIK3CD	rs28730677	3.82 (1.47,10.12)	0.6683
COL4A3	rs10178458	4.12 (1.61,10.83)	0.8571
COL4A3	rs6436669	4.12 (1.61,10.83)	0.8571
COL4A3	rs80109666	3.98 (1.54,10.55)	0.8571
COL4A3	rs55703767	4.09 (1.60,10.73)	0.8571
COL4A3	rs10205042	4.07 (1.59,10.70)	0.8686
COL4A3	rs34505188	4.21 (1.64,11.20)	0.84
COL4A3	rs11677877	4.19 (1.62,11.14)	0.8571
COL4A3	rs34019152	4.21 (1.64,11.20)	0.84
COL4A3	rs28381984	4.16 (1.62,10.98)	0.84

Fig. 1 Forest plots for the ORs in the Han population

to regulate erythrocyte production, possibly to prevent or reduce erythrocyte growth [18–22]. Recently, significant progress has been made in the study of the genetic basis of HAPC in Tibetans and Han, and some studies have confirmed that many genes are associated with HAPC. Namely, integrin subunit alpha 6 (ITGA6), erb-b2 receptor tyrosine kinase 4 (ERBB4), EPH receptor A2 (EPHA2), angiotensinogen (AGT), and endothelial PAS domain protein 1 (EPAS1) have been reported to play important roles in HAPC in Tibetans and Han [23–26]. Of these genes, EPHA2 can affect erythrocyte production by regulating EPO production and EPAS1 has been implicated as making the greatest contribution to genetic adaptation to high altitude and to the low Hb concentrations observed in the Tibetan population [18, 21]. Some research have shown that genetic variants selected for adaptation at extreme environmental conditions not only increase cancer risk later on age but may also be the downregulation of erythropoiesis in Tibetans in high altitude [22, 27, 28]. In our study, we found rs2230735, rs28730671, rs28730674, rs371870925, rs775 71929, rs117226273, rs28730676, rs28730677, and rs283 81984 in *PIK3CD* and *COL4A3* were significantly associated with decreased HAPC risk in the Tibetan population. However, in the Han population, we did not find any significant association. Inspired by the development of genome research and the genetic findings of high-altitude natives, we consider that genetic factors may be involved in the formation of such kind of disease.

Our study revealed an association of HAPC with SNPs in *PIK3CD* and *COL4A3* in the Tibetan population.

PIK3CD gene encodes P110δ catalytic subunit that is expressed predominantly in leukocytes and plays a vital role in the phosphoinositide 3-kinase (PI3K)/Akt signaling pathway. According to recent reports, p110δ contributes to the activation of Akt and cell proliferation in primary AML (acute myeloid leukemia) cells [29, 30]. PI3K signaling contributes to many processes, including cell cycle progression, proliferation and differentiation, survival, and migration [8, 9, 31]. PI3K/Akt pathways are critical to HIF-1α transcriptional activity in hypoxia. HIF-1, which is basically a heterodimer transcription factor, composed of HIF-1α and HIF-1β subunits, serves as a central regulator of metabolic adaptation to low oxygen [32]. The HIF-1α subunit is stabilized under hypoxia, translocating to the nucleus, forming a heterodimer with HIF-1β, and transactivating its target genes including EPO. HIF-1α is a factor that was originally thought to be bound to the 3′ enhancer region of the EPO genes, controlling for 100–200 genes that are involved in angiogenesis, glycolysis, and erythropoiesis [33]. The main organ for EPO production is the liver during the fetus stage, whereas it becomes the kidney after birth. However, there is small amount of expression in the other organs of the body, such as the brain, spleen, lungs, testis, and placenta. Further, it is a necessary glycoprotein, which does not only promote the maturation of red blood cell from erythroid progenitors but also mediates

Table 3 Basic information of candidate SNPs in Tibetan subjects

SNP_ID	Gene	Alleles A/B	Case (N)			Control (N)			OR (95% CI)	P	P1	P2
			AA	AB	BB	AA	AB	BB				
rs7518602	PIK3CD	C/T	5	29	36	1	10	19	1.043 (0.438–2.490)	0.612	0.240	0.238
rs7516138	PIK3CD	G/A	11	26	33	3	13	14	1.015 (0.428–2.411)	0.992	0.735	0.733
rs7516214	PIK3CD	G/A	11	26	32	3	13	14	0.992 (0.416–2.366)	0.982	0.688	0.691
rs11805716	PIK3CD	T/C	15	27	17	6	8	13	1.061 (0.416–2.718)	0.555	0.207	0.206
rs11806839	PIK3CD	G/C	5	7	4	2	9	3	1.205 (0.270–5.393)	0.893	0.593	0.612
rs79190623	PIK3CD	C/T	58	10	1	18	11	1	0.862 (0.349–2.106)	0.081	0.018	0.018
rs72633866	PIK3CD	G/A	57	8	1	25	2	0	1.071 (0.434–2.656)	0.791	0.366	0.367
rs2230735	PIK3CD	A/G	59	10	1	17	12	1	0.844 (0.337–2.079)	0.046	0.008	0.008
rs182137610	PIK3CD	A/C	57	10	1	18	9	1	0.764 (0.301–1.897)	0.150	0.050	0.045
rs188191807	PIK3CD	G/A	53	5	1	22	5	0	0.685 (0.266–1.726)	0.791	0.454	0.396
rs28730671	PIK3CD	C/T	63	6	1	19	10	1	0.821 (0.324–2.035)	0.046	0.007	0.007
rs111888887	PIK3CD	T/C	61	6	1	21	8	1	0.906 (0.368–2.205)	0.130	0.034	0.034
rs9430220	PIK3CD	T/C	29	34	5	12	14	4	0.940 (0.395–2.234)	0.851	0.536	0.535
rs28730674	PIK3CD	A/G	63	6	1	19	10	1	0.821 (0.324–2.035)	0.046	0.007	0.007
rs371870925	PIK3CD	T/C	64	4	1	20	9	1	0.812 (0.320–2.017)	0.046	0.007	0.007
rs199962152	PIK3CD	A/G	58	4	1	19	6	1	0.685 (0.256–1.766)	0.146	0.045	0.040
rs77571929	PIK3CD	T/C	63	5	1	19	10	1	0.814 (0.320–2.024)	0.046	0.005	0.005
rs117226273	PIK3CD	G/T	63	6	1	19	10	1	0.821 (0.324–2.035)	0.046	0.007	0.007
rs28730676	PIK3CD	T/C	63	6	1	19	10	1	0.821 (0.324–2.035)	0.046	0.007	0.007
rs10864435	PIK3CD	C/T	55	15	0	25	4	1	1.011 (0.423–2.417)	0.992	0.879	0.878
rs28730677	PIK3CD	G/A	63	6	1	19	10	1	0.821 (0.324–2.035)	0.046	0.007	0.007
rs10178458	COL4A3	T/C	4	21	45	4	7	19	1.026 (0.432–2.442)	0.851	0.539	0.537
rs6436669	COL4A3	A/G	4	21	45	4	7	19	1.026 (0.432–2.442)	0.851	0.539	0.537
rs80109666	COL4A3	G/A	60	9	1	28	2	0	1.070 (0.449–2.559)	0.655	0.271	0.267
rs55703767	COL4A3	G/T	47	21	2	18	8	4	0.990 (0.415–2.360)	0.524	0.184	0.184
rs10205042	COL4A3	C/T	0	23	47	4	8	18	1.017 (0.425–2.437)	0.305	0.102	0.102
rs34505188	COL4A3	G/A	42	20	8	10	14	6	0.948 (0.390–2.292)	0.115	0.028	0.028
rs11677877	COL4A3	A/G	42	21	7	10	13	7	0.941 (0.385–2.290)	0.070	0.013	0.013
rs34019152	COL4A3	G/A	42	20	8	10	13	7	0.928 (0.380–2.254)	0.081	0.018	0.018
rs28381984	COL4A3	C/T	24	39	7	23	6	1	0.761 (0.294–1.928)	0.035	0.001	0.001

The abbreviations were the same as Table 2

erythropoiesis. It is identified as an inducer of erythropoiesis and can promote excessive cell production. In addition, previous studies showed that inhibited PI3K/Akt signaling pathway led to decreased hematopoietic stem cell (HSC) proliferation. This suggests that such kind of pathway is important for HSC proliferation. HSC is involved in the formation of HAPC, expansion of the population, and enforcement of erythroid lineage-committed differentiation [34]. Therefore, we speculate that PIKCD may affect the generation of EPO and the decrease of HSC appreciation through the PI3K/Akt signaling pathway. In this study, we show here for the first time that the *PIK3CD* gene plays a crucial role in the production of erythrocyte, so *PIK3CD* has a significant influence on the formation of HAPC.

COL4A3 is an important risk gene for HAPC that is also linked to many diseases such as the Alport syndrome, focal segmental glomerulosclerosis, and type 2 diabetes [35–37]. Furthermore, it is important to the structure and function of various cell types and contributes to a variety of processes. Although the functional effects of the polymorphisms have not yet been elucidated fully, our current results show that the variants may have an effect on *COL4A3* expression or activity. Therefore, it may play an important role in modulating the susceptibility to HAPC. By searching the KEGG pathway database, we found that

Gene	RS	OR (95% CI)		P value
PIK3CD	rs7518602	1.04 (0.44,2.49)		0.3572
PIK3CD	rs7516138	1.01 (0.43,2.41)		0.7587
PIK3CD	rs7516214	0.99 (0.42,2.37)		0.7406
PIK3CD	rs11805716	1.06 (0.42,2.72)		0.3247
PIK3CD	rs11806839	1.20 (0.27,5.39)		0.6799
PIK3CD	rs79190623	0.86 (0.35,2.11)		0.045
PIK3CD	rs72633866	1.07 (0.43,2.66)		0.4999
PIK3CD	rs2230735	0.84 (0.34,2.08)		0.0257
PIK3CD	rs182137610	0.76 (0.30,1.90)		0.0834
PIK3CD	rs188191807	0.68 (0.27,1.73)		0.5159
PIK3CD	rs28730671	0.82 (0.32,2.03)		0.0255
PIK3CD	rs111888887	0.91 (0.37,2.20)		0.072
PIK3CD	rs9430220	0.94 (0.40,2.23)		0.6196
PIK3CD	rs28730674	0.82 (0.32,2.03)		0.0255
PIK3CD	rs371870925	0.81 (0.32,2.02)		0.0255
PIK3CD	rs199962152	0.68 (0.26,1.77)		0.081
PIK3CD	rs77571929	0.81 (0.32,2.02)		0.0255
PIK3CD	rs117226273	0.82 (0.32,2.03)		0.0255
PIK3CD	rs28730676	0.82 (0.32,2.03)		0.0255
PIK3CD	rs10864435	1.01 (0.42,2.42)		0.8777
PIK3CD	rs28730677	0.82 (0.32,2.03)		0.0255
COL4A3	rs10178458	1.03 (0.43,2.44)		0.6196
COL4A3	rs6436669	1.03 (0.43,2.44)		0.6196
COL4A3	rs80109666	1.07 (0.45,2.56)		0.3813
COL4A3	rs55703767	0.99 (0.42,2.36)		0.3074
COL4A3	rs10205042	1.02 (0.43,2.44)		0.1794
COL4A3	rs34505188	0.95 (0.39,2.29)		0.0638
COL4A3	rs11677877	0.94 (0.38,2.29)		0.039
COL4A3	rs34019152	0.93 (0.38,2.25)		0.045
COL4A3	rs28381984	0.76 (0.29,1.93)		0.0193

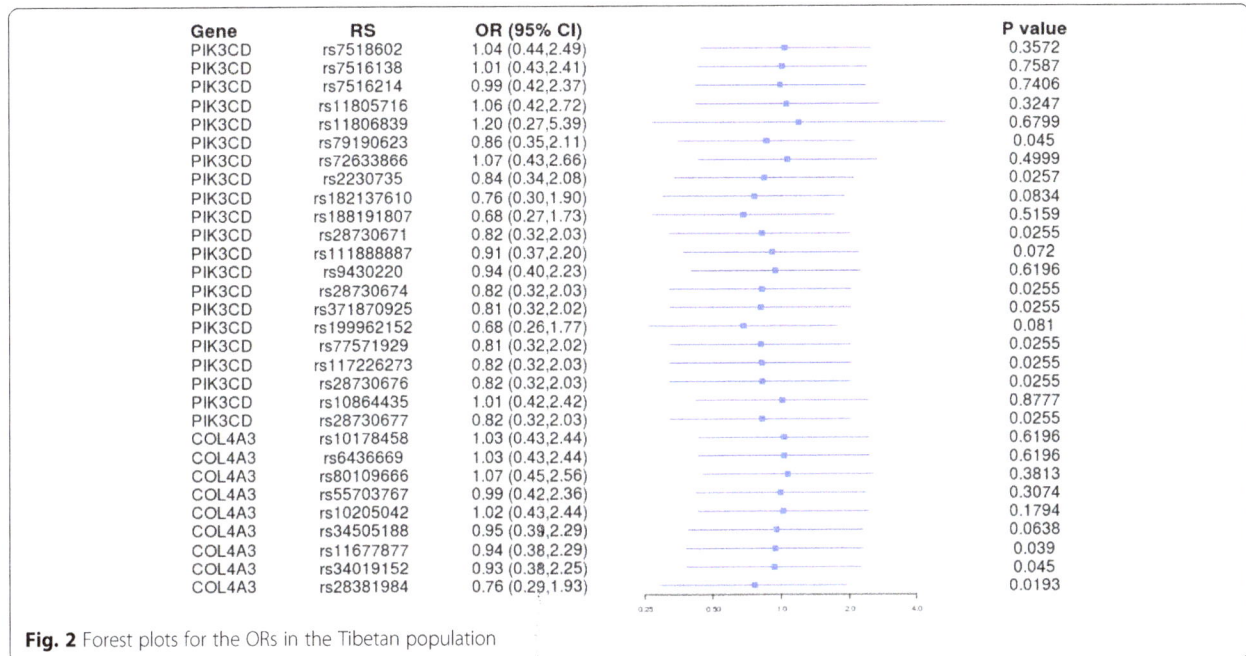

Fig. 2 Forest plots for the ORs in the Tibetan population

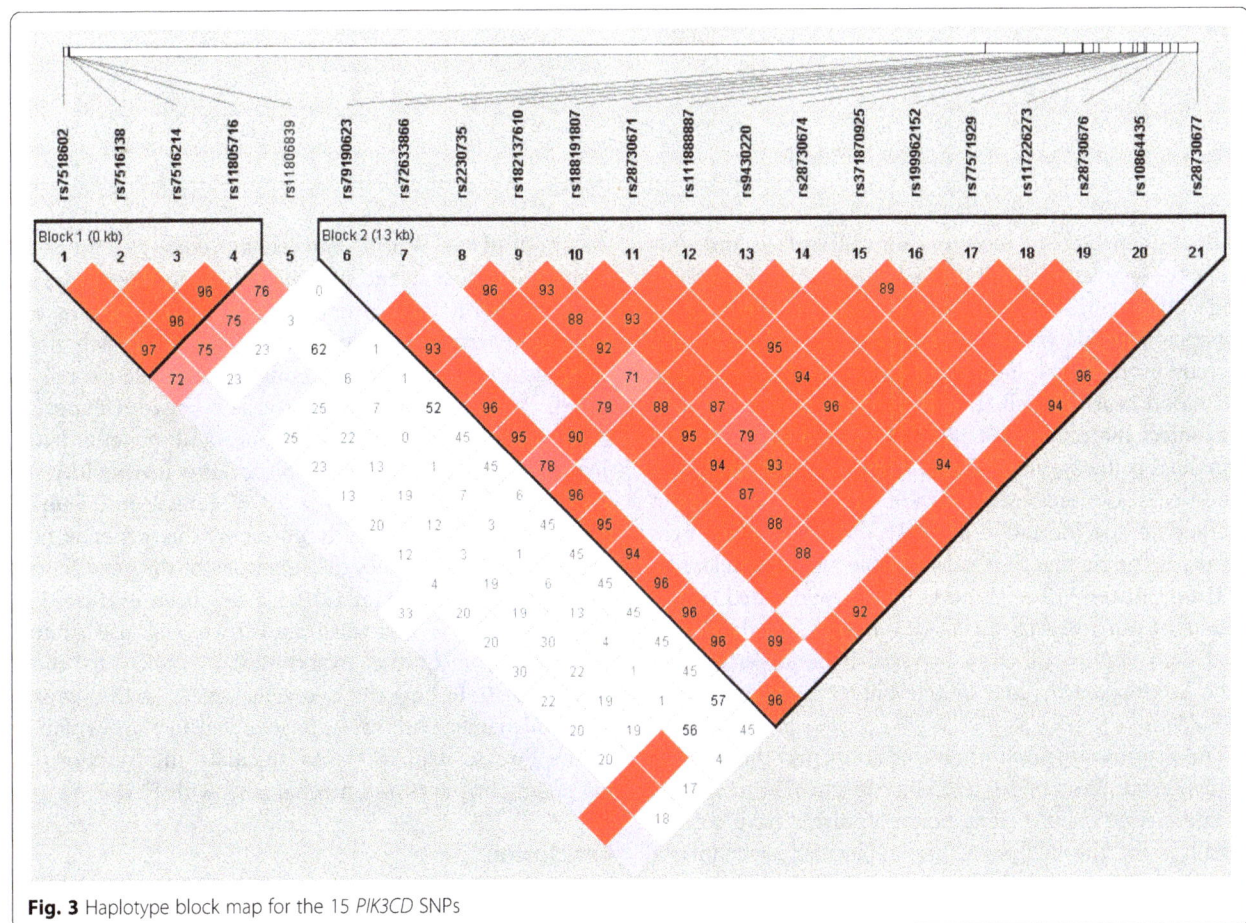

Fig. 3 Haplotype block map for the 15 *PIK3CD* SNPs

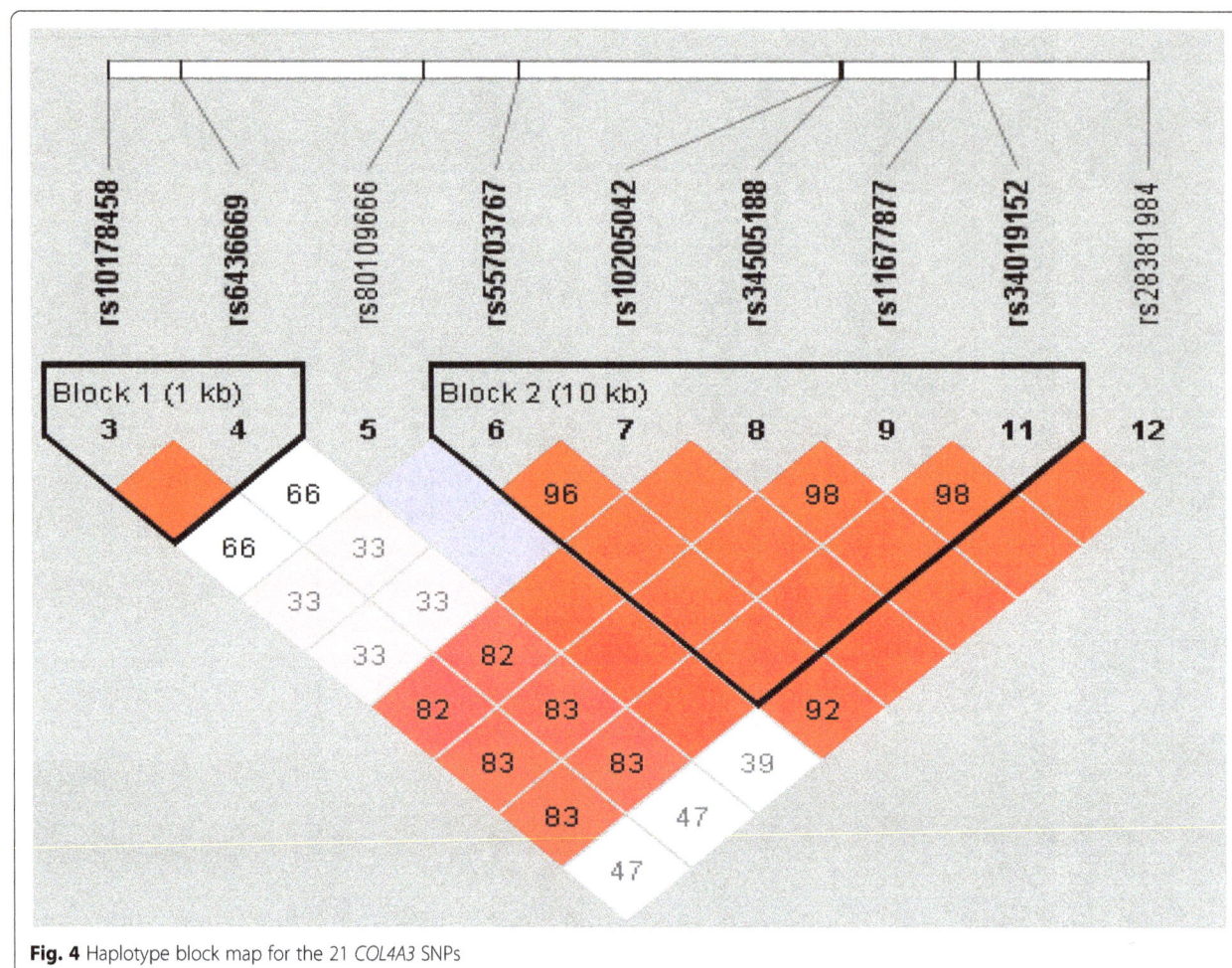

Fig. 4 Haplotype block map for the 21 *COL4A3* SNPs

COL4A3 can bind to receptors on cell surface and promote the activation of PI3K/Akt. Under hypoxic conditions, this pathway can promote the production of hypoxia-inducible factor and increase the cell cycle, and thereby promote the increase of EPO and the amount of red blood cells. Therefore, it is speculated that *COL4A3* may affect the production of EPO through the PI3K/Akt signaling pathway, thus affecting the production of red blood cells. Consequently, *COL4A3* gene may be a useful marker for the formation of HAPC. We also show here for the first time that the *COL4A3* gene plays a crucial role in the production of erythrocyte. Meanwhile, based on the results of our research, *COL4A3* was significantly associated with erythropoiesis in hypoxia. It is suggested that gene polymorphisms may be relevant to the susceptibility to HAPC.

The genome research era has also opened the road to studying the basis of susceptibility to chronic mountain sickness (CMS) [38]. Gene polymorphisms have set the platform for the analysis of the molecular mechanisms of adaptation to life at high altitudes [39]. Tibet, an average elevation above 4000 m, is commonly regarded as

the "Roof of the World" and has a unique genetic background and dietary and lifestyle habits. In this study, we have suggested that several genetic polymorphisms are associated with susceptibility to HAPC and each polymorphism may contribute to only a small relative risk of HAPC. It shows a complex interplay between exposure to hypoxic environmental stimuli and genetic background. There are important discoveries revealed by the studies, but there are still a lot of limitations. Due to these limitations, the study power of this paper is limited. On the other hand, the functions of the genetic variants and their mechanisms have not been evaluated in this study. In a following study, we will use animal models to verify the experimental results, to more clearly illustrate how the two genes affect erythrocytosis, which signaling pathways are involved in the formation of the disease, and to try to elucidate the functions of the genetic variants and mechanisms with HAPC.

Conclusion

We analyzed SNPs in *PIK3CD* and *COL4A3* and identified a relationship between genetic polymorphisms and

HAPC in the Tibetan people. This study sets out to improve the quality of life of people living in the Qinghai-Tibet Plateau, determines paramount insights into the etiology of HAPC, and may provide more guidance for such people with regard to prolonged and healthy living. However, additional genetic risk factors and functional investigations should be identified in order to further confirm our results.

Materials and methods

Study populations

A total of 140 patients (70 Han and 70 Tibetan) with HAPC and 60 healthy control subjects (30 Han and 30 Tibetan) were recruited for a case-control association study. The 200 subjects who participated in this research had resided at an altitude of above 4000 m, and these samples were collected from the General Hospital in Tibet Military Region and the second People's Hospital of Tibet Autonomous Region. Written informed consent was obtained from each individual. Patients met the diagnostic criteria for HAPC, i.e., males with hemoglobin ≥ 21 g/dL or females with hemoglobin ≥ 19 g/dL, and had no high-altitude cerebral edema and chronic respiratory disorders or secondary polycythemia due to hypoxia caused by certain chronic diseases. Moreover, subjects have no endocrinological, nutritional, and metabolic diseases. Healthy individuals were randomly selected as controls. The experimental protocol was established by the Ethics Committee of the Xizang Minzu University.

Epidemiological and clinical data

We used a standardized epidemiological questionnaire to collect demographic and clinical data, including information on gender, age, residential region, ethnicity, family history of cancer, and education status. Furthermore, the patient information was collected through physicians or from medical chart review. All participants signed informed consent, and 5 ml of peripheral blood was taken from each participant in this study.

Selection of SNPs and methods of genotyping

Thirty SNPs from *PIK3CD* and *COL4A3* were chosen for analysis in this study, including 21 SNPs in *PIK3CD* and 9 SNPs in *COL4A3* with minor allele frequency (MAF) > 0.05 in the Asian population HapMap database, and SNP genotyping was performed utilizing Illumina sequencing platform for exon sequencing of PIKCD and COL4A3. Because the genetic background of Han and Tibetan populations has not been compared yet, we selected these two candidate genes based on their relations to the oxygen metabolism in red blood cells, which were related to high-altitude adaptation in the Chinese Han and Tibetan populations.

Statistical analysis

The data were analyzed using an R program, Haploview, and Excel. Unconditional logistic regression analysis was used to calculate odds ratios (ORs), 95% confidence intervals (CIs), and *P* values for comparisons between cases and controls. Multiple comparisons were corrected using FDR, and FDR-corrected $P < 0.05$ was considered to indicate a significant difference.

Abbreviations

95%CI: 95% confidence intervals; AGT: Angiotensinogen; AML: Acute myeloid leukemia; CMS: Chronic mountain sickness; COL4A3: Collagen type IV α3 chain gene; ECM: Extracellular matrix; EPAS1: Endothelial PAS domain protein 1; EPHA2: EPH receptor A2; ERBB4: Erb-b2 receptor tyrosine kinase 4; FDR: False discovery rate; HAPC: High-altitude polycythemia; HIF-1α: Hypoxia-inducible factors-1α; HSC: Hematopoietic stem cell; ITGA6: Integrin subunit alpha 6; OR: Odds ratio; PIK3CD: Catalytic subunit delta gene

Acknowledgements

We are grateful to those who collected samples in the Tibetan Plateau, and we thank those who participated in the study and worked hard on the research. This work was supported by the National Natural Science Foundation of China (No. 31460286; 31660307; 31260252; 31330038), the Natural Science Foundation of Xizang (Tibet) Autonomous Region (No. Z2014A09G2-3), the Innovation Support Program for Young Teachers of Tibet Autonomous Region (No. QCZ2016-27; QCZ2016-29; QCZ2016-34), and the Science and Technology Department Project of Tibet Autonomous Region (No. 2016ZR-MQ-06; 2015ZR- 13-19).

Funding

This work was supported by the National Natural Science Foundation of China (No. 31460286; 31660307; 31260252; 31330038), the Natural Science Foundation of Xizang (Tibet) Autonomous Region (No. Z2014A09G2-3), the Innovation Support Program for Young Teachers of Tibet Autonomous Region (No. QCZ2016-27; QCZ2016-29; QCZ2016-34), and the Science and Technology Department Project of Tibet Autonomous Region (No. 2016ZR-MQ-06; 2015ZR- 13-19).

Authors' contributions

LK conceived and designed the study, supervised the project, and drafted the manuscript. XF participated in the design of study and data analysis and helped to draft the manuscript. LM, ZZhang, YL, MH, LL, YZ, FL, PC, and YL contributed to the sample collection and experiments. XL helped in the English language editing. ZZhao contributed to sample collection and experiments. All authors have read and approved the final manuscript.

Competing interests

The authors declare that they have no competing interests.

Author details

[1]Key Laboratory for Molecular Genetic Mechanisms and Intervention Research on High Altitude Disease of Tibet Autonomous Region, School of Medicine, Xizang Minzu University, Xianyang 712082, Shaanxi, China. [2]Key Laboratory of High Altitude Environment and Genes Related to Diseases of Tibet Autonomous Region, School of Medicine, Xizang Minzu University, Xianyang 712082, Shaanxi, China. [3]Ministry of Education Key Laboratory of

Contemporary Anthropology, Collaborative Innovation Center for Genetics and Development, School of Life Sciences, Fudan University, Shanghai 200433, China. [4]Division of Human Genetics, Department of Psychiatry, Yale University School of Medicine, New Haven, CT 06510, USA. [5]Six Industrial Research Institute, Fudan University, Shanghai 200433, China.

References

1. Leon-Velarde F, et al. Consensus statement on chronic and subacute high altitude diseases. High Alt Med Biol. 2005;6(2):147–57.
2. Otten, E.J., High altitude: an exploration of human adaptation.: edited by Hornbein TF and Schoene RB. New York, Marcel Dekker, Inc. 2001, 982 pages, $235. J Emerg Med, 2003. 25(3): p. 345-346.
3. Reeves JT, Leon-Velarde F. Chronic mountain sickness: recent studies of the relationship between hemoglobin concentration and oxygen transport. High Altitude Medicine & Biology. 2004;5(2):147.
4. Guan W, et al. Sleep disturbances in long-term immigrants with chronic mountain sickness: a comparison with healthy immigrants at high altitude. Respir Physiol Neurobiol. 2015;206:4–10.
5. Jiang C, et al. Gene expression profiling of high altitude polycythemia in Han Chinese migrating to the Qinghai-Tibetan plateau. Mol Med Rep. 2012; 5(1):287–93.
6. Wu TY. Chronic mountain sickness on the Qinghai-Tibetan plateau. Chin Med. 2005;118(2):161–8.
7. Vanhaesebroeck B, et al. P110delta, a novel phosphoinositide 3-kinase in leukocytes. Proc Natl Acad Sci U S A. 1997;94(9):4330.
8. Chantry D, et al. p110delta, a novel phosphatidylinositol 3-kinase catalytic subunit that associates with p85 and is expressed predominantly in leukocytes. J Biol Chem. 1997;272(31):19236.
9. Kok K, Geering B, Vanhaesebroeck B. Regulation of phosphoinositide 3-kinase expression in health and disease. Trends Biochem Sci. 2009;34(3):115.
10. Gaber T, et al. Hypoxia inducible factor (HIF) in rheumatology: low O2! See what HIF can do! Ann Rheum Dis. 2005;64(7):971.
11. Dayan F, et al. A dialogue between the hypoxia-inducible factor and the tumor microenvironment. Cancer Microenvironmen. 2008;1(1):53–68.
12. Tanaka T, Nangaku M. Recent advances and clinical application of erythropoietin and erythropoiesis-stimulating agents. Exp Cell Res. 2012; 318(9):1068–73.
13. Stabuc-Silih M, et al. Polymorphisms in COL4A3 and COL4A4 genes associated with keratoconus. Mol Vis. 2009;15(300-01):2848–60.
14. Osman OS, et al. A novel method to assess collagen architecture in skin. Bmc Bioinformatics. 2013;14(1):1–10.
15. Khan T, et al. Metabolic dysregulation and adipose tissue fibrosis: role of collagen VI. Mol Cell Biol. 2009;29(6):1575–91.
16. Wu T, Kayser B. High altitude adaptation in Tibetans. High Alt Med Biol. 2006;7(3):193.
17. Pennisi, E., Research funding. Are epigeneticists ready for big science? Science, 2008. 319(5867): p. 1177.
18. Yi X, et al. Sequencing of fifty human exomes reveals adaptation to high altitude. Science. 2010;329(5987):75–8.
19. Crawford JE, et al. Natural selection on genes related to cardiovascular health in high-altitude adapted Andeans. Am J Hum Genet. 2017;101(5): 752–67.
20. Simonson TS, et al. Genetic evidence for high-altitude adaptation in Tibet. Science. 2010;329(5987):72–5.
21. Beall CM, et al. Natural selection on EPAS1 (HIF2alpha) associated with low hemoglobin concentration in Tibetan highlanders. Proc Natl Acad Sci U S A. 2010;107(25):11459–64.
22. Bigham A, et al. Identifying signatures of natural selection in Tibetan and Andean populations using dense genome scan data. PLoS Genet. 2010;6(9): e1001116.
23. Xu J, et al. EPAS1 gene polymorphisms are associated with high altitude polycythemia in Tibetans at the Qinghai-Tibetan Plateau. Wilderness Environ Med. 2015;26(3):288–94.
24. Chen Y, et al. An EPAS1 haplotype is associated with high altitude polycythemia in male Han Chinese at the Qinghai-Tibetan plateau. Wilderness Environ Med. 2014;25(4):392–400.
25. Zhao Y, et al. Associations of high altitude polycythemia with polymorphisms in EPAS1, ITGA6 and ERBB4 in Chinese Han and Tibetan populations. Oncotarget. 2017;8(49):86736.
26. Liu L, et al. Associations of high altitude polycythemia with polymorphisms in EPHA2 and AGT in Chinese Han and Tibetan populations. Oncotarget. 2017;8(32):53234–43.
27. Macinnis MJ, Koehle MS, Rupert JL. Evidence for a genetic basis for altitude illness: 2010 update. High Alt Med Biol. 2010;11(4):349–68.
28. Voskarides K. Combination of 247 genome-wide association studies reveals high cancer risk as a result of evolutionary adaptation. Mol Biol Evol. 2017; 35(2):473–85.
29. Billottet C, et al. A selective inhibitor of the p110||[delta]|| isoform of PI 3-kinase inhibits AML cell proliferation and survival and increases the cytotoxic effects of VP16. Oncogene. 2006;25(50):6648.
30. Sujobert P, et al. Essential role for the p110delta isoform in phosphoinositide 3-kinase activation and cell proliferation in acute myeloid leukemia. Blood. 2005;106(3):1063.
31. Vanhaesebroeck B, et al. p110δ, a novel phosphoinositide 3-kinase in leukocytes. Proc Natl Acad Sci U S A. 1997;94(9):4330.
32. Zhou J, et al. PI3K/Akt is required for heat shock proteins to protect hypoxia-inducible factor 1α from pVHL-independent degradation. J Biol Chem. 2004;279(14):13506–13.
33. Tanaka T, Nangaku M. Recent advances and clinical application of erythropoietin and erythropoiesis-stimulating agents. Exp Cell Res. 2012; 318(9):1068.
34. Li P, et al. Regulation of bone marrow hematopoietic stem cell is involved in high-altitude erythrocytosis. Exp Hematol. 2011;39(1):37–46.
35. Jingyuan X, et al. COL4A3 mutations cause focal segmental glomerulosclerosis. J Mol Cell Biol. 2014;6(6):498–505.
36. Guo L, et al. Mutation analysis of COL4A3 and COL4A4 genes in a Chinese autosomal-dominant Alport syndrome family. J Genet. 2017;96(2):389.
37. Saravani S, et al. Association of COL4A3 (rs55703767), MMP-9 (rs17576) and TIMP-1 (rs6609533) gene polymorphisms with susceptibility to type 2 diabetes. Biomed Rep. 2017;6(3):329–34.
38. Thomas PK, et al. Neurological manifestations in chronic mountain sickness: the burning feet-burning hands syndrome. J Neurol Neurosurg Psychiatry. 2000;69(4):447–52.
39. Cohen J. DNA duplications and deletions help determine health. Science. 2007;317(5843):1315–7.

19

Associations between hypertension and the peroxisome proliferator-activated receptor-δ (*PPARD*) gene rs7770619 C>T polymorphism in a Korean population

Minjoo Kim[1], Minkyung Kim[1], Hye Jin Yoo[2], Jayoung Shon[2,3] and Jong Ho Lee[1,2,3]*

Abstract

Background: Oxidative stress is associated with the increased risk of hypertension (HTN). This cross-sectional study is aimed to identify the association between the peroxisome proliferator-activated receptor-δ (*PPARD*) polymorphism and plasma malondialdehyde (MDA), an oxidative stress marker which is related to HTN development, and to determine whether *PPARD* gene is a candidate gene for HTN.

Results: One thousand seven hundred ninety-three individuals with normal blood pressure (BP) and HTN were included in this cross-sectional study. The Korean Chip was used to obtain genotype data. Through the analysis, the ten most strongly associated single-nucleotide polymorphisms (SNPs) were nominated for an MDA-related SNP. Among them, the rs7770619 polymorphism was identified in the *PPARD* gene. The CT genotype of the *PPARD* rs7770619 C>T polymorphism was associated with a lower risk of HTN before and after adjustments for age, sex, body mass index, smoking, and drinking. Significant associations were observed between plasma MDA and the *PPARD* rs7770619 C>T polymorphism and between systolic BP and the *PPARD* rs7770619 SNP in the controls. The CT controls showed significantly lower systolic BP and plasma MDA than the CC controls. Additionally, in both controls and HTN patients, the CT subjects showed significantly lower serum glucose and higher adiponectin levels than the CC subjects. Furthermore, the CT subjects showed significantly higher serum free fatty acid levels than the CC subjects among the HTN patients.

Conclusion: This is a new finding that the *PPARD* rs7770619 C>T SNP is a novel candidate variant for HTN based on the association between *PPARD* and plasma MDA in a Korean population.

Keywords: Peroxisome proliferator-activated receptor-δ gene, Genetic polymorphism, Blood pressure, Hypertension, Malondialdehyde

Background

Oxidative stress is defined as a sustained increase in the levels of reactive oxygen species (ROS), such as hydrogen peroxide, superoxide anion radicals, and other free radicals. Lipids have been reported as one of the primary targets of ROS. Lipid peroxidation produces highly reactive aldehydes, including malondialdehyde (MDA), which has been reported as a primary biomarker of free radical-mediated lipid damage and oxidative stress [1]. Increased MDA levels as a marker of oxidative stress were higher in hypertensive patients than in normotensive individuals [2, 3]. Additionally, a positive correlation between serum MDA levels and systolic and diastolic blood pressure (BP) has been reported [4].

Hypertension (HTN) is a multifactorial disorder involving both genetic and environmental factors [5]. Therefore, genetic factors affecting oxidative stress may include a common genetic basis of susceptibility to HTN. Although some studies have focused on the association between peroxisome proliferator-activated receptor

* Correspondence: jhleeb@yonsei.ac.kr
[1]Research Center for Silver Science, Institute of Symbiotic Life-TECH, Yonsei University, Seoul 03722, Korea
[2]Department of Food and Nutrition, Brain Korea 21 PLUS Project, College of Human Ecology, Yonsei University, 50 Yonsei-ro, Seodaemun-gu, Seoul 03722, Korea
Full list of author information is available at the end of the article

(PPAR) and HTN [6–8], the association between PPAR-δ (PPARD) and HTN has not been extensively studied previously. Indeed, PPARD has been suggested to regulate BP by modulating risk factors of HTN, including obesity and fatty acid catabolism [9]. Since a close relationship was observed between BP and MDA levels in HTN [2, 3], the MDA-related single-nucleotide polymorphisms (SNPs) analyzed with the Korean Chip (K-CHIP) could also be novel SNPs associated with HTN risk. The K-CHIP is a customized chip optimized for genetic studies on diseases and complex traits in the Korean population. Therefore, the objective of this study was to determine whether the PPARD gene is a candidate gene for HTN by identifying any association between PPARD and MDA, which is increased in HTN [2, 3].

Methods

Study population

All individuals who visited the Health Service Center (HSC) at National Health Insurance Corporation Ilsan Hospital, Goyang, Korea, for their routine checkups (from January 2010 to March 2015) were potential study subjects for this research. Based on the data screened from HSC, men and women aged over 20 years (adult subjects) with nondiabetic normotension (systolic BP < 140 mmHg and diastolic BP < 90 mmHg) or HTN (systolic BP ≥ 140 mmHg or diastolic BP ≥ 90 mmHg) were asked to participate in this study and were given detailed explanation regarding the study, and then, individuals who agreed to take part in the study were recruited. These potential subjects were referred to the Department of Family Medicine, and their health and BP were reexamined. Finally, individuals who met the study criteria were included ($n = 2167$). The exclusion criteria were a current diagnosis or history of cardiovascular disease, liver disease, renal disease, pancreatitis, or cancer; pregnancy or lactation; and regular use of any medication except for HTN treatments. The inclusion criteria were men and women adults (aged over 20 years), nondiabetic (fasting glucose < 126 mg/dL and no use of glucose-lowering medication), and individuals who do not correspond to the exclusion criteria (Additional file 1: Figure S1). The aim of the study was carefully explained to all participants, who provided their written informed consent. The Institutional Review Board of Yonsei University and the National Health Insurance Corporation Ilsan Hospital approved the study protocol, which complied with the Declaration of Helsinki.

Blood sample collection

Venous blood samples were collected following an overnight fast for at least 12 h. The fasting blood specimens were collected in EDTA-treated tubes and serum tubes (BD Vacutainer; Becton, Dickinson and Company,

Franklin Lakes, NJ, USA) and were then centrifuged (1200 rpm, 20 min, 4 °C) to obtain plasma and serum. The plasma and serum sample aliquots were stored at − 80 °C prior to analysis.

BP measurement

Systolic and diastolic BP were measured using a random-zero sphygmomanometer (HM-1101, Hico Medical Co., Ltd., Chiba, Japan) with appropriately sized cuffs after a rest period of at least 20 min in a seated position. BP was measured three times in both arms. The differences among the three systolic BP measurements were always less than 2 mmHg. Participants were instructed not to smoke or drink alcohol for at least 30 min before each BP measurement.

Clinical and biochemical assessments

Body weight (UM0703581; Tanita, Tokyo, Japan) and height (GL-150; G-tech International, Uijeongbu, Korea) were measured after subjects removed their shoes, and the body mass index (BMI) was calculated (kg/m^2).

The serum fasting triglyceride (TG) and total cholesterol (TC) levels were measured enzymatically using TG and CHOL Kits (Roche, Mannheim, Germany), respectively. Serum fasting high-density lipoprotein (HDL)-cholesterol was measured by a selective inhibition method with an HDL-C Plus Kit (Roche, Mannheim, Germany). The resulting color reactions of the assays were monitored using a Hitachi 7600 autoanalyzer (Hitachi, Tokyo, Japan). Low-density lipoprotein (LDL)-cholesterol values were obtained indirectly using the Friedewald formula: LDL-cholesterol = TC − [HDL-cholesterol + (TG/5)].
Serum fasting free fatty acid was measured with enzymatic assays using an NEFA-M Kit (Shinyang Diagnostics, Gyeonggi, Korea), and the resulting color reactions of the assays were monitored with a Hitachi 7600 autoanalyzer (Hitachi, Tokyo, Japan).

The serum fasting glucose level was measured by a hexokinase method using a GLU Kit (Roche, Mannheim, Germany). The serum fasting insulin was measured by an immunoradiometric assay using an Insulin IRMA Kit (DIAsource, Louvain, Belgium). The resulting color reaction was monitored with a Hitachi 7600 autoanalyzer (Hitachi, Tokyo, Japan) and an SR-300 system (Stratec, Birkenfeld, Germany), respectively. To calculate insulin resistance (IR), the equation for homeostatic model assessment (HOMA) was used: HOMA-IR = [fasting insulin (μIU/mL) × fasting glucose (mg/dL)]/405. Plasma adiponectin was measured via an enzyme immunoassay using a Human Adiponectin ELISA Kit (B-Bridge International Inc., San Jose, CA, USA), and the resulting color reaction was monitored with a Victor2 (PerkinElmer Life Sciences, Turku, Finland).

Serum high-sensitivity C-reactive protein (hs-CRP) levels were measured using a CRP Kit (Roche, Mannheim, Germany), and the resulting colorimetric reaction was monitored with a Hitachi 7600 autoanalyzer (Hitachi, Tokyo, Japan). Plasma MDA was measured from thiobarbituric acid reactive substances (TBARS) using a TBARS Assay Kit (ZeptoMetrix Co., Buffalo, NY, USA).

Affymetrix Axiom™ KORV1.0-96 Array hybridization and SNP selection

The detailed information for this protocol is described in our previous study [10]. A total of 2167 samples were genotyped according to the manufacturer's protocol, which recommended the Axiom® 2.0 Reagent Kit (Affymetrix Axiom® 2.0 Assay User Guide; Affymetrix, Santa Clara, CA, USA). The genotype data were produced using the K-CHIP, which was available through the K-CHIP consortium. The K-CHIP was designed by the Center for Genome Science at the Korea National Institute of Health (4845-301, 3000-3031).

Samples that revealed the following features were excluded during the quality control process: sex inconsistency, markers with a high missing rate (> 5%), individuals with a high missing rate (> 10%), minor allele frequency < 0.01, and a significant deviation from Hardy-Weinberg equilibrium (HWE) ($p < 0.001$). In addition, SNPs were excluded if they were related to each other in linkage disequilibrium. Consequently, among a total of 833,535 SNPs on the arrays and 2167 samples, 395,787 SNPs and 2158 samples remained, and they were used in subsequent association analyses.

Statistical analysis

HWE and association assessments between SNPs and MDA using linear regression analysis were performed in PLINK version 1.07 (http://zzz.bwh.harvard.edu/plink); for issues of multiple comparisons between SNPs and MDA, false discovery rate (FDR) correction was used. Descriptive statistical analyses were conducted using SPSS version 23.0 (IBM, Chicago, IL, USA). Logarithmic transformation was used for the skewed variables, and a two-tailed p value of < 0.05 was considered statistically significant. An independent t test was performed on the continuous variables. Sex distribution, smoking and drinking status, and genotype frequency were tested using the chi-squared test. The association of HTN with a genotype was calculated using the odds ratio (OR) [95% confidence interval (CI)] of a logistic regression model with an adjustment for confounding factors.

Results

Through the subsequent analysis using 395787 SNPs and 2158 samples, the ten SNPs that were most strongly associated with plasma MDA were nominated

(Additional file 1: Table S1). Among them, one SNP, rs7770619, was identified in the *PPARD* gene. Therefore, we conducted an association analysis of *PPARD* rs7770619 polymorphism. Among 2158 subjects, 313 and 52 subjects did not have data of plasma MDA and rs7770619, respectively; thus, a total of 1793 subjects who had both plasma MDA and rs7770619 data were finally included in the final analysis (Additional file 1: Figure S1).

The clinical and biochemical characteristics of the normotensive controls ($n = 1359$) and HTN patients ($n = 434$) are shown in Table 1. HTN patients included those who use antihypertensive medication (35.9%). Thus, we subdivided HTN patients into two groups: those not treated with antihypertensive drugs (HTN without treatment, $n = 278$) and those treated with antihypertensive drugs (HTN with treatment, $n = 156$). Compared with normotensive controls, both HTN subgroups were older and heavier. After adjusting for age, sex, BMI, smoking, and drinking, the patients in both HTN subgroups showed higher systolic and diastolic BP and plasma MDA than normotensive controls. Serum TG was higher in HTN patients without treatment than in normotensive controls. The HTN with treatment subgroup showed lower TC and LDL-cholesterol and higher glucose than normotensive controls (Table 1).

Distribution of the *PPARD* rs7770619 C>T polymorphism

The observed and expected frequencies of the *PPARD* rs7770619 C>T polymorphism were in HWE in the entire population and in the control and patient groups. The relative *PPARD* rs7770619 C>T genotypes in the HTN patients differed significantly from those in the normotensive controls (Table 2). There was no homozygous mutation TT genotype in either the normotensive controls or the HTN patients. Frequencies of the T allele of the *PPARD* rs7770619 C>T polymorphism in the HTN patients (0.012) were significantly lower than those in the normotensive controls (0.028) ($p = 0.007$) (Table 2).

The presence of the CT genotype of the *PPARD* rs7770619 C>T SNP was associated with a lower risk of HTN [OR 0.404 (95% CI 0.207–0.788), $p = 0.008$] (Table 3). The significance of the association remained after adjusting for age, sex, BMI, smoking, and drinking [OR 0.478 (95% CI 0.238–0.960), $p = 0.038$], and the p value of Hosmer-Lemeshow goodness-of-fit test was 0.700 for this model implying that our model is well-fitted.

Associations of plasma MDA, systolic BP, serum glucose, free fatty acids, and adiponectin with the *PPARD* rs7770619 C>T polymorphism

A significant association was observed between plasma MDA and the *PPARD* rs7770619 C>T polymorphism in the normotensive controls. The CT carriers showed

Table 1 Clinical and biochemical characteristics in normotensive controls and HTN patients

	Normotensive controls ($n = 1359$)	HTN patients ($n = 434$)		
		Total ($n = 434$)	HTN without treatment ($n = 278$)	HTN with treatment ($n = 156$)
Age (year)	48.4 ± 0.28	53.8 ± 0.52***	51.5 ± 0.66***	57.9 ± 0.73***
Male/female, n (%)	499 (36.7)/860 (63.3)	229 (52.8)/205 (47.2)***	153 (55.0)/125 (45.0)***	76 (48.7)/80 (51.3)**
Current smoker, n (%)	193 (14.2)	74 (17.1)	55 (19.8)*	19 (12.2)
Current drinker, n (%)	824 (60.6)	259 (59.7)	177 (63.7)	82 (52.6)
BMI (kg/m²)	23.8 ± 0.08	25.4 ± 0.15***	25.3 ± 0.19***	25.5 ± 0.23***
Systolic BP (mmHg)	116.5 ± 0.31	$139.2 \pm 0.75^{\dagger\dagger\dagger}$	$144.4 \pm 0.75^{\dagger\dagger\dagger}$	$129.9 \pm 1.31^{\dagger\dagger\dagger}$
Diastolic BP (mmHg)	72.9 ± 0.23	$88.3 \pm 0.49^{\dagger\dagger\dagger}$	$92.6 \pm 0.46^{\dagger\dagger\dagger}$	$80.6 \pm 0.77^{\dagger\dagger\dagger}$
Triglyceride (mg/dL)$^{\int}$	119.2 ± 1.88	$148.3 \pm 4.24^{\dagger}$	$152.3 \pm 5.62^{\dagger\dagger}$	141.2 ± 6.20
Total cholesterol (mg/dL)$^{\int}$	199.4 ± 0.98	$199.3 \pm 1.73^{\dagger}$	202.9 ± 2.14	$192.8 \pm 2.86^{\dagger\dagger\dagger}$
HDL-cholesterol (mg/dL)$^{\int}$	54.4 ± 0.37	51.2 ± 0.60	51.1 ± 0.74	51.5 ± 1.05
LDL-cholesterol (mg/dL)$^{\int}$	122.0 ± 0.90	$119.2 \pm 1.58^{\dagger\dagger\dagger}$	122.3 ± 1.98	$113.7 \pm 2.55^{\dagger\dagger\dagger}$
Glucose (mg/dL)$^{\int}$	95.4 ± 0.55	$102.5 \pm 1.10^{\dagger}$	100.9 ± 1.39	$105.3 \pm 1.80^{\dagger\dagger}$
Insulin (μIU/mL)$^{\int}$	8.92 ± 0.12	9.59 ± 0.28	9.83 ± 0.38	9.11 ± 0.36
Free fatty acids (μEq/L)$^{\int}$	552.8 ± 6.65	567.9 ± 12.6	560.9 ± 16.0	581.8 ± 20.4
HOMA-IR$^{\int}$	2.09 ± 0.03	2.46 ± 0.10	2.54 ± 0.14	2.30 ± 0.10
hs-CRP (mg/dL)$^{\int}$	1.28 ± 0.08	1.60 ± 0.15	1.59 ± 0.16	1.61 ± 0.28
Adiponectin (ng/mL)$^{\int}$	6.49 ± 0.10	5.98 ± 0.17	5.94 ± 0.22	6.06 ± 0.27
Malondialdehyde (nmol/mL)$^{\int}$	8.89 ± 0.09	9.78 ± 0.27	$9.33 \pm 0.35^{\dagger\dagger}$	$10.6 \pm 0.43^{\dagger\dagger}$

Mean ± SE. $^{\int}$Tested following logarithmic transformation. *$p < 0.05$, **$p < 0.01$, and ***$p < 0.001$ derived from an independent t test between normotensive controls and each subgroup of hypertensive patients. $^{\dagger}p < 0.05$, $^{\dagger\dagger}p < 0.01$, and $^{\dagger\dagger\dagger}p < 0.001$ derived after adjusting for age, sex, BMI, smoking, and drinking

significantly lower MDA than the CC carriers (CC 8.98 ± 0.09 nmol/mL, CT 7.31 ± 0.20 nmol/mL; $p < 0.001$) (Fig. 1). Similarly, in the HTN patients, the CT carriers showed lower MDA than the CC carriers, but the difference was not statistically significant. Systolic BP and the *PPARD* rs7770619 C>T polymorphism were significantly associated in the normotensive controls (CC 116.7 ± 0.32 mmHg, CT 113.0 ± 1.36 mmHg; $p = 0.007$), and there was a trend toward an association between systolic BP and the *PPARD* rs7770619 C>T polymorphism in the HTN patients (CC 139.4 ± 0.76 mmHg, CT 130.9 ± 3.43 mmHg; $p = 0.090$). In the normotensive controls, the CT carriers showed significantly lower systolic BP than the CC carriers (Fig. 1). Additionally, in both normotensive controls and HTN patients, the CT carriers showed lower glucose and higher adiponectin than the CC carriers. In the HTN patients, compared with the CC carriers,

the CT carriers showed higher free fatty acid. In the normotensive controls, there was a trend toward an increase of free fatty acids in the CT carriers compared with the CC carriers (Fig. 1).

Discussion

The major finding of the present study was that the frequency of the *PPARD* rs7770619 CT genotype was significantly lower in patients with HTN than in the normotensive controls, suggesting that there was an association between the *PPARD* rs7770619 C>T SNP and HTN. This observation correlated with recent findings that the *PPARD* polymorphism has a key role for HTN development [9]. The significance of the present observations was established by the identification of the human polymorphism in the *PPARD* locus with altered BP and plasma MDA levels, which are reliable oxidative stress markers in HTN [2, 3].

Table 2 Frequencies of the *PPARD* rs7770619 genotypes in the normotensive controls and the HTN patients

PPARD rs7770619	Normotensive controls ($n = 1359$)		HTN patients ($n = 434$)		p values
	n	%	n	%	
CC	1284	94.5	424	97.7	0.006
CT	75	5.5	10	2.3	
T allele frequency	75	2.8	10	1.2	0.007

A chi-squared test was used to calculate the p values

Table 3 Unadjusted and adjusted odds ratios (ORs) for all the HTN patients according to the *PPARD* rs7770619 genotypes

	HTN patients ($n = 434$)	*p* values
PPARD rs7770619	OR (95% CI)	
Model 1		
C[‡] compared with T	0.411 (0.211 to 0.798)	0.009
CC[‡] compared with CT	0.404 (0.207 to 0.788)	0.008
Model 2		
C[‡] compared with T	0.486 (0.243 to 0.970)	0.041
CC[‡] compared with CT	0.478 (0.238 to 0.960)	0.038

Model 1: unadjusted; Model 2: adjusted for age, sex, BMI, smoking, and drinking. *CI* confidence interval. [‡]Reference

Patients with HTN tend to have several conditions that accelerate the atherogenic process, including an increase in free radicals. ROS are the most important free radicals in the human body and cause increased oxidative stress and tissue injury under pathological conditions [11, 12]. Several studies have reported evidence for enhanced ROS production and decreases in the antioxidant reserves in the plasma and tissues of hypertensive animals and humans [13, 14]. MDA is produced during the attack of ROS upon membrane lipoproteins and polyunsaturated fatty acids. Kashyap et al. [15] have reported increased MDA levels in hypertensive subjects compared with those in normotensive subjects and suggested that elevated lipid peroxidation reflected increased oxidative stress in patients with HTN. In a recent study, similar results were obtained in terms of MDA [3]. The authors found significantly higher MDA levels in the essential HTN group than in the control group. Similarly, this study also showed higher MDA levels in the HTN group regardless of whether they were taking antihypertensive medication than in the control group.

In the present study, subjects with the *PPARD* rs7770619 CT genotype showed significantly lower systolic BP than those with the CC genotype in the normotensive controls. Additionally, the significantly lower

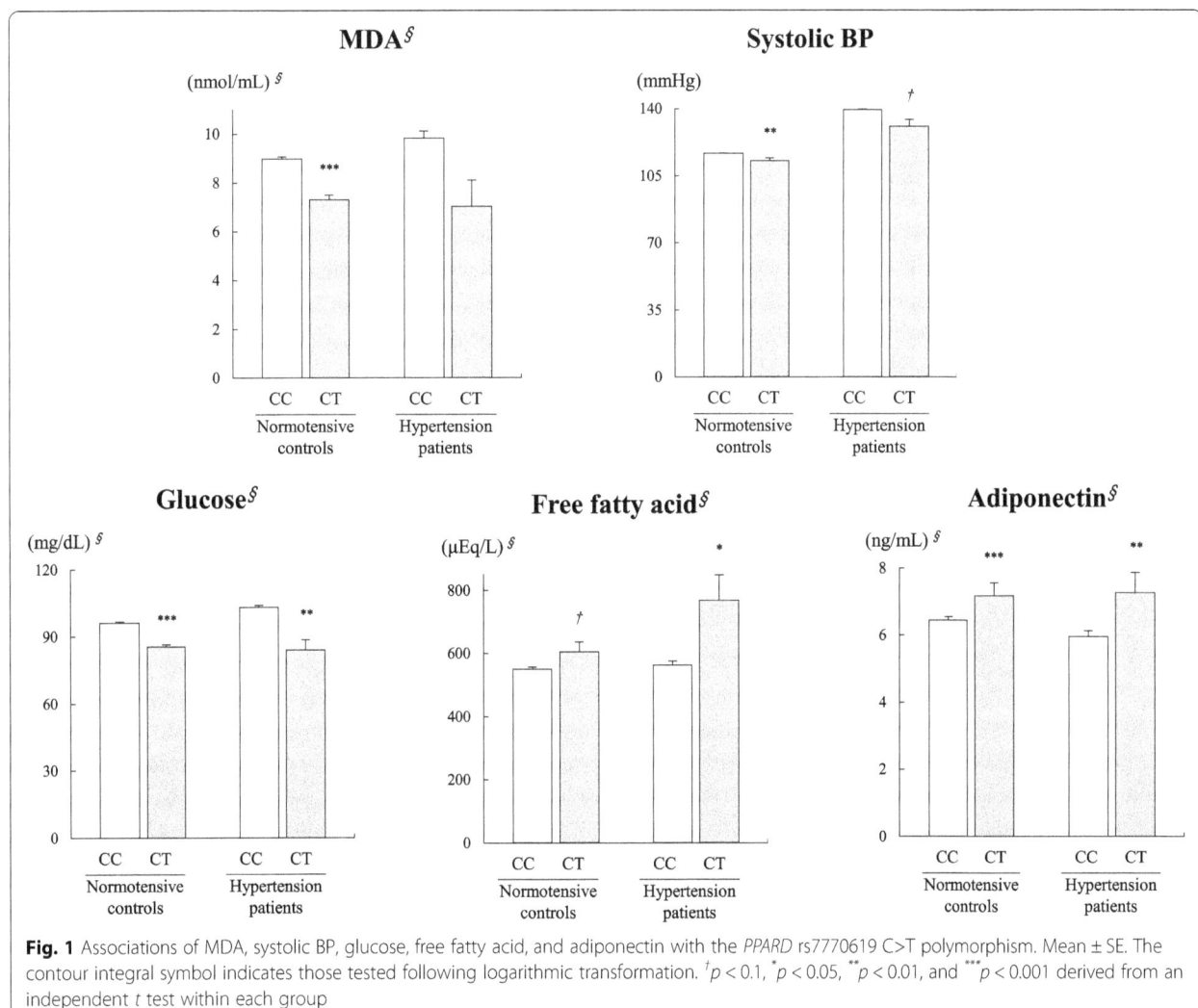

Fig. 1 Associations of MDA, systolic BP, glucose, free fatty acid, and adiponectin with the *PPARD* rs7770619 C>T polymorphism. Mean ± SE. The contour integral symbol indicates those tested following logarithmic transformation. [†]$p < 0.1$, [*]$p < 0.05$, [**]$p < 0.01$, and [***]$p < 0.001$ derived from an independent *t* test within each group

concentrations of plasma MDA in the subjects carrying the *PPARD* rs7770619 CT genotype than in the subjects with the CC genotype in the normotensive controls and the tendency toward a decrease in the HTN patients were found in this study. Recently, Li et al. [9] have observed associations between rs2016520 and the rs9794 minor allele of *PPARD* and decreased risk of HTN and additional interactions between these two SNPs. Although the *PPARD* rs7770619 SNP is not equivalent to the SNPs identified in other studies [9], the results of this study indicate that the *PPARD* rs7770619 SNP may represent a critical locus that negatively influences HTN and oxidative stress.

The *PPARD* rs7770619 C>T SNP is considered functional since serum glucose and the *PPARD* rs7770619 C>T polymorphism were significantly associated in both normotensive controls and HTN patients in this study. *PPARD* activation in the liver appears to decrease hepatic glucose output, which contributes to improved glucose control [16]. *PPARD* also appears to have a role in the regulation of fatty acid oxidation in several tissues, including skeletal muscle and adipose tissue [17]. It has been suggested that the mechanisms of action of this gene involve redistribution of the non-esterified fatty acid (NEFA) flux. The increasing oxidative capability draws the NEFA to the muscle to be preferentially oxidized rather than stored in adipose tissue, which leads to a decrease in adipocyte size, enhanced lipolysis, and increased adiponectin secretion [18]. In this study, subjects with the *PPARD* rs7770619 CT genotype showed significantly higher adiponectin concentrations than those with the CC genotype in both the normotensive controls and the HTN patients. Additionally, HTN patients with the CT genotype showed an increase in serum free fatty acid compared with subjects with the CC genotype.

The rs7770619 SNP, showing the features above in this study, is an intron mutation located at chromosome 6:35382265 (GRC38p.12 assembly of the human genome). Introns are involved in regulation of alternative splicing and gene expression [19]; therefore, the rs7770619 C>T polymorphism "may" affect the *PPARD* gene splicing, *PPARD* splice variants generation, and/or PPARD function. So far, however, there is a lack of studies on rs7770619, and studies about an impact of rs7770619 on *PPARD* gene splicing do not exist. Thus, at the present stage of knowledge and information, it is difficult to prove that the intron mutation of rs7770619 "really" influences splicing of *PPARD* gene. Moreover, to the best of our knowledge, no literatures that investigated altered risk of HTN, oxidative stress, or MDA levels according to *PPARD* splice variants exist. Our study only approached the association between *PPARD* rs7770619 C>T polymorphism and the risk of HTN in the Korean cohort; thus, the exact mechanism on

development of HTN through the SNP is still unknown. Therefore, attempts to verify the underlying mechanism is needed in the future.

According to the dbSNP (http://www.ncbi.nlm.nih.gov/snp), MAF for rs7770619 SNP is 7.5% in the 1000 Genomes Project (phase 3) and 10.5% in TOPMED. In the present study, MAF of rs7770619 was 2.4% in the whole participants (2.8% and 1.2% for normotensive controls and HTN patients, respectively); somewhat low MAF was shown in the Korean cohort compared to the world's average. Indeed, MAFs for rs7770619 vary based on ethnic groups. Many African populations have high rs7770619 MAF (> 20%), whereas in Asian populations (especially East Asians such as Korean, Chinese, and Japanese), rs7770619 MAF is generally low; based on the 1000 Genomes Project (phase3) (https://www.ncbi.nlm.nih.gov/variation/tools/1000genomes), in the population of Han Chinese in Beijing (HCB population) and Japanese in Tokyo (JPT population), MAF is 1.5% and 0.5%, respectively. Therefore, considering ethnic origin, MAF for rs7770619 observed in our cohort is not exclusively low. Many studies have reported the ethnic-dependent differences of HTN prevalence; studies have shown that black people are under higher risk of HTN than white people [20–23]. Moreover, Cappuccio et al. [24] showed that the South Asian population had two- to three-fold higher prevalence of HTN than white people, and Holly et al. [23] also showed significant higher odds ratio of HTN in the Chinese population compared with the white population after adjusting confounding factors. In dbSNP, the Caucasian population (CAUC1) shows 8.1% of MAF for rs7770619. Since our results demonstrated that rs7770619 minor T allele is associated with lower risk of HTN, higher risk of HTN in Asian populations whose MAF for rs7770619 is lower than white people makes sense; however, higher prevalence of HTN was also observed in the black population, thus, our results do not entirely correspond with other researches in terms of ethnicity. HTN can be caused by various risks such as genetic, metabolic, and environmental (e.g., dietary habit and physical activity) factors. A complex interaction of these risk factors induces HTN; thus, risk of HTN according to ethnic groups cannot be explained by only one polymorphism. At least, in a Korean population, rs7770619 was found as a novel SNP for HTN risk via a connection with oxidative stress (MDA). In addition, rs7770619 C>T polymorphism has not been studied with regard to oxidative stress and HTN, and this is the first study to identify association between rs7770619 SNP and HTN risk. Therefore, based on the results of our study, gradual expansion of the HTN study in respect of rs7770619 polymorphism is needed.

There are several limitations. First, when interpreting the findings of this study, it should be considered that our results share the limitations of cross-sectional observational studies becuase we evaluated only an association rather than prospective prediction. Second, in terms of conventional genome-wide association study (GWAS), this study did not share the exact analysis method of conventional GWAS, because (1) imputation could not be conducted due to the limit of equipment's calculation capacity and (2) when we selected SNPs, we used FDR correction instead of Bonferroni correction, widely used in conventional GWAS. Bonferroni correction has a very conservative threshold ($p < 5 \times 10^{-8}$) so that it can cause decrease of statistical power [25, 26]. Recently, indeed, not only Bonferroni correction but also FDR correction has been used in common practice [27, 28]. Third, unexpectedly, low MAF generated a too small sample size of individuals with rs7770619 CT genotype; thus, in Fig. 1, a subset analysis with the HTN without treatment group (for control of HTN medication effects) according to the rs7770619 genotypes could not be performed due to a problem of statistical power. Lastly, we specifically focused on a representative group of Korean subjects. Therefore, our results cannot be generalized to other ethnicities, age groups, or geographical groups. Taken together, further study needs to be conducted by exact manner of GWAS with a cohort having a much larger sample size to confirm replication of the results observed in this study. Despite these limitations, our results show interesting associations between the *PPARD* rs7770619 CT genotype, a decreased risk of HTN, and decreased oxidative stress. These results suggest that the *PPARD* rs7770619 C>T SNP is a novel candidate gene for HTN through the association between *PPARD* and MDA, a biomarker of oxidative stress.

Conclusion

According to the individuals' *PPARD* rs7770619 genotype, the risk of HTN development is predictable via association between *PPARD* rs7770619 SNPs and MDA. Reducing MDA in subjects with *PPARD* rs7770619 CC genotype is necessary to decrease the risk of HTN development. Therefore, by analyzing personal genetic background, MDA, the oxidative stress marker, can be considered as a therapeutic target of HTN in a Korean population.

Abbreviations
BP: Blood pressure; CI: Confidence interval; FDR: False discovery rate; GWAS: Genome-wide association study; HDL: High-density lipoprotein; HOMA: Homeostatic model assessment; hs-CRP: High-sensitivity C-reactive protein; HTN: Hypertension; HWE: Hardy-Weinberg equilibrium; IR: Insulin resistance; K-CHIP: Korean Chip; LDL: Low-density lipoprotein; MDA: Malondialdehyde; NEFA: Non-esterified fatty acid; OR: Odds ratio; PPAR: Peroxisome proliferator-activated receptor; PPARD: Peroxisome proliferator-activated receptor-δ; ROS: Reactive oxygen species; SNP: Single-nucleotide polymorphism; TC: Total cholesterol; TG: Triglyceride

Acknowledgements
The genotype data were generated using the Korean Chip (K-CHIP), which is available through the K-CHIP consortium. The K-CHIP was designed by the Center for Genome Science at the Korea National Institute of Health, Korea (4845-301, 3000-3031). We appreciate Dr. Sang-Hyun Lee, who belongs to the Department of Family Practice, National Health Insurance Corporation, Ilsan Hospital, Goyang, Korea, for collaborating on the acquisition of the valuable data.

Funding
This study was funded by the Mid-career Researcher Program (NRF-2016R1A2B4011662) of the Ministry of Science and ICT through the National Research Foundation of Korea, Republic of Korea.

Authors' contributions
All authors contributed to the conception and design of the study. MJK and JHL were responsible for the analysis and interpretation of the data and preparation of the manuscript. MKK and HJY took part in the analysis of the data and preparation of the manuscript. JS carried out the acquisition and analysis of the data. All authors contributed to the critical revisions of the paper and have approved the study for publication.

Competing interests
The authors declare that they have no competing interests.

Author details
[1]Research Center for Silver Science, Institute of Symbiotic Life-TECH, Yonsei University, Seoul 03722, Korea. [2]Department of Food and Nutrition, Brain Korea 21 PLUS Project, College of Human Ecology, Yonsei University, 50 Yonsei-ro, Seodaemun-gu, Seoul 03722, Korea. [3]Department of Food and Nutrition, National Leading Research Laboratory of Clinical Nutrigenetics/Nutrigenomics, College of Human Ecology, Yonsei University, Seoul 03722, Korea.

References
1. Tiwari BK, Pandey KB, Abidi AB, Rizvi SI. Markers of oxidative stress during diabetes mellitus. J Biomark. 2013;2013:378790.
2. Armas-Padilla MC, Armas-Hernández MJ, Sosa-Canache B, Cammarata R, Pacheco B, Guerrero J, et al. Nitric oxide and malondialdehyde in human hypertension. Am J Ther. 2007;14:172–6.
3. Gönenç A, Hacışevki A, Tavil Y, Çengel A, Torun M. Oxidative stress in patients with essential hypertension: a comparison of dippers and non-dippers. Eur J Intern Med. 2013;24:139–44.
4. Uzun H, Karter Y, Aydin S, Curgunlu A, Simşek G, Yücel R, et al. Oxidative stress in white coat hypertension; role of paraoxonase. J Hum Hypertens. 2004;18:523–8.
5. Yagil Y, Yagil C. The search for the genetic basis of hypertension. Curr Opin Nephrol Hypertens. 2005;14:141–7.

6. Zhu Q, Guo Z, Hu X, Wu M, Chen Q, Luo W, et al. Haplotype analysis of *PPARγ* C681G and intron CT variants. Positive association with essential hypertension. Herz. 2014;39:264–70.

7. Gu SJ, Guo ZR, Wu M, Ding Y, Luo WS. Association of peroxisome proliferator-activated receptor γ polymorphisms and haplotypes with essential hypertension. Genet Test Mol Biomarkers. 2013;17:418–23.

8. Usuda D, Kanda T. Peroxisome proliferator-activated receptors for hypertension. World J Cardiol. 2014;6:744–54.

9. Li Y, Sun G. Case-control study on association of peroxisome proliferator-activated receptor-δ and SNP-SNP interactions with essential hypertension in Chinese Han population. Funct Integr Genomics. 2016;16:95–100.

10. Kim M, Kim M, Yoo HJ, Yun R, Lee S-H, Lee JH. Estrogen-related receptor γ gene (*ESRRG*) rs1890552 A>G polymorphism in a Korean population: association with urinary prostaglandin-$F_{2\alpha}$ concentration and impaired fasting glucose or newly diagnosed type 2 diabetes. Diabetes Metab. 2017; 43:385–8.

11. Ischiropoulos H, Beckman JS. Oxidative stress and nitration in neurodegeneration: cause, effect, or association? J Clin Invest. 2003;111:163–9.

12. Schopfer FJ, Baker PR, Freeman BA. NO-dependent protein nitration: a cell signaling event or an oxidative inflammatory response? Trends Biochem Sci. 2003;28:646–54.

13. Dhalla NS, Temsah RM, Netticadan T. Role of oxidative stress in cardiovascular diseases. J Hypertens. 2000;18:655–73.

14. Touyz RM, Schiffrin EL. Reactive oxygen species in vascular biology: implications in hypertension. Histochem Cell Biol. 2004;122:339–52.

15. Kashyap MK, Yadav V, Sherawat BS, Jain S, Kumari S, Khullar M, et al. Different antioxidants status, total antioxidant power and free radicals in essential hypertension. Mol Cell Biochem. 2005;277:89–99.

16. Villegas R, Williams S, Gao Y, Cai Q, Li H, Elasy T, et al. Peroxisome proliferator-activated receptor delta (*PPARD*) genetic variation and type 2 diabetes in middle-aged Chinese women. Ann Hum Genet. 2011;75:621–9.

17. Fredenrich A, Grimaldi PA. Roles of peroxisome proliferator-activated receptor delta in skeletal muscle function and adaptation. Curr Opin Clin Nutr Metab Care. 2004;7:377–81.

18. Schulze MB, Hu FB. Primary prevention of diabetes: what can be done and how much can be prevented? Annu Rev Public Health. 2005;26:445–67.

19. Jo BS, Choi SS. Introns: the functional benefits of introns in genomes. Genomics Inform. 2015;13:112–8.

20. Ortega LM, Sedki E, Nayer A. Hypertension in the African American population: a succinct look at its epidemiology, pathogenesis, and therapy. Nefrologia. 2015;35:139–45.

21. Lackland DT. Racial differences in hypertension: implications for high blood pressure management. Am J Med Sci. 2014;348:135–8.

22. Brown MJ. Hypertension and ethnic group. BMJ. 2006;332:833–6.

23. Kramer H, Han C, Post W, Goff D, Diez-Roux A, Cooper R, et al. Racial/ethnic differences in hypertension and hypertension treatment and control in the multi-ethnic study of atherosclerosis (MESA). Am J Hypertens. 2004;17:963–70.

24. Cappuccio FP, Cook DG, Atkinson RW, Strazzullo P. Prevalence, detection, and management of cardiovascular risk factors in different ethnic groups in south London. Heart. 1997;78:555–63.

25. Nakagawa S. A farewell to Bonferroni: the problems of low statistical power and publication bias. Behav Ecol. 2004;15:1044–5.

26. Benjamini Y, Hochberg Y. Controlling the false discovery rate: a practical and powerful approach to multiple testing. J R Statist Soc B. 1995;57:289–300.

27. Li S, Xie L, Du M, Xu K, Zhu L, Chu H, et al. Association study of genetic variants in estrogen metabolic pathway genes and colorectal cancer risk and survival. Arch Toxicol. 2018. https://doi.org/10.1007/s00204-018-2195-y.

28. Duan B, Hu J, Liu H, Wang Y, Li H, Liu S, et al. Genetic variants in the platelet-derived growth factor subunit B gene associated with pancreatic cancer risk. Int J Cancer. 2018;142:1322–31.

20

A novel *LRAT* mutation affecting splicing in a family with early onset retinitis pigmentosa

Yabin Chen[1†], Li Huang[2†], Xiaodong Jiao[1], Sheikh Riazuddin[3,4,5], S. Amer Riazuddin[6†] and J. Fielding Hetmancik[1*†]

Abstract

Background and purpose: Retinitis pigmentosa is an important cause of severe visual dysfunction. This study reports a novel splicing mutation in the lecithin retinol acyltransferase (*LRAT*) gene associated with early onset retinitis pigmentosa and characterizes the effects of this mutation on mRNA splicing and structure.

Methods: Genome-wide linkage analysis followed by dideoxy sequencing of the linked candidate gene *LRAT* was performed in a consanguineous Pakistani family with autosomal recessive retinitis pigmentosa. In silico prediction and minigene assays were used to investigate the effects of the presumptive splicing mutation.

Results: ARRP in this family was linked to chromosome 4q31.21-q32.1 with a maximum LOD score of 5.40. A novel homozygous intronic mutation (NM_004744.4: c.541-15T>G) was detected in *LRAT*. In silico tools predicted that the AG-creating mutation would activate an intronic cryptic acceptor site, but cloning fragments of wild-type and mutant sequences of *LRAT* into Exontrap Cloning Vector pET01 and Expression Cloning Vector pCMV-(DYKD$_4$K)-C showed that the primary effect of the sequence change was to weaken the nearby authentic acceptor site and cause exon skipping, with only a small fraction of transcripts utilizing the acceptor site producing the reference transcript.

Conclusions: The c.541-15T>G mutation in *LRAT* results in aberrant splicing and is therefore predicted to be causal for the early onset retinitis pigmentosa in this family. In addition, this work suggests that minigenes adapted to the specific gene and exon may need to be designed for variants in the first and last exon and intron to mimic the authentic splicing mechanism in vivo.

Keywords: Retinitis pigmentosa, *LRAT*, Splicing mutation, Cryptic splice site, Minigene assay, Exon splicing, Linkage

Introduction

Retinitis pigmentosa (RP, [MIM 268000]) is a clinically and genetically heterogeneous disorder affecting approximately 1 in 4000 individuals worldwide [1]. Clinically, patients initially exhibit night blindness followed by progressive loss of peripheral visual fields and eventually complete loss of central vision. Typical fundus changes include bone spicule-like pigmentation in the mid-peripheral retina, waxy pallor of the optic discs, and attenuation of retinal blood vessels. Since RP initially affects the rod photoreceptors, followed by the degeneration of cone photoreceptors, patients often have severely diminished or extinguished rod response in electroretinography (ERG) recordings even in early stages, while the cone response is relatively preserved initially but becomes undetectable as the disease progresses [2]. The genetic inheritance patterns of RP include autosomal-dominant (about 30–40% of cases), autosomal-recessive (50–60%), and X-linked (5–15%) [3, 4] inheritance. More than 82 causative genes have been identified for RP so far, of which 58 genes have been identified in families with autosomal recessive RP (arRP; RetNet).

Lecithin retinol acyltransferase (LRAT) is a retinyl ester synthase, catalyzing the formation of fatty acid retinyl

* Correspondence: hejtmancikj@nei.nih.gov

†Yabin Chen, Li Huang, S. Amer Riazuddin and J. Fielding Hetmancik contributed equally to this work.

[1]Ophthalmic Genetics and Visual Function Branch, National Eye Institute, National Institutes of Health, Bethesda, MD 20892, USA

Full list of author information is available at the end of the article

esters, a crucial step in the retinoid cycle. In the eye, it is specifically expressed in the retinal pigmented epithelium (RPE), so that LRAT dysfunction leads to diminished visual chromophores and eventual retinal degeneration [5]. Mutations in the *LRAT* gene can cause Leber congenital amaurosis, juvenile retinitis pigmentosa, and early-onset severe retinitis pigmentosa with autosomal recessive inheritance (MIM 604863). Leber congenital amaurosis is the most severe retinal dystrophic disease. Patients usually present in the first decade of life with severe visual impairment and pendular nystagmus [6].

It is estimated that about 10% of disease-causing mutations affect splicing [7]. Most of the splice site mutations affect the invariant GT or AG dinucleotides in the 3′ and 5′ splice sites, respectively [8, 9]. However, mutations involving other positions of the 5′ or 3′ splice sites can also impair splicing and typically lead to exon skipping, activation of a cryptic splice site, or intron retention [10]. This study demonstrates that single base pair substitution in the intron even 15 bases upstream of 3′ splice site can disrupt spliceosomal recognition of the splice site.

Materials and methods
Clinical assessment
This study was approved by the Institutional Review Boards (IRB) of the National Centre of Excellence in Molecular Biology, Lahore, Pakistan, and the CNS IRB at the National Institutes of Health. Participating individuals or their guardians gave written informed consent consistent with the tenets of the Declaration of Helsinki before the study. Family 61254 is a consanguineous Pakistani family with non-syndromic RP. All participants underwent a thorough family, ophthalmic, and medical history, and selected individuals were assessed by best-corrected visual acuity, slit-lamp biomicroscopy, fundus photography, and electroretinography (ERG). Blood samples were collected from potentially informative family members, and genomic DNA was extracted from leukocytes according to standard protocols [11].

Genome-wide linkage analysis
We designed linkage mapping panels to complete a genome-wide scan for family 61254. Primer sequences and PCR conditions are shown in Additional file 1: Table S1. Based on the initial results of the linkage analysis, markers with logarithm of the odds (LOD) scores greater than 2 were selected for further fine mapping by microsatellite markers closely spaced 1–2 cM apart.

Two-point linkage analyses were performed with alleles of family 61254 obtained through the genome-wide scan and fine mapping using the FASTLINK modification of the MLINK program in the LINKAGE program package [12, 13] using the pedigree file shown in

Additional file 2. Maximum LOD scores were calculated using ILINK. Autosomal recessive RP was analyzed as a fully penetrant trait with an affected allele frequency of 0.0001. Haplotypes were drawn by the Cyrillic 2.1 program (Cyrillic Software, Wallingford, Oxfordshire, UK) and confirmed by inspection.

Mutation screening
Primer pairs for the coding exons and 100 bp of flanking intronic regions of *LRAT* were designed using the Primer 3 program (http://primer3.ut.ee/) and are shown in Additional file 3: Table S3. Amplifications were completed in 10 μl reactions containing 40 ng of genomic DNA, 0.5 μl of 5 μM of each primer, 1 μl GeneAmp 10×PCR Gold buffer (Applied Biosystems), 0.6 μl of 25 mM MgCl2, 0.8 μl of 2.5 mM dNTP mixture, and 1 μl of 5 U/μl Taq DNA polymerase. PCR reactions consisted of a denaturation step at 95 °C for 5 min followed by a two-step touchdown procedure. The first 15 cycles consisted of denaturation at 95 °C for 30 s, followed by a touchdown annealing step for 30 s in which the annealing temperature was initially set at 64 °C and decreased by 0.5 °C per cycle, and an elongation step at 72 °C for 30 s. The second step of 20 cycles consisted of denaturation at 95 °C for 30 s followed by annealing at 57 °C for 30 s and elongation at 72 °C for 30 s. These were followed by a final elongation at 72 °C for 10 min. PCR products were purified using the AMPure XP system (Beckman coulter Biomek NX, Brea, CA). The PCR primers for each exon were used for bidirectional sequencing using the BigDye Terminator Ready Reaction mix (Applied Biosystems), according to the manufacturer's instructions. The sequencing products were purified using the Agencourt CleanSEQ system (Beckman Coulter Biomeck NX). Sequencing was performed on an ABI PRISM 3130 Automated sequencer (Applied Biosystems, Foster City, CA). Sequencing results were analyzed using Mutation Surveyor (SoftGenetics, State College, PA) and Seqman software Lasergene 12.2.0 (DNASTAR, Madison, WI).

In silico splice site prediction
To evaluate the potential pathogenicity of the splice site variation, several in silico splice site prediction programs were used, including Human Splice Finder (http://www.umd.be/HSF3/), SpliceView (http://bioinfo.itb.cnr.it/oriel/splice-view.html), Berkeley Drosophila Genome Project Neural Network (BDGP: http://www.fruitfly.org/), and NetGene2 (http://www.cbs.dtu.dk/services/NetGene2/). Default settings are applied for all analyses.

Generation of vector constructs
Minigene assays were performed to confirm the predicted pathogenic effects of the *LRAT* mutation. Since mutation c.541-15T>G (NM_004744.4) was in intron 2,

a 5228-bp genomic DNA fragment that included exon 2, intron 2, and part of exon 3 of *LRAT* was amplified using primers LRAT-gDNA-F and LRAT-gDNA-R. Because limited minigene amplicon length can be included in the minigene assay, and exon 3 is 4136-bp long with 153-bp coding sequence and 3983-bp 3′ UTR sequence, only part of exon 3 (402-bp) containing the coding region and several predicted downstream cryptic splice donor and acceptor sites were included in the 5228-bp fragment used for the minigene assay. The wildtype and mutant DNA fragments were amplified from genomic DNA of unaffected sibling 6125441 and patient 6125408 carrying the wild-type and homozygous mutant alleles, respectively. PCR products were cloned into a TA vector (pCR®II TOPO) and then subcloned into Exontrap cloning Vector pET01 (MoBiTec GmbH, Göttingen, Germany) via BamHI and NotI restriction sites to generate the wild-type WT-LRAT-pET01 and mutant Mut-LRAT-pET01 constructs.

Because exon 3 is the last exon of *LRAT*, to mimic authentic splicing mechanism in vivo, we also used a Q5 Site-Directed Mutagenesis Kit (New England Biolabs, Ipswich, MA) to abolish the splice acceptor site of 3′ exon on pET01 by altering the final acceptor AG to AT, creating the modified empty construct pET01-2, modified wildtype construct WT-2-LRAT-pET01, and modified mutant construct Mut-2-LRAT-pET01. In

addition, the same 5228-bp genomic DNA fragment was also amplified by PCR with primers containing the appropriate restriction enzyme sites (LRAT-gDNA-F-SalI and LRAT-gDNA-R-KpnI) and then cloned into the expression vector pCMV-(DYKD$_4$K)-C (Clontech Laboratories, Inc. CA, USA), which has no vector exons before and behind the inserted PCR products. SalI and KpnI restriction sites were used to insert the PCR products and construct wildtype construct WT-LRAT-pCMV and mutant construct Mut-LRAT-pCMV.

The primers used for PCR amplification and mutagenesis are listed in Table 1. The sequences and correct orientations of all constructs were validated using Sanger sequencing.

Cell culture and transfection

Human embryonic kidney 293T cells and human retinal pigment epithelial cells (ARPE-19) were maintained in Dulbecco's modified Eagle medium supplemented with 10% fetal bovine serum in 5% CO_2 at 37 °C. The Exontrap cloning vectors pET01, WT-LRAT-pET01, Mut-LRAT-pET01, pET01-mut, WT-2-LRAT-pET01, and Mut-2-LRAT-pET01 were transfected into 293T cells using PolyJet In Vitro DNA Transfection Reagent (SignaGen Laboratories, MD). The expression vectors pCMV-(DYKD$_4$K)-C, WT-LRAT-pCMV, and Mut-LRAT-pCMV were transfected into 293T cells and

Table 1 Two-point LOD scores of markers around 4q31.21-q32.1

Marker	CM	Mb	0	0.01	0.05	0.1	0.2	0.3	0.4	Z_{max}	θ_{max}
D4S1615	128.31	128.21	− 3.81	− 2.00	− 0.36	0.15	0.30	0.17	0.03	0.30	0.20
D4S429	131.00	133.11	− 2.05	− 1.19	− 0.08	0.25	0.31	0.17	0.04	0.31	0.20
D4S1575	132.05	134.79	4.90	4.80	4.40	3.89	2.82	1.72	4.90	4.90	0.00
D4S3039	132.72	135.96	1.26	2.78	3.10	2.93	2.24	1.42	3.10	3.10	0.05
D4S1576	135.57	138.99	− 5.19	− 2.27	− 1.14	− 0.74	− 0.38	− 0.17	− 0.17	− 0.17	0.30
D4S1579	140.64	140.73	− ∞	− 0.01	1.01	1.17	0.89	0.42	1.17	1.17	0.10
D4S2939	142.24	141.15	− ∞	− 0.92	1.99	2.13	1.74	1.06	0.36	2.13	0.09
D4S424	144.56	142.20	− ∞	− 3.69	− 0.19	0.30	0.51	0.39	0.19	0.51	0.20
D4S2998	145.98	145.57	5.40	5.39	4.89	4.36	3.25	2.08	0.94	5.40	0.00
D4S1586	147.06	146.78	5.13	5.12	4.61	4.08	2.99	1.88	0.83	5.13	0.00
D4S3008	152.98	150.30	2.72	2.72	2.54	2.29	1.70	1.04	0.43	2.72	0.00
D4S1548	153.51	152.14	1.74	1.74	1.63	1.46	1.05	0.62	0.25	1.74	0.00
D4S3021	154.63	154.94	4.08	4.08	3.77	3.39	2.52	1.57	0.68	4.08	0.00
D4S3049	155.19	154.77	4.54	4.53	4.03	3.51	2.41	1.29	0.35	4.54	0.00
D4S2976	155.31	155.80	3.99	3.98	3.57	3.15	2.29	1.45	0.66	3.99	0.00
LRAT c.541-15T>G		155.67	6.57	6.47	6.04	5.48	4.28	2.94	1.49	6.57	0.00
D4S2934	155.41	154.05	4.89	4.88	4.40	3.90	2.86	1.81	0.83	4.89	0.00
D4S2918	157.99	160.33	2.77	2.76	2.45	2.14	1.51	0.91	0.39	2.77	0.00
D4S1585	157.99	157.51	3.05	3.04	2.74	2.42	1.78	1.13	0.52	3.05	0.00
D4S2982	158.65	161.09	− ∞	0.98	2.30	2.20	1.71	1.11	0.52	2.30	0.05

ARPE-19 cells, respectively, using PolyJet In Vitro DNA Transfection Reagent. For nonsense-mediated decay inhibition studies, non-transfected and transfected ARPE19 cells were treated with 0, 5 μM, and 10 μM PTC124 separately (Enzo Life Sciences, Inc., NY) for 24 h. Cells were harvested 24 h after transfection.

RNA isolation, cDNA synthesis, PCR, and sequencing

Total cellular RNA was extracted using Trizol reagent (Life Technologies), and cDNA was synthesized using a reverse transcriptase kit (Invitrogen, Carlsbad, CA) with oligo $(dT)_{20}$ primers. Primers used for PCR amplification for cDNA are listed in Additional file 2: Table S2. The amplified products were separated by electrophoresis on 10% Novex TBE gels (Invitrogen) and stained with ethidium bromide. Visualized bands were extracted from the gels, and the same primers were used for sequencing to validate the splice effects in the in vitro assays.

Results

RP in family 61254 showed an autosomal recessive inheritance pattern, and all affected individuals are offspring of first-cousin matings (Fig. 1a). The medical records of affected members in family 61254 reported signs of retinal degeneration early in life. Fundus photographs and ERGs were available only for individuals 5, 8, and 32 (Figs. 2 and 3). Affected individual 8, who was 35 years old at the time of examination, showed typical signs of RP, including waxy pale optic discs, attenuation of retinal arteries, bone spicule-like pigment deposits in the midperiphery of the retina, and macular changes. Affected individual 32, who was 10 years old at the time of examination, only showed attenuation of retinal arteries in fundus photographs. But both individual 8 and 32 had extinguished ERGs, consistent with extensive loss of rod and cone function typical of advanced arRP. Unaffected individual 5 showed no retinal abnormalities in fundus photographs and normal ERG recordings, although his fundus appears cloudy due to age-related cataracts.

During a genome-wide scan for family 61254, a LOD score greater than 2.0 was found only for markers D4S1575, D4S413, D14S261, and D17S921. Except for a single chromosome 4 locus, which was narrowed from D4S429 to D4S424, other regions were excluded by fine mapping markers at 1–2 cM intervals and haplotype inspection. Among the markers selected for fine mapping of the chromosome 4 locus, D4S2998 obtained a maximum LOD score of 5.40 at $\theta = 0$ (Table 1). Thus, two-point linkage mapping in family 61254 identified a linked region of 14.09 cM (18.89 Mb) on chromosome 4q31.21-q32.1 flanked by markers D4S424 and D4S2982 (Table 1, Fig. 1a).

LRAT is the only known candidate gene for inherited retinal diseases in the linked region. Sequencing of all coding exons and exon-intron boundaries detected a single novel splicing site variation in *LRAT*. All affected individuals in family 61254 carry a homozygous T>G change 5′ of exon 3 (c.541-15T>G, rs779487944), which cosegregates with the phenotype in the family (Fig. 1). The frequency of this change was 0.000004 as reported in the gnomAD database (http://gnomad.broadinstitute.org/about) with a single heterozygous individual in the South Asian population. In silico splice prediction tools including Human Splice Finder and SpliceView predicted that the AG-creating mutation would activate an intronic cryptic acceptor site, causing retention of an additional 14 bases from intron 2 in the transcript, leading to a frameshift in the translation reading frame, and resulting in a truncated protein p.(F181Ifs*10). The SpliceView program also predicted minimal weakening of the authentic acceptor site. However, the predicted new intronic cryptic acceptor site was not identified by BDGP or NetGene2, which only showed minimal weakening of the authentic acceptor site (Fig. 4).

To test these predictions, we carried out a minigene assay with Exontrap Cloning Vector pET01 to examine the potential pathogenic effects of this mutation (Fig. 5a). The 293T cells transfected with empty plasmid (pET01) produced a 242-bp band, consistent with correct transcript splicing with excision of the intron flanked by pre-proinsulin 5′ and 3′ exons (Fig. 5c). Cells transfected with WT-LRAT-pET01 produced a faint 242-bp band and another 865-bp band. Direct sequencing of the PCR products revealed that the 865-bp band was consistent with correct mRNA splicing at the end 5′ of exon 3, which also utilized a cryptic donor site in the coding region of exon 3 of *LRAT* to join to the 3′ exon in pET01 (Fig. 5b, d). In contrast, cells transfected with Mut-LRAT-pET01 containing the c.541-15T>G mutation produced a shorter band that skipped exon 3 of LRAT. These findings are consistent with disruption of the authentic acceptor site of exon 3 by the c.541-15T>G change.

Because there is no exon following exon 3 in human genomic DNA of *LRAT*, we abolished the splice acceptor site of the pre-proinsulin 3′ exon on pET01 to reduce its effect on mRNA splicing of the inserted sequence of *LRAT*. Cells transfected with WT-2-LRAT-pET01 still produced mRNA with correct splicing at the 5′ end of exon 3, and cells transfected with Mut-2-LRAT-pET01 still produced mRNA skipping the exon 3. However, because the authentic acceptor site of the pre-proinsulin 3′ exon was abolished, the transcription utilized a cryptic acceptor site within the 3′ exon (Fig. 5).

To further mimic the splicing mechanism in vivo, we inserted the same 5228-bp genomic DNA fragment of *LRAT* into expression vector pCMV-$(DYKD_4K)$-C which

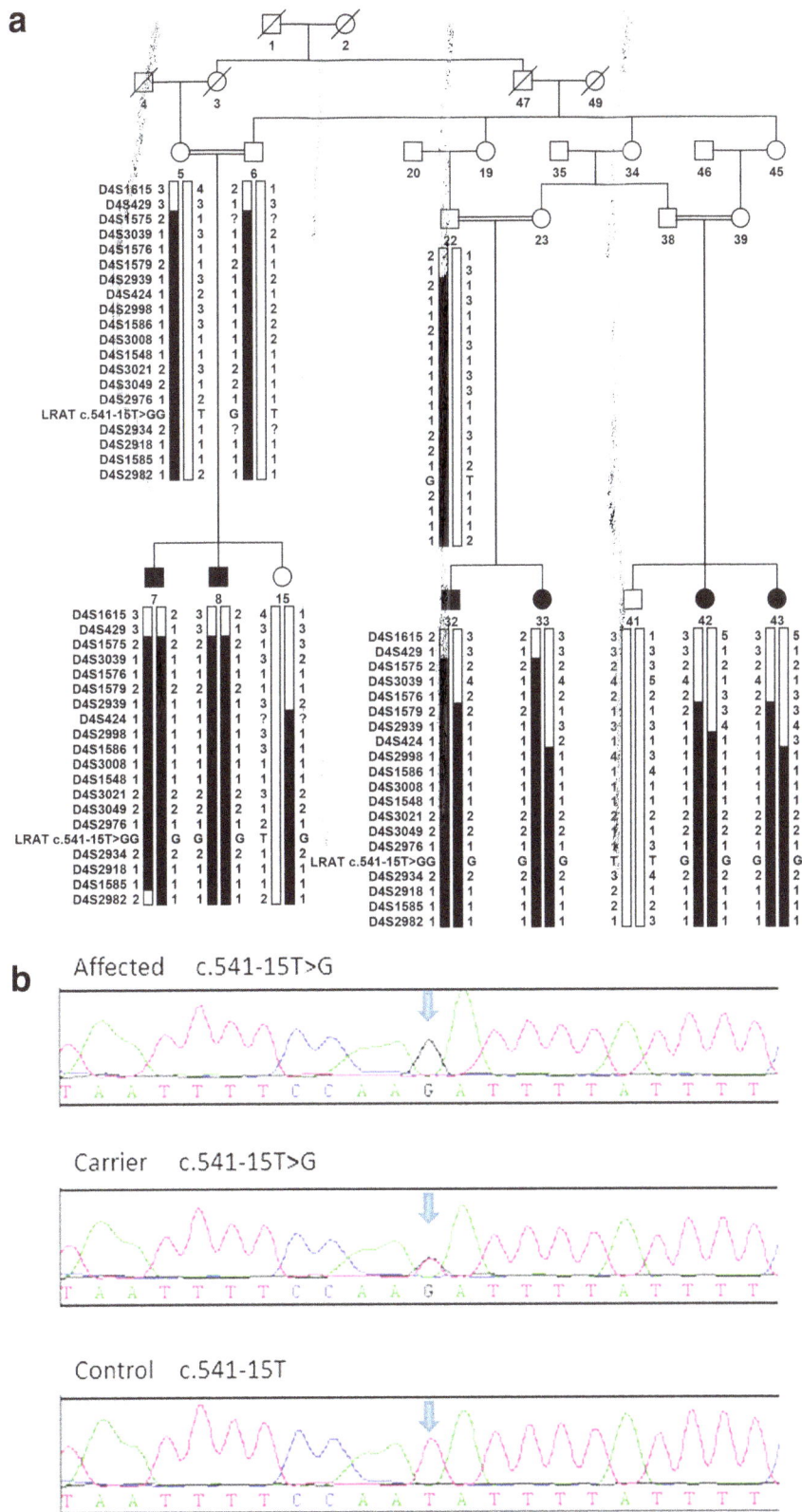

Fig. 1 Pedigree, *LRAT* Region, and sequence. **a** Haplotypes of the *LRAT* region of family 61254 showing the *LRAT* c.541-15T>G mutation and surrounding microsatellite markers included in Table 1. The risk haplotype is marked in black. **b** Electropherograms of the *LRAT* homozygous mutation c.541-15T>G (up, individual 7), carrier sequence (middle, individual 22), and wildtype alleles (down, individual 41)

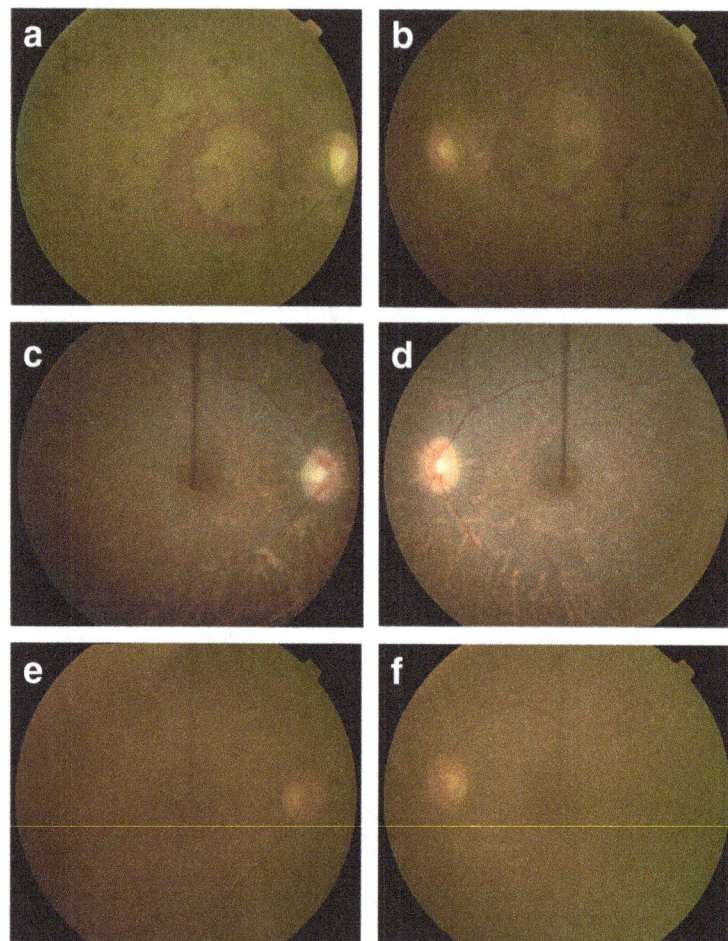

Fig. 2 Fundus photographs of family 61254. **a**, **b** Oculus dexter (OD) and oculus sinister (OS) of an affected 35-year-old individual (08), which show waxy pale optic discs, attenuation of retinal arteries, bone spicule-like pigment deposits in the midperiphery of the retina, and macular changes. **c**, **d** OD and OS of an affected 10-year-old individual (32), which show attenuation of retinal arteries. **e**, **f** OD and OS of an unaffected 60-year-old individual (05), which show no signs of retinal dystrophy but does show haziness secondary to age-related cataracts

has no exons before or behind the inserted region and used it to transfect both 293T cells and ARPE19 cells (Fig. 6a). Cells transfected with WT-LRAT-pCMV produced a 723 bp cDNA with correct splicing at the 5′ end of exon 3 (Fig. 6b, d). Both 293T cells and ARPE19 cells transfected with Mut-LRAT-pCMV produced a much fainter band of the same size, as well as a shorter 379 bp fragment skipping the authentic splice acceptor site at the 5′ of exon 3 and utilizing a cryptic acceptor site in the 3′ UTR instead. In contrast to the results in 293T cells, ARPE19 cells transfected with Mut-LRAT-pCMV also produced an extremely faint 513 bp fragment skipping the authentic splice site at the 5′ of exon 3 and utilizing another cryptic acceptor site in the 3′ UTR. To investigate whether the mutation caused mis-splicing events which would lead to nonsense-mediated decay, non-transfected and transfected ARPE19 cells were treated with PTC124 for 24 h to inhibit nonsense-mediated decay, and no extra transcripts were identified (Fig. 6c).

Discussion

We have identified a c.541-15T>G mutation in *LRAT* that results in aberrant splicing as the cause of autosomal recessive early-onset retinitis pigmentosa in a Pakistani family. The mammalian 3′ splice site consensus consists of three critical parts: YAG (Y = pyrimidine) at positions −1 to −3 relative to the first nucleotide of exon, a polypyrimidine tract (PPT) starting at position −5 and extending 10 or more nucleotides into the intron, and the branch point sequence (BPS; mammalian consensus YNCURAY, where Y = pyrimidine, R = purine, and N = any nucleotide) located upstream of the PPT, usually 11–40 nucleotides from the YAG [14, 15]. The PPT is a crucial recognition element for branch site definition prior to splicing, and the factor responsible for this early PPT recognition is U2AF[65] a subunit of the U2 snRNP auxiliary factor (U2AF) [14]. Since the c.541-15T>G mutation replaces a pyrimidine with a purine at the 5′ end of the PPT, it might possibly affect the interaction of the U2AF[65] with the PPT, thus

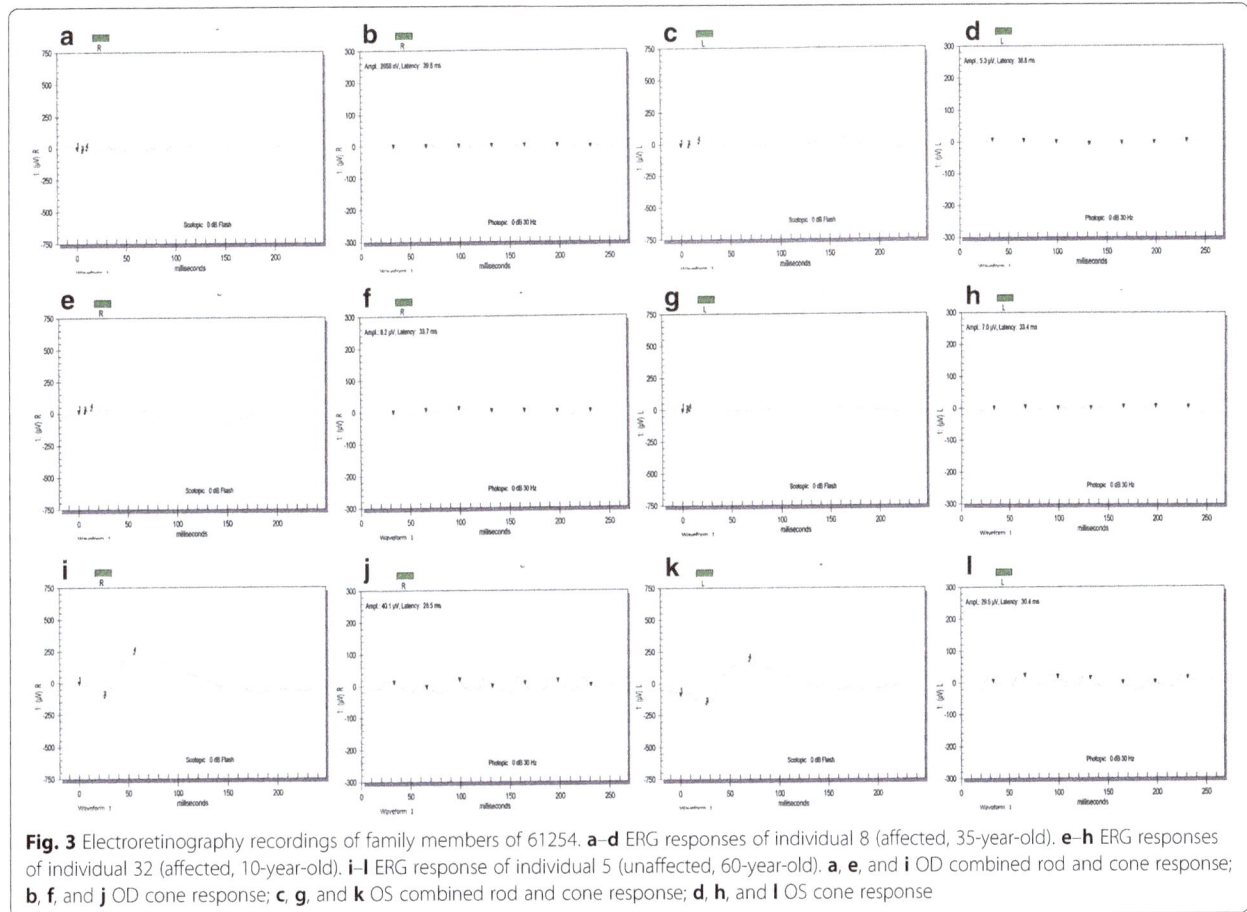

Fig. 3 Electroretinography recordings of family members of 61254. **a–d** ERG responses of individual 8 (affected, 35-year-old). **e–h** ERG responses of individual 32 (affected, 10-year-old). **i–l** ERG response of individual 5 (unaffected, 60-year-old). **a**, **e**, and **i** OD combined rod and cone response; **b**, **f**, and **j** OD cone response; **c**, **g**, and **k** OS combined rod and cone response; **d**, **h**, and **l** OS cone response

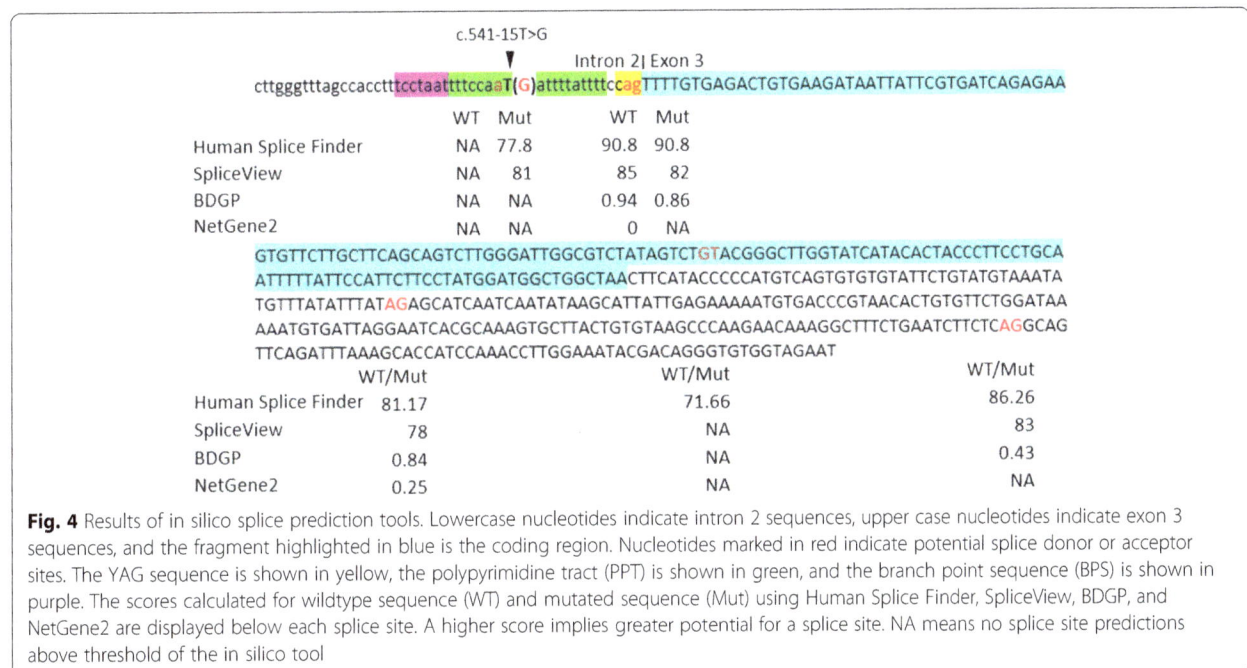

Fig. 4 Results of in silico splice prediction tools. Lowercase nucleotides indicate intron 2 sequences, upper case nucleotides indicate exon 3 sequences, and the fragment highlighted in blue is the coding region. Nucleotides marked in red indicate potential splice donor or acceptor sites. The YAG sequence is shown in yellow, the polypyrimidine tract (PPT) is shown in green, and the branch point sequence (BPS) is shown in purple. The scores calculated for wildtype sequence (WT) and mutated sequence (Mut) using Human Splice Finder, SpliceView, BDGP, and NetGene2 are displayed below each splice site. A higher score implies greater potential for a splice site. NA means no splice site predictions above threshold of the in silico tool

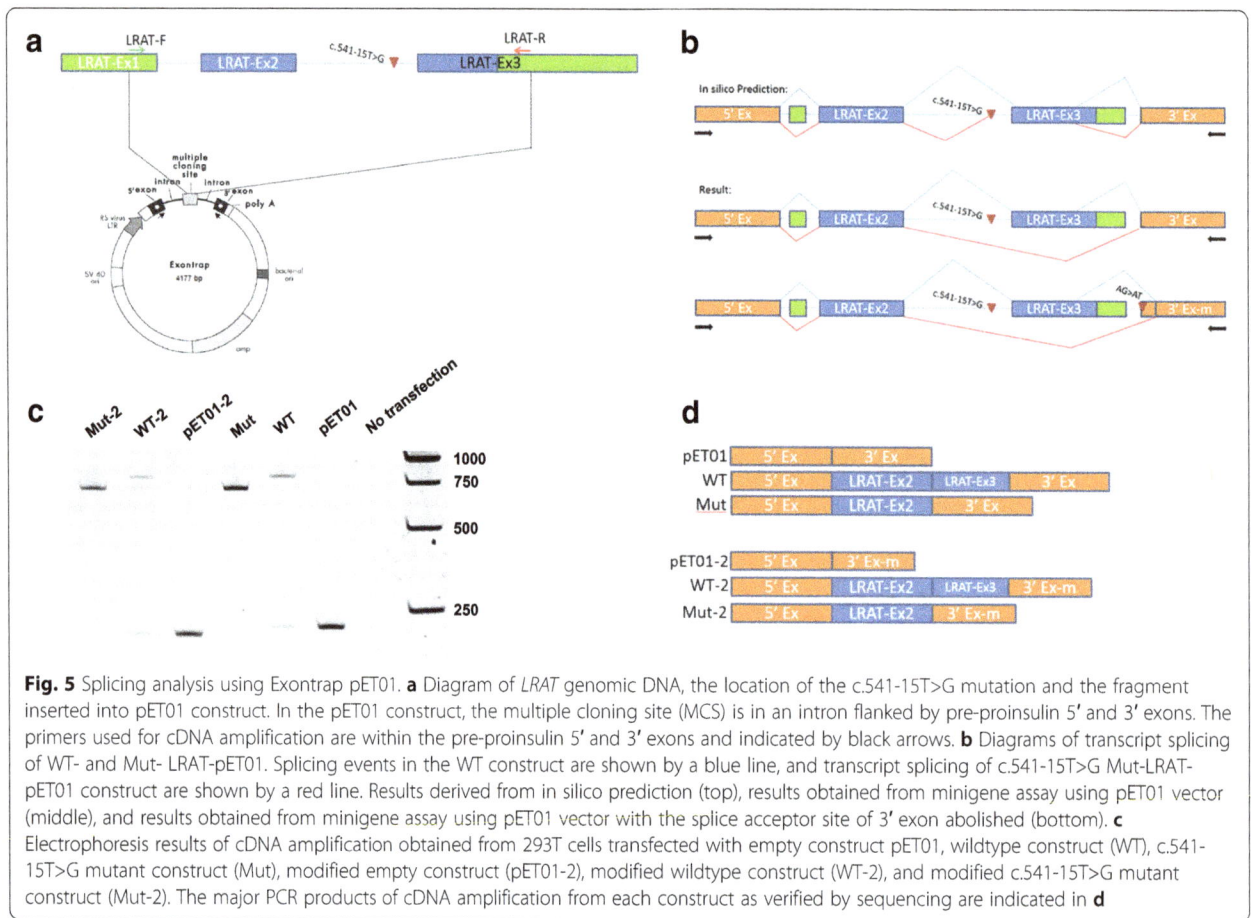

Fig. 5 Splicing analysis using Exontrap pET01. **a** Diagram of *LRAT* genomic DNA, the location of the c.541-15T>G mutation and the fragment inserted into pET01 construct. In the pET01 construct, the multiple cloning site (MCS) is in an intron flanked by pre-proinsulin 5′ and 3′ exons. The primers used for cDNA amplification are within the pre-proinsulin 5′ and 3′ exons and indicated by black arrows. **b** Diagrams of transcript splicing of WT- and Mut- LRAT-pET01. Splicing events in the WT construct are shown by a blue line, and transcript splicing of c.541-15T>G Mut-LRAT-pET01 construct are shown by a red line. Results derived from in silico prediction (top), results obtained from minigene assay using pET01 vector (middle), and results obtained from minigene assay using pET01 vector with the splice acceptor site of 3′ exon abolished (bottom). **c** Electrophoresis results of cDNA amplification obtained from 293T cells transfected with empty construct pET01, wildtype construct (WT), c.541-15T>G mutant construct (Mut), modified empty construct (pET01-2), modified wildtype construct (WT-2), and modified c.541-15T>G mutant construct (Mut-2). The major PCR products of cDNA amplification from each construct as verified by sequencing are indicated in **d**

weakening activity of the authentic splice acceptor site. Both bioinformatic tools and minigene assays showed that the novel c.541-15T>G mutation in the *LRAT* gene causes aberrant splicing and is therefore causal for early onset retinitis pigmentosa, further broadening the mutation spectrum in the *LRAT* gene.

Two in silico prediction tools, Human Splice Finder and SpliceView, predicted creation of a new splice acceptor site by the mutation, consistent with the AG/GT rule. Minigene assays using both vector pET01 and pCMV-(DYKD$_4$K)-C based constructs showed that the resulting mutant cDNA skipped exon 3 of *LRAT*. The wild-type transcript was absent in 293T cells transfected with the pET01 construct containing the mutant fragment of *LRAT*, and identified at reduced levels in 293T cells transfected with mutated pCMV-(DYKD$_4$K)-C construct compared with cells transfected with the wildtype pCMV construct. This suggests that the mutation does not completely inactivate the authentic splice site but rather suppresses it so that some WT *LRAT* RNA might be present, consistent with the concept of leaky splicing [16]. This RNA level might not be sufficient to maintain adequate *LRAT* function in the retina so that patients

homozygous for this mutation might manifest a RP phenotype. Although the minigene assays are not in perfect accordance with the in silico predictions about splicing patterns, all indicated that the mutation would result in aberrant splicing.

Minigene assays provide a rapid way to evaluate the impact of splice site mutations, especially when isolation and characterization of mRNA from the original source is technically difficult or ethically impossible. *LRAT* is expressed in RPE cells and is important for the retinoid cycle [5]. Since it is not expressed in peripheral blood cells and retinal biopsy is too invasive for patients, minigene assays provided an optimal approach to studying the in vitro effect of *LRAT* spice site mutations. However, the system also does not always reflect the exact splicing patterns of in vivo studies. While it allows prediction of whether a mutation is going to influence splicing, several studies have found occasional differences in splice patterns between minigene and RNA analyses in patient samples [17–19]. This might well relate to differences between the vector sequence surrounding the cloned insert and the genomic DNA in vivo. In an attempt to address this, we abolished the splice acceptor site of 3′

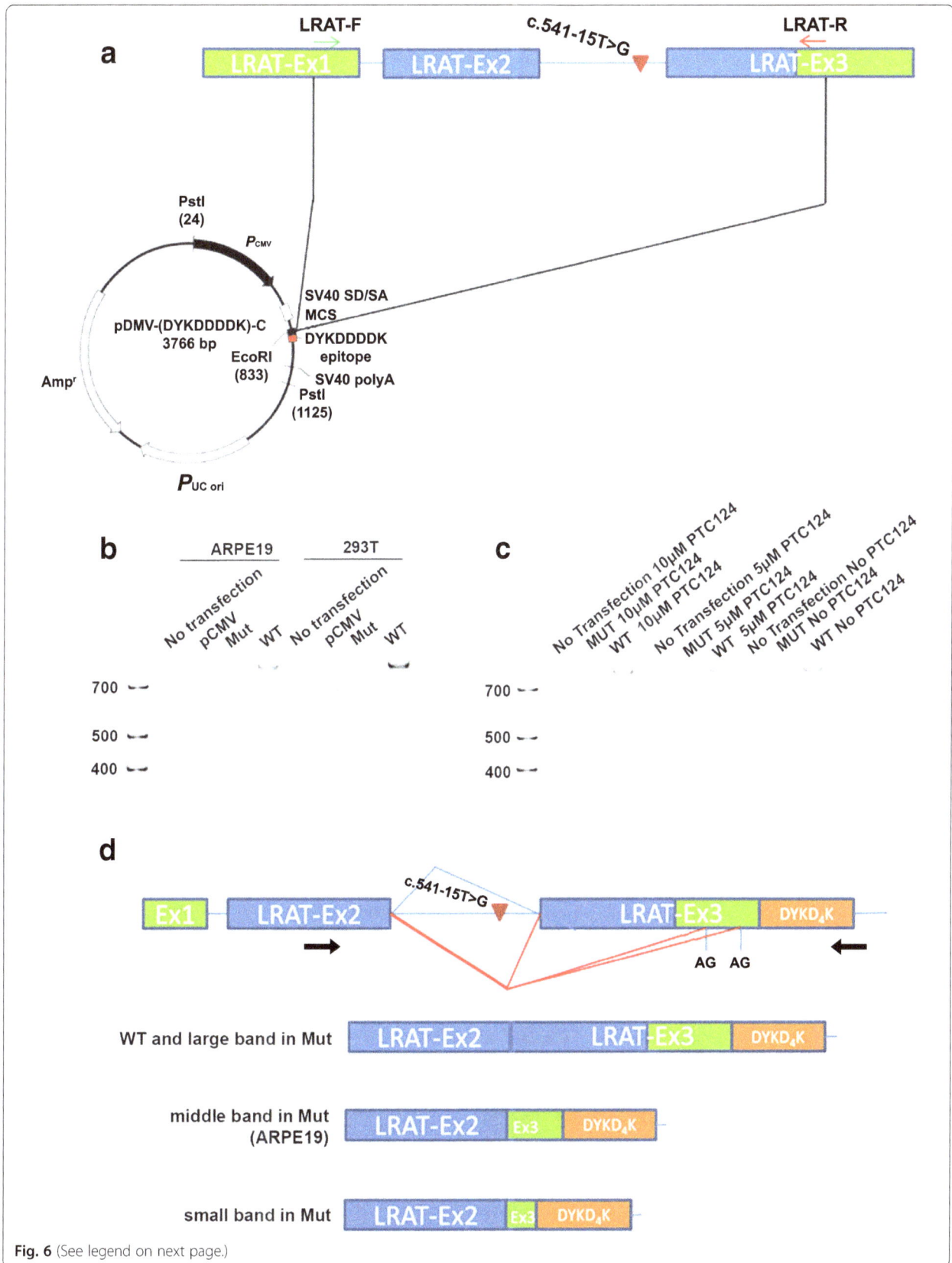

Fig. 6 (See legend on next page.)

(See figure on previous page.)
Fig. 6 a Diagram of the *LRAT* gene showing the location of the c.541T>G variation and the fragment inserted into the pCMV-(DYKD$_4$K)-C construct. **b** Electrophoresis results of cDNA amplification obtained from 293T cells and ARPE-19 cells transfected with the wildtype construct WT, mutated construct Mut, and empty construct pCMV. **c** Non-transfected and transfected ARPE19 cells were treated with 0, 5 μM, and 10 μM PTC124 separately for 24 h. There were no extra transcripts under PTC124 treatment. **d** Diagram of transcript in which splicing of WT-LRAT-pCMV is shown by a blue line; transcript splicing of Mut-LRAT-pCMV is shown by a red line. The forward primer used in cDNA amplification is within the exon 2 of *LRAT* and the reverse primer binds to the construct sequence of DYKD$_4$K epitope, which are indicated by arrows (the AG shown in the 3′ UTR of LRAT refers to the last two AG in Fig. 4). A diagram of the PCR product of cDNA amplification from each construct is also shown in **d**

exon on pET01 and also used the pCMV-(DYKD$_4$K)-C vector to investigate further the splicing effect of the mutation, aiming to weaken the influence of vector sequence on the cloned insert. The results confirmed that the mutation could cause splicing impairment compared with the wildtype sequence.

In conclusion, bioinformatics tools may be useful for predicting the pathogenicity of variants, but minigene assays are more reliable in the evaluation of the potential effects of splice-site mutations. Adapted minigenes may need to be designed for variants in the first and last exon and introns to mimic the authentic splicing mechanism in vivo. Despite the limitations of both in silico predictions and minigene assays, it is likely that this mutation c.541-15T>G is pathogenic, when all the information including linkage and co-segregation in the pedigree excluding other candidates, the known role of LRAT in retinal degeneration, in silico analyses predicting splicing impairment, and two minigene assays are consistent with weakening of the authentic splice acceptor site resulting in a truncated LRAT protein and arRP.

Acknowledgements
The authors are thankful to all the family members for their participation in this study.

Funding
This work was supported by NEI project EYE000272.

Authors' contributions
YC carried out the experiments, assisted with the analysis, and helped write the manuscript. LH carried out the experiments, assisted with the analysis, and helped write the manuscript. XDJ carried out the experiments, assisted with the analysis, and helped write the manuscript. SR helped plan the project. SAR helped plan the project, conceive of the experiments, analyze the data, and write the manuscript. JFH helped plan the project, conceive of the experiments, analyze the data, and write the manuscript. All authors read and approved the final manuscript.

Competing interests
The authors declare that they have no competing interests.

Author details
[1]Ophthalmic Genetics and Visual Function Branch, National Eye Institute, National Institutes of Health, Bethesda, MD 20892, USA. [2]State Key Laboratory of Ophthalmology, Zhongshan Ophthalmic Center, Sun Yat-Sen University, Guangzhou, Guangdong, China. [3]National Centre of Excellence in Molecular Biology, University of the Punjab, Lahore, Pakistan. [4]Allama Iqbal Medical College, University of Health Sciences, Lahore, Pakistan. [5]National Centre for Genetic Diseases, Shaheed Zulfiqar Ali Bhutto Medical University, Islamabad, Pakistan. [6]The Wilmer Eye Institute, Johns Hopkins University School of Medicine, Baltimore, MD, USA.

References
1. Hartong DT, Berson EL, Dryja TP. Retinitis pigmentosa. Lancet. 2006;368: 1795–809.
2. Bird AC. Retinal photoreceptor dystrophies LI. Edward Jackson memorial lecture. AmJOphthalmol. 1995;119:543–62.
3. Bunker CH, Berson EL, Bromley WC, Hayes RP, Roderick TH. Prevalence of retinitis pigmentosa in Maine. AmJOphthalmol. 1984;97:357–65.
4. Rivolta C, Sharon D, DeAngelis MM, Dryja TP. Retinitis pigmentosa and allied diseases: numerous diseases, genes, and inheritance patterns. HumMolGenet. 2002;11:1219–27.
5. Sears AE, Palczewski K. Lecithin:retinol acyltransferase: a key enzyme involved in the retinoid (visual) cycle. Biochemistry. 2016;55:3082–91.
6. Koenekoop RK. An overview of Leber congenital amaurosis: a model to understand human retinal development. SurvOphthalmol. 2004;49:379–98.
7. Lopez-Bigas N, Audit B, Ouzounis C, Parra G, Guigo R. Are splicing mutations the most frequent cause of hereditary disease? FEBS Lett. 2005;579:1900–3.
8. Krawczak M, Thomas NS, Hundrieser B, Mort M, Wittig M, Hampe J, Cooper DN. Single base-pair substitutions in exon-intron junctions of human genes: nature, distribution, and consequences for mRNA splicing. Hum Mutat. 2007;28:150–8.
9. Krawczak M, Reiss J, Cooper DN. The mutational spectrum of single base-pair substitutions in mRNA splice junctions of human genes: causes and consequences. Hum Genet. 1992;90:41–54.
10. Ward AJ, Cooper TA. The pathobiology of splicing. J Pathol. 2010;220:152–63.
11. Smith RJH, Holcomb JD, Daiger SP, Caskey CT, Pelias MZ, Alford BR, Fontenot DD, Hejtmancik JF. Exclusion of Usher syndrome gene from much of chromosome 4. CytogenetCell Genet. 1989;50:102–6.
12. Lathrop GM, Lalouel JM. Easy calculations of lod scores and genetic risks on small computers. AmJ Hum Genet. 1984;36:460–5.
13. Schaffer AA, Gupta SK, Shriram K, Cottingham RW. Avoiding recomputation in genetic linkage analysis. Hum Hered. 1994;44:225–37.
14. Moore MJ. Intron recognition comes of AGe. Nat Struct Biol. 2000;7:14–6.
15. Peled-Zehavi H, Berglund JA, Rosbash M, Frankel AD. Recognition of RNA branch point sequences by the KH domain of splicing factor 1 (mammalian branch point binding protein) in a splicing factor complex. Mol Cell Biol. 2001;21:5232–41.
16. Caminsky N, Mucaki EJ, Rogan PK. Interpretation of mRNA splicing mutations in genetic disease: review of the literature and guidelines for information-theoretical analysis. F1000Res. 2014;3:282.
17. Schneider B, Koppius A, Sedlmeier R. Use of an exon-trapping vector for the evaluation of splice-site mutations. Mamm Genome. 2007;18:670–6.
18. Bonnet C, Krieger S, Vezain M, Rousselin A, Tournier I, Martins A, Berthet P, Chevrier A, Dugast C, Layet V, et al. Screening BRCA1 and BRCA2 unclassified variants for splicing mutations using reverse transcription PCR on patient RNA and an ex vivo assay based on a splicing reporter minigene. J Med Genet. 2008;45:438–46.
19. Acedo A, Sanz DJ, Duran M, Infante M, Perez-Cabornero L, Miner C, Velasco EA. Comprehensive splicing functional analysis of DNA variants of the BRCA2 gene by hybrid minigenes. Breast Cancer Res. 2012;14:R87.

21

Whole-exome sequencing identifies novel pathogenic mutations and putative phenotype-influencing variants in Polish limb-girdle muscular dystrophy patients

Jakub Piotr Fichna[1*] (iD), Anna Macias[2], Marcin Piechota[3], Michał Korostyński[3], Anna Potulska-Chromik[2], Maria Jolanta Redowicz[4] and Cezary Zekanowski[1]

Abstract

Background: Limb girdle muscular dystrophies (LGMD) are a group of heterogeneous hereditary myopathies with similar clinical symptoms. Disease onset and progression are highly variable, with an elusive genetic background, and around 50% cases lacking molecular diagnosis.

Methods: Whole exome sequencing (WES) was performed in 73 patients with clinically diagnosed LGMD. A filtering strategy aimed at identification of variants related to the disease included integrative analysis of WES data and human phenotype ontology (HPO) terms, analysis of genes expressed in muscle, analysis of the disease-associated interactome and copy number variants analysis.

Results: Genetic diagnosis was possible in 68.5% of cases. On average, 36.3 rare variants in genes associated with various muscle diseases per patient were found that could relate to the clinical phenotype. The putative causative mutations were mostly in LGMD-associated genes, but also in genes not included in the current LGMD classification (*DMD*, *COL6A2*, and *COL6A3*). In three patients, mutations in two genes were suggested as the joint cause of the disease (*CAPN3+MYH7*, *COL6A3+CACNA1S*, *DYSF+MYH7*). Moreover, a variety of phenotype-influencing variants were postulated, including in patients with an identified already known primary pathogenic mutation.

Conclusions: We hypothesize that LGMD could be better described as oligogenic disorders in which dominant clinical presentation can result from the combined effect of mutations in a set of genes. In this view, the inter- and intrafamilial variability could reflect a specific genetic background and the presence of sets of phenotype-influencing or co-causative mutations in genes that either interact with the known LGMD-associated genes or are a part of the same pathways or structures.

Keywords: Limb-girdle muscular dystrophy, LGMD, Skeletal muscle, Exome, Next generation sequencing, NGS, WES

Background

Limb girdle muscular dystrophies (LGMD) are a heterogeneous group of genetic disorders with similar clinical features, and a diverse and partially unknown genetic background. LGMD are characterized clinically by progressive muscle weakness and atrophy, predominantly or primarily of the pelvic and shoulder girdle muscles, without facial muscle dysfunction. The clinical course of the disease may be variable, ranging from severe forms with early onset and rapid progression to milder forms with later onset and minor physical disability. In the majority of cases, serum creatine kinase (CK) is elevated and a dystrophic pattern with necrosis and regeneration is observed on muscle biopsy [1, 2]. Most patients show a definable phenotype, but there are numerous exceptions as well as intrafamilial variability. LGMD are very rare disorders, fulfilling the criteria for orphan diseases with an estimated prevalence of 1/44000–1/123000 [3, 4].

* Correspondence: jfichna@imdik.pan.pl
[1]Department of Neurodegenerative Disorders, Mossakowski Medical Research Centre, Polish Academy of Sciences, 5 Pawinskiego St., 02-106 Warsaw, Poland
Full list of author information is available at the end of the article

Numerous studies performed world-wide in the last two decades have led to the identification of mutations in 30 genes (and one associated *locus*) causally involved in LGMD pathophysiology [5]. Current LGMD classification is based on the mode of inheritance and the particular gene involved. The two general categories, autosomal dominant LGMD1 and autosomal recessive LGMD2, are divided into subgroups with different alphabetic designators, each caused by mutations in a specific gene.

To date, eight LGMD1 and 23 LGMD2 subtypes have been recognized [6–8]. This list is still expanding, with seven subtypes added in the last 3 years. The diagnosis of muscular dystrophies (including within the LGMD group) is difficult due to the presence of a number of different conditions with similar clinical phenotypes, including limb-girdle muscle weakness, e.g., myofibrillar myopathies, Bethlem myopathy, Becker muscular dystrophy, facioscapulohumeral muscular dystrophy, and Emery-Dreifuss muscular dystrophy. In fact, some of the latter have been considered a form of LGMD [1, 6].

According to the latest guidelines, the precise diagnosis of LGMD should rely on a detailed clinical examination, muscle biopsy, and genetic analysis to detect the causative mutations [9]. However, muscle biopsy findings are often not sufficiently specific; therefore, genetic testing is considered the most reliable tool in LGMD diagnosis.

The molecular pathophysiology of LGMD is heterogeneous, with mechanisms ranging from defects in the dystrophin-dystroglycan complex, through abnormal localization of components of the muscle cytoskeleton and enzymatic defects, to sarcomeric and nuclear lamina dysfunctions. Different mutations in the same gene can cause widely different phenotypes (e.g., individual *FKRP* mutations cause a form of muscle-eye brain disease, a congenital severe muscular dystrophy, and a classical, adult LGMD form [10, 11]). The functional diversity of the protein products of the disease-causing genes makes the diagnosis very difficult and complex, requiring deep phenotyping.

It should be emphasized that despite intensive research, especially on the identification of novel causative genes, up to 50% of clinically defined LGMD cases are still without genetic diagnosis. Furthermore, the treatment of LGMD remains supportive and palliative, although it is expected that early diagnosis of the disease subtypes, based mainly on genetic testing, will allow the development of therapeutic strategies preventing or delaying the pathological process in the foreseeable future [12, 13]. Proactive multidisciplinary care and genetic counseling of LGMD patients is recommended, preferably immediately after diagnosis.

Since not all genetic risk factors of LGMD have been identified, further studies into the genetic background of the disease are necessary. Whole exome sequencing (WES) and, even more so, whole genome sequencing (WGS) provide a non-biased approach towards discovery of potentially causative mutations [14]. Subsequent comprehensive bioinformatic analyses of the resulting list of genomic variants could not only pinpoint novel genes that could be associated with the disease, but also reveal mutations in genes related to other disorders explaining some of the as-yet molecularly undiagnosed cases. Additionally, apart from the causative mutations, variants that could be called phenotype-influencing, or even co-causative, could add up to the clinical phenotype.

Here, we report genetic variants identified using WES and comprehensive bioinformatic analyses in a fairly large group of Polish patients with clinically diagnosed LGMD. We found putative pathogenic mutations in known myopathy-related genes in 68.5% of cases. In all the cases, we propose numerous possibly phenotype-influencing or even co-causative mutations, including in genes not previously related to LGMD.

Methods

Patients

The study involved 72 cases (73 patients including a pair of siblings) with clinically diagnosed limb-girdle muscular dystrophy from a single neuromuscular diagnosis and treatment medical center. LGMD was defined as a progressive muscle weakness and atrophy of the pelvic and shoulder girdle muscles, as well as proximal limb muscles, without an involvement of facial muscles. The diagnosis was made on the basis of clinical assessment and muscle biopsy. Childhood cases with early-onset asymptomatic persistent hyperCKemia were included when the muscle biopsy showed evident features of muscular dystrophy. Miyoshi myopathy phenotypes (muscular dystrophy with predominant calf atrophy and high CK level) were also included because of their considerable genetic and phenotypic overlap with LGMD2B and 2L. Other types of muscular dystrophies (Duchenne muscular dystrophy, Becker muscular dystrophy, facioscapulohumeral muscular dystrophy, Emery-Dreifuss muscular dystrophy, and myotonic dystrophy type 1 and 2) and other myopathies (congenital, metabolic, mitochondrial, myofibrillar, and inflammatory) were excluded on the base of their clinical, electrophysiological, and morphological characteristics. To avoid Becker muscular dystrophy cases, we included male patients who had either similarly affected female siblings or previous negative MLPA (multiplex ligation-dependent probe amplification) results (which excluded large deletions or duplications in the dystrophin gene) together with normal muscle immunofluorescence staining for dystrophin.

The mean age of the patients was 26 years (range 3–78). The basic clinical data are shown in a supplementary file (see Additional file 1). Thirty-nine probands had one or more affected siblings. Two patients (no. 243 and 407) had a positive family history suggesting autosomal dominant inheritance; however, no parent was available for clinical assessment. In four patients, there was a background of second-degree parental consanguinity.

We also performed WES for 12 patients with non-classic muscular disease phenotypes where an LGMD diagnosis could not be definitively excluded (see Additional file 1). Data from these cases, and from an additional 16 patients from seven families with non-muscular neurological diseases, were used for comparison during the bioinformatic assessment of WES results.

Genetic analyses

DNA was extracted from peripheral blood using standard methods [15]. Whole exome sequencing (WES) was performed commercially at BGI Tech Solutions (Hong Kong) using a SureSelect Human All Exon v5+UTR enrichment kit and paired-end 100-nt sequencing on the Illumina HiSeq2000 platform. Fast read files were generated from the sequencing platform via the Illumina pipeline. Adapter sequences in the raw data were removed and low-quality reads with low base quality discarded. On average, 240,451,900 "clean" paired-end reads per sample were aligned to the human reference genome hg19 using the Burrows-Wheeler Alignment (BWA) package [16]. Duplicate reads were removed with Picard and base quality Phred scores were recalibrated using GATK's covariance recalibration [17]. The obtained 15 Giga-bases of aligned sequence data resulted in 125x median coverage of the target capture regions with 97.4% of target bases covered at least 10×. Capture performance statistics were calculated using CollectHsMetrics in Picard 2.17.10. The alignments were viewed with an Integrative Genomics Viewer [18]. SNVs (single-nucleotide variants) and indels (small insertion/deletion) variants were called using the GATK Unified Genotyper. Annovar was used for initial variant annotation [19] with further annotation, filtering, and analysis performed on Galaxy (on PL-Grid Infrastructure) and GeneTraps (Intelliseq) platforms.

Copy number variant analysis

Copy number variants (CNVs) were called using CODEX software (version 1.8) [20]. The analysis was performed within technical batches of samples. CNVs were annotated with allele frequencies using best-matching CNVs from 1000 genomes, and all the CNVs matching common CNVs (MAF > 1%) were removed. Genes overlapping each CNV in patients were identified using Ensembl version 86. The genes assigned to CNVs were annotated using diseases and phenotypes from Human Phenotype Ontology (HPO) [21] and tissue expression scores obtained from the GeneAtlas.

Bioinformatic analyses

Whole exome sequencing identified on average 125,000 SNVs and 23,000 indels in each sample, of which 76,000 and 15,000, respectively, were off target (defined as intergenic or intronic, but not affecting splice sites) and therefore removed from further consideration. Only variants with an impact on coding regions were retained: missense, nonsense, frameshift, and essential splice site mutations. Further filtering was based on Phred quality scores, allele frequency in the ExAC (Exome Aggregation Consortium) database (< 3% for variants in genes already associated with LGMD, and < 1% for variants in other genes), association with HPO terms and predicted pathogenicity [22]. The HPO terms used were: "muscular_dystrophy," "muscle_weakness," "limb-girdle," "myopathy," "muscular_atrophy," "muscle_atrophy," and "creatine phosphokinase." Variants predicted to be pathogenic by at least one of the following programs were taken into further consideration: Mutation Taster, PolyPhen2, and SIFT. In total, among all the samples, 1880 variants were analyzed further (see Additional file 2). Prioritization was based on the following: the predicted effect, with truncating and elongating variants being evaluated more carefully; the predicted pathogenicity; and, finally, known association with myopathic phenotypes. All these variants were individually assessed by a board of geneticists and clinicians according to the guidelines of the American College of Medical Genetics and Genomics [23], with emphasis on the actual phenotype of each patient. Variants were then categorized as putative pathogenic (fit the phenotype effect very well) or potentially phenotype-influencing (could be responsible for naturally occurring variability of symptoms in frame of a typical LGMD clinical phenotype), with other variants assessed as unlikely to be related to the disease.

Independently, additional analyses were carried out with Exomiser2, PhenIX and Exome walker, with prioritization of variants based on possible association with limb-girdle muscular dystrophy (HP:0006785), and (based) on random-walk analysis of protein interaction networks with proteins already associated with the LGMD phenotype [24].

Additionally, in a second approach, rare (< 1% in ExAC database) variants in genes expressed in the human muscle, and in genes whose mouse homologs are expressed in muscle, were analyzed. Further analysis included ultra-rare variants (< 0.1% in ExAC), highly damaging mutations (including nonsense, frameshift, splice site mutations), interactome and association with pathways and structures that could play a role in LGMD pathogenesis. Known LGMD-associated genes were used to query the Biological General Repository for Interaction Datasets (BioGRID, version 3.4.151, accessed 3 August 2017) and Kyoto Encyclopedia of Genes and

Genomes (KEGG, release 83.1, accessed 3 August 2017), which yielded potential interactors and muscle related pathways. Variants in genes that either interact with known LGMD-associated genes or are in the same pathway (as suggested by BioGRID and KEGG databases) were selected (see Additional file 3). Again, at the end of this discrimination pipeline (Fig. 1.), extracted variants were also correlated with patient phenotype and results of clinical examinations.

Selected variants (including all the putative causative mutations) were confirmed using direct fluorescence-based sequencing (ABI 3130 Genetic Analyzer, Applied Biosystems, USA). Segregation analysis including confirmation of trans configuration of compound heterozygotes could not always be performed because of the limited availability of DNA samples of the relatives.

Results

Using whole exome sequencing, we found putative pathogenic mutations (*pathogenic* or *likely pathogenic* according to ACMG criteria) in known myopathy genes in 50 of the 72 LGMD cases (68.5%). In 43 cases, the identified variants were known to be pathogenic (found in OMIM, ClinVar, HGMD, or LOVD databases, or already described). These were associated mainly with the LGMD phenotype, but also with collagen-related myopathy and MYH-7 related myopathy. Putative causative mutations were found not only in LGMD-related genes (45 cases, 62.5%) but also in other myopathy-related genes (5 cases, 8%), highlighting the clinical overlap between muscular disorders. The latter cases had mutations in collagen myopathy-related genes (4 cases) and Becker's muscular dystrophy (1 case). Selected

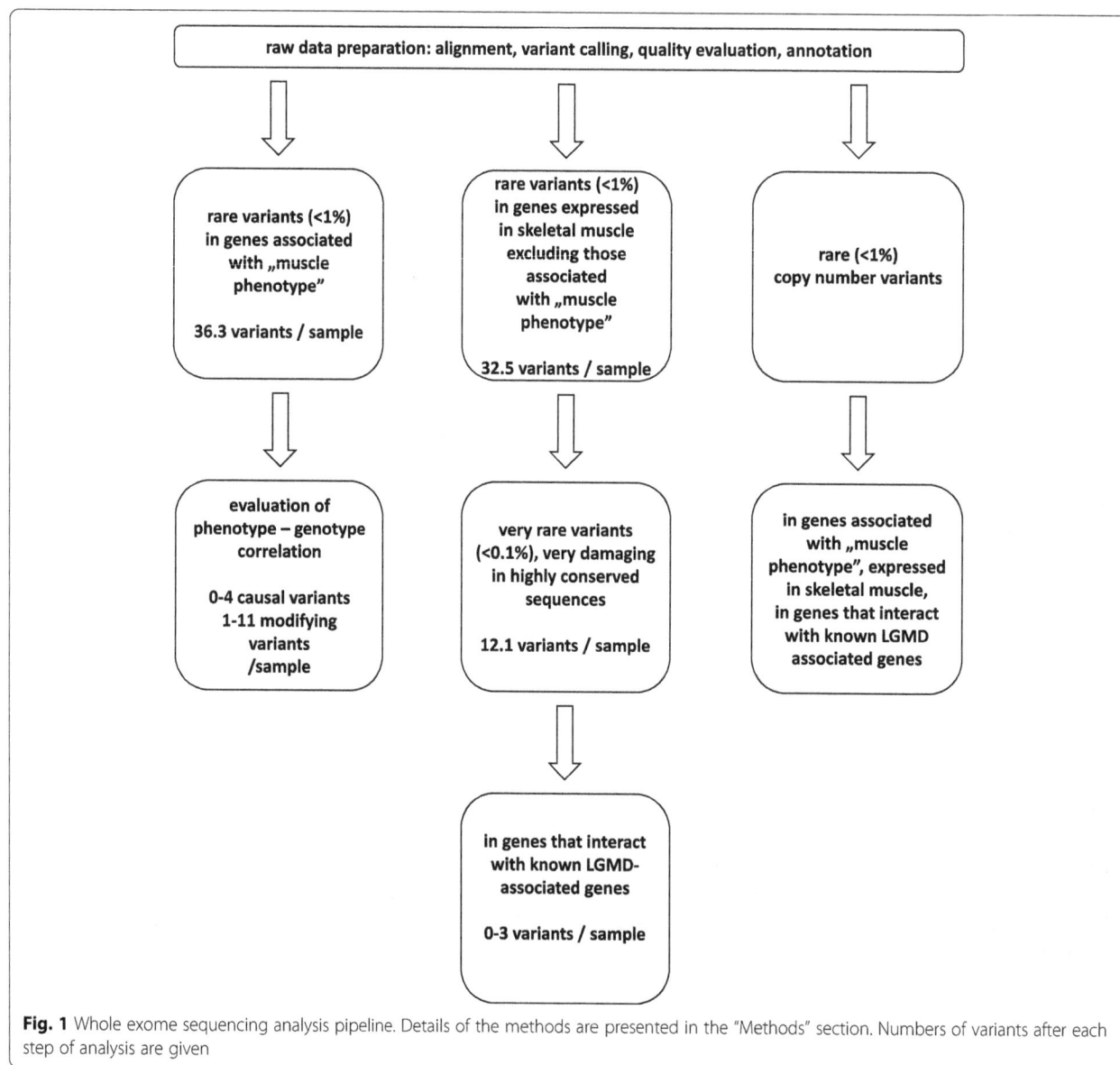

Fig. 1 Whole exome sequencing analysis pipeline. Details of the methods are presented in the "Methods" section. Numbers of variants after each step of analysis are given

variants most probably influencing the phenotype are presented in Table 1. A full version of the table including basic clinical data and evidence of pathogenicity is provided in a supplementary table (see Additional file 1).

The dominant forms of LGMD were relatively uncommon, with only one case each of LGMD1B (patient19) and LGMD1E (patient 275B). In two cases, mutations in *MYOT* (patient 175d) and *CAV3* (patient 196) could also be considered responsible for the disease, but mutations in other genes (*CAPN3* and *COL6A2*, respectively) were assessed as better explaining the patients' phenotypes. It is noteworthy that all four mutations, G523R in *LMNA*, G77E in *DNAJB6*, R126H in *CAV3*, and R370C in *MYOT*, are ultra-rare, with a prevalence of < 0.02% in the European population according to the ExAC database.

In 22 cases, we found homozygous or compound heterozygous mutations in *CAPN3*. Additionally, in 13 cases, we found only a single heterozygous putative pathogenic mutation in *CAPN3*, and 11 of these cases were in the group of patients without an identified causative mutation. These cases were familial and clearly autosomal recessive.

Mutations in *DYSF* (homozygous or compound heterozygous) were found to be responsible for the disease in six patients from five families. Interestingly, we found the same compound heterozygous mutations in the *DYSF* gene in siblings with discordant phenotypes (LGMD in the sister, Miyoshi myopathy in the brother). In seven cases, we found mutations in *FKRP*; sarcoglycanopathies were represented by four families: two cases with mutations in *SGCA* and two in *SGCB*. Another two cases had *ANO5* mutations.

In five cases, we found putative causative mutations in genes typically associated with other forms of myopathy. Four families had mutations in *COL6A2* and *COL6A3*, typically associated with Bethlem myopathy, but recently also found in LGMD-like cases. In one male proband, a single known pathogenic deletion of three nucleotides was found in the *DMD* gene.

In all the cases, additional variants that could relate to case-specific muscle weakness phenotypes were found. Possible causes of phenotypic overlap, and of inter- and intrafamilial (patients 24 and 3) differences, were mutations in other LGMD-associated genes, and mutations in genes associated with myofibrillar myopathy, congenital muscular dystrophy, collagen myopathy, Duchenne / Becker muscular dystrophy, Emery-Dreifuss muscular dystrophy, or cardiomyopathy. A number of other variants in muscle pathogenesis-related genes were found, with uncertain significance. Filtering of the variants annotated with myopathy phenotype-related HPO terms returned between 21 and 59 variants per sample, with an average of 36.3 per sample.

Analysis of genes expressed in muscle (based on the Geneatlas database) gave 2036 variants (total for all analyzed patients), of which 1271 were ultra-rare (< 0.1%) and 214 had a putative high impact on the protein (nonsense, frameshift, splice site mutations). Interactome-based analysis of these variants reduced their number to 83 in 20 genes associated with known LGMD-related genes (Table 2). A supplementary table lists variants found in genes whose products interact with myopathy-related proteins (see Additional file 3).

Rare copy number variants in LGMD-related genes were found in 18 cases. A supplementary file shows detected CNVs in detail, not only in LGMD-related genes but also in the interactome of those genes, in other myopathy-related genes, and in genes expressed in muscles (see Additional file 4). It must be stressed that CNV predictions from WES data are not completely reliable [25, 26] and are presented in the supplementary material for indicative purposes only.

Discussion

We performed the first comprehensive genetic analysis of patients with clinically defined LGMD in the Polish population.

On average, 36.3 rare variants per sample possibly related to the myopathic phenotype were identified. These variants were located in genes previously implicated in diverse muscle diseases (not just LGMD). These genes can be grouped according to the functional or structural association of their products: (i) dystrophin glycoprotein complex (*SGCA*, *SGCB*, *SGCD*, *SGCG*, *DAG1*), (ii) sarcomere structure (*TCAP*, *TTN*, *PLEC*, *DES*, *MYOT*) or assembly (*CAPN3*, *DNAJB6*), (iii) glycosylation (*FKRP*, *POMT1*, *POMT2*, *POMGNT1*, *ISPD*), (iv) signal transduction (*CAV3*, *DAG1*, *BVES*), (v) trafficking (*TRAPPC11*, *CAV3*, *DYSF*, *BVES*), and (vi) splicing (*TNPO3*, *HNRPDL*). After confirming the consistency of these results with the clinical and pathological characteristics of the patients, highly probable pathogenic genotypes could be identified in 50 out of 72 cases (68.5%). The above results gave a similar diagnostic rate to other recent NGS (next-generation sequencing) studies in genetically undiagnosed cohorts of LGMD: 47% in the Czech Republic, 62% in China, and 76% in Saudi Arabia [27–29]. Lower yields have been reported in studies involving patients pre-screened by targeted gene sequencing: 33% in Germany, 40% in the USA, and 45% in Australia [30–32]. The distribution of LGMD subtypes was similar to those observed in Germany [30] and Italy [33], with *CAPN3* being the most frequent main putative pathogenic cause, and frequent cases with *FKRP* and *DYSF* mutations.

It should be noted that putative causative mutations in genes not included in the LGMD classification, *COL6A2*, *COL6A3*, and *DMD*, have also been reported by other authors in their LGMD cohorts [27–31], indicating

Table 1 Putative causative mutations and genes with potentially phenotype-influencing variants identified by WES in 73 LGMD patients

Patient no.	Putative causative gene(s)	Genotype	Genes with mutations putatively influencing clinical phenotype
20	*ANO5*	p.D81G/p.R758C	*NEB, DES, TTN*
10	*ANO5*	p.D81G/p.W401X*	*BAG3, FLNC, CHRNE, CACNA1S, TTN x2*
173a	*CAPN3*	c.1193+1G>A (splice site)/c.598-612delGTTCTGGAGTGCTCT	*NEB x2, DNM2, TTN x2, CACNA1S*
424	*CAPN3*	c.598-612delGTTCTGGAGTGCTCT/p.G221S*	*COL12A1, PLEC, DNM2TTN*
186a	*CAPN3*	c.550delA/p.A609E	*LDB3/ZASP x2, COL6A2, COL6A3, SGCD, POMT1, DYSF, SYNE2, MYH6, B3GALNT2*
175d	*CAPN3*	c.550delA/c.598-612delGTTCTGGAGTGCTCT	*MYOT, SGCB, RYR1, NEB, SYNE2, TTN*
12	*CAPN3*	c.550delA/c.550delA	*COL6A3, FLNC, NEB,TTN x2*
144	*CAPN3*	c.550delA/c.550delA	*DNM2, TMEM5, TTN x2*
212	*CAPN3*	c.550delA/c.550delA	*DYSF, TTN x6*
127	*CAPN3*	c.550delA/c.550delA	*RYR1, FLNC, SYNE2, TTN x4*
184a	*CAPN3*	c.550delA/c.550delA	*HSPG2, TTN*
6	*CAPN3*	c.550delA/c.550delA	*TRAPPC11, RYR1, LAMA2, FLNC, NEB, PPARGC, TTN, MYF6*
764	*CAPN3*	c.550delA/c.1722delC	*LDB3/ZASP x2, POMT1, TMEM43*
18	*CAPN3* *MYH7*	c.550delA/p.E566K p.R204H	*LDB3/ZASP x2, GBE1, TTN x4,*
TO	*CAPN3*	c.550delA/p.G221S*	*TRAPPC11, LIPE, GBE1, HSPG2, TTN x3*
8	*CAPN3*	c.550delA/p.P82L	*NEB x2, COL6A3, SYNE1 x2, TTN x5, LDB3/ZASP, HSPG2*
13	*CAPN3*	c.550delA/p.R147X	*COL12A1, NEB*
4	*CAPN3*	c.550delA/p.R355W	*FLNC, SYNE1, DCTN1, TTN x3*
433	*CAPN3*	c.550delA/p.R448C	*COL6A3, TARDBP, TTN x2*
668	*CAPN3*	c.550delA/p.T560A	*PLEC x 3, SYNE1 x2, CCDC78, COL9A3, HSPG2*
193a	*CAPN3*	c.550delA/p.W130R*	*COL6A3, NEB, HSPG2, TTN x2, GNE*
113	*CAPN3*	p.R748X/c.1722delC	*COL6A3, RYR1, HSPG2, SYNE1 x2, DCTN1, TTN x2*
144a	*CAPN3*	p.R748X/c.598-612delGTTCTGGAGTGCTCT	*COL6A1, COL6A3, HNRNPDL, RYR1 x2, SYNE1, MYH7, TTN x5*
225	*CAPN3*	p.P102L/p.S606L	*MYH3, SYNE1, SYNE2, TTN*
196	*COL6A2*	p.G277E*	*CAV3, LAMA2, ANO5 – ITGA7, RYR1, SYNE2, TTN x3*
901	*COL6A3* *CACNA1S*	p.E1386K/p.R2420W p.T349I*	*NEB, TTN*
7	*COL6A3*	p.R2142X*/p.K2483E	*FLNC*
275	*COL6A3*	p.T1368M/p.V2398I	*DAG1, NEB, SYNE1, TTN*
135	*DMD*	c.678-681delCTT*	*RYR1, ITGA7, DYSF, CCDC78, COL9A3*
275B	*DNAJB6*	p.G77E	*COL6A2, DAG1, DYSF, ISPD, NEB, RYR1, SYNE1, CHRNE, TTN x3*
192	*DYSF*	c.4821delG*/c.5058-1G>T* (splice site)	*LDB3/ZASP, ANO5, PLEC, SYNE1, TTN*
16	*DYSF*	p.D1876N/p.D1876N / c.5179delA*/c.5179delA*	*FLNC, DMD, MYH6, COL9A3, NIPA1, HSPG2, TTN x2*
219	*DYSF*	p.D1876N/p.E1763D/c.5179del*A	*PLEC x2, LDB3/ZASP x2, COL6A2, FKRP, COL12A1, TTN x3*
24 (family A)	*DYSF*	p.Q1323E/c.5237delG*	*COL6A3, MYH3, LDB3/ZASP*
3 (family A)	*DYSF*	p.Q1323E/c.5237delG*	*PLEC, COL6A3*
407	*DYSF* *MYH7*	p.V374L/c.5946G>A (splice site) p.A1487T	*ANO5, NEB*
15	*FKRP*	p.L276I/c.253+2T>C (splice site)	*PLEC x2, LARGE, KBTBD13, DCTN1, MYPN, TTN x2*
198	*FKRP*	p.L276I/c.650-667del CGCCCGCTATGTGGTGGG*	*COL6A3, COL4A1, NEB x2, TTN*
KW	*FKRP*	p.L276I/p.L276I	*ISPD, DYSF, ITGA7, SYNE1, TTN x2*
5	*FKRP*	p.L276I/p.L276I	*PLEC x2, COL6A3 x2, DYSF, POMGNT2, FLNC, TTN x3*

Table 1 Putative causative mutations and genes with potentially phenotype-influencing variants identified by WES in 73 LGMD patients (Continued)

Patient no.	Putative causative gene(s)	Genotype	Genes with mutations putatively influencing clinical phenotype
102	*FKRP*	p.L276I/p.L276I	*COL12A1, MYH2, SYNE2, TTN*
84e	*FKRP*	p.L276I/p.P217Q*	*TCAP, COL6A2, TTN x2*
CM	*FKRP*	p.L93P/p.R270C	*CAPN3, DMD, NEB, SYNE1 x2, CCDC78, TTN x4*
19	*LMNA*	p.G523R	*CAPN3, COL6A3, PLEC x3, RYR1, HSPG2, SYNE1, MYH3, LMOD3, RBM20, TNNI3K*
21	*SGCA*	p.V247M/p.V250L* (splice site)	*COL6A1, COL6A2, MYH2, LDB3/ZASP, POMT1*
84a	*SGCA*	p.V250L* (splice site) / p.R284C	*LDB3/ZASP x2, RYR1, COL6A2, COL6A3, SYNE1*
157	*SGCB*	p.S114F/p.I119N*	*PLEC x2, TRAPPC11, HSPG2 x2, TTN*
201	*SGCB*	p.S114F/p.S114F	*PLEC x2, TRAPPC11, B3GALNT2, HSPG2, SYNE1*
270a	*TCAP*	c.358-359delGA*/c.358-359delGA*	*NEB X3, SYNE1, BVES, TTN x2*
229a	*TRAPPC11*	p.D26G*/p.D26G*	*NEB, ITGA7, POMGNT1*
448a			*CAPN3, TTN (likely pathogenic fs),*
179			*CAPN3, COL6A2, DNM2, -BVES, TTN x4*
214			*CAPN3, COL6A3, POMT2, COL12A1, TTN x2*
191			*CAPN3, FKRP, TTN x3*
658			*CAPN3,, MYPN, TARDBP, TTN x2*
752			*CAPN3, POMT2, FLNC x5, NEB, HSPG2, SYNE2, TTN*
170			*CAPN3, SGCA, RYR1, CACNA1S, LDB3/ZASP,*
250a			*CAPN3, SGCD, HSPG2, TTN*
130a			*CAPN3, PLEC x2, SYNE1 x2, SYNE2, CACNA1S, TTN*
160a			*CAPN3, BAG3, DES, NEB x2, TTN x2, CACNA1S*
128a			*RYR1 x2, COL6A3*
243			*BVES x2, SYNE1, TTN, HSPG2, HACD1*
592			*BAG3, TMEM43, TTN x3, HSPG2*
197			*COL6A3, ANO5, NEB, COL12A1, MYH3, SYNE1, TTN x2, SCN4A, LMNB2*
17			*DMD, PLEC x2, LAMA2, ITGA7, MYH6, SYNE2, CACNA1S, NEB*
195			*DNM2, TRIM32, POMGNT1, FLNC, NEB,*
14			*FLNC x2, TTN x2*
1038			*DYSF, PLEC, SYNE1, SYNE2, TTN x2*
9			*RYR1 x2, NEB, MYH7, FLNC, TTNx2*
155			*RYR1, ISPD, POMGNT2, COL6A2 DYSF, NEB, MYH3, TTN x3*
11			*TRAPPC11, NEB, HSPG2*
194			*HSPG2, TTN*
859			*CACNA1S*

*Indicates novel variants; RefSeq transcript reference sequences as in the LOVD database: ANO5 - NM_213599.2, CACNA1S - NM_000069.2, CAPN3 - NM_000070.2, COL6A2 - NM_001849.3, COL6A3 - NM_004369.3, DMD - NM_004006.2, DNAJB6 - NM_058246.3, DYSF - NM_003494.3, FKRP - NM_024301.4, LMNA - NM_170707.3, MYH7 - NM_000257.2, SGCA - NM_000023.2, SGCB - NM_000232.4, TCAP - NM_003673.3, TRAPPC11 - NM_021942.5

phenotypic overlap between LGMD and other myopathies, making clinical diagnosis difficult in some cases. As a result of WES analysis, a diagnosis correction was made in the case of patient 135 to Becker muscular dystrophy. In the case of patients with causative mutations in *COL6* genes, the diagnosis was also changed to suspected collagen myopathy (as *COL6* genes mutations are not included in the current LGMD classification). In other cases, including those that were genetically unsolved, we upheld the clinical diagnosis of LGMD.

In the unsolved cases, the pathogenic mutations or copy number variants could be located in noncoding, regulatory or deep intronic regions. This could explain, for instance, the excess of single *CAPN3* mutation

Table 2 Genes expressed in muscle and components of the interactomes of known LGMD genes

Gene	Protein	Interactive partner
ANK1	ankyrin 1	RYR1, TTN
ANKRD23	ankyrin repeat domain 23	TTN
ATP1B4	ATPase beta 4 polypeptide	POMT1, POMT2
C1QTNF9	C1q and tumor necrosis factor protein 9	COL6A1, COL6A2
C1QTNF9	C1q and tumor necrosis factor protein 9B	COL6A1, COL6A2
EVC2	Ellis-van Creveld syndrome 2	TOR1AIP1
FYCO1	FYVE and coiled-coil containing 1	LMNA
HECW2	HECT, C2 and WW containing E3 ubiquitin	DYSF
HSPB2	heat shock protein 2	BAG3, CRYAB, FLNC, TCAP, TTN
MLIP	muscular LMNA-interacting protein	LMNA
MYOZ1	myozenin 1	FLNC, TCAP
MYOZ2	myozenin 2	FLNC, TCAP
MYOZ3	myozenin 3	FLNC, TCAP
OPRM1	opioid receptor mu 1	TNPO3
PDLIM7	PDZ and LIM domain 7	BAG3, PLEC
RXRA	retinoid x receptor alpha	TRIM32
SIRT2	sirtuin 2	DMD, DNAJB6
SRRM2	serine/arginine repetitive matrix 2	LMNA, PLEC
SVIL	Supervillin	LMNA
TRIM63	tripartite motif containing 63, E3 ubiquitin protein ligase	DES, FLNC, MYOT, TCAP, TTN

carriers as compared to population-wide data. It is also likely that additional co-responsible *CAPN3* mutations are located in the regulatory regions of the gene and therefore missed by exome sequencing. In sporadic or first cases in a family, a post-zygotic mutation event in the muscle could also be the cause of the disease [34].

In at least three cases, the patient's clinical phenotype could be plausibly explained by mutations in more than one gene (*CAPN3* + *MYH7*, *COL6A3* + *CACNA1S*, *DYSF* + *MYH7*). In these cases apart from clinical phenotype of LGMD, additional features included the following: considerable distal weakness with early onset typical for MYH7-related myopathies (patient 18, *CAPN3* + *MYH7*), early disease onset not typical for LGMD2B and possible autosomal dominant inheritance (patient 407, *DYSF* + *MYH7*), and almost exclusively type 1 fibers in biopsy unexpected for LGMD or Bethlem myopathy, whereas encountered in CACNA1S-related myopathies (patient 901, *COL6A3* + *CACNA1S*). In these cases, a clinical diagnosis was upheld with possible co-existing MYH7 and CACNA1S-related myopathy. Likewise, in the majority of cases, additional

variants in other genes apart from the highly probable major pathogenic mutations could at least add to the phenotypic manifestation; however, selecting co-causative variants from those classified as potentially modifying was not possible. Discrimination between possible phenotype-influencing variants and thousands of insignificant variants harbored by each individual became one of the most difficult novel challenges. Indeed, in all the studied cases, we encountered novel and rare variants related to LGMD and other myopathies, but their relevance could not be established based on the inheritance mode, patient's phenotype, and known effect of mutations in these genes.

Here, we adopted a strategy for identifying the phenotype-influencing variants that linked the genes bearing found variants with any of the terms from the HPO database pointing to muscle physiology or structures. However, this approach could result in missing variants located in genes not yet associated with muscle disease, or missing variants coding for an interactome of the known causative proteins. Therefore, we additionally tried to identify putative phenotype-influencing variants by comprehensively analyzing those with MAF < 0.1%, expressed in muscle (human and/or murine) and markedly influencing the structure/function of the encoded protein (human and/or murine), but with no known association with the myopathy clinical phenotype (therefore excluding variants identified in the first approach). These variants were analyzed further based on the association of respective genes with known LGMD-related genes or pathways in which LGMD-related genes are involved. This reduced the overall number of such variants to 68 in 19 genes (0–3 per case). In light of their inheritance pattern, their presence in our in-house WES/WGS control group as well, and the presence of other variants that seem to explain the phenotype well in many cases, it is unlikely that the aforementioned 68 variants are causative. Still, putative phenotype-influencing variants could be within those in genes expressed in skeletal muscle.

By using various filtering approaches to WES results, one can gain insight into the possible influence of new genes on the disease. A list of such selected genes previously not associated with LGMD, but, according to our analysis, with a likely effect on the disease, is presented in Table 3.

All the genes listed in Table 3 have already been examined in the context of muscular disorders, as well as muscle structure and functioning (see Additional file 5).

Numerous genetic muscular disorders phenotypically overlap with LGMD, as limb-girdle weakness is one of their common symptoms. NGS-based genetic analyses can resolve clinical dilemmas and facilitate exact diagnosis [35–37]. Additionally, with the reporting of new cases, the spectrum of clinical manifestations of

Table 3 Selected genes with reported skeletal muscle expression which could contribute to LGMD

Gene	Protein	Interacts with
OBSCN	Obscurin	TTN
MAP4	microtubule-associated protein 4	BAG3, TARDBP
MAST2	Microtubule-associated serine/threonine kinase 2	DMD
CACNA1S	calcium channel, voltage-dependent, L type, alpha 1S subunit	–
MYH7	myosin heavy chain 7	TPM2

mutations in a given gene is likely to expand. Moreover, recent mass sequencing results show that the genetic background is more complex than previously considered [5, 6]. Also, our data suggest that mutations in more than one gene in a single patient can result in the LGMD phenotype. Taking into account the phenotypic variability within a given LGMD subtype or even between patients with the same causative mutation [38–40], one should expect a strong influence of disease-modifying genes, although no specific modifier or co-causative genes have been described to date. In our patients with identified primary causative mutations, at least a dozen additional variants that could influence or modify the phenotype were found, even when only genes known to be associated with muscle pathology were taken into consideration. It is therefore likely that the spectrum of genetic factors influencing the disease is substantially wider than previously recognized.

Indeed, a common polymorphism in the *LTPB4* gene has been shown to be a disease-modifying factor in dystrophinopathy [41]. Moreover, in some cases, mutations in more than one gene could be necessary to cause the disease [42]. Thus, digenic inheritance has been proven for a subtype of facioscapulohumeral muscular dystrophy [43] found in congenital myasthenic syndrome [44], and it has also been suggested for calpainopathy [45].

Proteins of the muscle cell form a complex machinery where structural or functional impairment of any of its components can result in progressive muscle dysfunction and eventual destruction. The mutational burden in the numerous genes involved in muscular diseases must not be overlooked, as accumulation of minor defects, even those without an apparent overall effect when present in isolation, could result in a similar phenotype. Indeed, oligogenic etiology may be most easily observable in unsolved, sporadic LGMD cases, where the main putative causative mutation has not been identified. Interestingly, two of our "double trouble" cases were found precisely in sporadic patients.

On the other hand, some of the mutations described as disease-causing prior to the NGS era might only have a modifying effect, incomplete penetrance, and require

additional variants to bring about pathology [40, 46]. The overrepresentation of single heterozygous CAPN3 mutations in our group may also indicate digenic or oligogenic inheritance.

Multiple annotation tools have become available using various algorithms and databases to predict the functional effects of genomic variants. One should bear in mind, however, that the functional scores of a given variant may differ substantially between different databases and prediction tools as they can be based on different functional aspects and prior knowledge. The superiority of high-scale bioinformatic analysis over focused genetic studies lies in the possibility of repeating the analysis and making use of novel knowledge [47].

Ideally, genetic testing should be combined not only with deep phenotyping but also with comprehensive analyses of transcripts and protein isoforms to pinpoint novel causative, co-causative, and phenotype-modifying variants.

Conclusions

The availability of exome and whole genome data for various conditions, including LGMD, challenges the classical definition of genetic causality and the concept of strictly monogenic disorders [48] and underlines the heterogeneity and complexity of the human genome [49]. Our results show a range of phenotypes associated not only with genes previously and typically associated with LGMD but also with genes related to similar muscular disorders, such as Bethlem myopathy, myofibrillar myopathy, or congenital muscle dystrophy, as well as with genes not previously considered in the context of myopathies. Even if it is not always possible to prove the effect of putative modifying variants on the phenotype, aggregate analysis of mutations suggests that the sheer "variant burden" contributes to phenotypic variability.

Based on the obtained exomic data, we propose that LGMD could be better defined as a group of oligogenic disorders, in which variable clinical symptoms result from the combined effects of mutations in a set of genes and can result in a broad spectrum of clinical presentation rather than distinct disease entities. This could explain the fact that NGS methods fail to identify a single main causative gene in many LGMD cases, but indicate a range of possibly pathogenic and/or co-causative mutations in almost every case.

This could also explain the clinical heterogeneity not only of LGMD or within subtypes but also among individuals harboring the same known pathogenic mutations, and even between affected members of the same family. While a considerable proportion of LGMD cases can be easily attributed clinically to a single gene, the high number of variants that could relate to myopathy and sometimes to specific phenotype features in cases with mutations in known LGMD-associated genes suggests that the oligogenic nature of the disease may be important even in patients with a well-defined primary pathogenic cause.

However, unequivocal identification of such modifying variants requires comprehensive bioinformatic analyses integrated with deep phenotyping to make a final diagnosis [50]. It should be remembered, nevertheless, that it is practically impossible to ascertain the causality even of a single gene in a single subject or a risk-family [51]. Identification of all risk or co-causative factors requires bioinformatical analysis of combined genomic and clinical data on large groups of ethnically diverse patients with various muscle diseases followed by functional in vitro studies.

We expect that with the appearance of genomic data from large groups of patients with a large spectrum of myopathies, it will become possible to examine not just a limited number of genes and variants, but groups of genes encoding entire pathways and modules [52]. As a result, the traditional descriptive classification of muscle diseases will transform into a systemic and pathway-based view of clinical phenotypes [53]. The presented results are the first and indispensable step towards this goal of translational medicine.

Abbreviations
BWA: Burrows-Wheeler alignment (software); CK: Serum creatine kinase; CNV: Copy number variant; ExAC: The exome aggregation consortium (database); GATK: Genome analysis toolkit (software); HGMD: Human gene mutation database; HPO: The human phenotype ontology (database); indel : Small insertion/deletion; LGMD: Limb-girdle muscular dystrophy; LOVD: Leiden open variation database; MLPA: Multiplex ligation-dependent probe amplification; NGS: Next-generation sequencing; OMIM: Online Mendelian inheritance in man (database); PCR: Polymerase chain reaction; SIFT: Sorting intolerant from tolerant (software); SNV: Single-nucleotide variation; WES: Whole exome sequencing; WGS: Whole genome sequencing

Funding
This work was supported by National Science Centre, Poland grants (NCN, 2013/09/B/NZ4/03258 and 2015/19/N/NZ2/02915), and by the KNOW-MMRC project financed by the Ministry of Science and Higher Education (to JPF). The bioinformatics part of the study (JPF) was supported by PL-Grid Infrastructure financed by the Polish Ministry of Science and Higher Education and co-funded by the European Regional Development Fund as part of the

Innovative Economy program. The funding sources had no involvement in the experiment design, analysis, data interpretation, and manuscript preparation.

Authors' contributions
JPF, AM, and MP contributed equally. The study was designed by JPF and CZ. MK supervised the bioinformatic part and CZ the genetic part of the research. AM and APC recruited the patients and conducted clinical phenotyping. MP performed the bioinformatic analysis. JPF performed the analysis of the pre-filtered datasets and analyzed putative influence on phenotype of variants with AM. JPF performed the PCR and Sanger sequencing validation experiments. JPF, AM, MJR, and CZ drafted and edited the manuscript. All authors reviewed and commented on the manuscript. All authors read and approved the final manuscript.

Competing interests
The authors declare that they have no competing interests.

Author details
[1]Department of Neurodegenerative Disorders, Mossakowski Medical Research Centre, Polish Academy of Sciences, 5 Pawinskiego St., 02-106 Warsaw, Poland. [2]Department of Neurology, Medical University of Warsaw, 1a Banacha St., 02-097 Warsaw, Poland. [3]Department of Molecular Neuropharmacology, Institute of Pharmacology, Polish Academy of Sciences, 31-344 Krakow, Poland. [4]Laboratory of Molecular Basis of Cell Motility, Department of Biochemistry, Nencki Institute of Experimental Biology, 3 Pasteur St., 02-093 Warsaw, Poland.

References
1. Mitsuhashi S, Kang PB. Update on the genetics of limb girdle muscular dystrophy. Semin Pediatr Neurol. 2012;19(4):211–8. https://doi.org/10.1016/j.spen.2012.09.008.
2. Bushby K. Diagnosis and management of the limb girdle muscular dystrophies. Pract Neurol. 2009;9:314–23. https://doi.org/10.1136/jnnp.2009.193938.
3. Norwood FL, Harling C, Chinnery PF, Eagle M, Bushby K, Straub V. Prevalence of genetic muscle disease in Northern England: in-depth analysis of a muscle clinic population. Brain. 2009;132:3175–86. https://doi.org/10.1093/brain/awp236.
4. van der Kooi AJ, Barth PG, Busch HF, de Haan R, Ginjaar HB, van Essen AJ et al. The clinical spectrum of limb girdle muscular dystrophy. A survey in The Netherlands. Brain. 1996;119(Pt 5): 1471–1480 doi: https://doi.org/10.1093/brain/119.5.1471.
5. Nigro V, Savarese M. Genetic basis of limb-girdle muscular dystrophies: the 2014 update. Acta Myol. 2014;33(1):1–12.
6. Vissing J. Limb girdle muscular dystrophies: classification, clinical spectrum and emerging therapies. Curr Opin Neurol. 2016;29(5):635–41. https://doi.org/10.1097/WCO.0000000000000375.
7. Ghaoui R, Benavides T, Lek M, Waddell LB, Kaur S, North KN, et al. TOR1AIP1 as a cause of cardiac failure and recessive limb-girdle muscular dystrophy. Neuromuscul Disord. 2016;26(8):500–3. https://doi.org/10.1016/j.nmd.2016.05.013.
8. Servián-Morilla E, Takeuchi H, Lee TV, Clarimon J, Mavillard F, Area-Gómez E, et al. A POGLUT1 mutation causes a muscular dystrophy with reduced Notch signaling and satellite cell loss. EMBO Mol Med. 2016;8(11):1289–309. https://doi.org/10.15252/emmm.201505815.
9. Narayanaswami P, Weiss M, Selcen D, David W, Raynor E, Carter G, et al. Evidence-based guideline summary: diagnosis and treatment of limb-girdle and distal dystrophies: report of the Guideline Development Subcommittee of the American Academy of Neurology and the Practice Issues Review Panel of the American Association of Neuromuscular & Electrodiagnostic medicine. Neurology. 2014;83(16):1453–63. https://doi.org/10.1212/WNL.0000000000000892.
10. Beltran-Valero de Bernabé D, Voit T, Longman C, Steinbrecher A, Straub V, Yuva Y, et al. Mutations in the FKRP gene can cause muscle-eye-brain disease and Walker-Warburg syndrome. J Med Genet. 2004;41:e61. https://doi.org/10.1136/jmg.2003.013870.
11. Chan YM, Keramaris-Vrantsis E, Lidov HG, Norton JH, Zinchenko N, Gruber HE, et al. Fukutin-related protein is essential for mouse muscle, brain and eye development and mutation recapitulates the wide clinical spectrums of dystroglycanopathies. Hum Mol Genet. 2010;19:3995–4006. https://doi.org/10.1093/hmg/ddq314.
12. Qiao C, Wang CH, Zhao C, Lu P, Awano H, Xiao B, et al. Muscle and heart function restoration in a limb girdle muscular dystrophy 2I (LGMD2I) mouse model by systemic FKRP gene delivery. Mol Ther. 2014;22:1890–9. https://doi.org/10.1038/mt.2014.141.
13. Sondergaard PC, Griffin DA, Pozsgai ER, Johnson RW, Grose WE, Heller KN, et al. AAV dysferlin overlap vectors restore function in dysferlinopathy animal models. Ann Clin Transl Neurol. 2015;2:256–70. https://doi.org/10.1002/acn3.172.
14. Lek M, MacArthur D. The challenge of next generation sequencing in the context of neuromuscular diseases. J Neuromuscul Dis. 2014;1:135–49. https://doi.org/10.3233/JND-140032

15. Miller SA, Dykes DD, Polesky HF. A simple salting out procedure for extracting DNA from human nucleated cells. Nucleic Acids Res. 1988;16: 1215. https://doi.org/10.1093/nar/16.3.1215.

16. Li H, Durbin R. Fast and accurate short read alignment with Burrows-Wheeler transform. Bioinformatics. 2009;25:1754–60. https://doi.org/10.1093/bioinformatics/btp324.

17. McKenna A, Hanna M, Banks E, Sivachenko A, Cibulskis K, Kernytsky A, et al. The Genome Analysis Toolkit: a MapReduce framework for analyzing next-generation DNA sequencing data. Genome Res. 2010;20:1297–303. https://doi.org/10.1101/gr.107524.110.

18. Robinson JT, Thorvaldsdóttir H, Winckler W, Guttman M, Lander ES, Getz G, et al. Integrative genomics viewer. Nat Biotechnol. 2011;29:24–6. https://doi.org/10.1038/nbt.1754.

19. Wang K, Li M, Hakonarson H. ANNOVAR: functional annotation of genetic variants from high-throughput sequencing data. Nucleic Acids Res. 2010;38: e164. https://doi.org/10.1093/nar/gkq603.

20. Jiang Y, Oldridge DA, Diskin SJ, Zhang NR. CODEX: a normalization and copy number variation detection method for whole exome sequencing. Nucleic Acids Res. 2015;43(6):e39. https://doi.org/10.1093/nar/gku1363.

21. Köhler S, Schoeneberg U, Czeschik JC. Clinical interpretation of CNVs with cross-species phenotype data. J Med Genet. 2014;51(11):766–72. https://doi.org/10.1136/jmedgenet-2014-102633.

22. Masino AJ, Dechene ET, Dulik MC, Wilkens A, Spinner NB, Krantz ID, et al. Clinical phenotype-based gene prioritization: an initial study using semantic similarity and the human phenotype ontology. BMC Bioinformatics. 2014;15: 248. https://doi.org/10.1186/1471-2105-15-248.

23. Richards S, Aziz N, Bale S, Bick D, Das S, Gastier-Foster J, et al. Standards and guidelines for the interpretation of sequence variants: a joint consensus recommendation of the American College of Medical Genetics and Genomics and the Association for Molecular Pathology. Genet Med. 2015; 17(5):405–24. https://doi.org/10.1038/gim.2015.30.

24. Smedley D, Robinson PN. Phenotype-driven strategies for exome prioritization of human Mendelian disease genes. Genome Med. 2015;7(1): 81. https://doi.org/10.1186/s13073-015-0199-2.

25. Khateb S, Hanany M, Khalaileh A, Beryozkin A, Meyer S, Abu-Diab A, et al. Identification of genomic deletions causing inherited retinal degenerations by coverage analysis of whole exome sequencing data. J Med Genet. 2016; 53(9):600–7. https://doi.org/10.1136/jmedgenet-2016-103825.

26. Belkadi A, Bolze A, Itan Y, Cobat A, Vincent QB, Antipenko A, et al. Whole-genome sequencing is more powerful than whole-exome sequencing for detecting exome variants. Proc Natl Acad Sci U S A. 2015;112(17):5473–8. https://doi.org/10.1073/pnas.1418631112.

27. Stehlíková K, Skálová D, Zídková J, Haberlová J, Voháňka S, Mazanec R, et al. Muscular dystrophies and myopathies: the spectrum of mutated genes in the Czech Republic. Clin Genet. 2017;91(3):463–9. https://doi.org/10.1111/cge.12839.

28. Yu M, Zheng Y, Jin S, Gang Q, Wang Q, Yu P, et al. Mutational spectrum of Chinese LGMD patients by targeted next-generation sequencing. PLoS One. 2017;12(4):e0175343. https://doi.org/10.1371/journal.pone.0175343.

29. Monies D, Alhindi HN, Almuhaizea MA, Abouelhoda M, Alazami AM, Goljan E, et al. A first-line diagnostic assay for limb-girdle muscular dystrophy and other myopathies. Hum Genomics. 2016;10(1):32. https://doi.org/10.1186/s40246-016-0089-8.

30. Kuhn M, Gläser D, Joshi PR, Zierz S, Wenninger S, Schoser B, et al. Utility of a next-generation sequencing-based gene panel investigation in German patients with genetically unclassified limb-girdle muscular dystrophy. J Neurol. 2016;263(4):743–50. https://doi.org/10.1007/s00415-016-8036-0.

31. Reddy HM, Cho KA, Lek M, Estrella E, Valkanas E, Jones MD, et al. The sensitivity of exome sequencing in identifying pathogenic mutations for LGMD in the United States. J Hum Genet. 2017;62(2):243–52. https://doi.org/10.1038/jhg.2016.116.

32. Ghaoui R, Cooper ST, Lek M, Jones K, Corbett A, Reddel SW, et al. Use of whole-exome sequencing for diagnosis of limb-girdle muscular dystrophy: outcomes and lessons learned. JAMA Neurol. 2015;72(12):1424–32. https://doi.org/10.1001/jamaneurol.2015.2274.

33. Magri F, Nigro V, Angelini C, Mongini T, Mora M, Moroni I, et al. The italian limb girdle muscular dystrophy registry: relative frequency, clinical features, and differential diagnosis. Muscle Nerve. 2017;55(1):55–68. https://doi.org/10.1002/mus.25192

34. Acuna-Hidalgo R, Bo T, Kwint MP, van de Vorst M, Pinelli M, Veltman JA, et al. Post-zygotic point mutations are an underrecognized source of de novo genomic variation. Am J Hum Genet. 2015;97(1):67–74. https://doi.org/10.1016/j.ajhg.2015.05.008

35. Simeoni S, Russo V, Gigli GL, Scalise A. Facioscapulohumeral muscular dystrophy and limb-girdle muscular dystrophy: "double trouble" overlapping syndrome? J Neurol Sci. 2015;348(1–2):292–3. https://doi.org/10.1016/j.jns.2014.12.009.

36. Ciafaloni E, Chinnery PF, Griggs RC. Evaluation and Treatment of myopathies. Oxford: Oxford University Press; 2014.

37. Pegoraro E and Hoffman EP, Limb-Girdle Muscular Dystrophy Overview. In Pagon RA, Bird TD, Dolan CR, eds. GeneReviews, University of Washington, Seattle, WA, USA, 2012.

38. Weiler T, Bashir R, Anderson LV, Davison K, Moss JA, Britton S, et al. Identical mutation in patients with limb girdle muscular dystrophy type 2B or Miyoshi myopathy suggests a role for modifier gene(s). Hum Mol Genet. 1999;8:871–7. https://doi.org/10.1093/hmg/8.5.871.

39. Illarioshkin SN, Ivanova-Smolenskaya IA, Greenberg CR, Nylen E, Sukhorukov VS, Poleshchuk VV, et al. Identical dysferlin mutation in limb-girdle muscular dystrophy type 2B and distal myopathy. Neurology. 2000;55:1931–3. https://doi.org/10.1212/WNL.55.12.1931.

40. Fee DB, So YT, Barraza C, Figueroa KP, Pulst SM. Phenotypic variability associated with Arg26Gln mutation in caveolin3. Muscle Nerve. 2004;30(3): 375–8. https://doi.org/10.1002/mus.20092.

41. Flanigan KM, Ceco E, Lamar KM, Kaminoh Y, Dunn DM, Mendell JR, et al. LTBP4 genotype predicts age of ambulatory loss in Duchenne muscular dystrophy. Ann Neurol. 2013;73(4):481–8. https://doi.org/10.1002/ana.23819.

42. Posey JE, Harel T, Liu P, Rosenfeld JA, James RA, Coban Akdemir ZH, et al. Resolution of disease phenotypes resulting from multilocus genomic variation. N Engl J Med. 2017;376(1):21–31. https://doi.org/10.1056/NEJMoa1516767.

43. Lemmers RJ, Tawil R, Petek LM, Balog J, Block GJ, Santen GW, et al. Digenic inheritance of an SMCHD1 mutation and an FSHD-permissive D4Z4 allele causes facioscapulohumeral muscular dystrophy type 2. Nat Genet. 2012; 44(12):1370–4. https://doi.org/10.1038/ng.2454.

44. Lam CW, Wong KS, Leung HW, Law CY. Limb girdle myasthenia with digenic RAPSN and a novel disease gene AK9 mutations. Eur J Hum Genet. 2017;25(2):192–9. https://doi.org/10.1038/ejhg.2016.162.

45. Saenz A, Lopez de Munain A. Dominant LGMD2A: alternative diagnosis or hidden digenism? Brain. 2017;140(Pt 2):e7. https://doi.org/10.1093/brain/aww281.

46. Di Fruscio G, Garofalo A, Mutarelli M, Savarese M, Nigro V. Are all the previously reported genetic variants in limb girdle muscular dystrophy genes pathogenic? Eur J Hum Genet. 2016;24(1):73–7. https://doi.org/10.1038/ejhg.2015.76.

47. Need AC, Shashi V, Schoch K Petrovski S, Goldstein DB. The importance of dynamic re-analysis in diagnostic whole exome sequencing. J Med Genet. 2017;54:155–6. https://doi.org/10.1136/jmedgenet-2016-104306.

48. Katsanis N. The continuum of causality in human genetic disorders. Genome Biol. 2016;17:233. https://doi.org/10.1186/s13059-016-1107-9.

49. Gao F, Keinan A. High burden of private mutations due to explosive human population growth and purifying selection. BMC Genomics. 2014;15:S3. https://doi.org/10.1186/1471-2164-15-S4-S3.

50. Hennekam RC, Biesecker LG. Next-generation sequencing demands next-generation phenotyping. Hum Mutat. 2012;33(5):884–6. https://doi.org/10.1002/humu.22048.

51. Marian AJ. The case of "missing causal genes" and the practice of medicine. Circ Res. 2016;119:21–4. https://doi.org/10.1161/CIRCRESAHA.116.308830.

52. McCarthy MI, MacArthur DG. Human disease genomics: from variants to biology. Genome Biol. 2017;30(18):20. https://doi.org/10.1186/s13059-017-1160-z.

53. Thompson R, Straub V. Limb-girdle muscular dystrophies—international collaborations for translational research. Nat Rev Neurol. 2016;12(5):294–309. https://doi.org/10.1038/nrneurol.2016.35.

Permissions

All chapters in this book were first published in HG, by BioMed Central; hereby published with permission under the Creative Commons Attribution License or equivalent. Every chapter published in this book has been scrutinized by our experts. Their significance has been extensively debated. The topics covered herein carry significant findings which will fuel the growth of the discipline. They may even be implemented as practical applications or may be referred to as a beginning point for another development.

The contributors of this book come from diverse backgrounds, making this book a truly international effort. This book will bring forth new frontiers with its revolutionizing research information and detailed analysis of the nascent developments around the world.

We would like to thank all the contributing authors for lending their expertise to make the book truly unique. They have played a crucial role in the development of this book. Without their invaluable contributions this book wouldn't have been possible. They have made vital efforts to compile up to date information on the varied aspects of this subject to make this book a valuable addition to the collection of many professionals and students.

This book was conceptualized with the vision of imparting up-to-date information and advanced data in this field. To ensure the same, a matchless editorial board was set up. Every individual on the board went through rigorous rounds of assessment to prove their worth. After which they invested a large part of their time researching and compiling the most relevant data for our readers.

The editorial board has been involved in producing this book since its inception. They have spent rigorous hours researching and exploring the diverse topics which have resulted in the successful publishing of this book. They have passed on their knowledge of decades through this book. To expedite this challenging task, the publisher supported the team at every step. A small team of assistant editors was also appointed to further simplify the editing procedure and attain best results for the readers.

Apart from the editorial board, the designing team has also invested a significant amount of their time in understanding the subject and creating the most relevant covers. They scrutinized every image to scout for the most suitable representation of the subject and create an appropriate cover for the book.

The publishing team has been an ardent support to the editorial, designing and production team. Their endless efforts to recruit the best for this project, has resulted in the accomplishment of this book. They are a veteran in the field of academics and their pool of knowledge is as vast as their experience in printing. Their expertise and guidance has proved useful at every step. Their uncompromising quality standards have made this book an exceptional effort. Their encouragement from time to time has been an inspiration for everyone.

The publisher and the editorial board hope that this book will prove to be a valuable piece of knowledge for researchers, students, practitioners and scholars across the globe.

List of Contributors

Neven Maksemous, Robert A. Smith, Larisa M. Haupt and Lyn R. Griffiths
Genomics Research Centre, Institute of Health and Biomedical Innovation (IHBI), School of Biomedical Sciences, Queensland University of Technology (QUT), Q Block, 60 Musk Ave, Kelvin Grove Campus, Brisbane 4059, Queensland, Australia

Hye Jin Yoo
National Leading Research Laboratory of Clinical Nutrigenetics/ Nutrigenomics, Department of Food and Nutrition, College of Human Ecology, Yonsei University, 50 Yonsei-ro, Seodaemun-gu, Seoul 03722, South Korea
Department of Food and Nutrition, Brain Korea 21 PLUS Project, College of Human Ecology, Yonsei University, Seoul 03722, South Korea

Jong Ho Lee
National Leading Research Laboratory of Clinical Nutrigenetics/ Nutrigenomics, Department of Food and Nutrition, College of Human Ecology, Yonsei University, 50 Yonsei-ro, Seodaemun-gu, Seoul 03722, South Korea
Department of Food and Nutrition, Brain Korea 21 PLUS Project, College of Human Ecology, Yonsei University, Seoul 03722, South Korea
Research Center for Silver Science, Institute of Symbiotic Life-TECH, Yonsei University, Seoul 03722, South Korea

Minjoo Kim, Minkyung Kim and Jey Sook Chae
Research Center for Silver Science, Institute of Symbiotic Life-TECH, Yonsei University, Seoul 03722, South Korea

Sang-Hyun Lee
Department of Family Practice, National Health Insurance Corporation, Ilsan Hospital, Goyang 10444, South Korea

Shrey Gandhi
GN Ramachandran Knowledge Center for Genome Informatics, CSIR Institute of Genomics and Integrative Biology (CSIR-IGIB), Mathura Road, Delhi 110 025, India

Saakshi Jalali and Vinod Scaria
GN Ramachandran Knowledge Center for Genome Informatics, CSIR Institute of Genomics and Integrative Biology (CSIR-IGIB), Mathura Road, Delhi 110 025, India

Academy of Scientific and Innovative Research (AcSIR), CSIR-IGIB South Campus, Mathura Road, Delhi 110025, India

Charlotte Philpott, Hannah Tovell, Ian M. Frayling, David N. Cooper and Meena Upadhyaya
Division of Cancer and Genetics, Institute of Medical Genetics, Cardiff University, Heath Park, Cardiff CF14 4XN, UK

Hung-Lun Chiang
Institute of Clinical Medicine, National Yang-Ming University, Taipei, Taiwan
Institute of Biomedical Sciences, Academia Sinica, Taipei, Taiwan

Yuan-Tsong Chen
Institute of Clinical Medicine, National Yang-Ming University, Taipei, Taiwan
Institute of Biomedical Sciences, Academia Sinica, Taipei, Taiwan
Department of Pediatrics, Duke University Medical Center, Durham, USA

Jer-Yuarn Wu
Institute of Biomedical Sciences, Academia Sinica, Taipei, Taiwan
Graduate Institute of Chinese Medical Science, China Medical University, Taichung, Taiwan

Jianxin Wang
School of Information Science and Engineering, Central South University, Changsha 410083, China

Xueyong Li
School of Information Science and Engineering, Central South University, Changsha 410083, China
Department of Information and Computing Science, Changsha University, Changsha 410003, China

Bihai Zhao
Department of Information and Computing Science, Changsha University, Changsha 410003, China

Fang-Xiang Wu
Department of Mechanical Engineering and Division of Biomedical Engineering, University of Saskatchewan, Saskatoon, SK S7N 5A9, Canada

Yi Pan
Department of Computer Science, Georgia State University, Atlanta, GA 30302-4110, USA

Tine Descamps, Els Delporte, Nancy H. C. Roosens, Sigrid C. J. De Keersmaecker, Vanessa De Wit, Jean Tafforeau, Stefaan Demarest and Marc Van den Bulcke
Scientific Institute of Public Health, Brussels, Belgium

Jimmy Van den Eynden
Scientific Institute of Public Health, Brussels, Belgium
Department of Medical Biochemistry and Cell Biology, Institute of Biomedicine, The Sahlgrenska Academy, University of Gothenburg, Gothenburg, Sweden

Herman Van Oyen
Scientific Institute of Public Health, Brussels, Belgium
Department of Public Health, Ghent University, Ghent, Belgium

Joris Robert Vermeesch
Laboratory of Cytogenetics and Genome Research, Department of Human Genetics, KU Leuven, Leuven, Belgium

Els Goetghebeur
Department of Applied Mathematics, Computer Science and Statistics, Ghent University, Ghent, Belgium

Jubin Osei-Mensah and Yusif Mubarik
Kumasi Centre for Collaborative Research in Tropical Medicine, Kumasi, Ghana

Linda Batsa Debrah
Kumasi Centre for Collaborative Research in Tropical Medicine, Kumasi, Ghana
Department of Clinical Microbiology, Kwame Nkrumah University of Science and Technology, Kumasi, Ghana

Achim Hoerauf, Kenneth Pfarr, Andrea Hofmann and Anna Albers
Institute for Medical Microbiology, Immunology and Parasitology, University Hospital Bonn, Sigmund-Freud-Str. 25, 53127 Bonn, Germany

Alexander Yaw Debrah
Faculty of Allied Health Sciences of Kwame Nkrumah University of Science and Technology, Kumasi, Ghana

Felix F. Brockschmidt
Institute of Human Genetics, University of Bonn, Bonn, Germany
Department of Genomics, Life and Brain Center, University of Bonn, Bonn, Germany

Tim Becker and Christine Herold
Institute for Medical Biometry, Informatics and Epidemiology, University of Bonn, Bonn, Germany

Holger Fröhlich
Bonn-Aachen International Center for Information Technology (B-IT), University of Bonn, Bonn, Germany

Anna Sundby and Ole Mors
Department of Clinical Medicine, Psychosis Research Unit, Aarhus University Hospital, Skovagervej 2, 8240 Risskov, Denmark
The Lundbeck Foundation Initiative for Integrative Psychiatric Research, iPSYCH, Copenhagen, Denmark

Merete Watt Boolsen
Department of Political Science, Copenhagen University, Copenhagen, Denmark

Kristoffer Sølvsten Burgdorf and Henrik Ullum
Department of Clinical Immunology, Copenhagen University Hospital, Copenhagen, Denmark

Thomas Folkmann Hansen
The Lundbeck Foundation Initiative for Integrative Psychiatric Research, iPSYCH, Copenhagen, Denmark
Institute for Biological Psychiatry, Mental Health Centre Sct. Hans, Copenhagen University Hospital, Copenhagen, Denmark
Danish Headache Center, Department of Neurology, Rigshospitalet-Glostrup, Copenhagen, Denmark

Gorjana Robevska and Jocelyn A. van den Bergen
Murdoch Childrens Research Institute, Melbourne, Victoria, Australia

Katie L. Ayers and Andrew H. Sinclair
Murdoch Childrens Research Institute, Melbourne, Victoria, Australia
Department of Paediatrics, University of Melbourne, Melbourne, Victoria, Australia

Aurore Bouty
Murdoch Childrens Research Institute, Melbourne, Victoria, Australia
The Royal Children's Hospital, Melbourne, Victoria, Australia

Sultana M. H. Faradz, Achmad Zulfa Juniarto and Nurin Aisyiyah Listyasari
Division of Human Genetics, Centre for Biomedical Research, Faculty of Medicine, Diponegoro University (FMDU), JL. Prof. H. Soedarto, SH, Tembalang, Semarang 50275, Central Java, Indonesia

Jarrett D. Morrow, Xiaobo Zhou, Weiliang Qiu and Kimberly Glass
Channing Division of Network Medicine, Brigham and Women's Hospital, 181 Longwood Avenue, Boston, MA 02115, USA

Edwin K. Silverman, Craig P. Hersh, Dawn L. DeMeo and Michael H. Cho
Channing Division of Network Medicine, Brigham and Women's Hospital, 181 Longwood Avenue, Boston, MA 02115, USA
Division of Pulmonary and Critical Care Medicine, Brigham and Women's Hospital, Boston, MA 02115, USA

Bartholome Celli and George R. Washko
Division of Pulmonary and Critical Care Medicine, Brigham and Women's Hospital, Boston, MA 02115, USA

John Platig and John Quackenbush
Department of Biostatistics and Computational Biology, Dana-Farber Cancer Institute, Boston, MA 02115, USA

Nathaniel Marchetti and Gerard J. Criner
Division of Pulmonary and Critical Care Medicine, Temple University, Philadelphia, PA 19140, USA

Raphael Bueno
Division of Thoracic Surgery, Brigham and Women's Hospital, Boston, MA 02115, USA

Fida K. Dankar
College of IT, UAEU, Al Ain, UAE

Andrey Ptitsyn
Gloucester Marine Genomics Institute, Gloucester, MA, USA

Samar K. Dankar
Faculty of Sciences, University of Balamand, Souk El Ghareb, Lebanon

Teresa Requena and Alvaro Gallego-Martinez
Otology & Neurotology Group CTS495, Department of Genomic Medicine, GENYO - Centre for Genomics and Oncological Research – Pfizer/University of Granada/ Junta de Andalucía, PTS, 18016 Granada, Spain

Jose A. Lopez-Escamez
Otology & Neurotology Group CTS495, Department of Genomic Medicine, GENYO - Centre for Genomics and Oncological Research – Pfizer/University of Granada/ Junta de Andalucía, PTS, 18016 Granada, Spain

Department of Otolaryngology, Complejo Hospitalario Universidad de Granada (CHUGRA), ibs.granada, 18014 Granada, Spain

Jin-Woo Park, Jae-Mok Lee and Jo-Young Suh
Department of Periodontology, School of Dentistry, Kyungpook National University, Daegu 41940, Korea

Yong-Gun Kim
Department of Periodontology, School of Dentistry, Kyungpook National University, Daegu 41940, Korea
Institute for Hard Tissue and Bone Regeneration, Kyungpook National University, Daegu 41940, Korea

Jae-Young Kim and Youngkyun Lee
Institute for H.ard Tissue and Bone Regeneration, Kyungpook National University, Daegu 41940, Korea
Department of Biochemistry, School of Dentistry, Kyungpook National University, 2177 Dalgubeol-daero, Joong-gu, Daegu 41940, Korea

Minjung Kim
Department of Life and Nanopharmaceutical Sciences, Kyung Hee University, Seoul 02447, Korea

Jae-Hyung Lee
Department of Life and Nanopharmaceutical Sciences, Kyung Hee University, Seoul 02447, Korea
Department of Maxillofacial Biomedical Engineering, School of Dentistry, Kyung Hee University, 26 Kyunghee-daero, Dongdaemun-gu, Seoul 02447, Korea

Ji Hyun Kang and Hyo Jeong Kim
Department of Biochemistry, School of Dentistry, Kyungpook National University, 2177 Dalgubeol-daero, Joong-gu, Daegu 41940, Korea

Muna Monther Abdullah Al-Breacan
Department of Genetics, King Faisal Specialist Hospital, and Research Centre, PO Box 3354, Riyadh 11211, Saudi Arabia

Dorota Monies, Ewa A. Goljan, Banan Al-Younes, Salma M. Wakil and Brian F. Meyer
Department of Genetics, King Faisal Specialist Hospital, and Research Centre, PO Box 3354, Riyadh 11211, Saudi Arabia
Saudi Human Genome Program, King Abdulaziz City for Science and Technology, Riyadh, Saudi Arabia

Saeed Bohlega
Saudi Human Genome Program, King Abdulaziz City for Science and Technology, Riyadh, Saudi Arabia
Department of Neurosciences, King Faisal Specialist Hospital and Research Centre, PO Box 3354, Riyadh 11211, Saudi Arabia

Hussam Abou Al-Shaar
Department of Neurosciences, King Faisal Specialist Hospital and Research Centre, PO Box 3354, Riyadh 11211, Saudi Arabia

Maher Mohammed Al-Saif and Khalid S. A. Khabar
Biomolecular Medicine, Research Centre, King Faisal Specialist Hospital and Research Centre, Riyadh, Saudi Arabia

Bihai Zhao, Sai Hu, Xueyong Li, Fan Zhang, Qinglong Tian and Wenyin Ni
Department of Mathematics and Computing Science, Changsha University, Changsha, Hunan 410022, China

Ron Shamir
Blavatnik School of Computer Science, Tel Aviv University, 6997801 Tel Aviv, Israel

Kobi Perl
Blavatnik School of Computer Science, Tel Aviv University, 6997801 Tel Aviv, Israel
Department of Human Molecular Genetics and Biochemistry, Sackler Faculty of Medicine and Sagol School of Neuroscience, Tel Aviv University, 6997801 Tel Aviv, Israel

Karen B. Avraham
Department of Human Molecular Genetics and Biochemistry, Sackler Faculty of Medicine and Sagol School of Neuroscience, Tel Aviv University, 6997801 Tel Aviv, Israel

Xiaowei Fan, Lifeng Ma, Zhiying Zhang, Zhipeng Zhao, Yiduo Zhao, Fang Liu, Lijun Liu, Peng Cai, Yansong Li and Longli Kang
Key Laboratory for Molecular Genetic Mechanisms and Intervention Research on High Altitude Disease of Tibet Autonomous Region, School of Medicine, Xizang Minzu University, Xianyang 712082, Shaanxi, China
Key Laboratory of High Altitude Environment and Genes Related to Diseases of Tibet Autonomous Region, School of Medicine, Xizang Minzu University, Xianyang 712082, Shaanxi, China

Meng Hao
Ministry of Education Key Laboratory ofContemporary Anthropology, Collaborative Innovation Center for Genetics and Development, School of Life Sciences, Fudan University, Shanghai 200433, China

Yi Li
Ministry of Education Key Laboratory ofContemporary Anthropology, Collaborative Innovation Center for Genetics and Development, School of Life Sciences, Fudan University, Shanghai 200433, China

Six Industrial Research Institute, Fudan University, Shanghai 200433, China

Xingguang Luo
Division of Human Genetics, Department of Psychiatry, Yale University School of Medicine, New Haven, CT 06510, USA

Minjoo Kim and Minkyung Kim
Research Center for Silver Science, Institute of Symbiotic Life-TECH, Yonsei University, Seoul 03722, Korea

Jong Ho Lee
Research Center for Silver Science, Institute of Symbiotic Life-TECH, Yonsei University, Seoul 03722, Korea
Department of Food and Nutrition, Brain Korea 21 PLUS Project, College of Human Ecology, Yonsei University, 50 Yonsei-ro, Seodaemun-gu, Seoul 03722, Korea
Department of Food and Nutrition, National Leading Research Laboratory of Clinical Nutrigenetics Nutrigenomics, College of Human Ecology, Yonsei University, Seoul 03722, Korea

Hye Jin Yoo
Department of Food and Nutrition, Brain Korea 21 PLUS Project, College of Human Ecology, Yonsei University, 50 Yonsei-ro, Seodaemun-gu, Seoul 03722, Korea

Jayoung Shon
Department of Food and Nutrition, Brain Korea 21 PLUS Project, College of Human Ecology, Yonsei University, 50 Yonsei-ro, Seodaemun-gu, Seoul 03722, Korea
Department of Food and Nutrition, National Leading Research Laboratory of Clinical Nutrigenetics Nutrigenomics, College of Human Ecology, Yonsei University, Seoul 03722, Korea

Yabin Chen, Xiaodong Jiao and J. Fielding Hetmancik
Ophthalmic Genetics and Visual Function Branch, National Eye Institute, National Institutes of Health, Bethesda, MD 20892, USA

Li Huang
State Key Laboratory of Ophthalmology, Zhongshan Ophthalmic Center, Sun Yat-Sen University, Guangzhou, Guangdong, China

Sheikh Riazuddin
National Centre of Excellence in Molecular Biology, University of the Punjab, Lahore, Pakistan
Allama Iqbal Medical College, University of Health Sciences, Lahore, Pakistan

National Centre for Genetic Diseases, Shaheed Zulfiqar Ali Bhutto Medical University, Islamabad, Pakistan

S. Amer Riazuddin
The Wilmer Eye Institute, Johns Hopkins University School of Medicine, Baltimore, MD, USA

Jakub Piotr Fichna and Cezary Zekanowski
Department of Neurodegenerative Disorders, Mossakowski Medical Research Centre, Polish Academy of Sciences, 5 Pawinskiego St., 02-106 Warsaw, Poland

Anna Macias and Anna Potulska-Chromik
Department of Neurology, Medical University of Warsaw, 1a Banacha St., 02-097 Warsaw, Poland

Marcin Piechota and Michał Korostyński
Department of Molecular Neuropharmacology, Institute of Pharmacology, Polish Academy of Sciences, 31-344 Krakow, Poland

Maria Jolanta Redowicz
Laboratory of Molecular Basis of Cell Motility, Department of Biochemistry, Nencki Institute of Experimental Biology, 3 Pasteur St., 02-093 Warsaw, Poland

Index